Frontiers of Medical Imaging

Frontiers of Medical Imaging

editor

C H Chen

University of Massachusetts Dartmouth, USA
Information Research Foundation, Dartmouth, USA

World Scientific

NEW JERSEY • LONDON • SINGAPORE • BEIJING • SHANGHAI • HONG KONG • TAIPEI • CHENNAI

Published by

World Scientific Publishing Co. Pte. Ltd.
5 Toh Tuck Link, Singapore 596224
USA office: 27 Warren Street, Suite 401-402, Hackensack, NJ 07601
UK office: 57 Shelton Street, Covent Garden, London WC2H 9HE

Library of Congress Cataloging-in-Publication Data
Frontiers of medical imaging / [edited by] C. H. Chen.
p. ; cm.
Includes bibliographical references and index.
ISBN 978-9814611091 (hardcover : alk. paper)
I. Chen, C. H. (Chi-hau), 1937– editor.
[DNLM: 1. Diagnostic Imaging. 2. Image Processing, Computer-Assisted. WN 180]
RC78.7.D53
616.07'54--dc23

2014018386

British Library Cataloguing-in-Publication Data
A catalogue record for this book is available from the British Library.

In-house Editor: Darilyn Yap

Typeset by Stallion Press
Email: enquiries@stallionpress.com

Printed by FuIsland Offset Printing (S) Pte Ltd Singapore

Preface

Medical imaging has experienced significant growth in terms of both methodologies and instrumentation in recent years. It has played a major role in modern medicine for providing important and often essential information for medical diagnosis and treatment as well as preventive healthcare. Since the area is very broad and fast-growing, it is not possible for a single volume to cover every aspect of medical imaging. The book places emphasis only on frontier development in medical imaging with three parts: (1) theory, techniques and physics, (2) image processing, (3) emerging methods and medical imaging systems. Some chapters may belong to more than one of the three parts. The book has a broader coverage of medical imaging than the companion volume *Computer Vision in Medical Imaging* (hereafter noted as CVMI Book) edited by myself and recently published (Nov. 2013) also by World Scientific Publishing with table of content attached to the Preface.

In Part 1, Chapter 1 by Prociask *et al.* deals with minimal invasive coronary angiography by multi-slice computed tomography (MSCT-CA). This chapter focuses on the feasibility to derive quantitative tissue composition measurements from the plaque Hounsfield Units (HU) distribution and shows the first steps towards further development of the method for clinical use. MSCT-CA does have the advantage over intravascular ultrasound (IVUS) in that the complete coronary artery tree is visualized. Chapter 2 by Szirmay-Kalos *et al.* presents Monte Carlo estimates to compute forward and back projections in iterative PET reconstruction and proposed two techniques to improve the accuracy. Chapter 3 by Majumdar reviews the online dynamic MRI reconstruction techniques. In general, any online reconstruction technique consists of two steps: prediction and correction. Broadly, there are two classes of techniques: the compressive sensing based method and the Kalman filtering based techniques. A hybrid method is proposed that can better meet the online reconstruction need. The theory of longitudinal brain image registration is well-developed. Chapter 4 by Fletcher surveys the current literature and then proposes an approach for enhancing specificity using prior information. It has demonstrated increased ability to distinguish between Alzheimer's disease and normal subjects, as well as increased statistical power, reflected in decreased sample size needed to detect change beyond normal aging. While X-ray computer tomography (CT) has been popular in diagnosis and treatment planning of cancer, it lacks the ability to image multiple processes at the molecular level and thus may be difficult to differentiate benign from cancerous modules. Chapter 5 by Li and Kuang presents, as a proof-of-concept, an X-ray fluorescence computed tomography (XHCT) system as a promising modality for multiplexed imaging of high atomic numbers probes. Chapter 6 by Xu *et al.* presents a dictionary learning based approach for low dose CT data that tends to be noisy and incomplete. The dictionary learning approach aims at capturing localized structural information and suppressing noise so that image reconstruction with a sparse representation in terms of dictionary can perform well. Chapter 7 by Lu *et al.* describes algorithms for diagnosis of psoriasis severity using only 2D digital skin images. Segmenting the symptoms in a digital image and using the segmented image to make a diagnosis can both be implemented using statistical machine learning involving support vector machine in conjunction with Markov random fields.

Part 2 begins with Chapter 8 by Honorio that studies the conditions for the reasonably good performance of linear support vector machines (SVMs) on brain functional magnetic resonance imaging (fMRI) data. To this end, a synthetic method is proposed that is based on a number of Gaussian-distributed regions with Gaussian spatially correlated noise. Such model introduces many intuitions from neuroscience. Several synthetic experiments were performed to analyze the different aspects of brain fMRI data. In comparison with other feature extraction methods, original features and PCA features, the generalization accuracy of linear SVMs using most discriminative feature is significantly better. It is interesting to note that with 50 or more samples per class, the classification accuracy is nearly 90% or slightly above. For other pattern classification work on MRI data using SVMs, the readers are referred to Chapter 16 of the CVMI book. Another approach to the analysis of the fMRI data is presented in Chapter 9 by Oikonomou and Blekas. The basic element of the fMRI data which is noisy is called voxel and represents a value on a grid in 3D. By taking the values of voxels over time, we create a set of time series. A regression mixture model is used as a probabilistic modeling tool for data analysis. The model is trained by expectation-maximization (EM) algorithm so that each voxel can be assigned to one of K-clusters. To take into account the spatial dependence among 8 neighboring voxels, a Markov

Random Field (MRF) analysis is performed by constructing a design matrix for each cluster from a linear combination of S kernel matrices. The EM algorithm is further applied to estimate the parameters. Finally, the activation-based and resting state applications clearly demonstrated experimentally the superiority of approach presented. Chapter 10 by Lee *et al.* presents a new framework for automatic analysis of dermoscopic images. It is a novel approach inspired by the analysis of the growth pattern of skin lesions. In this approach, a dermoscopic image is decomposed using a simple growth model estimated using a single image; then a tree-structure is constructed to represent the growth model. Both segmentation and diagnosis programs return good and promising results. The tree structure framework is also useful for other skin image analysis tasks. Both Chapters 11 and 12 deal with eye images. Retinal imaging is nowadays a mainstay of the clinical care and management of patients with retinal as well as systemic diseases. Segmentation of retina structure is a fundamental component of most automatic retinal disease screening systems. Chapter 11 by Morales *et al.* is focused on detection methods of the vascular tree and the optic disc, by using a combination of several morphological operators and by making use of stochastic watershed transformation. For both the detection of the main retinal structure and optic disc segmentation, the method proposed shows significant improvement over the previously reported results. Chapter 12 is focused on glaucoma screening by introducing the Automatic RetinA cup to disc Ratio AssessmenT (ARARAT) derived from optic disc and cup segmentation using fast superpixel based methods. The ROC plots show that ARARAT consistently outperformed over other methods. For enhancement of retinal images, the readers may consult the deconvolution method presented in Chapter 12 of the CVMI Book. Chapter 13 by Mehrabian presents an algorithm using adaptive complex independent component analysis as a blind source separation method to identify and separate the intravascular signal from the dynamic contrast enhanced (DCE)-MRI data at the tissue of interest. Pharmacokinetic modeling of tumor tissues using their DCE-MRI requires information about the contrast agent concentration in the intravascular space. The signal is inseparable from the DCE-MRI data, but the algorithm presented is shown to be effective to perform the desired separation. The work is useful for prostate cancer assessment. Chapter 14 deals with an automated ultrasonic breast screening system. Ultrasound can improve cancer detection compared with using mammography alone and it is radiation-free. The algorithms of the computer aided detection include speckle noise reduction, multi-scale blob detection, tumor candidate extraction, feature extraction, region classification and statistical evaluation. The analysis shows that breast tumors known as ellipse-like shape and hypo-echogenic in the automated ultrasound images were successfully discovered with 100% sensitivity in the experiment. The author noted that the system needs to be improved to detect tumor sizes smaller than 1 cm.

Part 3 begins with a review (Chapter 15) by Veltri and Madabshi *et al.* that demonstrates how prostate cancer quantitative histomorphometry can be used to extract and employ computer-assisted image features and hence serve as a potentially new and innovative predictive tool to improve the determination of aggressive phenotypes of cancer. Additional development and validation of the tools presented are expected to help the pathologist to predict severe outcomes early so that appropriate interventions can be made by the urologist and patient. Chapter 16 by Aquino provides a comprehensive overview of the automated detection of diabetic retinopathy (DR), from medical point of view followed by screening systems using automated segmentation. It is encouraging to state that automated DR detection systems have achieved comparable performance to a single DR human expert. Chapter 17 by Roujo *et al.* presents the different techniques which have been developed to alleviate the problem of physiological motion for magnetic resonance guided high intensity focused ultrasound ablation of abdominal organs. Advanced motion correction strategies which enable continuous monitoring of the thermal dose and continuous sonication under free breathing conditions have been demonstrated in a few pre-clinical studies. Additional pre-clinical studies are needed to fully demonstrate the accuracy, safety and robustness of these techniques. Chapter 18 by Su *et al.* reviews proton therapy physics, sources of proton-range uncertainties, and the advanced imaging technologies used to minimize these uncertainties before, during and after proton therapy. Chapter 19 by Prakash *et al.* presents a continuation of research effort on intravascular ultrasound image processing and analysis as reported in Chapter 20 of the CVMI Book. A robust and fully automated IVUS segmentation using meta-algorithm is presented to work on a large database which contains some manual segmentation results for comparison with automated segmentation. The entire system consists of a library of preprocessors, a library of segmentation algorithms some of which employ neural networks, and an algorithm selector in an effort to reach a 95% segmentation accuracy as compared with manual segmentation. The preliminary results shown indicate that the method is very promising to achieve an automated IVUS segmentation with desired accuracy objective. Chapter 20 by Mendizabal-Ruiz and Kakadiaris examines a broader scope of computation methods and issues including such as segmentation, plaque characterization, nonlinear IVUS and differential imaging for the IVUS data. Chapter 21 by Savoia and Caliano shows that capacitive micromachined ultrasonic transducer

(CMUTs) can be popular in medical ultrasound in the future because it enables a realization of extremely low-cost and high-performance device. Characterization and imaging results are used to assess the performance of CMUTs with respect to conventional piezoelectric transducers. The last chapter, Chapter 22 by Shen and Chen provides a descriptive discussion of picture archiving communication system and medical imaging cloud. Good record keeping of medical images and rapid retrieval of such image history are important issues facing healthcare industry. The advances of cloud computing greatly enhance the capability of working with enormous amount of medical image data. The "Big Data" is an area that touches many fields and can be of much interest to medical imaging researchers with strong computer science background.

Medical imaging is indeed a very broad and highly interdisciplinary area that requires collaboration among medical, engineering, physics and computer science professions as demonstrated in this book. Researchers in pattern recognition and computer vision may find that Chapters 7, 8, 10, 14 and 19 to be particularly informative. All chapters provide good introduction of the topic considered and extensive list of reference articles, which are helpful to a broad range of readers.

In my nearly forty years of editing different technical books, I am indebted greatly to many professional friends for their help. I like to mention in particular of the help of Prof. Ching-Chung Li of University of Pittsburgh, a leading expert in biomedical pattern recognition, who brought to my attention the important work of Dr. Robert Veltri, whose chapter is in the book. Prof. Li was also helpful to contribute to all four books, *Handbook of Pattern Recognition and Computer Vision* (1993, 1999, 2005, 2010) which I edited for World Scientific publication. With the rapid progress in technical fields, edited books play an increasingly important role to deliver the most up-to-date technical knowledge to a wide range of audience along with other publication methods.

I am most grateful to all authors for their outstanding contributions to the book. With their valuable inputs, I am convinced that much has been achieved with medical imaging, while much more have yet to be done in this challenging area. It is useful to keep in mind that the problems considered can be very complex and highly complicated and we can only make incremental progresses rather than expect for major breakthroughs. The new and more powerful medical devices and instrumentation only bring in additional challenges to researchers. We look forward to the continued progress on medical imaging for many years to come.

C.H. Chen
May 4, 2014

Table of Contents of ***Computer Vision in Medical Imaging***, edited by C.H. Chen; World Scientific Publishing, Nov. 2013; ISBN 978-981-4460-93-4.

Chapter 10: "Three-dimensional Reconstruction Methods in Near-field Coded Aperture for SPECT Imaging System"
Stephen Baoming Hong

Chapter 11: "An Alternative Volume Reconstruction Based on Direct Frame Interpolation"
Sergei Koptenko, Rachel Remlinger, Martin Lachaine, Tony Falco and Ulrich Scheipers

Chapter 12: "Deconvolution Technique for Enhancing and Classifying the Retinal Images"
Uvais A. Qidwai and Umair A. Qidwai

Chapter 13: "Medical Ultrasound Digital Signal Processing in the GPU Computing Era"
Marcin Lewandowski

Chapter 14: "Designing Medical Imaging Processing Algorithms for GPU Assisted Parallel Computation"
Mathias Broxvall and Marios Daout

Part 3 Specific Image Processing and Computer Vision Methods for Different Imaging Modalities

Chapter 15: "Computer Vision in Interventional Cardiology"
Kendall R. Waters

Chapter 16: "Pattern Classification on Brain Diffusion MRI: Application to Schizopherenia Diagnosis"
Ali Tabesh, Maththew J. Hoptman, Debra D'Angelo and Babak A. Ardekani

Chapter 17: "On Compressive Sensing in Magnetic Resonance Imaging"
Benjamin Paul Berman, Sagar Mandava, and Ali Bilgin

Chapter 18: "On Hierarchical Statistical Shape Models with Application to Brain MRI"
Juan J. Cerrolaza, Arantxa Villanueva and Rafael Cabeza

Chapter 19: "Advanced PDE Based Methods for Automatic Quantification of Cardiac Function and Scar from Magnetic Resonance Imaging"
Durco Turco and Cristiana Corsi

Chapter 20: "On Automated IVUS Segmentation Using a Deformable Template Model with Feature Tracking"
Prakash Manandhar and Chi Hau Chen

Subject Index

Contents

Part 1

Theory, Techniques and Physics

Chapter 1

Coronary Plaque Quantification by Multi-slice Computed Tomography

Elzbieta Pociask,[*,†] *Klaudia Proniewska*[*,†] *and Nico Bruining*[†,‡]

[*]*AGH University of Science and Technology, Krakow, Poland*
[†]*Thoraxcenter, Department of Cardiology, Erasmus MC, Rotterdam, The Netherlands*
[‡]*E-mail: n.bruining@erasmusmc.nl*

Coronary artery disease (CAD) is one of the main causes of human deaths in the western world. Usually, patients are being diagnosed by ECG analysis first, after which for asymptomatic patients additional tests are necessary. Ultimately an imaging procedure might be necessary to image the coronary arteries. Until a decade ago invasive coronary angiography was the standard imaging method for this. Since then, minimal invasive coronary angiography by multi-slice computed tomography (MSCT-CA) became available and has been a highly investigated imaging technique and may become a standard imaging tool for the diagnosis of coronary artery disease (CAD). The three-dimensional (3D) nature of MSCT-CA allows 3D image reconstruction from which quantitative parameters of the coronary arteries and plaques can be derived.

1. Introduction

Multi-slice computed tomography of coronary arteries (MSCT-CA) has gained large interest as a diagnostic imaging tool for patients suspected of coronary artery disease (CAD).[1–3] The three-dimensional (3D) nature of MSCT-CA allows 3D image reconstruction of the coronary artery tree[4] with the advantage over standard coronary angiography to show not only luminal obstructions but also plaque formation.[5] Quantitative MSCT-CA (QMSCT-CA) has been developed[6–9] and most manufacturers are currently implementing computer-assisted analysis tools in their MSCT-CA analysis consoles.

Since plaque composition is one of the important predictors of future events, quantification of its composition by a non-invasive imaging method would have advantages.[10,11] Early attempts by MSCT showed mixed results.[5,12]

This could be explained by the lack of a robust dedicated MSCT-CA plaque compositional analysis method.[5,13–15] There are also technical difficulties comparing *in-vivo* MSCT-CA data to reference methods, such as intravascular ultrasound (IVUS) or histology. Despite the rapid technical developments of MSCT-CA, the thickness of reconstructed cross-sectional images is currently 400 to 600 micron and is significantly below that of IVUS (approximately 200 micron) and histology (6 micron). Since plaque components are mostly heterogeneously distributed, straightforward comparison of a single individual cross-sectional MSCT-CA image against a single individual cross-section of one of these two reference methods (e.g. a straightforward 2D comparison) may also lead to divergent results.

This book chapter describes a possible computer-assisted volumetric method for quantitative plaque compositional measurements by MSCT-CA which was tested on *ex-vivo* human coronary specimen data.

2. MSCT Procedure

The developments in coronary MSCT imaging are advancing fast. Until a few years ago 4 and 16-slice scanners were the standard, today 320 slice scanners capable of acquiring multi-phases of the heart cycle are available. However, concerning the detection of coronary plaques and the evaluation of their composition, nothing much has changed as the image resolution, e.g. the voxel resolution did not change. So, those principles are overall still similar compared to the previous generations of MSCT scanners.

Patients who underwent MSCT scanning were in sinus rhythm with a heart rate <70 beats/min (spontaneously or after oral β-blockade). A bolus of 120 ml of iodinated contrast medium (Visipaque 320, Amersham Health, Little Chalfont, United Kingdom) was administered through an arm vein (4 ml/s). Scan parameters were a detector collimation of 16×0.75 mm, a table feed of 3.0 mm/rotation, a gantry rotation time of 0.42 second, and a tube voltage of 120 kV. Datasets of reconstructed coronary vessels were created at different points of the cardiac phase, e.g. 350-, 400- and 450 ms before the next R-wave, using a retrospectively ECG-gated reconstruction algorithm (Siemens, Forchheim, Germany). This algorithm uses data of a single heartbeat obtained in half gantry rotation time resulting in a temporal resolution of 188 ms. Datasets reconstructed within the middle- and later phase of diastole provided nearly motion-free image quality. All MSCT datasets were uploaded to an MSCT-Picture Archiving and Communication System (CT-PACS).

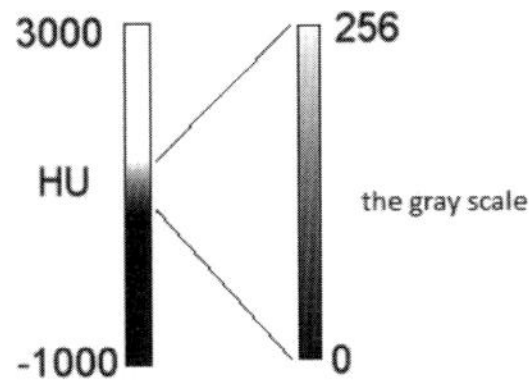

Fig. 1. The CT Hounsfield scale, air is assigned a value of −1000, and bone +3000. The grayscale color corresponding HU values, depending on the window setting selected.

3. Coronary Plaque Segmentation

3.1. *MSCT-CA Image Processing*

MSCT identifies different human tissues by their various ability to absorb X-ray. Attenuation variability measured in Hounsfield Units (HU) is given by:

$$HU = \frac{\mu_{tissue} - \mu_{water}}{\mu_{water}} \cdot 1000 \qquad (1)$$

Where μ_{water} and μ_{tissue} are the linear attenuation coefficients of water and tissue of interest. Next Hounsfield scale is converted to values of greyscale (Fig. 1). Changes of these regions are larger than 256 values, which makes it impossible to visualize all values of grayscale simultaneously on a computer display. Images are generated by the defined window of HU values.

Parameters of window are described using the terms center (L) and a width (W). In this way, referring to the brightness (center) and to contrast (width) of the image. Frame image sets range: from L − 1/2 W to L + 1/2 W.

All pixels of the image smaller than L − 1/2 or larger $L + 1/2$ are either white or black.

The figure below (Fig. 2) shows the same image, but displayed with different parameters for L and W. There is a noticeable change in image brightness and contrast.

Dense tissue attenuates X-rays much more compared to softer tissues and is displayed as bright structures identifying the so-called high HU values.

Standard coronary plaque compositional measurements by MSCT-CA is often performed by retrieving absolute HU values at a limited number of positions within a coronary plaque at a typical individual cross-sectional location, mostly with the largest visible amount of plaque, within the coronary vessel. This makes it difficult to derive a comprehensive overview of the coronary plaque in the complete affected region of interest. The proposed method in this chapter derives the total plaque composition from the HU distribution in an arbitrary coronary plaque segment.

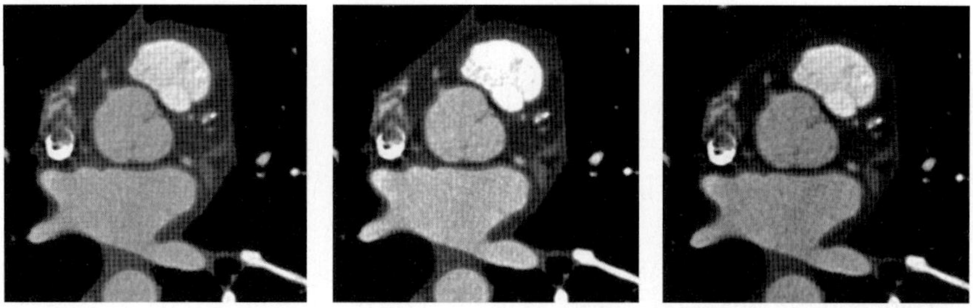

(a) (b) (c)

Fig. 2. These three images are of the same section, viewed at different windows settings. (a) a window center of 140 and a window width of 900, (b) a window center is 140 and a window width 700 and (c) a window center 240 and a window width 700 Hounsfield units. This enables details of plaque in coronary vessel.

After the MSCT scan the image data were stored in the DICOM format onto a DVD, today it is stored onto a picture archiving and communication system (PACS). From the MSCT-CA scanned volume, the coronary arteries can be semi-automatically extracted by dedicated vessel extraction software (MSCT Extractor, CURAD BV, Amsterdam, Netherlands)[8] (Fig. 3), which allows one to present the data in a similar fashion as if performing a pullback of a coronary catheter such as intravascular ultrasound (IVUS) or optical coherence tomography (OCT). Using this approach, longitudinally reconstructed coronary vessels (L-Views) originating from different imaging modalities can be simultaneously displayed for accurate comparison and matching such as IVUS and/or OCT.[16,17]

3.2. *Quantitative MSCT-CA and Validation*

The golden reference method to quantify coronary plaques has been up until today IVUS. Therefore to validate the MSCT-CA quantitative analysis method, there is a need to perform the analysis of the two different modalities as similar as possible. Quantitative IVUS analyses are mostly performed on longitudinal reconstructed L-views and the best match of the MSCT derived coronary vessel data to compare to intracoronary imaging methods is to perform a similar analysis. This can be achieved by preparing the MSCT data so that a sort of "virtual" IVUS pullback can be performed extracting the vessels and regions of interests (ROI) by dedicated software algorithms. Each ROI was extracted from the 3D MSCT-CA dataset by semi-automated vessel extraction software (CURAD) (Fig. 3 A–D). Matching was performed by identifying side-branches visible in both datasets (e.g. MSCT-CA and IVUS). After extraction, the ROI was visualized, similarly to the IVUS L-mode views. This allows

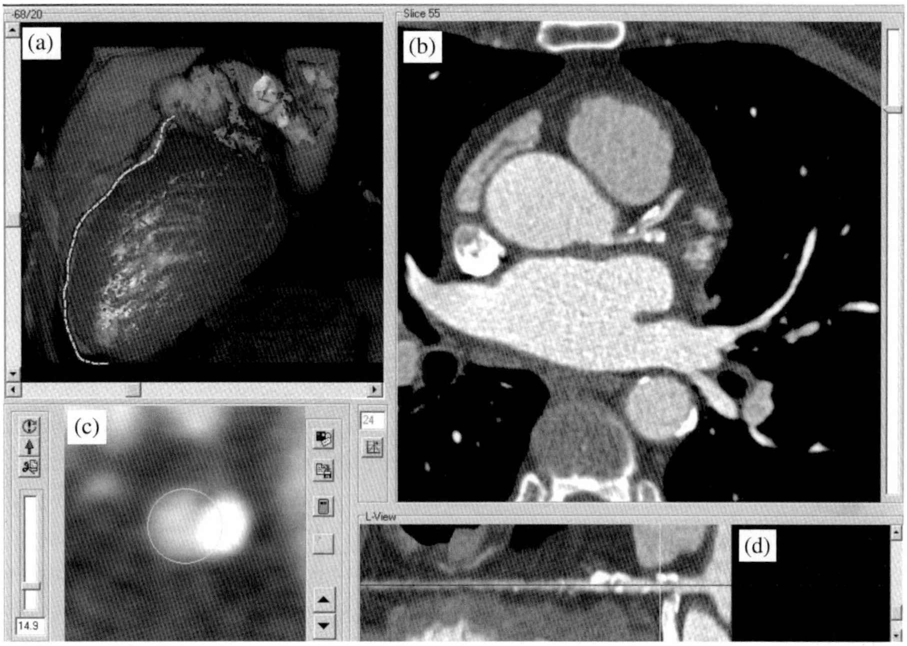

Fig. 3. Panels A–D show the MSCT coronary vessel extractor interface. In panel A, after loading the DICOM data from DVD or from the PACS a three-dimensional (3D) reconstruction is created automatically. The line is the later extracted virtual IVUS catheter path. The individual original MSCT-CA cross-sectional images can be viewed in panel B, which can be scrolled up and down to view the other cross-sections. Panel C, shows a reconstructed cross-sectional view of the vessel, in this case a right coronary artery RCA and its surrounding tissue, perpendicular to the virtual IVUS path. After identification of one point in the center of the coronary lumen and by giving a direction (by example from distal to proximal), the software automatically extracts the centerline of the contrast-enhanced coronary lumen. The detected centerline is visualized in the 3D reconstruction by the white line with its control points (presented as dots). Those can be interactively corrected if necessary (by example in areas of heavy calcification). Finally, the vessel is extracted from the dataset and visualized similar to IVUS, as presented in panel D.

direct comparison of the two imaging modalities onto one individual computer display for accurate matching. Furthermore, errors introduced by artificially straightening of the vessels in the L-views are now avoided as the same analytic method is applied for both modalities. Previous research showed that this method decreases volumetric measurement errors by $\pm 5\%$.[18] However, there are still motion induced artifacts which are caused by possible breathing of the patient during the MSCT scan. During the extraction procedure, the MSCT-CA image quality was qualitatively scored as poor = multiple breathing artifacts, moderate = 1 or 2 breathing artifacts, good = no artifact or a breathing artifact in a region outside of the ROI.

For further quantitative analyses, dedicated software was applied (CURAD).[17] At first, manual identification was applied for the lumen-intima interface and the adventitia-fat boundary in the MSCT data. After the ROI's were matched between the two modalities, the MSCT-CA derived segments were qualitatively scored for the amount of calcium presence as follows: none = no calcification, little = some spots, moderate = < half of the ROI calcified, high = half to > half calcified and very high = complete calcification.

An automated lumen detector algorithm semi-automatically detected the lumen-intima interface, and this algorithm is described in detail elsewhere.[17] Briefly, this automated-lumen-detector applies an edge-detection method, using a digital Deriche filter. This filter calculates the gradient of the image while applying a smoothing operator to the data in such a way that possible presence of noise is reduced and that the true boundaries are enhanced. The subsequent edge-thinning and edge-linking method exploits the continuity of the longitudinal contours as well as knowledge of the gradient directions of the structure boundaries of interest. In calcified areas, the lumen contour was adjusted in L-views by interpolation of the contour between the last distal non-calcified lumen border and the most proximal non-calcified lumen border. This protocol was followed to minimize the blooming effect of calcium on MSCT images with concern to luminal measurements. Unfortunately, this automated edge-detection cannot be used to identify the adventitia-fat border in MSCT-CA images. This was therefore only applied for lumen detection in addition to manually performed measurements. The standard window- and level-settings used during the MSCT-CA acquisition were also applied in the manual analyses. However, the investigators were allowed to alter these settings for the quantification process.

3.3. *Results of QMSCT-CA Validation*

Applying the above-described methodology, the results in a validation study were good and showed that contrast enhanced QMSCT-CA allows reproducible measurements of coronary artery dimensions.[8] When compared to IVUS, the current reference method for coronary plaque quantification, a systematic underestimation was found for both lumen- and vessel dimensions. However, for plaque measurements this underestimation was ruled out, although the regions of agreement are somewhat wide. It was also found that motion artifacts and amount of calcification did not affect the reproducibility. Most respirations motion artifacts occurs mostly in parts of the scan near the distal sections of the coronaries and will be diminished in the newer scanner types capable of acquiring dynamic MSCT-CA images. The fact that calcium also did not significantly influence the results could have been caused by the approach to minimize the effects of calcium on the quantitative measurements.

Therefore, other possible causes must be considered. A possible explanation for the smaller absolute differences of the vessel dimensions and larger differences of the lumen dimensions is that the accuracy of MSCT improves when more voxels are included in a larger area. Since the voxels at (sharp) interface borders have diminished intensity, the radius measurement is on average underestimated by half a voxel size. For 16-slice CT scans, the voxel size is approximately $0.6 * 0.6 * 0.6$ mm. Consequently, a lumen diameter of 3 mm results in an area measurement underestimation of about 50%, compared to 30% for a vessel of 5 mm. Another factor, which could have caused the larger lumen diameters as measured by IVUS, is the injection of isosorbide dinitrate before the IVUS examination to prevent possible coronary spasms. A 10% increase in lumen surface area has been described after injection of vasodilators, although in diseased vessels this could be considerably less.[19,20] Furthermore, in IVUS image data the vessel border is taken at the external elastic membrane (EEM). In contrast within MSCT-CA the vessel border will be most likely the adventitia-fat border, since this border has theoretically the largest HU-value difference in the outer vessel region. This could possibly result in a systematic deviation (e.g. an overestimation of plaque dimensions by QMSCT-CA). The exact magnitude of this deviation is still unknown.

The fact that the intra- and the inter-investigator reproducibility results are better in the matched ROI's than in the total extracted coronary segments by QMSCT-CA, is most likely caused by the fact that the matched ROI's were mostly found in the proximal part of the coronary vessels, including larger lumen-, and vessel areas in which QMSCT-CA has a higher sensitivity and accuracy as compared to more distal and thus smaller coronary dimensions. There is also a remarkable difference in the outcome of the intra- and inter-observer variability measurements in the lumen volume detection. This could have been caused by a learning effect.

4. MSCT-CA Plaque Composition

4.1. *MSCT Derived Tissue Component Information*

Identification and quantification of plaque composition are important prognostic indicators in patients with suspected CAD.

The HU scale is used to identify different human tissues. Softer tissue, as by example lipids do have a low HU value (around zero) and calcium at the other end of the tissue spectrum shows values >200 up to 800. Calcium is also often presented in coronary plaques and is a predictor of severity of the atherosclerotic process, although there is still large scientific debate if it is a predictor of vulnerability or stabilization of the plaques. Also IVUS is capable of identifying human coronary plaque components, although limited and is identified mostly qualitatively by "soft", "fibrotic" and "calcified" and is therefore the most used reference imaging methodology to compare/validate MSCT derived coronary plaque composition measurements methods.[16,21] Of course, there are much more of these studies published of which some are discussed in more detail in the next sub-chapter.

There are two major possible factors which potentially could affect plaque compositional measurements by MSCT and these are: (1) the applied convolution kernel when extracting the MSCT data from the scanner and translate it into the DICOM image format, and thus to grey values, to store it on the DVD's or PACS and to prepare it for further processing and analysis,[22] and (2) even more importantly, the used contrast HU levels are influencing the absolute HU levels of the coronary plaque as well as the identification of the lumen border when segmenting the image to identify the plaques.[16] These two very influential parameters have been thoroughly evaluated and this validation is described in Chapter 4.2.

4.1.1. *Literature overview*

Feasibility and validation studies of QMSCT-CA have been reported[5,12,23–27] as well as those evaluating coronary plaque composition based on HU Hounsfield unit distribution.[5,9,28] However, most of these studies (Table 1) were performed with limited software tools and/or validation was performed not always using histology, the golden reference method to assess tissue composition, but by cross-referencing their new methods to another limited method with respect to assessment of tissue composition such as IVUS.[9]

If histology is used as reference method then one of most difficult tasks is the localization of the acquired histology sections with respect to their location before they were acquired within the MSCT-CA image data. A direct visual 1-to-1 comparison of the reconstructed cross-sectional images from the MSCT-CA data to the histology sections is impossible due to the large differences in image resolution. Therefore, OCT, with its excellent image resolution, lateral approximately 7 μm (resembling the one from histology), and in-plane approximately 5 μm, was applied to act as the link between the two modalities.[21] In addition, the OCT imaging catheter is also very small, certainly with respect

Table 1. Literature overview.

Authors	Title	Journal	Year
Miszalski-Jamka *et al.*[29]	*The composition and extent of coronary artery plaque detected by multislice computed tomographic angiography provides incremental prognostic value in patients with suspected coronary artery disease.*	*Cardiovasc Imaging* 28:621–631	2012
Pundzuite *et al.*[30]	*Assessment with multislice computed tomography and gray-scale and virtual histology intravascular ultrasound of gender-specific differences in extent and composition of coronary atherosclerotic plaques in relation to age*	*Journal of the American College of Cardiology* 105:480–486	2010
Bruining *et al.*[21]	*Compositional volumetry of non-calcified coronary plaques by multislice computed tomography: An ex vivo feasibility study.*	*Eurointervention* 5:558–564	2009
Bruining *et al.*[8]	*Reproducible coronary plaque quantification by multislice computed tomography.*	*Catheter Cardiovasc Interv.* 69:857–865	2007
Cademartiri *et al.*[22]	*Influence of convolution filtering on coronary plaque attenuation values: observations in an ex vivo model of multislice computed tomography coronary angiography*	*Eur Radiol* 17:1842–1849	2007
De Weert *et al.*[28]	*In Vivo characetrisation and quantification of atherosclerotic cartoid plaque components with multidetector computed tomography and histopathological correlation*	*Arteriosclerosis, Thrombosis, and Vascular Biology.* 26:2366–2372	2006
Leber *et al.*[9]	*Quantification of obstructive and nonobstructive coronary lesions by 64-slice computed tomography*	*Journal of the American College of Cardiology* 46:147–154	2005
Cademartiri *et al.*[16]	*Influence of intracoronary attenuation on coronary plaque measurements using multislice computed tomography: observations in an ex vivo model of multislice computed tomography coronary angiography*	*Eur Radiol* 15:1426–1431	2005
Leber *et al.*[5]	*Accuracy of multidetector spiral computed tomography in identyfing and differentiating the composition of coronary atherosclerotic plaques*	*Journal of the American College of Cardiology* 43:1241–1247	2004
Schoeder *et al.*[27]	*Accuracy and reliability of quantitative measurements in coronary arteries by multi-slice computed tomography: Experimental and initial clinical results.*	*Clinical Radiology* 56:466–474	2001

to an IVUS catheter, avoiding the possible risk of altering the geometry of the artery lumen, by dilating the lumen, in severe lesions with narrow lumens.

In many instances a rough qualitative scoring system was developed and the image-based gated IVUS technology Intelligate® used in our institute allows a comparison between MSCT-CA and IVUS images, with smooth L-mode views of the coronaries without motion artifacts, hence providing more consistent and reproducible results (an image can be found in the discussion section). Furthermore, it has been reported that ECG-gated QCU yields significantly different volumetric results than non-gated QCU.[31] The matching of the coronary ROI's based on the identification of side-branches in both image modalities on a single computer screen provides an optimal set-up. A ROI-based analysis that uses side-branches, which are unambiguously identifiable landmarks, must result in a more accurate plaque volume assessment than measurements of a limited stack of non-ECG-gated single two-dimensional cross-sections.

4.2. *Quantitative MSCT-CA Plaque Composition Measurements*

As described above, most plaque compositional methods are using absolute cut-off or threshold HU values to identify the three defined basic tissue types: (1) soft, (2) hard and (3) calcium. However as shown by Cademartiri *et al.*[16] this is not appropriate as the HU value of the contrast, which easily could be around the same levels as expected from the tissue components in the coronary plaques, influences the absolute HU values of the coronary plaque adjacent to the coronary lumen. This could only be overcome by imaging the coronary arteries without contrast, however, such a scan makes it impossible to identify the coronary lumens in a 3D MSCT dataset. An *ex-vivo* explanted coronary artery study, with histology as reference method, showed this very well (Fig. 4).[8]

The authors of this study suggested to identify also three regions, as similar to the other studies, but using the Hounsfield units distribution,[8] which is independent of the absolute HU value distribution. It showed that the influence of the use of contrast agents must be evaluated. These are needed to visualize the coronary arteries *in-vivo* and have an effect on the plaque HU distribution (Fig. 5).

The HU value distributions of the voxels within the segmented coronary plaque were calculated for each reconstructed cross-sectional image and the 3D sub-segments. The resulting histograms typically show a Gaussian distribution,

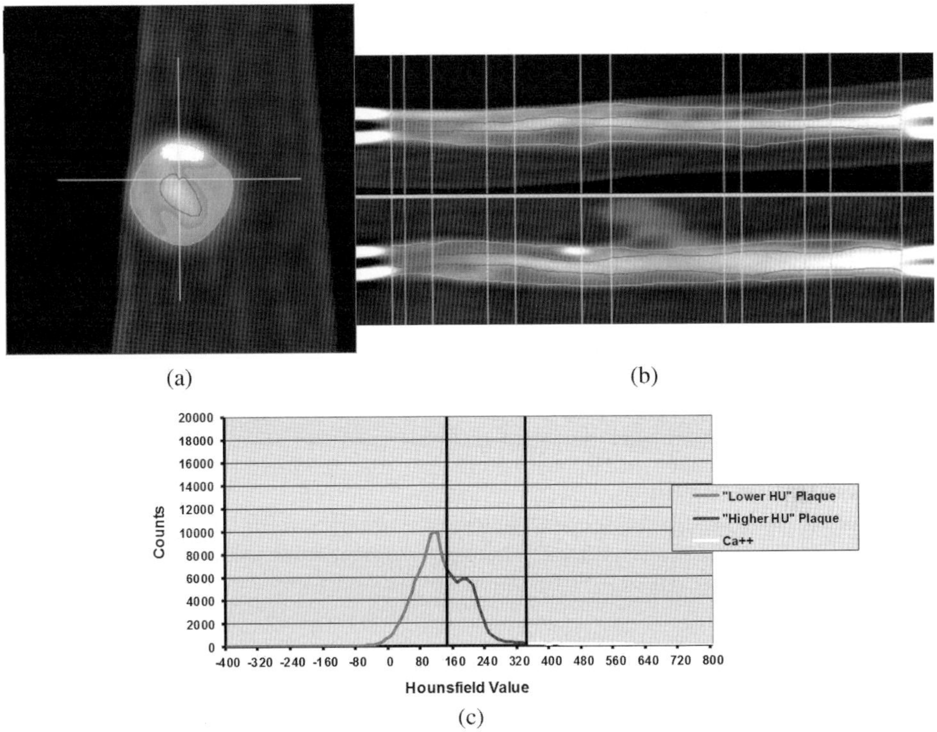

Fig. 4. Panel A shows a cross-section with low HU values displayed as light gray (between 0–150) and higher values as darker grey (between 150–330) and calcium as white (>330) Panel C. Panel B shows and longitudinal view of an explanted specimen were between the horizontal lines the coronary plaque is segmented.

depends strongly on the administered contrast concentration which is shown by elevation at right hand side (Fig. 5B). The peaked distribution was subdivided into two parts comprising the same HU range. "Soft tissue" was determined as belonging to the left area (relatively lower HU values) and "hard tissue" to the right area (relatively higher HU values). The voxels containing HU values in the high HU tail were identified as calcium.

This complies with the results of Cademartiri *et al.*[16] who found a nearly linear relation of the measured HU values in a plaque as a function of luminal contrast. Consequently, the plaque HU distribution broadens with increasing luminal contrast and shows more structure. Although absolute HU values should therefore be used with caution, the discriminating power of the HU distribution seems to improve by the luminal contrast. This is supported by received result that the contrast-enhanced scan shows a closer match to histology than the saline scan. The mechanistic details of this contrast influence,

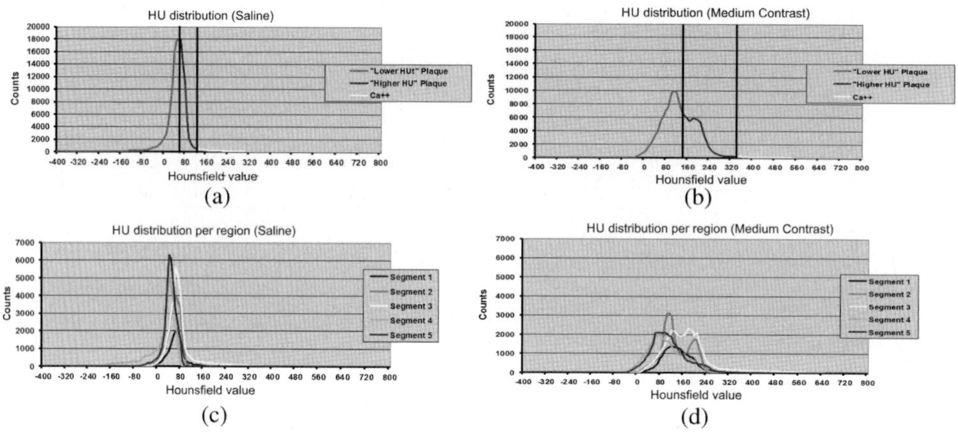

Fig. 5. Panels A and B show the Hounsfield unit (HU) distribution for the total plaque volume of the coronary specimen with no contrast (a) and medium contrast levels (b). Panels C and D are showing also the HU distribution with saline and medium contrast conditions but now for 5 sub-segments within the coronary plaque. These sub-segments are presented in the longitudinal reconstructed view of Fig. 4B.

taking into account scanner resolution, applied CT reconstruction algorithms and convolution kernels needs to be further explored.

5. Discussion

The different studies show the feasibility of volumetric plaque tissue composition analysis by MSCT-CA. However, it is easy to determine on hand calcium at one side and non-calcified tissue components on the other side (Fig. 6). It is however, much more challenging to identify the other tissue types which are non-calcified such as lipids, necrotic core and more fibrotic tissues.

In contrast, other MSCT-CA plaque compositional studies reported mostly disappointing results.[5,6,13,15] The deviation in outcomes could have been caused by application of different methods. MSCT-CA imaging of a rapidly moving coronary artery *in-vivo* causes much more possible artifacts than *ex-vivo* imaging of a coronary specimen. Furthermore, most other studies are applying IVUS as reference method, which presents plaque compositional results differently than histology, making comparison of the different studies difficult. Also, and maybe even more importantly, most of these studies applied a limited MSCT-CA plaque compositional measurement method, by measuring manually HU values at a very limited number of positions within a coronary plaque at a given individual cross-sectional location in the coronary vessel.

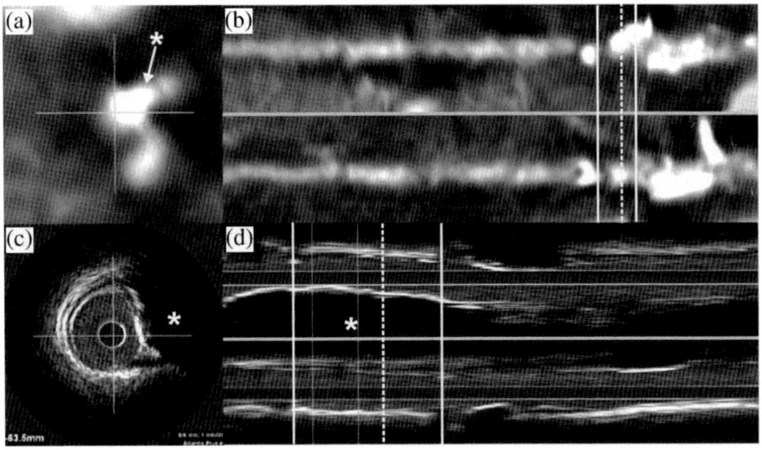

Fig. 6. Panel A shows a reconstructed cross-sectional image of a calcified segment of the coronary artery of which the longitudinal reconstructed view (L-view) is presented in panel B. In panel C, a cross-sectional intravascular ultrasound image is presented at approximately the same position as panel A. The calcium causes a so-called acoustic shadow which is visible from 12 to 3 o'clock in panel A in which the asterisk shows the shadow. The thick white lines in both panels B and D identifies the same coronary segment of interest in both MSCT (panel A) as well as in the IVUS reconstruction (panel D).

Furthermore, they did not take into account the influence of the administered contrast medium.[16]

Another possible cause of error in the other studies could be an erroneous identification (e.g. segmentation) of the plaque since correct delineation of the boundaries in an *in-vivo* situation is difficult. The coronary plaque composition can be determined from the HU distribution. The choice of the definition of three sub-classes of tissue components (e.g. soft, hard and calcium) is perhaps rather crude and has limitations, however, the commonly used IVUS derived compositional techniques also show only a limited number of different tissue components.[32,33] *In-vivo* validation of these approaches most likely will be performed by using IVUS as reference method and derived compositional techniques such as virtual histology[33] and/or echogenicity.[34]

6. Future Developments

This chapter focuses on the feasibility to derive quantitative tissue composition measurements from the plaque HU distribution and shows the first steps towards further development of the method for clinical use. An *in-vivo* plaque segmentation method and consequently a plaque dimensional measurement method is clinically necessary.[8] Good correlations with quantitative IVUS was found. However, tracing both the luminal- and external vessel boundaries *in-vivo* is far more difficult due to artifacts caused by the cardiac and respiratory motion of the patient. The reproducibility of the proposed methods depends on the accuracy of the delineation of the plaque within the original MSCT-CA images. Previous work showed that the reproducibility for dimensional MSCT-CA measurements was reasonable using previous generation scanners and with the current rapid technological developments of the MSCT-CA scanners, which are much faster in acquisition, reducing motion artifacts, and with increasing imaging resolution, the reproducibility is expected to increase.[8] This, although more research is necessary, could provide the opportunity to study plaque compositional changes under influence of new treatment methods non-invasively applying the proposed method.

Although MSCT-CA has a lower image resolution than IVUS, the results of these studies indicate that when significant plaque burden exists, its composition can be measured from the HU distribution. Definition of more tissue sub-classes will be the subject of further research when scanner technology improves (e.g. higher spatial resolution).

7. Conclusions

Assessment of coronary plaques is currently performed mostly invasively. Follow-up examinations thus require additional angiography with subsequent risks and discomfort to the patients. A non-invasive imaging procedure such as MSCT-CA could therefore be a major step forward in the research of CAD. MSCT-CA also has the advantage over IVUS that the complete coronary artery tree is visualized. However, there is still need for more in-depth evaluations and computer assisted analyses methods. Furthermore, one great concern about the use of MSCT-CA imaging still remains — the radiation exposure. This will be significantly reduced by using new technologies in the future.[35]

References

1. P.J. de Feyter, K. Nieman, "Noninvasive multi-slice computed tomography coronary angiography: An emerging clinical modality," *J Am Coll Cardiol* **44**, 1238–1240 (2004).
2. G.L. Raff, M.J. Gallagher, W.W. O'Neill, J.A. Goldstein, "Diagnostic accuracy of noninvasive coronary angiography using 64-slice spiral computed tomography," *J Am Coll Cardiol* **46**, 552–557 (2005).
3. S. Leschka, H. Alkadhi, A. Plass, L. Desbiolles, J. Grunenfelder, B. Marincek, S. Wildermuth, "Accuracy of msct coronary angiography with 64-slice technology: First experience," *Eur Heart J* **26**, 1482–1487 (2005).

4. K. Nieman, M. Oudkerk, B.J. Rensing, P. van Ooijen, A. Munne, R.J. van Geuns, P.J. de Feyter, "Coronary angiography with multi-slice computed tomography," *Lancet* **357**, 599–603 (2001).
5. A.W. Leber, A. Knez, A. Becker, C. Becker, F. von Ziegler, K. Nikolaou, C. Rist, M. Reiser, C. White, G. Steinbeck, P. Boekstegers, "Accuracy of multidetector spiral computed tomography in identifying and differentiating the composition of coronary atherosclerotic plaques: A comparative study with intracoronary ultrasound," *J Am Coll Cardiol* **43**, 1241–1247 (2004).
6. K. Nikolaou, C.R. Becker, M. Muders, G. Babaryka, J. Scheidler, T. Flohr, U. Loehrs, M.F. Reiser, Z.A. Fayad, "Multidetector-row computed tomography and magnetic resonance imaging of atherosclerotic lesions in human ex vivo coronary arteries," *Atherosclerosis* **174**, 243–252 (2004).
7. F. Moselewski, D. Ropers, K. Pohle, U. Hoffmann, M. Ferencik, R.C. Chan, R.C. Cury, S. Abbara, I.K. Jang, T.J. Brady, W.G. Daniel, S. Achenbach, "Comparison of measurement of cross-sectional coronary atherosclerotic plaque and vessel areas by 16-slice multidetector computed tomography versus intravascular ultrasound," *Am J Cardiol* **94**, 1294–1297 (2004).
8. N. Bruining, J.R. Roelandt, A. Palumbo, L.L. Grutta, F. Cademartiri, P.J. de Feijter, N. Mollet, R.T. van Domburg, P.W. Serruys, R. Hamers, "Reproducible coronary plaque quantification by multislice computed tomography," *Catheter Cardiovasc Interv* **69**, 857–865 (2007).
9. A.W. Leber, A. Knez, F. von Ziegler, A. Becker, K. Nikolaou, S. Paul, B. Wintersperger, M. Reiser, C.R. Becker, G. Steinbeck, P. Boekstegers, "Quantification of obstructive and nonobstructive coronary lesions by 64-slice computed tomography: A comparative study with quantitative coronary angiography and intravascular ultrasound," *J Am Coll Cardiol* **46**, 147–154 (2005).
10. M. Schmid, T. Pflederer, I.K. Jang, D. Ropers, K. Sei, W.G. Daniel, S. Achenbach, "Relationship between degree of remodeling and ct attenuation of plaque in coronary atherosclerotic lesions: An *in-vivo* analysis by multi-detector computed tomography," *Atherosclerosis* **197**, 457–464 (2008).
11. E. Falk, "Why do plaques rupture?" *Circulation* **86**, III30–42 (1992).
12. A.W. Leber, A. Becker, A. Knez, F. von Ziegler, M. Sirol, K. Nikolaou, B. Ohnesorge, Z.A. Fayad, C.R. Becker, M. Reiser, G. Steinbeck, P. Boekstegers, "Accuracy of 64-slice computed tomography to classify and quantify plaque volumes in the proximal coronary system: A comparative study using intravascular ultrasound," *J Am Coll Cardiol* **47**, 672–677 (2006).
13. C.R. Becker, K. Nikolaou, M. Muders, G. Babaryka, A. Crispin, U.J. Schoepf, U. Loehrs, M.F. Reiser, "*Ex vivo* coronary atherosclerotic plaque characterization with multi-detector-row ct," *Eur Radiol* **13**, 2094–2098 (2003).
14. K. Pohle, S. Achenbach, B. Macneill, D. Ropers, M. Ferencik, F. Moselewski, U. Hoffmann, T.J. Brady, I.K. Jang, W.G. Daniel, "Characterization of non-calcified coronary atherosclerotic plaque by multi-detector row ct: Comparison to ivus," *Atherosclerosis* **190**, 174–180 (2007).
15. S. Schroeder, A. Kuettner, T. Wojak, J. Janzen, M. Heuschmid, T. Athanasiou, T. Beck, C. Burgstahler, C. Herdeg, C.D. Claussen, A.F. Kopp, "Non-invasive evaluation of

atherosclerosis with contrast enhanced 16 slice spiral computed tomography: Results of *ex vivo* investigations," *Heart* **90**, 1471–1475 (2004).

16. F. Cademartiri, N.R. Mollet, G. Runza, N. Bruining, R. Hamers, P. Somers, M. Knaapen, S. Verheye, M. Midiri, G.P. Krestin, P.J. de Feyter, "Influence of intracoronary attenuation on coronary plaque measurements using multislice computed tomography: Observations in an *ex vivo* model of coronary computed tomography angiography," *Eur Radiol* **15**, 1426–1431 (2005).
17. R. Hamers, N. Bruining, M. Knook, M. Sabate, J.R.T.C. Roelandt, "A novel approach to quantitative analysis of intravascular ultrasound images," *Comp Cardiol* 589–592 (2001).
18. C. von Birgelen, A. van der Lugt, A. Nicosia, G.S. Mintz, E.J. Gussenhoven, E. de Vrey, M.T. Mallus, J.R. Roelandt, P.W. Serruys, P.J. de Feyter, "Computerized assessment of coronary lumen and atherosclerotic plaque dimensions in three-dimensional intravascular ultrasound correlated with histomorphometry," *Am J Cardiol* **78**, 1202–1209 (1996).
19. J.C. Kaski, D. Tousoulis, A.W. Haider, S. Gavrielides, F. Crea, A. Maseri, "Reactivity of eccentric and concentric coronary stenoses in patients with chronic stable angina," *J Am Coll Cardiol* **17**, 627–633 (1991).
20. J.M. Hodgson, S.P. Graham, H. Sheehan, A.D. Savakus, "Percutaneous intracoronary ultrasound imaging: Initial applications in patients," *Echocardiography* 7:403–413 (1990).
21. N. Bruining, J.R. Roelandt, S. Verheye, M. Knaapen, Y. Onuma, E. Regar, F. Cademartiri, S. de Winter, G. Van Langenhove, P.W. Serruys, R. Hamers, P.J. de Feyter, "Compositional volumetry of non-calcified coronary plaques by multislice computed tomography: An *ex vivo* feasibility study," *EuroIntervention* **5**, 558–564 (2009).
22. F. Cademartiri, L. La Grutta, G. Runza, A. Palumbo, E. Maffei, N.R. Mollet, T.V. Bartolotta, P. Somers, M. Knaapen, S. Verheye, M. Midiri, R. Hamers, N. Bruining, "Influence of convolution filtering on coronary plaque attenuation values: Observations in an ex vivo model of multislice computed tomography coronary angiography," *Eur Radiol* **17**, 1842–1849 (2007).
23. A.F. Kopp, S. Schroeder, A. Baumbach, A. Kuettner, C. Georg, B. Ohnesorge, M. Heuschmid, R. Kuzo, C.D. Claussen, "Non-invasive characterisation of coronary lesion morphology and composition by multislice ct: First results in comparison with intracoronary ultrasound," *Eur Radiol* **11**, 1607–1611 (2001).
24. S. Achenbach, F. Moselewski, D. Ropers, M. Ferencik, U. Hoffmann, B. MacNeill, K. Pohle, U. Baum, K. Anders, I.K. Jang, W.G. Daniel, T.J. Brady, "Detection of calcified and noncalcified coronary atherosclerotic plaque by contrast-enhanced, submillimeter multidetector spiral computed tomography: A segment-based comparison with intravascular ultrasound," *Circulation* **109**, 14–17 (2004).
25. C. Caussin, A. Ohanessian, S. Ghostine, L. Jacq, B. Lancelin, G. Dambrin, A. Sigal-Cinqualbre, C.Y. Angel, J.F. Paul, "Characterization of vulnerable nonstenotic plaque with 16-slice computed tomography compared with intravascular ultrasound," *Am J Cardiol* **94**, 99–104 (2004).
26. P. Schoenhagen, E.M. Tuzcu, A.E. Stillman, D.J. Moliterno, S.S. Halliburton, S.A. Kuzmiak, J.M. Kasper, W.A. Magyar, M.L. Lieber, S.E. Nissen, R.D. White, "Non-invasive assessment of plaque morphology and remodeling in mildly stenotic coronary segments: Comparison of 16-slice computed tomography and intravascular ultrasound," *Coron Artery Dis* **14**, 459–462 (2003).

27. S. Schroeder, A.F. Kopp, B. Ohnesorge, T. Flohr, A. Baumbach, A. Kuettner, C. Herdeg, K.R. Karsch, C.D. Claussen, "Accuracy and reliability of quantitative measurements in coronary arteries by multi-slice computed tomography: Experimental and initial clinical results," *Clin Radiol* **56**, 466–474 (2001).
28. T.T. de Weert, M. Ouhlous, E. Meijering, P.E. Zondervan, J.M. Hendriks, M.R. van Sambeek, D.W. Dippel, A. van der Lugt, "*In vivo* characterization and quantification of atherosclerotic carotid plaque components with multidetector computed tomography and histopathological correlation," *Arterioscler Thromb Vasc Biol* **26**, 2366–2372 (2006).
29. T. Miszalski-Jamka, P. Klimeczek, R. Banys, M. Krupinski, K. Nycz, K. Bury, M. Lada, R. Pelberg, D. Kereiakes, W. Mazur, "The composition and extent of coronary artery plaque detected by multislice computed tomographic angiography provides incremental prognostic value in patients with suspected coronary artery disease," *Int J Cardiovasc Imaging* **28**, 621–631 (2012).
30. G. Pundziute, J.D. Schuijf, J.E. van Velzen, J.W. Jukema, J.M. van Werkhoven, G. Nucifora, F. van der Kley, L.J. Kroft, A. de Roos, E. Boersma, J.H. Reiber, M.J. Schalij, E.E. van der Wall, J.J. Bax, "Assessment with multi-slice computed tomography and gray-scale and virtual histology intravascular ultrasound of gender-specific differences in extent and composition of coronary atherosclerotic plaques in relation to age," *Am J Cardiol* **105**, 480–486 (2010).
31. N. Bruining, C. von Birgelen, P.J. de Feyter, J. Ligthart, W. Li, P.W. Serruys, J.R. Roelandt, "Ecg-gated versus nongated three-dimensional intracoronary ultrasound analysis: Implications for volumetric measurements," *Cathet Cardiovasc Diagn* **43**, 254–260 (1998).
32. C.A. Van Mieghem, N. Bruining, J.A. Schaar, E. McFadden, N. Mollet, F. Cademartiri, Mastik F, J.M. Ligthart, G.A. Granillo, M. Valgimigli, G. Sianos, W.J. van der Giessen, B. Backx, M.A. Morel, G.A. Van Es, J.D. Sawyer, J. Kaplow, A. Zalewski, A.F. van der Steen, P. de Feyter, P.W. Serruys, "Rationale and methods of the integrated biomarker and imaging study (ibis): Combining invasive and non-invasive imaging with biomarkers to detect subclinical atherosclerosis and assess coronary lesion biology," *Int J Cardiovasc Imaging* **21**, 425–441 (2005).
33. A. Nair, B.D. Kuban, E.M. Tuzcu, P. Schoenhagen, S.E. Nissen, D.G. Vince, "Coronary plaque classification with intravascular ultrasound radiofrequency data analysis," *Circulation* **106**, 2200–2206 (2002).
34. S.A. de Winter, I. Heller, R. Hamers, P.J. de Feijter, P.W. Serruys, J.R.T.C. Roelandt, N. Bruining, "Computer assisted three-dimensional plaque charcterization in intracoronary ultrasound studies," *Comp Cardiol* **30**, 73–76 (2003).
35. T.F. Jakobs, C.R. Becker, B. Ohnesorge, T. Flohr, C. Suess, U.J. Schoepf, M.F. Reiser, "Multislice helical ct of the heart with retrospective ecg gating: Reduction of radiation exposure by ecg-controlled tube current modulation," *Eur Radiol* **12**, 1081–1086 (2002).

Chapter 2

On-The-Fly Monte Carlo Methods In Iterative Pet Reconstruction

László Szirmay-Kalos, Milán Magdics and Balázs Tóth*

Department of Control Engineering and Information Technology, Budapest University of Technology and Economics, Hungary
http://cg.iit.bme.hu
**E-mail: szirmay@iit.bme.hu*

Iterative Positron Emission Tomography (PET) reconstruction computes projections between the voxel space and the LOR space, which are mathematically equivalent to the evaluation of multi-dimensional integrals. These integrals are elements of the System Matrix (SM) and can be obtained either by deterministic quadrature or Monte Carlo (MC) methods. Due to the enormous size of the SM, it cannot be stored but integral estimation should be repeated whenever matrix elements are needed. In this paper we show that it is worth using random SM estimates, because this way errors caused by the projectors of different iteration steps can compensate each other, and do not accumulate to unacceptable values, which can happen in case of deterministic approximation. MC quadrature, however, introduces a random noise in the iteration process, which will not be convergent but iterated values will fluctuate around the real solution. We also propose methods to reduce the scale of this fluctuation and force the iteration to concentrate on the real solution.

1. Introduction

In Positron Emission Tomography (PET) we need to find the spatial positron emission density.[9] At a positron–electron annihilation, two oppositely directed 511 keV photons are generated. As these photons fly in the medium, they might collide with the particles of the material before they leave the tomograph or get captured by the detectors. During such collisions the photon may get absorbed or scattered either coherently or incoherently, but in [100, 700] keV energy range typical in PET, only incoherent, i.e. Compton scattering is relevant.

A PET/CT collects the numbers $\mathbf{y} = (y_1, y_2, \ldots, y_{N_{\mathrm{LOR}}})$ of simultaneous photon incidents in detector pairs, also called *Lines Of Responses* or *LORs*, and obtains the *material map* of the examined object by a CT scan. The output of the reconstruction method is the *tracer density* function $x(\vec{v})$, which is approximated in a *finite function series* form:

$$x(\vec{v}) = \sum_{V=1}^{N_{\text{voxel}}} x_V b_V(\vec{v}) \tag{1}$$

where $\mathbf{x} = (x_1, x_2, \ldots, x_{N_{\text{voxel}}})$ are the unknown coefficients called *voxel values* and $b_V(\vec{v})$ ($V = 1, \ldots, N_{\text{voxel}}$) are pre-defined basis functions, which can be piece-wise constant, tri-linear or even of higher order.[3]

The correspondence between the coefficients of the tracer density function (voxel values) and the LOR hits is established by the *system sensitivity* $\mathcal{T}(\vec{v} \to L)$ defining the probability that a radioactive decay happened in $\vec{v}$ is detected by LOR L.

The Maximum Likelihood Expectation Maximization (ML-EM) scheme searches tracer density coefficients $x_1, \ldots, x_{N_{\text{voxel}}}$ that maximize the probability of measurement results $y_1, \ldots, y_{N_{\text{LOR}}}$ by an iterative algorithm,[10] which alternates simulations, called forward projections, and corrective steps based on the computed and measured values, which are called back projections.

Forward projection computes the expectation value of the number of hits $\tilde{\mathbf{y}} = (\tilde{y}_1, \tilde{y}_2, \ldots, \tilde{y}_{N_{\text{LOR}}})$ in each LOR L:

$$\tilde{y}_L = \int_{\mathcal{V}} x(\vec{v})\mathcal{T}(\vec{v} \to L)\mathrm{d}v = \sum_{V=1}^{N_{\text{voxel}}} \mathbf{A}_{LV} x_V \tag{2}$$

where $\mathcal{V}$ is the domain of the reconstruction, and $\mathbf{A}_{LV}$ is the *System Matrix* (*SM*):

$$\mathbf{A}_{LV} = \int_{\mathcal{V}} b_V(\vec{v})\mathcal{T}(\vec{v} \to L)\mathrm{d}v. \tag{3}$$

Taking into account that the measured hits follow a Poisson distribution, after the forward projection of iteration step n, the ML-EM scheme executes a *back projection* correcting the voxel estimates based on the ratios of measured y_L and computed $\tilde{y}_L^{(n)}$ LOR values:

$$x_V^{(n+1)} = x_V^{(n)} \cdot \frac{\sum_L \mathbf{A}_{LV} \frac{y_L}{\tilde{y}_L^{(n)}}}{\sum_L \mathbf{A}_{LV}}, \tag{4}$$

where

$$\tilde{y}_L^{(n)} = \sum_{V'=1}^{N_{\text{voxel}}} \mathbf{A}_{LV'} x_{V'}^{(n)}$$

is the result of forward projecting the current estimate. With a more compact matrix notation, we can also write

$$\mathbf{x}^{(n+1)} = \langle x_V^{(n)} \rangle \cdot \bar{\mathbf{A}}^T \cdot \frac{\mathbf{y}}{\mathbf{A} \cdot \mathbf{x}^{(n)}} \tag{5}$$

where $\langle x_V^{(n)} \rangle$ is a diagonal matrix of current voxel values,

$$\bar{\mathbf{A}}_{LV} = \frac{\mathbf{A}_{LV}}{\sum_{L'} \mathbf{A}_{L'V}}$$

is the *normalized SM*, and vector division is interpreted in an element-wise manner.

If the iteration is convergent, then this iteration converges to a fixed point $\mathbf{x}^*$ where voxel values are not modified by this formula, i.e. the iteration solves the following equation:

$$\bar{\mathbf{A}}^T \cdot \frac{\mathbf{y}}{\mathbf{A} \cdot \mathbf{x}^*} = \mathbf{1}.$$

In order to study the convergence properties, let us express the activity estimate in step n as $\mathbf{x}^{(n)} = \mathbf{x}^* + \Delta\mathbf{x}^{(n)}$, i.e. with the difference from the fixed point. Substituting this into the iteration formula and replacing the terms by first order Taylor's approximations, we obtain[6]:

$$\Delta\mathbf{x}^{(n+1)} \approx \left(\mathbf{1} - \langle x_V^* \rangle \cdot \bar{\mathbf{A}}^T \cdot \left\langle \frac{y_L}{\tilde{y}_L^2} \right\rangle \cdot \mathbf{A} \right) \cdot \Delta\mathbf{x}^{(n)}$$

where $\left\langle \frac{y_L}{\tilde{y}_L^2} \right\rangle$ is a diagonal matrix of ratios $\frac{y_L}{\tilde{y}_L^2}$. The iteration is convergent if matrix

$$\mathbf{T} = \mathbf{1} - \langle x_V^* \rangle \cdot \bar{\mathbf{A}}^T \cdot \left\langle \frac{y_L}{\tilde{y}_L^2} \right\rangle \cdot \mathbf{A}$$

is a *contraction*.

2. Error Analysis

To compute forward and back projections, we should consider all points where positrons can be generated and all possible particle paths that can lead to an event in LOR L. A particle path can be described by a sequence of particle–matter interaction points, thus potential contribution $\mathcal{T}(\vec{v} \to L)$ of positron emission point $\vec{v}$ to LOR L is a high-dimensional integral, so are the expected LOR hits in Eq. (2) and SM elements in Eq. (3).

In tomography the size of the SM is enormous since both N_{voxel} and N_{LOR} may exceed 10^8, thus matrix elements cannot be pre-computed and stored, but must be re-computed each time when a matrix element is needed. The standard ML-EM reconstruction scheme is based on the assumption that SM elements and expected number of hits $\tilde{y}_L$ can be precisely computed. However, this is not the case since SM computation involves numerical quadrature. Deterministic quadrature results in estimations of deterministic error while MC methods result in random values involving random approximation error. To show why MC methods offer a better solution, we first analyze the application of deterministic approximations.

2.1. *Deterministic Approximation*

Deterministic approximation makes a similar error in each iteration step, and errors may accumulate during the iteration. To formally analyze this issue, let us first consider that SM estimations may be different in forward projection and back projection, and due to the numerical errors, both differ from exact matrix $\mathbf{A}$. Let us denote the forward projection SM by $\mathbf{F} = \mathbf{A} + \Delta\mathbf{F}$ where $\Delta\mathbf{F}$ represents its calculation error. The back projector matrix $\mathbf{B}$ also differs from the real SM, so is the normalized back projector

$$\bar{\mathbf{B}}_{LV} = \frac{\mathbf{B}_{LV}}{\sum_{L'} \mathbf{B}_{L'V}}$$

from the real normalized SM $\bar{\mathbf{A}}$. The approximate normalized back projector is $\bar{\mathbf{B}} = \bar{\mathbf{A}} + \Delta\bar{\mathbf{B}}$ where $\Delta\bar{\mathbf{B}}$ is the error.

The ML-EM iteration scheme using the approximate matrices is

$$\mathbf{x}^{(n+1)} = \langle x_V^{(n)} \rangle \cdot \bar{\mathbf{B}}^T \cdot \frac{\mathbf{y}}{\mathbf{F} \cdot \mathbf{x}^{(n)}}. \tag{6}$$

The question is how the application of approximate matrices modifies the fixed point $\mathbf{x}^*$ of the iteration scheme using the exact SM. Let us express the activity estimate in step n as $\mathbf{x}^{(n)} = \mathbf{x}^* + \Delta\mathbf{x}^{(n)}$. Substituting this into the iteration formula and replacing the terms by first order Taylor's approximations, we obtain:

$$\Delta\mathbf{x}^{(n+1)} \approx \mathbf{T} \cdot \Delta\mathbf{x}^{(n)} + \langle x_V^* \rangle \cdot (\Delta\mathbf{b} - \Delta\mathbf{f})$$

where

$$\Delta\mathbf{f} = \bar{\mathbf{A}}^T \cdot \left\langle \frac{y_L}{\tilde{y}_L^2} \right\rangle \cdot \Delta\mathbf{F} \cdot \mathbf{x}$$

is the error due to the forward projection estimation, and

$$\Delta\mathbf{b} = \Delta\bar{\mathbf{B}}^T \cdot \frac{\mathbf{y}}{\tilde{\mathbf{y}}}$$

is the error due to the back projection estimation.

The limiting value will be different from $\mathbf{x}^*$ due to the errors of forward and back projections:

$$\Delta\mathbf{x}^{(\infty)} = \left(\mathbf{A}^T \cdot \left\langle \frac{y_L}{\tilde{y}_L^2} \right\rangle \cdot \mathbf{A} \right)^{-1} \cdot (\Delta\mathbf{b} - \Delta\mathbf{f}). \tag{7}$$

According to this formula, matrix $\left(\mathbf{A}^T \cdot \left\langle \frac{y_L}{\tilde{y}_L^2} \right\rangle \cdot \mathbf{A} \right)^{-1}$ expresses *error accumulation*, i.e. how the error made in a single step is scaled up during the iteration. If $\mathbf{A}^T \cdot \mathbf{A}$ is far from the identity matrix, or many LORs have small or even zero measured value y_L, then error accumulation can be prohibitively large even if the error of a single step is acceptable.

2.2. *Random Approximation*

The error accumulation problem of deterministic approximations can be attacked by applying Monte Carlo quadrature to re-compute projections, because an unbiased Monte Carlo quadrature has a random error of zero mean, so errors made in different iteration steps can hopefully compensate each other. In this case, projector matrices $\mathbf{F}^{(n)}$ and $\bar{\mathbf{B}}^{(n)}$ are realizations of random variables and have a different value in each iteration step. Note that as we have to re-compute the matrix elements anyway, the costs of repeating the previous computation or obtaining a statistically independent new estimation are the same.

If projections are computed with *unbiased estimators*, then the expectations of the random projection matrices will be equal to the exact ones:

$$E[\mathbf{F}] = \mathbf{A}, \quad E[\bar{\mathbf{B}}] = \bar{\mathbf{A}}.$$

Using a random approximation instead of a deterministic approximation of expected LOR value $\tilde{y}_L$, we obtain a random variable $\hat{y}_L$ that only approximates the expected value. This random variable depends on the pseudo-random numbers used to compute the MC estimate, thus it can change in every iteration step.[12] This random and varying error makes the iteration not convergent but the iterated value will fluctuate around the exact solution. To get an accurate reconstruction, the center of the fluctuation should be identical or close to the real solution and its amplitude should be small when actual estimate $\mathbf{x}$ is close to fixed point $\mathbf{x}^*$.

2.2.1. *Center of the fluctuation*

The center of the fluctuation is the real solution if iterating from the fixed point, the expectation of executing a forward and a back projection for the real solution is still the real solution, i.e.

$$E\left[\bar{\mathbf{B}}^T \cdot \frac{\mathbf{y}}{\mathbf{F} \cdot \mathbf{x}^*}\right] = \bar{\mathbf{A}}^T \cdot \frac{\mathbf{y}}{\mathbf{A} \cdot \mathbf{x}^*}.$$

Unfortunately, this requirement is not met even by unbiased projectors.

If the forward projector and the back projector are statistically independent, then the expectation of their product is the product of their expectations:

$$E\left[\bar{\mathbf{B}}^T \cdot \frac{\mathbf{y}}{\mathbf{F} \cdot \mathbf{x}^*}\right] = E[\bar{\mathbf{B}}^T] \cdot E\left[\frac{\mathbf{y}}{\mathbf{F} \cdot \mathbf{x}^*}\right] = \bar{\mathbf{A}}^T \cdot E\left[\frac{\mathbf{y}}{\mathbf{F} \cdot \mathbf{x}^*}\right]. \tag{8}$$

Note that the second factor is generally not equal to $\frac{\mathbf{y}}{\mathbf{A} \cdot \mathbf{x}}$ even for unbiased forward and back projectors since the forward projection result is in the denominator, thus its non-linear, reciprocal function determines the expectation value:

$$E\left[\frac{\mathbf{y}}{\mathbf{F} \cdot \mathbf{x}}\right] \neq \frac{\mathbf{y}}{E[\mathbf{F}] \cdot \mathbf{x}} = \frac{\mathbf{y}}{\mathbf{A} \cdot \mathbf{x}}.$$

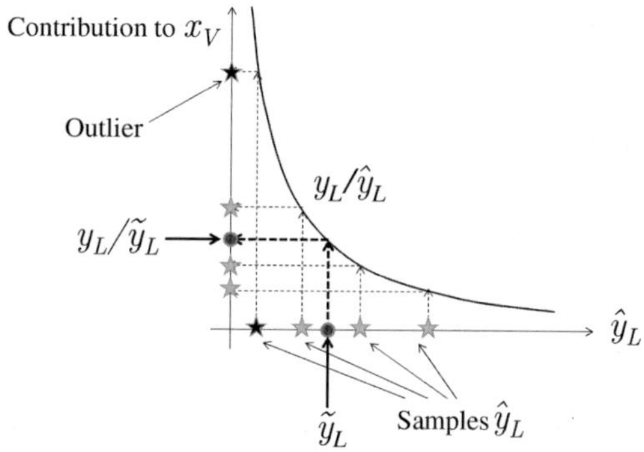

Fig. 1. Expected LOR hit number $\tilde{y}_L$ is approximated by random samples $\hat{y}_L$, which have mean $\tilde{y}_L$. These random samples are shown on the horizontal axis. Back projection computes ratio $y_L/\hat{y}_L$ to obtain voxel updates, which is a non-linear, convex function, resulting in voxel values that may be much higher than the correct value $y_L/\tilde{y}_L$. These overshooting samples are responsible for a positive bias and occasionally cause a large random increase in the voxel value.

To examine this for a single element of the vector, let us consider the expectation of the ratio of measured and computed hits, $y_L/\hat{y}_L$. According to the relation of harmonic and arithmetic means, or equivalently to the Jensen's inequality taking into account that $1/\hat{y}_L$ is a convex function, we obtain:

$$E\left[\frac{y_L}{\hat{y}_L}\right] \geq \frac{y_L}{E\left[\hat{y}_L\right]} = \frac{y_L}{\tilde{y}_L}. \tag{9}$$

This inequality states that $y_L/\tilde{y}_L$ has a random estimator of positive bias.[14] An intuitive graphical interpretation of this result is shown by Fig. 1. Here we assume that the iteration is already close to the fixed point, so different estimates are around the expected detector hit corresponding to the maximum likelihood. Note that the division in the back projection may amplify forward projection error causing large fluctuations, especially when $\tilde{y}_L$ is close to zero.

This bias can be tolerated if the forward projector has low variance, thus the generated values $\hat{y}_L$ are in a small interval where the application of a non-linear reciprocal function can be well approximated by a linear one. Another approach is the modification of the ML-EM scheme in order to correct the distorted sample distributions to restore unbiasedness even after the application of the reciprocal function.[14]

If the forward projector and the back projector are not statistically independent, even the factorization of Eq. (8) fails in addition to the problem of non-linear operations. From the point of view of having the random process oscillating around the real solution, we can conclude that the forward projector and the back projector should preferably be independent and the forward projector should have small variance.

2.2.2. *Amplitude of the fluctuation*

The second requirement of accurate reconstruction is that the fluctuation should have small amplitude, i.e. the variance of applying a complete iteration step is small, especially when the process is close to the fixed point.

To meet this requirement and get small variance, the following factors need to be taken into account. The forward projector should be of small variance especially where the LOR value is small, because this LOR value will be the denominator in the back projection formula. The slope of the $1/\hat{y}_L$ function is $-1/\hat{y}_L^2$, which scales up the variance of the forward projector especially when $\hat{y}_L$ is close to zero.

The variance of the back projector is included in the variance of the result without any amplification. As the back projector matrix elements are in the numerator and the forward projector matrix elements in the denominator of Eq. (6), the variance can also be reduced if they are made correlated. When, due to the random approximation of the forward projector a matrix element is overestimated, and thus the corresponding LOR value in the denominator gets greater than needed, the modified voxel value can be made more accurate by simultaneously increasing the matrix element in the numerator, which represents the back projector. So, from the point of view of the oscillation amplitude, it seems advantageous to use the same projector for back projection as used for forward projection of the same iteration step. Establishing such a correlation is easy if the same algorithm is used to compute the forward projection and the back projection, only the seed of the random number generator should be set to the same value before back projection as was set before forward projection of this iteration step.

2.2.3. *Optimal randomization*

Analyzing the mean and the variance of a single ML-EM step involving random projectors, we noted that the accuracy of forward projection is more crucial than that of the back projection. However, for the independence or correlation of forward and back projectors, unbiasedness and low variance resulted in different requirements. Unbiasedness prefers statistically *independent* forward and back projectors, but low variance due to error compensation needs *correlated* forward and back projectors.

Matrix elements are integrals of Eq. (2) where the integrand is a product of source intensity $x(\vec{v})$ and scanner sensitivity $\mathcal{T}(\vec{v} \to L)$, and the integration domain is the path space where a "point" corresponds to a path of particles from the emission to the absorption in the detectors. The variance of the MC quadrature depends on the number and distribution of the samples and on the variation of the integrand.[15] There are many possibilities to generate sample paths, which differ in the direction of path building and also in whether roughly the same number of samples is used for each LOR integral, or the sampling process prefers some LORs to others and allocates most of the samples to the preferred ones.

If natural phenomena are directly simulated, then annihilation points are sampled proportionally to their emission density, and each sample path is generated with its real probability and can cause a single hit. Thus, the number of samples in LORs will be proportional to the expected values that are computed. This method is called *voxel driven*.[13] Voxel driven approaches calculate different LORs with a similar absolute error. Voxel driven methods are particularly efficient when the activity distribution has high variation, for example, when the activity is concentrated in a few small point like features. However, voxel driven methods can lose a lot of samples and can thus be inefficient when the detector modules are seen just in a small solid angle from the voxels, which is typically the case in human PETs.

LOR driven methods initiate computation at LORs and for each LOR, they try to find contributing voxels. When roughly the same number of samples are allocated for each LOR, their error depends just on the variation of their corresponding integral. If the variation is proportional to the integrand, then different LORs are computed with the same relative error. Note that LOR driven methods build up paths indirectly and following directions that are opposite to those of nature, starting at the detectors and finding the point of emission just at the end of the exploration. Such indirect approach can also be imagined as shooting virtual particles from detectors, that deliver the contribution to their parents when they find active regions. LOR driven methods are unable to concentrate on active regions but all samples will contribute to some LOR, so these approaches are good at reconstructing homogeneous regions and work well even if the detector modules subtend just a small solid angle. Note that classical direct contribution calculation methods, like Siddon's[11] or Joseph's method,[5] or Watson's single scatter simulation[16] fall into the category of LOR driven approaches. Another advantage of LOR driven methods is that they are output driven in forward projection, which means that output values can be computed independently of each other, which improves the efficiency of parallel GPU implementations.[8]

Whether it is worth trading more bias for less variance, i.e. using correlated projectors rather than independent ones, depends on the level of fluctuation. This level can be very high when low contribution LORs are estimated with similar absolute error as high contribution LORs. In the extreme case it can happen that a LOR value is approximated by zero in forward projection, which results in an infinite fluctuation unless the matrix elements corresponding to this LOR are also zero in back projection. Thus, voxel driven methods seem to be better with correlated projectors, but LOR driven approaches prefer lower bias provided by independent projectors.

3. Photon Tracing

Photon tracing is an MC approach that directly simulates physical phenomena. In Photon Tracing, first annihilation point $\vec{v}$ is sampled, then the paths of the two annihilation photons are generated mimicking the free path length and scattering in the real material. If annihilation points are sampled proportional to the activity,[2] then we have a voxel driven approach. A voxel driven approach initiates

$$N_V = \frac{x_V N_{\mathrm{PT}}}{\sum_{V'=1}^{N_{\mathrm{voxel}}} x_{V'}}$$

number of photons from voxel V where N_{PT} is the total number of paths initiated from all photons.

Although photon tracing builds up paths from the emission to the point of absorption, we can consider it as a LOR-driven method if the same

$$N_V = \frac{N_{\mathrm{PT}}}{N_{\mathrm{voxel}}}$$

annihilation sample points are allocated to each voxel, since this sampling does not prefer some voxels to others and allocates roughly the same number of samples to each LOR.

Sampling point $\vec{v}$ in the voxel depends on the function series in Eq. (1). If piece-wise constant basis functions are used, i.e. activity $x(\vec{v})$ is assumed to be constant in each voxel and thus basis functions are box functions, then the three Cartesian coordinates of $\vec{v}$ are uniformly distributed independent random numbers inside the voxel. In case of tri-linear interpolation or higher order spline basis functions, we can take advantage of that these basis functions can be obtained as the self convolution of box functions,[2] i.e. a tent-like tri-linearly interpolating basis function is the convolution of the box with itself, a quadratic spline is the convolution of the tri-linear basis function and a box function, etc. As the probability density of the sum of two independent random variables is the convolution of the individual densities, samples can be generated with tri-linear density by adding two random samples obtained with constant density, with quadratic splines as adding three random samples of uniform distribution, etc.

The paths of the two annihilation photons are obtained with scanner sensitivity $\mathcal{T}(\vec{v} \to L)$. To do this, an initial direction is drawn from uniform distribution. Two photons are started from the annihilation point and their free paths are sampled to find the photon–material interaction points. As these photons fly in the medium, they might collide with the particles of the material. The probability that collision happens in unit distance is the *cross section* σ. When Compton scattering happens, there is a unique correspondence between the relative scattered energy and the cosine of the scattering angle, as defined by the *Compton formula*:

$$\epsilon = \frac{1}{1 + \epsilon_0(1 - \cos\theta)} \Longrightarrow \cos\theta = 1 - \frac{1-\epsilon}{\epsilon_0 \epsilon},$$

where $\epsilon = E_1/E_0$ expresses the ratio of the scattered energy E_1 and the incident energy E_0, and $\epsilon_0 = E_0/(m_e c^2)$ is the incident energy relative to the energy of the electron.

The phase function, i.e. the probability density that the photon is scattered from direction $\vec{\omega}$ to $\vec{\omega}'$, is given by the *Klein-Nishina formula*[18]:

$$P_{\mathrm{KN}}(\vec{\omega} \cdot \vec{\omega}') \propto \epsilon + \epsilon^3 - \epsilon^2 \sin^2\theta.$$

The ratio of proportionality can be obtained from the requirement that this is a probability density, thus integrating $\vec{\omega}'$ for the directional sphere, we should get 1.

When one of the photons leaves the detector or its energy drops below the discrimination threshold, the photon pair is lost and no LOR is contributed. If photons hit the detector surfaces of LOR L, the simulation of this path is terminated and the affected SM element A_{LV} is given a contribution equal to $1/N_V$.

Photon tracing, as MC methods in general, results in random SM elements, i.e. projections. The MC simulation is repeated in forward and back projections in each iteration step. The correlation or independence between the forward and back projections can be controlled by whether or not the seed of the pseudo random number generator is reset between these projections. As stated, the accuracy of forward projection is more important, therefore we propose two techniques to increase the accuracy of forward projections without increasing the number of samples, i.e. computation time.

4. Statistical Filtering

Recall that the classical ML-EM scheme works with two values in a LOR, the measured value y_L and its mean $\tilde{y}_L$ computed from the actual activity estimate.

The expected value is a scalar determined by the activity, the measured value is a realization of a random variable of Poisson distribution having mean $\tilde{y}_L$. Based on the concept of maximum likelihood estimation, the activity estimate is found so that the joint probability of measured values given the expectations obtained from the activity has a maximum.

This classical view should be altered and we should accept the fact that expectation $\tilde{y}_L$ cannot be accurately computed, we can only get random samples $\hat{y}_L$ approximating the expectation. When a LOR is processed we have two random samples: measured value y_L and random estimate $\hat{y}_L$ of its expectation. Fluctuations of the iterated activity can be suppressed if we replace those estimates $\hat{y}_L$ that are unacceptable outliers by some robust estimate.

To detect whether the pair of measured value y_L and expected value approximation $\hat{y}_L$ is acceptable or an outlier, we should check whether y_L could be a reasonable realization of a Poisson distributed random process of mean $\hat{y}_L$.

Given an observation y_L, the confidence interval for mean $\tilde{y}_L$ with confidence level $1 - \alpha$ is given by the following fairly sharp approximation[1,17]:

$$F(y_L) \leq \tilde{y}_L \leq F(y_L + 1)$$

where

$$F(y_L) = y_L \left(1 - \frac{1}{9y_L} - \frac{z_{\alpha/2}}{3\sqrt{y_L}}\right)^3$$

and $z_{\alpha/2}$ is the standard normal deviate with upper tail integral $\alpha/2$. It means that when our approximation of the expected value satisfies inequality

$$\hat{y}_L < y_L \left(1 - \frac{1}{9y_L} - \frac{z_{\alpha/2}}{3\sqrt{y_L}}\right)^3,$$

then we cannot be confident in this approximation and therefore we correct it. We set $z_{\alpha/2} = 2.1$ because it guarantees that $\hat{y}_L = 0$, which would lead to a division by zero, is outside of the confidence interval if measured value $y_L \geq 1$. This corresponds to 98% confidence.

When the current expected value approximation is out of the confidence interval, we should replace it with an acceptable value or completely ignore this LOR in this iteration step. We first try to substitute value $\hat{y}_L$ by the average of the approximations of this LOR in previous iteration cycles. Note that when the algorithm is close to the converged state, the expected LOR hit does not change too much, so averaging the previous estimates helps decrease the variance of the estimator by trading variance to a small bias. We accept the average when it is in the confidence interval. If even the average is out of the confidence interval, then this LOR is skipped during back projection.

5. LOR Space Blurring

The result of forward projection is the random estimation of LOR hits $\hat{y}_L$, which is usually an unbiased estimate having higher variance. As stated, low variance LOR values are essential especially when the expectation is close to zero. Thus, it is worth trading some bias for reduced variance. We can assume that neighboring LORs get similar number of hits, thus variance can be reduced by 4D spatial blurring, which means that each LOR value is replaced by the average of neighboring LOR values.

6. Flat-land Results

We examine a simple *flat-land* problem describing a 2D PET where $N_{\rm LOR} = 2115$ and $N_{\rm voxel} = 1024$ (Fig. 2). The reason of the application of the flat-land model is that the 2D planar case makes the SM of reasonable size, so the proposed methods can be compared to ground truth solutions when the SM is pre-computed and re-used in iteration steps (recall that this is not possible in fully-3D PET because of the prohibiting size). In order to test scattering in the flat-land model, the Compton law and the Klein-Nishina phase function should be modified to be consistent with the planar case. This means that we

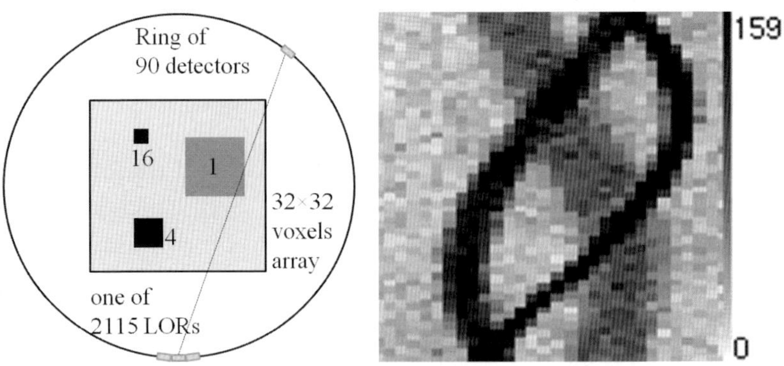

Fig. 2. 2D tomograph model: The detector ring contains 90 detector crystals and each of them is of size 2.2 in voxel units and participates in 47 LORs connecting this crystal to crystals being in the opposite half circle, thus the total number of LORs is $90 \times 47/2 = 2115$. The voxel array to be reconstructed is in the middle of the ring and has 32×32 resolution, i.e. 1024 voxels. The ground truth voxel array has three hot squares of activity densities 1, 4, and 16 [Bq/voxel] and of sizes 8^2, 4^2, and 2^2. The voxel array is measured for 260 seconds tracing $5 \cdot 10^4$ photon pairs, resulting in the sinogram of the right image.

use only the scattering angle θ and assume that photons remain in the flat-land even after scattering. In 3D, a uniform random rotation around the original direction is also involved, which is now replaced by a random mirroring of 0.5 probability, i.e. by a random decision whether or not θ is multiplied by -1.

The reference activity is a simple function defined by three hot rectangles of Fig. 2. The voxel array is measured tracing $5 \cdot 10^4$ photon pairs by Monte Carlo simulation, resulting in the sinogram of the right image.

The compared approaches are combinations of presented techniques. Path samples can be allocated proportionally to the activity, when the method is called voxel driven, and also uniformly, when the method is called LOR driven. When the SM is computed only once without assuming anything about the activity, and the same SM is applied in all forward and back projections, the method is *Deterministic*. The *Reference* reconstruction is also obtained by a Deterministic approach, but we took significantly higher number of samples in this case. Note that not even the Reference reconstruction is perfect since "measured values" have noise which prohibits ideal reconstruction.

In the *Independent* method the random number generator is not reset during the iterative process and SMs of each forward and back projection are built from scratch, so we can assume that they are statistically independent. In the *Correlated* approach, a different random number generator seed is taken in every iteration step, but in a single iteration the SM computations of both forward projection and back projection are started from the same seed, making the forward and back projections of an iteration correlated, but different iterations independent. *Filtered* reconstruction means the application of statistical filtering, and *Blurred* reconstruction involves LOR space blurring after forward projection.

The L_2 error curves are shown by Figs. 3 and 6 for voxel driven and LOR driven methods, respectively, and Figs. 4, 5, 7, and 8 show the reconstructed volumes. As the given tomograph model captures all events, here the voxel driven method is more accurate. Thus, we used $N_{\mathrm{PT}} = 10^4$ and $5 \cdot 10^4$ MC samples in the voxel driven method and $N_{\mathrm{PT}} = 10^5$ and $5 \cdot 10^5$ samples for the LOR driven method, respectively. The SM of the Reference reconstruction is obtained with $2 \cdot 10^6$ LOR driven samples.

Deterministic iteration, where the same matrix is used in all forward and back projections, has unacceptably poor accuracy if the number of samples is not particularly high. For voxel driven sampling, Correlated projectors provide better solution than Independent projectors. Independent projectors are significantly improved by either statistical filtering or blurring, but only blurring helps Correlated projectors.

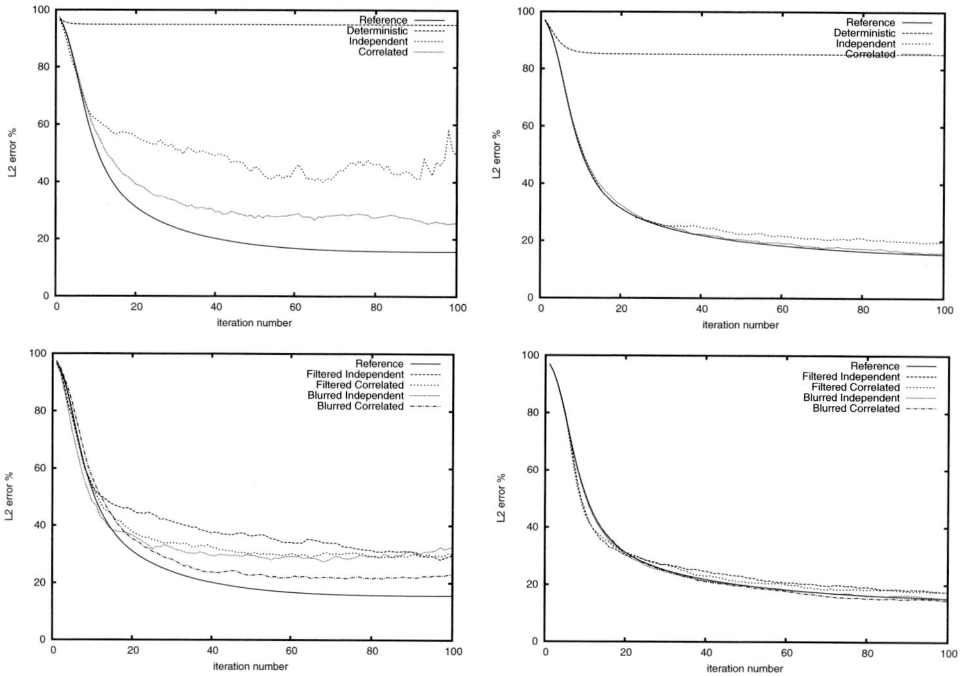

10^4 samples

5.10^4 samples

Fig. 3. L_2 errors of a voxel driven direct MC method.

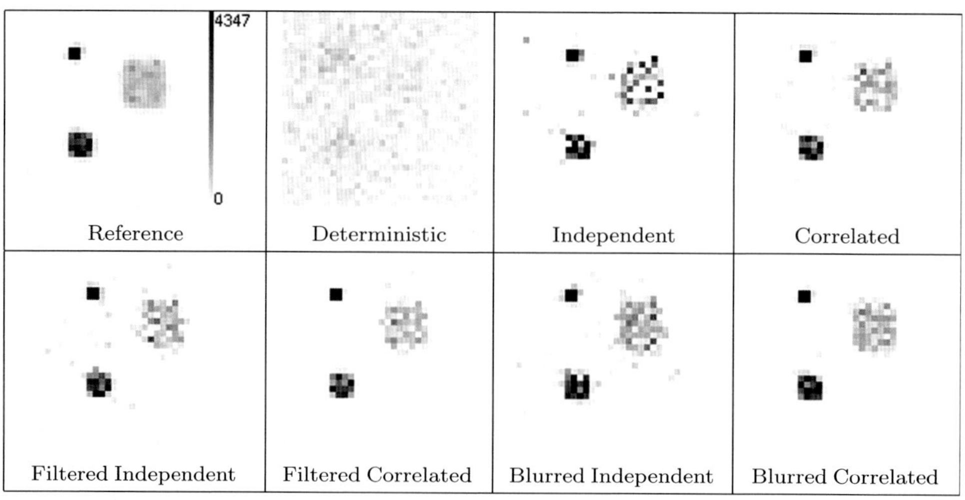

Fig. 4. Reconstructions of the voxel driven method using 10^4 samples.

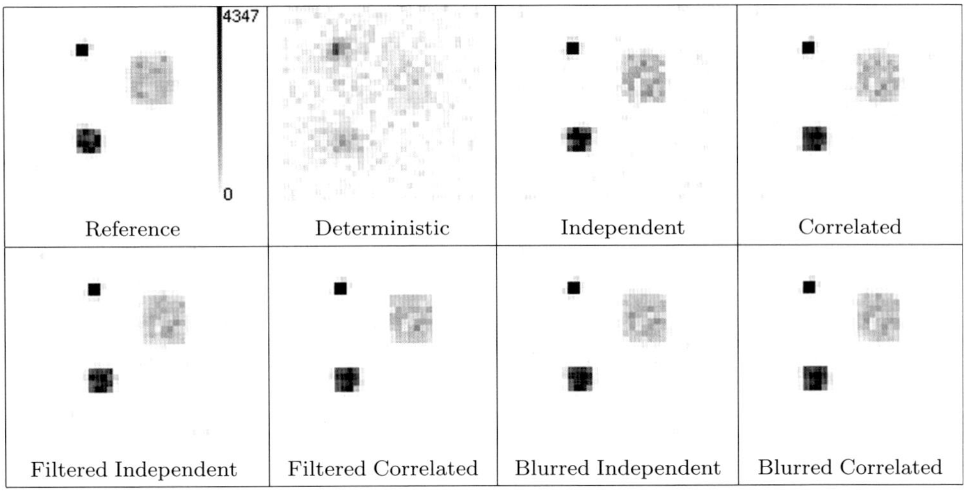

Fig. 5. Reconstructions of the voxel driven method using $5 \cdot 10^4$ samples.

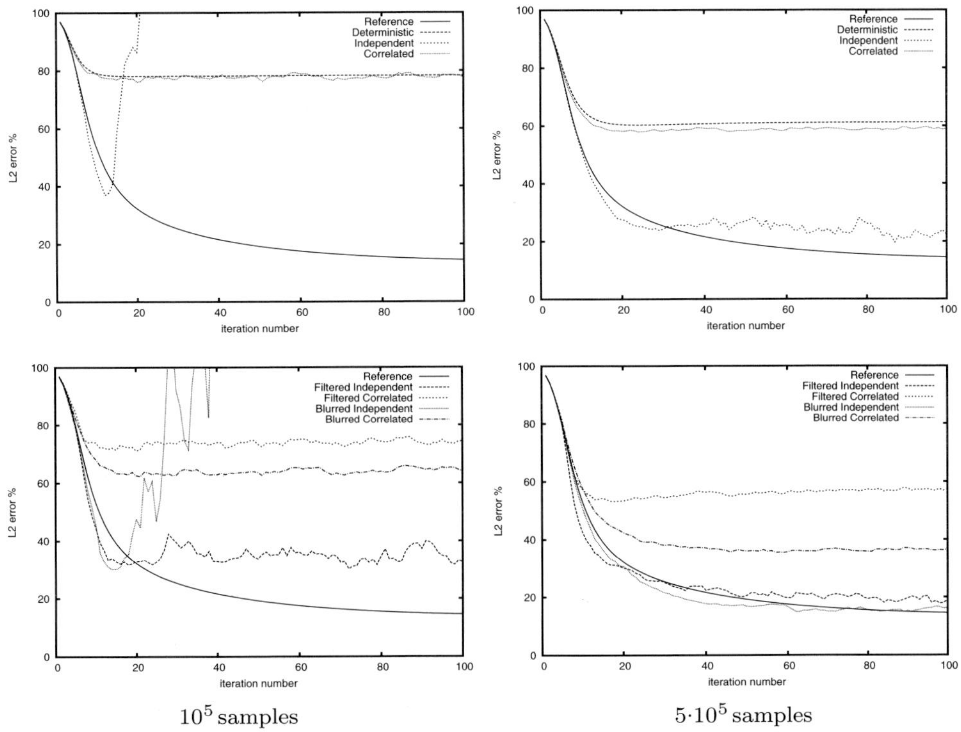

Fig. 6. L_2 errors of a LOR driven direct MC method.

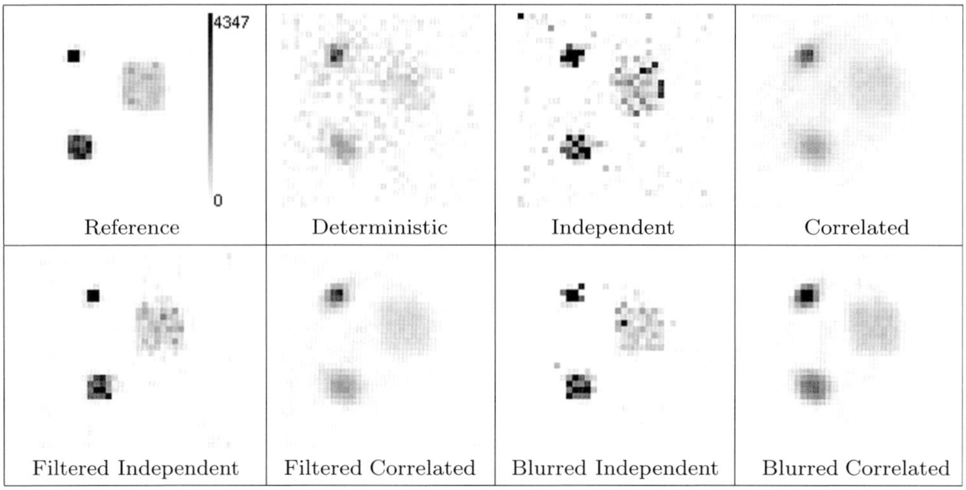

Fig. 7. Reconstructions of the LOR driven method using 10^5 samples.

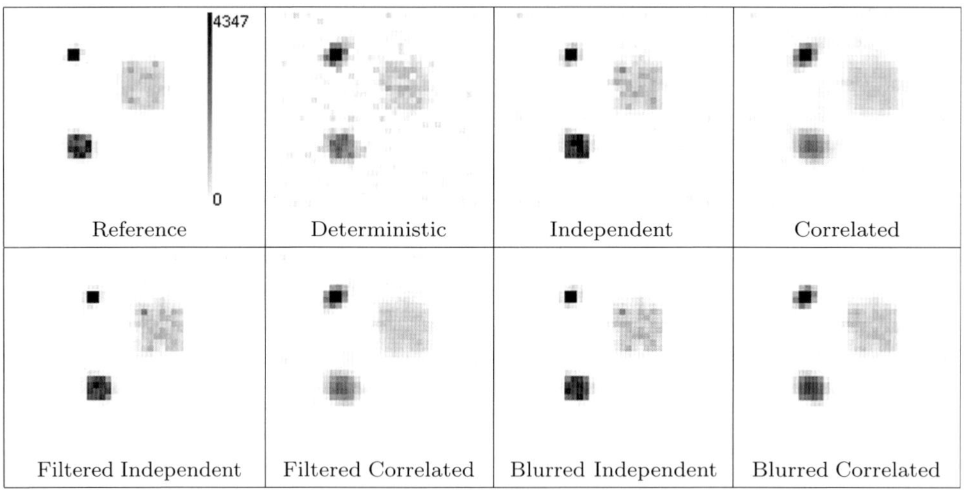

Fig. 8. Reconstructions of the LOR driven method using $5 \cdot 10^5$ samples.

In case of LOR driven sampling, Correlated projectors are almost as bad as Deterministic projectors due to the added bias. Here, blurring helps but filtering does not. The Independent projector is unstable if fewer samples are used. Interestingly, the initial convergence of the Independent projectors is faster than that of the Reference solution but later they cause very large fluctuations. The reason for faster initial convergence is that the convergence speed is determined by the contraction of the approximated matrix **T**, which is increased by the replacement of many non-zero matrix elements by zero in MC estimates. The high fluctuation caused by the Independent projector is moderately reduced by blurring but is efficiently addressed by statistical filtering. For higher sample numbers, Independent projectors are much better than Correlated methods. We can also observe that Correlated projectors result in noise free but blurred reconstructions while Independent projectors lead to sharper but noisier reconstructed activities.

7. Application in Fully-3D Reconstruction

The proposed LOR space blurring and statistical filtering can be plugged in any reconstruction algorithm that uses MC estimation during projections. As LOR space is four dimensional, the size of the blurring filter quickly increases with the number of considered neighbors. On the other hand, LOR space blurring trades variance with bias, but cannot reduce both at the same time. However, statistical filtering does not have these problems. It requires just a small modification of the back projection before the ratio of the measured and computed hit values are divided and has practically no added computational cost.

We built the Filtered Independent scheme into a small animal PET reconstruction application that is a part of the Tera-tomo package. We modeled Mediso's *nanoScan PET/CT*,[7] which consists of twelve detector modules of 81×39 crystals of surface size $1.12 \times 1.12\,\text{mm}^2$. To compare the Filtered Independent iteration to the standard Independent iteration, we took the *Derenzo* phantom with rod diameters $1.0, 1.1, \ldots, 1.5$ mm in different segments. To obtain measured value y_L, we assigned 5 MBq to the *Derenzo*, and simulated a 100 sec long measurement with GATE,[4] which mimics physical phenomena and thus obtains the measured data with realistic Poisson noise.

The phantom is reconstructed on a grid of $144^2 \times 128$ voxels of edge length 0.23 mm. The projector involves both LOR driven and voxel driven samples and combines them with multiple importance sampling.[13] The LOR driven method samples 9 discrete voxel points for each LOR. The voxel driven method initiates 5000 paths altogether from the volume. The reason for using so few sample paths is to emphasize the differences of not filtered and filtered versions.

Figure 9 shows the L_2 error curves of Independent iteration and the application of statistical filtering, and also a slice of the reconstructed data that is obtained with statistical filtering. Note that statistical filtering efficiently removes higher fluctuation.

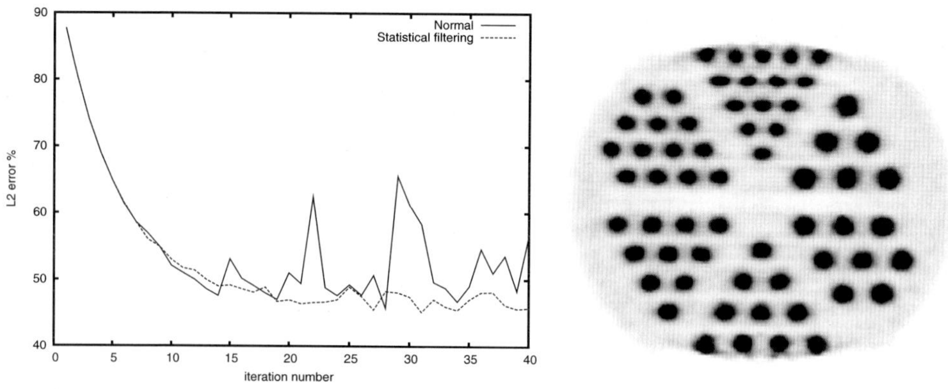

Fig. 9. L_2 error curves and reconstruction results obtained with statistical filtering.

8. Conclusions

This chapter examined why it is worth using MC estimates to compute forward and back projections in iterative PET reconstruction. We also analyzed the question whether forward and back projections should be statistically independent or correlated and proposed two techniques to improve the accuracy. These techniques are basically filtering, but statistical filtering operates in the time domain while blurring in the spatial LOR domain.

We concluded that voxel driven methods are worth combining with correlated sampling while LOR driven methods are combined with independent projections. In the future, we will examine how the benefits of both approaches can be obtained. Additionally, we will also develop more sophisticated LOR blurring methods and instead of applying the same kernel for all contributions, we plan to increase the kernel size depending on the number of scattering events occurred on the photon path.

Acknowledgement

This work has been supported by OTKA K–104476.

References

1. N. E. Breslow and N. E. Day, *Statistical Methods in Cancer Research: Volume 2 — The Design and Analysis of Cohort Studies*. International Agency for Research on Cancer. ISBN 978-92-832-0182-3 (1987).

2. B. Csébfalvi and L. Szirmay-Kalos, "Monte Carlo volume rendering," *Proc. of the 14th IEEE Visualization Conference (VIS'03)* 449–456 (2003).
3. M. Hadwiger, C. Sigg, H. Scharsach, K. Bühler, and M. Gross, "Real-time ray-casting and advanced shading of discrete isosurfaces," *Computer Graphics Forum* **22**, 303–312 (2005).
4. S. Jan and *et al.* "GATE: A simulation toolkit for PET and SPECT," *Physics in Med Biol* **49**, 4543–4561 (2004).
5. P. M. Joseph, "An improved algorithm for reprojecting rays through pixel images," *IEEE Trans Med Imaging* **1**, 192–196 (1982).
6. M. Magdics, L. Szirmay-Kalos, B. Tóth, and A. Penzov, "Analysis and control of the accuracy and convergence of the ML-EM iteration," *Lect Notes Comp Sci* **8353**, 147–154 (2014).
7. Mediso. NanoScan-PET/CT, www.mediso.com/products.php?fid=2,11&pid=86.
8. G. Pratx and L. Xing, "GPU computing in medical physics: A review," *Medical Physics* **38**, 2685 (2011).
9. A. J. Reader and H. Zaidi, "Advances in PET image reconstruction," *PET Clinics* **2**, 173–190 (2007).
10. L. Shepp and Y. Vardi, "Maximum likelihood reconstruction for emission tomography," *IEEE Trans Med Imaging* **1**, 113–122 (1982).
11. R. L. Siddon, "Fast calculation of the exact radiological path for a three-dimensional CT array," *Medical Physics* **12**, 252–257 (1985).
12. L. Szirmay-Kalos, "Stochastic iteration for non-diffuse global illumination," *Computer Graphics Forum* **18**, 233–244 (1999).
13. L. Szirmay-Kalos, M. Magdics, and B. Tóth, "Multiple importance sampling for PET," *IEEE Trans Med Imaging* **33**, 970–978 (2014).
14. L. Szirmay-Kalos, M. Magdics, B. Tóth, and T. Bükki, "Averaging and metropolis iterations for positron emission tomography," *IEEE Trans Med Imaging* **32**, 589–600 (2013).
15. L. Szirmay-Kalos and L. Szécsi, "Deterministic importance sampling with error diffusion," *Computer Graphics Forum* **28**, 1056–1064 (2009).
16. C. C. Watson, "New, faster, image-based scatter correction for 3D PET," *IEEE Trans Nucl Science* **47**, 1587–1594 (2000).
17. Wikipedia, http://en.wikipedia.org/wiki/poisson_distribution (2013).
18. C. N. Yang, "The Klein-Nishina formula & quantum electrodynamics," *Lect Notes Phys* **746**, 393–397 (2008).

Chapter 3

Advances In Online Dynamic MRI Reconstruction

Angshul Majumdar

Indraprastha Institute of Information Technology, Delhi, India
E-mail: angshul@iiitd.ac.in

In dynamic MRI reconstruction, the problem is to recover the sequence given partially sampled K-space of each frame. Traditionally, the reconstruction is offline. However such offline reconstruction precludes application of these techniques where real-time reconstruction is necessary, viz. image guided surgery, catheter tracking etc. To enable such applications, there is an interest in online reconstruction of dynamic MRI. This chapter reviews existing techniques in this area.

1. Introduction

Magnetic Resonance Imaging (MRI) is a versatile imaging modality. It is safe and can produce very high quality, though not as good as far as image quality goes. CT produces relatively good quality images but is not considered safe owing to its ionizing radiation. On the other hand, USG is very safe but yields very poor quality images. In spite of these advantages, the main shortcoming of MRI is its relatively longer acquisition time. One of the major problems in MRI, ever since its inception, has been to devise techniques to reduce data acquisition times.

The problem of slow acquisition exists both for static and dynamic scans. The issue is more pronounced for dynamic scans. Since the data acquisition time is lengthy, the number of frames that can be acquired in a unit of time is severely limited. If one wants to improve temporal resolution, there is a trade-off in temporal resolution and vice versa. Given the current techniques, it is not possible to produce high resolution scans that are able to capture fast transient phenomena.

The only way to reduce scan time is by acquiring less data. But this poses a challenge for reconstruction. Recovery from partially sampled K-space was made possible by recent advances in Compressed Sensing (CS); CS based methods can reduce the data acquisition times for both static[1] and dynamic

MRI.[2,3] For dynamic MRI, CS exploits the spatio-temporal redundancies in the sequence of frames in order to reconstruct it from partially sampled K-space.

Dynamic MRI sequences are mostly acquired for analysis, e.g. understanding brain excitation for functional MRI via BOLD signals. For such applications, it does not matter if the reconstruction is offline. There is no need to analyze MRI frames on-the-fly. Online MRI reconstruction is a challenging area, and will have crucial applications in the future; mostly in image-guided surgery. Even though the topic of discussion in this chapter is Online Dynamic MRI Reconstruction, the large bulk of work in dynamic MRI is still offline. Therefore, we will briefly discuss offline MRI reconstruction.

2. Offline Reconstruction

The dynamic MRI data acquisition model can be expressed succinctly. Let X_t, denote the MR image frame at the tth instant. We assume that the images are of size N × N and T is the total number of frames collected. Let y_t be the k-space data for the tth frame. The problem is to recover all X_t's (t=1...T) from the collected k-space data y_t's. The MR imaging equation for each frame is as follows,

$$y_t = RFx_t + \eta, \text{ define } x_t = vec(X_t) \tag{1}$$

Where R is the sub-sapling mask, F is the Fourier mapping from the spatial domain to the frequency domain (K-space) and η is white Gaussian noise.

A typical CS approach[2,3] employs wavelet transform for sparsifying the spatial redundancies in the image and Fourier transform for sparsifying along the temporal direction. This was a realistic assumption since both of them worked on dynamic imaging of the heart where the change over time is smooth and periodic, thereby leading to a compact (sparse) support in the frequency space.

The data from (1) can be organized in the following manner,

$$\Upsilon = RFX + \eta \tag{2}$$

where Υ and X are formed by stacking y_t's and x_t's as columns respectively.

In both Refs. [2, 3], the standard CS optimization problem is employed to reconstruct the dynamic MR image sequence from the k-space samples,

$$\min_x \| W \otimes F_{1D} vec(X)\|_1 \quad \text{subject to } \| \Upsilon - RFx\|_2^2 \leq \varepsilon \tag{3}$$

where $W \otimes F_{1D}$ is the Kronecker product of wavelet transform (for sparsifying in space) and 1D Fourier transform (for sparsifying along temporal direction).

In the original studies,[2,3] the Kronecker product was not used; we introduced it to make the notation more compact.

The 1D Fourier transform may not always be the ideal choice for sparsifying along the temporal direction (if the signal is not smooth or periodic); in such a case 1D wavelet transform can be used instead. Some other studies[4–6] assumed the image to be sparse in $x - f$ space, i.e. the signal was assumed to be sparse in $I \otimes F_{1D}$ basis (where I is just the Dirac basis). In these studies, the emphasis was on the solver for (3); they used the FOCUSS (FOCally Under-determined System Solver)[7] method for minimizing the l_1-norm. However, in practice any other state-of-the-art l_1-norm minimization solver (e.g. Spectral Projected Gradient L1 or Nesterov's Algorithm) will work.

Some other studies[8–11] either assumed the MR image frames to be spatially sparse or were only interested in the 'change' between the successive frames. These studies did not explicitly exploit the redundancy of the MR frames in the spatial domain, rather they only applied a Total Variation (TV) regularization in the temporal domain. The optimization problem is the following,

$$\min_{x} TV_t(x) \quad \text{subject to } \|y - RFx\|_2^2 \leq \varepsilon \tag{4}$$

where $TV_t = \sum_{i=1}^{N^2} \|\nabla_t x_i\|$ and ∇_t denotes the temporal differentiation for the ith pixel.

In essence the approach in Refs. [8–11] differs only slightly from Refs. [4–6]. In Refs. [4–6] it is assumed that the signal is smoothly varying over time, so that it is sparse in temporal Fourier transform. In Refs. [8–11], temporal Fourier transform is not directly employed, but is assumed that the signal is smoothly varying with time with only a finite number of discontinuities, so that it will be sparse in temporal differencing domain.

There is yet another class of methods that reconstruct the dynamic MRI sequence as a rank deficient matrix. In Refs. [12, 13], it is argued that the matrix X is rank deficient, and can be modeled as a linear combination of very few temporal basis functions. This is true because the columns of X, which are formed by stacking the frames of the sequence are temporally correlation; therefore X is a rank-deficient matrix. Based on this assumption, Refs. [12, 13] proposed solving the inverse problem (2) as follows,

$$\min_{X} \|X\|_* \quad \text{subject to } \|Y - RFX\|_F^2 \leq \varepsilon \tag{5}$$

where $\|.\|_*$ denotes the nuclear norm of the matrix and $\|.\|_F$ denotes the Frobenius norm of the matrix.

For recovering a rank deficient solution, one ideally has to minimize the rank of a matrix subject to data constraints. However, minimizing the rank is an NP hard problem. Thus, theoretical research in this area proposed substituting the NP hard rank by its tightest convex surrogate the nuclear norm. Following these studies, the inverse problem (2) is solved by nuclear norm minimization (5).

We have discussed two approaches for offline dynamic MRI reconstruction — sparsity based techniques and rank-deficiency exploiting methods. Later studies Refs. [14–17] improved upon these individual approaches by combining the two. For example in Refs. [16, 17], the reconstruction was carried out by solving:

$$\min_{X} \|X\|_* + \lambda \|I \otimes F_{1D} vec(X)\|_1 \quad \text{subject to } \|\Upsilon - RFX\|_F^2 \leq \varepsilon \tag{6}$$

Here X denotes the signal in $x - t$ space as arranged in (5) where as x denotes the signal in $x - t$ space as arranged in (2). It is assumed that the dynamic MRI sequence is sparse in $x-f$ space. The term λ balances the relative importance of rank deficiency and sparsity.

There is a recent work that used the Blind Compressed Sensing (BCS) framework for dynamic MRI reconstruction. BCS marries dictionary learning with CS. In standard CS, it is assumed that the signal is sparse in a known basis such as DCT, wavelet, etc. Dictionary learning techniques estimate the sparsifying basis empirically; this dictionary learning is offline. In BCS, the dictionary learning and signal reconstruction proceeds simultaneously. The signal is modeled as Refs. [18, 19]:

$$X = DZ \tag{7}$$

where both D and Z need to be estimated, D is the dictionary and Z is the sparse transform coefficients.

The reconstruction is framed as follows:

$$\min_{D,Z} \|\Upsilon - RFDZ\|_F^2 + \lambda_1 \|D\|_F^2 + \lambda_2 \|vec(Z)\|_1 \tag{8}$$

Recently an improvement over the BCS framework was suggested in Ref. [20]. The BCS does not explicitly exploit the fact that the signal X is low-rank.[14–17] Therefore it is possible to improve upon (8) by incorporating this information, leading to:

$$\min_{D,Z} \|\Upsilon - RFDZ\|_F^2 + \lambda_1 \|D\|_F^2 + \lambda_2 \|vec(Z)\|_1 + \lambda_3 \|Z\|_* \tag{9}$$

Both D and Z are variables. But D is the dictionary and we are minimizing its nuclear norm, therefore D cannot be low-rank, the only possibility is to impose low-rank constraint on (9) and hence the formulation.

3. Online Reconstruction

In the previous section, we discussed about offline reconstruction. The discussion was brief since it does not form the topic of this chapter. The rest of the chapter is dedicated to detailed discussion on online recovery. There are two approaches for online reconstruction. The first approach is to modify CS techniques in an online fashion. The second approach is to use well-known statistical dynamical models for reconstruction.

3.1. *Compressed Sensing Based Techniques*

3.1.1. *k-t FOCUSS*

The k-t FOCUSS method[4–6] was never designed to be an online technique; we discussed it in the previous section. However as we will now see, it indeed was the first online dynamic MRI reconstruction technique based on the principles of CS. This method expresses every frame in the following manner,

$$x_t = x_{ref} + \nabla x_t \tag{10}$$

Here x_{ref} is the reference/prediction for the t_{th} frame, and Δx_t is the difference/residual between the reference and the actual frame. The general idea is that, if the prediction is good, the residual will be sparse. Therefore, it will be possible to estimate the residual using CS recovery methods such as,

$$\nabla \hat{x}_t = \min_{\nabla x_t} \|\nabla x_t\|_p^p \quad \text{subject to } \|y_t - RF(x_{ref} + \nabla x_t)\|_2^2 \leq \varepsilon \tag{11}$$

This is a standard l_p-minimization problem. In the aforesaid works, the FOCUSS algorithm[7] was used to solve it (hence the name k-t FOCUSS); any other algorithm will work equally well.

Once the residual between the prediction and the actual frame is estimated, it is added to the predicted/reference frame to obtain the final estimate of the tth frame.

The prediction of the current frame (x_{ref}) should (ideally) be only dependent on prior frames. Thus to estimate the residual via (17) only the previous frames $(\mathrm{x}_1, \mathrm{x}_2, \ldots, \mathrm{x}_{t-1})$ are required; the reconstruction does not require frames from the future $(\mathrm{x}_{t+1}, \mathrm{x}_{t+2}, \ldots, \mathrm{x}_T)$. Thus, the final reconstruction (16) is causal and online.

The idea of separating a frame from a dynamic sequence into reference and residual follows from video processing. In video compression, all the frames are not transmitted; only the reference frames are transmitted and for the remaining frames, the residual/difference between the reference and those frames are transmitted.

It can be seen from (9) that computing the residual is straight forward. The interesting aspect of k-t FOCUSS is in estimating the reference frame. In Ref. [4], two techniques are proposed to estimate the reference frame. The first one is based on RIGR[18]; this is basically a frequency domain interpolation technique for estimating a frame.

The other technique proposed in Ref. [4] to estimate the reference frame follows from the motion estimation–motion compensation framework used in video processing. However, the basic challenge (and therefore the main difference from video processing) is that video coding is an offline technique so predicting the motion vectors by computing block difference between previous and current frame is straight-forward. Unfortunately this is not possible (ideally) for dynamic online MRI reconstruction; we want to reconstruct the current frame, we do not have it, therefore we cannot compute the motion vectors for this scenario. There is no logical way to overcome this problem, in Ref. [4] it is assumed that a crude estimate of the current frame is somehow available (may be from a low-resolution image, or from CS reconstruction of the full frame). This crude estimate can be used to compute the motion vectors between the previous and current frame. In the motion compensation stage, the computed motion vectors are used to predict the current frame (given the previous frame).

The experimental results shown here are from Ref. [5]. A cardiac cine MRI dataset was used for the experiments. The ground-truth is formed from fully sampled K-space data. For experiments, a six-fold acceleration factor is simulated by radial sampling of the K-space. The following reconstruction methods are used filtered back-projection (since the sampling is radial), Sliding Window (SW), k-t BLAST, k-t FOCUSS (with RIGR) and k-t FOCUSS with ME/MC. The reconstruction results are shown in Fig. 1. The figure is marked to notice deviations from the ground-truth.

Filtered backprojection shows severe streaking artifacts; the streaking is caused by radial sampling. SW shows some streaking artifacts; the heart wall and muscles are very blurred from SW reconstruction. k-t BLAST also shows some streaking artifacts and blurred vessels. However, k-t FOCUSS (with RIGR) and k-t FOCUSS with ME/MC show very clear texture and structures of the heart.

3.1.2. *Least Squared CS for dynamic MRI reconstruction*

In recent work called Least Squares Compressed Sensing (LS-CS),[21] it is assumed that the difference image is not sparse but is sparse in a transform domain (say wavelets), i.e. $\nabla\alpha_t = W\nabla x_t$ is sparse. Thus in LS-CS, the sparse

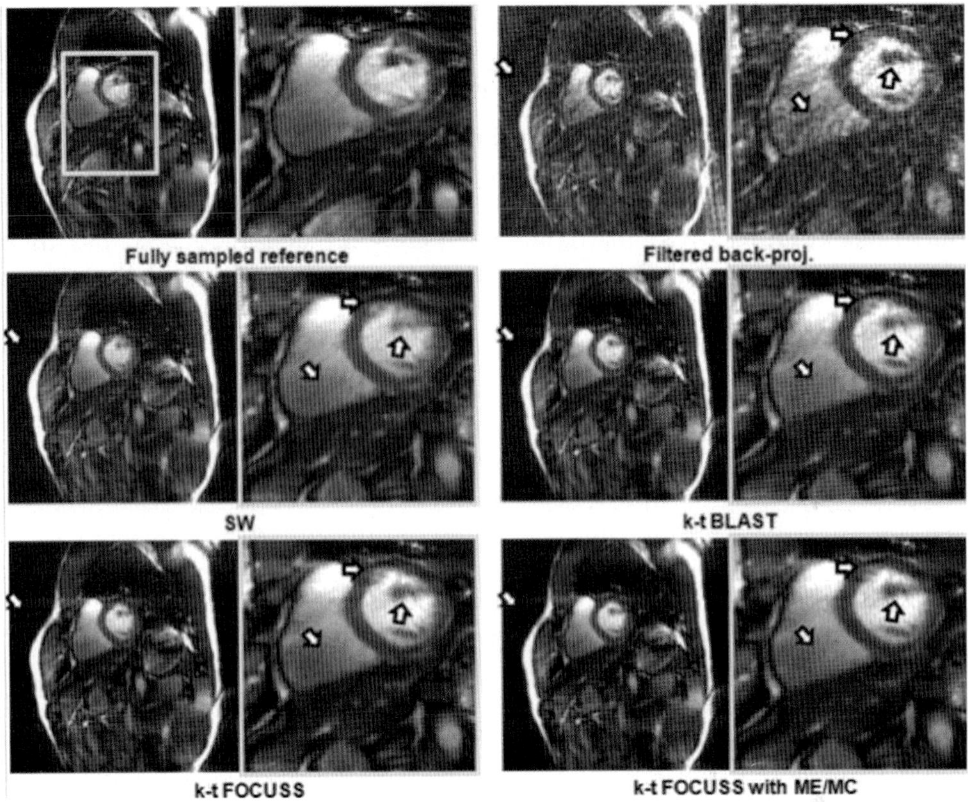

Fig. 1. Reconstructed images using various FOCUSS techniques and their comparison to others.

transform coefficients of the difference frame is solved for. The following optimization problem is employed for the purpose,

$$\nabla\hat{\alpha}_t = \min_{\nabla\alpha_t} \|\nabla\alpha_t\|_p^p \quad \text{subject to } \|y_t - RFx_{t-1} - RFW^T\nabla\alpha_t)\|_2^2 \leq \varepsilon \qquad (12)$$

where $x_{t-1}$is the reconstructed previous frame and $\nabla\alpha_t$ is the wavelet transform of the difference between the previous and the current frame.

Unlike k-t FOCUSS, the LS-CS does not stop here. It assumes that the sparsity pattern varies slowly with time. For each time frame, the difference of the wavelet transform coefficients $\nabla\alpha_t$ is computed, from which an intermediate estimate of the wavelet coefficients of current frame is obtained as,

$$\tilde{\alpha}_t = \alpha_{t-1} + \nabla\alpha_t \qquad (13)$$

The intermediate estimate is thresholded (via hard thresholding) and all the values below a certain threshold τ (depending on noise level) are discarded. The value of the thresholded wavelet coefficients are not of importance, but their indices are. Assuming that the set of indices having non-zero values after thresholding is Ω, the final value of the wavelet transform coefficient is estimated as,

$$\hat{\alpha}_t = (R_t F_{2D} W_{2D})^{\dagger}_{\Omega} y_t \tag{14}$$

where $(\cdot)^{\dagger}$ denotes the Moore-Penrose pseudo-inverse and $(\cdot)_{\Omega}$ indicates that only those columns of the matrix has been chosen that are indexed in Ω, $\hat{\alpha}_t$ is the estimated wavelet coefficient from the tth frame. The image is reconstructed from the wavelet coefficients via the synthesis equation.

We do not provide any results for LS-CS in this sub-section. This technique was not particularly developed for solving dynamic MRI problems, it was rather developed for solving more general problems where the purpose was to solve for a sequence of observations which was varying slowly with time and had a sparse representation in a transform domain. In Ref. [21], dynamic MRI was one application area for this technique; the authors felt that dynamic MRI reconstruction would benefit from their technique.

3.1.3. *Real-time CS based dynamic MRI reconstruction*

This work is similar to k-t FOCUSS. It assumes that the difference image between two consecutive frames is sparse and one does not need to be in the wavelet domain in order to sparsify it. This assumption is indeed true as can be verified from Figs. 2 and 3. Figure 10 visually corroborates the fact that the

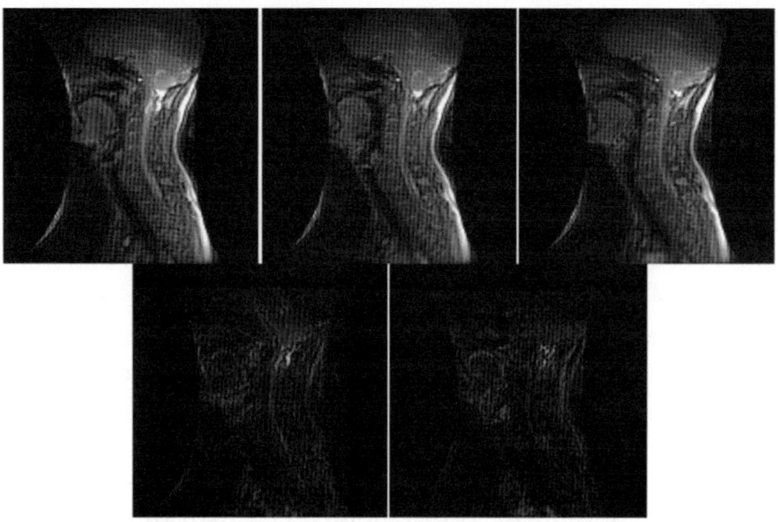

Fig. 2. Top: Three consecutive images from a larynx sequence; Bottom: Difference images between the three consecutive frames.

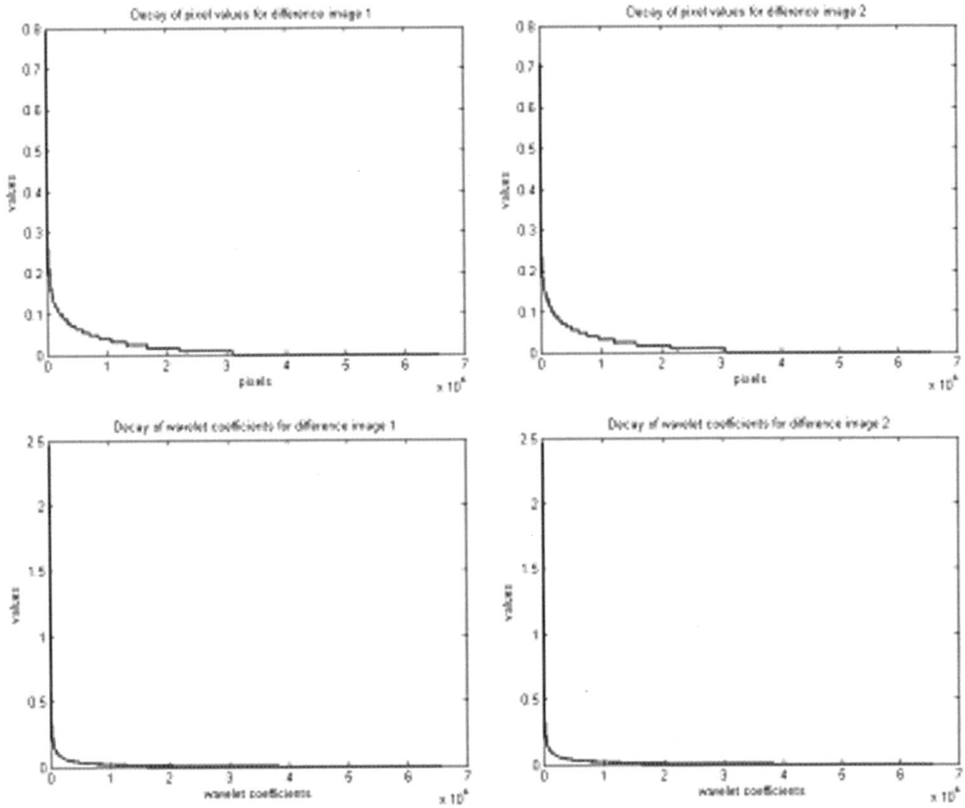

Fig. 3. Top: Sorted pixel values of the difference images; Bottom: Sorted wavelet coefficients of the difference image.

difference image between two consecutive frames is sparse. This is quantitatively supported in Fig. 3. It can be seen from this figure that both the pixel values of the difference image and the wavelet transform coefficients of the difference image have fast decays, i.e. most of the signal energy is confined in a relatively small number of high valued coefficients. The energy confined in the top 10% of the pixels in the difference image is 93% of the total energy and in the top 10% of the wavelet coefficients, it is 98%. Thus, the difference image has a slightly sparser representation in the wavelet domain than in pixel domain. However, the slim relative advantage of wavelets in terms of energy compaction in fewer coefficients will be offset by other factors as will be discussed now.

The fact that mutual coherence between the random Fourier ensembles and Dirac basis is the minimum, is well-known in CS based MR image reconstruction literature. Independent of the k-space (Fourier domain) under-sampling ratio, the mutual coherence is always 'unity' between the aforesaid two basis (the normalized mutual coherence is N^{-2}, N being the number of pixels in the image). The mutual coherence between Fourier and wavelet basis is always higher than unity.[20,21] Higher mutual coherence leads to worse signal reconstruction accuracy (when the number of measurement samples is fixed). In order to alleviate this problem in static MRI, 'spread spectrum CS' techniques were proposed in Refs. [22, 23]. In Ref. [22] it was reported that for an image of size 256 × 256, the mutual coherence between the Fourier measurement basis (*k*-space) and the Dirac basis (pixel domain) is 3.906×10^{-3}; and the mutual coherence between the Fourier measurement basis and the wavelet basis (sparsifying transform) is 2.272×10^{-2} for Daubechies wavelets with 4 vanishing moments at 3 levels of decomposition. Thus, if one uses wavelets for sparsifying the difference image, the mutual coherence increases by a factor of 5. Even though mutual coherence based bounds are pessimistic, it follows that the number of wavelet coefficients that can be recovered by CS algorithms will be less than number of pixel values recovered. Therefore, the modeling/reconstruction error for a CS recovery method using wavelet coefficients (such as Ref. [21]) will be more than our proposed method. The slim advantage wavelet transform coefficients have over pixel values in terms of energy compaction in fewer coefficients (see Fig. 3) is offset by the increased mutual coherence between the measurement basis and the sparsifying transform.

Working in the transform domain (like Ref. [21]) buys nothing — this is the reason, it was never successful in dynamic MRI reconstruction. It only increases computational cost. In Ref. [24], the aim was to develop an algorithm for real-time dynamic MRI reconstruction. Thus, computational complexity was at a premium. They proposed the following simple optimization problem to solve the difference frame,

$$\nabla \hat{x}_t = \min_{\nabla x_t} \|\nabla x_t\|_p^p \quad \text{subject to } \|y_t - RF(x_{t-1} + \nabla x_t)\|_2^2 \leq \varepsilon \tag{15}$$

This is similar to FOCUSS except for the fact that here the reference frame is just the previous frame — we have argued before why this is a realistic assumption (Figs. 2 and 3). Such a simplifying model cuts on unnecessary computational complexity. Furthermore, Ref. [24] does not use the FOCUSS algorithm to solve (15). FOCUSS is a second order algorithm and computationally expensive. A first order modified iterative soft thresholding algorithm is developed in Ref. [24] to solve the optimization problem. The parameters are tuned there to achieve super-linear convergence.

The experiments that were carried out on cardiac perfusion dataset. The data was collected on a 3T Siemens scanner. In this work, we simulated a radial sampling with 24 lines were acquired for each time frame; this corresponds

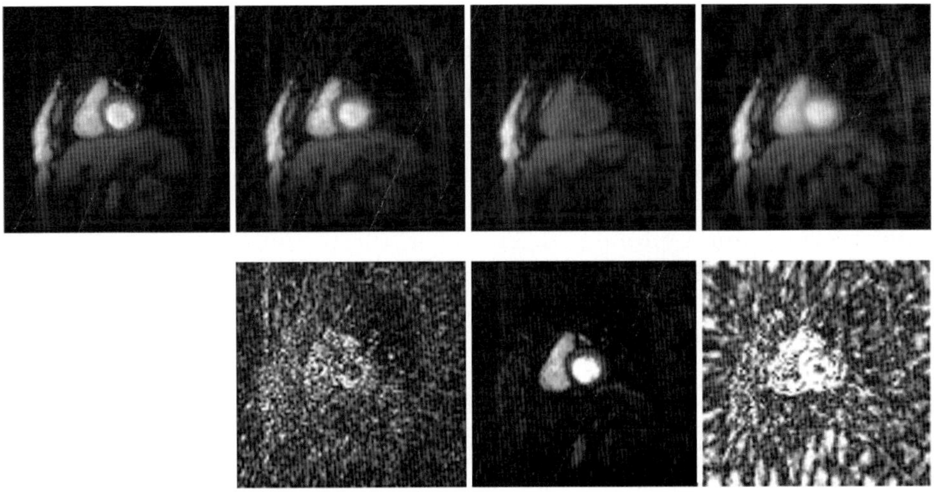

Fig. 4. Left to Right: Ground-truth, CS reconstruction, LS-CS and Kalman Filter. Top — reconstructed images; Bottom — difference images.

to an under-sampling ratio of 0.21. The full resolution of the dynamic MR images is 128×128. About 6.7 samples were collected per second. The scanner parameters for the radial acquisition were TR $= 2.5-3.0$ msec, TE $= 1.1$ msec, flip angle $= 12°$ and slice thickness $= 6$ mm. The reconstructed pixel size varied between 1.8 mm^2 and 2.5 mm^2. Each image was acquired in a ~62-msec readout, with radial field of view (FOV) ranging from 230 to 320 mm.

The results are shown in Fig. 4. The work was compared with LS-CS and another real-time dynamic MRI reconstruction technique based on the Kalman Filter model (will be discussed later). The LS-CS yields the worst reconstruction as is evident even from the reconstructed image. It completely misses to reconstruct a valve. One can see the valve in the difference image. This is unacceptable for any MRI application. The Kalman filter reconstruction shows a lot of streaking artifacts (difference image) but is slightly better than LS-CS since it does not lose any important structure. The simple CS based reconstruction technique[24] yields the best results.

Since this is real-time technique, it is supposed to reconstruct the frames as fast as they are acquired. The frames for cardiac perfusion are of size 128×128 and about 6 to 7 frames are acquired every second. The Kalman Filter yields the fastest reconstruction as it only requires a fixed number of re-gridding and Fourier transform operations to reconstruction each time frame. It is about 4 times faster than the CS based method; and the CS based method[24] is nearly a magnitude faster than LS-CS. The average reconstruction time per frame is

0.2 seconds; although this is not exactly real-time, the performance is close enough.

In a more recent work,[25] a rudimentary attempt was taken to accelerate reconstruction speeds by exploiting the massively multi-core architecture of new Graphical Processing Units (GPU). It was shown that for images of size 128 × 128, simple parallelization techniques are able to reduce the reconstruction time by four-fold. However, the technique used in Ref. [25] is not scalable and thus in future, new parallelized CS recovery algorithms will be needed to recover larger sized datasets.

3.2. *Kalman Filter Based Techniques*

So far we have studied CS based reconstruction techniques. It is surprising that there have only been a handful of studies that used conventional yet powerful techniques to model dynamic MRI reconstruction problems. Dynamical systems has been an interesting topic of research for both theoretical and applied statistics and machine learning researchers for the last four decades. There are powerful techniques in computational statistics that can be harnessed to solve the dynamic MRI reconstruction problem; and yet these techniques have not been widely explored.

Kalman Filtering is one of the simplest techniques in modeling dynamical systems. In recent studies,[26–28] Kalman Filtering has been proposed to solve

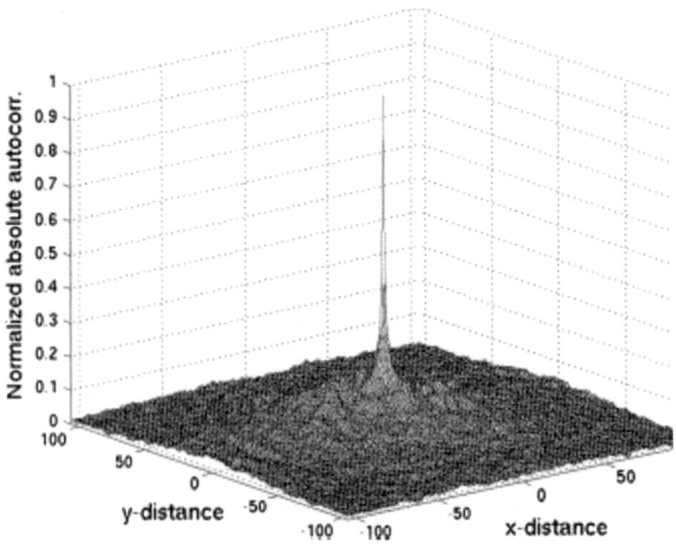

Fig. 5. Normalized absolute autocorrelation function estimate of the difference between two cardiac images.

the real-time dynamic MR reconstruction problem. The following model is proposed:

$$x_t = x_{t-1} + u_t \tag{16a}$$

$$y_t = RF_{2D}x_t + \eta_t \tag{16b}$$

where the pixel values x_t is the state variable, the K-space sample y_t is the observation, η_t is the observation noise and u_t is the innovation in state variables.

In general, the Kalman filter is computationally intensive since it requires explicit matrix inversion for computing the covariance matrix; this requires a computational complexity of the order of $O(n^3)$. For dynamic MRI frames of size 128×128, the covariance matrix of size $16,384 \times 16,384$. The memory requirement to invert such a huge matrix is beyond the capacity of a normal personal computer, and hence is not feasible. In Refs. [26, 27], this problem was alleviated by diagonalization of the covariance matrix; this reduces the complexity to $O(n)$. They argued that since the autocorrelation function is peaked around the central value (Fig. 13), the diagonalization assumption is realistic. However, this diagonalization assumption holds only for non-Cartesian trajectories.

Instead of looking at such plots (as Fig. 13), let us probe one level deeper. The diagonalization assumption means that pixel motion (u_t) is uncorrelated and changes independently with time, i.e. there is no relationship between pixel motion at one point and its adjacent point. This is an absurd assumption in any rigid/semi-rigid body dynamic problem! Moreover, Kalman Filter assumes that the innovation u_t is Gaussian. This is unlikely to be true in the present scenario; but this is a minor problem since we know even if motion is not Gaussian, the Kalman Filter estimated will be optimal in the least squares sense.

We mentioned before that the diagonalization assumption only holds for non-Cartesian trajectories. There are two problems with this — first, Cartesian trajectories are more predominantly used than non-Cartesian ones, thereby limiting the applicability of Refs. [26, 27]. The other problem is that, Refs. [26, 27] requires an almost uniform (density) sampling of the K-space. This requires re-gridding the K-space samples thereby adding extra computational cost to the reconstruction process.

The main forte of the Kalman Filtering technique proposed in Refs. [26, 27] is its superior reconstruction speed. They argue that the reconstruction for each frame takes only two forward and backward Fourier transform computations. But there is a catch. Computing and forward and backward inverses from a non-Cartesian grid is not as efficient as the Cartesian counterpart; to overcome the problem they re-grid the non-Cartesian samples on the Cartesian grid. However, they do not include the time required for re-gridding into the reconstruction time.

To overcome these issues, a simple solution is proposed in Ref. [28]. This work, proposed a technique to reconstruct images from Cartesian sampled K-space data. Kalman Filtering is applied on each row of the K-space to reconstruct the corresponding pixels in the image domain. The advantage of this method is that it has a lower computational complexity — simply because the size of the problem is now smaller. Also, the different rows can be processed in parallel.

Unfortunately, there is no major benefit from this study Ref. [28]. They just proposed a technique to process the frames piecemeal – one row at a time. In a fashion similar to Refs. [26, 27], the covariance matrix is approximated to be diagonal. Unlike, Refs. [26, 27], there is no intuitive or empirical justification of why such an assumption will hold for Cartesian sampling.[28] The only advantage in terms of the covariance matrix in Ref. [28] is that, since it is smaller, it is easier to estimate from limited amount of data and therefore will yield better reconstruction results.

The results from Ref. [28] are shown here. Free-breathing, untriggered dynamic cardiac imaging experiments were performed on a 1.5-T GE Signa system. Scans were taken for approximately 10 seconds. The reconstruction result is shown in Fig. 6. Kalman Filter reconstruction[28] is compared with the sliding window technique. The results are shown in Fig. 6. The arrow points to the location where sliding window fails but Kalman Filter succeeds. The experiments were carried out on spiral trajectories with 6 times acceleration factor. The K-space was sampled on a spiral trajectory and therefore does not have a fully sampled ground-truth. However, the quality of reconstruction is visible from the reconstructed images.

3.3. *Hybrid Methods*

The idea of using predicted frames was introduced in k-t FOCUSS.[4–6] In Ref. [6], motion estimation concepts developed in video coding was used for predicting MRI frames. The k-t FOCUSS method was not intended for online reconstruction, and hence was not focused on reducing complexity. But for real-time reconstruction, we would like the reconstruction to be fast; thus we require smarter motion estimation techniques than offered by video coding.

In general, any online reconstruction technique consists of two steps:

(1) Prediction — the current frame (the frame to be reconstructed) is estimated based on information from previous frames.

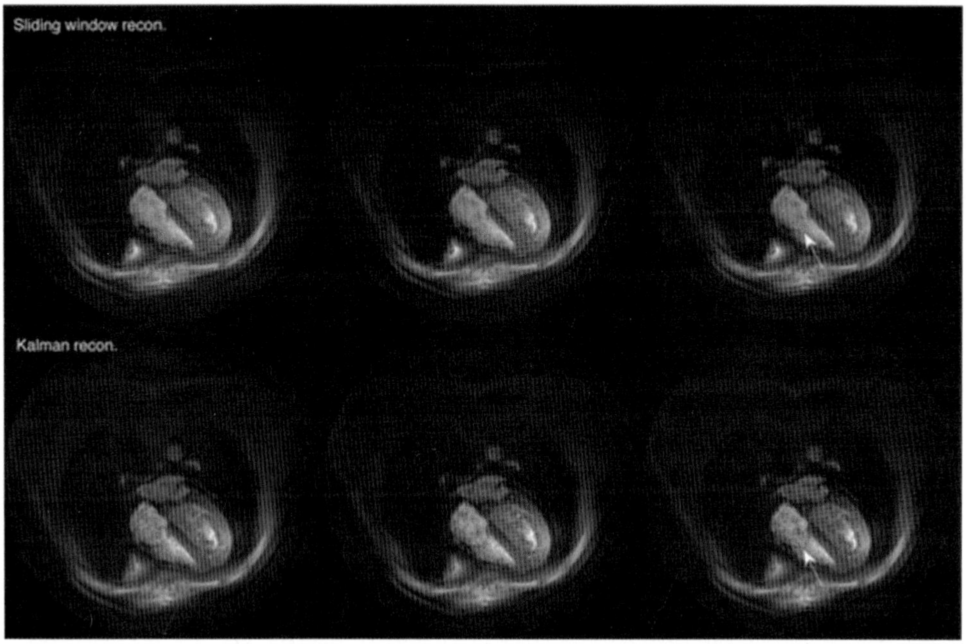

Fig. 6. Reconstruction of three consecutive frames.

(2) Correction — the difference between the predicted and the actual frame is computed based on the collected K-space samples for the current frame; the final reconstruction is obtained by adding the computed difference to the predicted image.

The framework for the hybrid model is slightly different from (16); the prediction model is expressed as follows,

$$x_t = x_{t-1} + \nabla x_t \tag{17}$$

where $\tilde{x}_t$ is the predicted frame and $\nabla \tilde{x}_t$ is the estimated motion.

The problem is to estimate $\nabla \tilde{x}_t$. The estimation of $\nabla \tilde{x}_t$ will be based on the actual motions from two previous frames — ∇x_{t-1} and ∇x_{t-2}. In Ref. [29], a simple linear dynamical model is used for predicting motions for subsequent frames, which is given by,

$$\nabla x_{t-1} = \beta \cdot \nabla x_{t-2} + \delta \tag{18}$$

Here '·' denotes component wise product and δ is the estimation error assumed to be distributed Normally. This (28) is actually an Auto-Regressive process of order 1. In general an AR(1) process is expressed as,

$$\nabla x_{t-1} = B \nabla x_{t-2} + \delta \tag{19}$$

where B is a matrix.

In Ref. [29] the assumptions are the same as in Refs. [26, 27], i.e. motion at a particular point is independent of the motions at points surrounding it. This allows for diagonal B, which we have expressed in (19) as a component wise product.

Based on this simple model and if β is known, one can estimate the motion for the current frame as,

$$\nabla \tilde{x}_t = \beta \cdot \nabla x_{t-1} \tag{20}$$

The assumption here is that motion in the subsequent frames is slow and the value of β remains the same for motions of two consecutive frames. The problem is to estimate β. In Ref. [29], it is estimated using the following Tikhonov regularized least squares minimization problem,

$$\min_{\beta} \|\nabla x_{t-1} - \beta \cdot \nabla x_{t-2}\|_2^2 + \lambda \|\beta\|_2^2 \tag{21}$$

The aforesaid problem has an analytical solution which is,

$$\beta = \nabla x_{t-1} \cdot \nabla x_{t-2} / \cdot (\nabla x_{t-2} \cdot \nabla x_{t-2} + \lambda) \tag{22}$$

Here '$\cdot$' denotes component wise multiplication and '$/\cdot$' denotes component wise division. Computing β is fast, since it has a complexity of $O(n)$.

Once β has been solved, the motion for the predicted frame can be computed using (20). The predicted frame is estimated by adding the predicted motion to the previous frame.

This is the prediction step; the next step is the correction step. Here, the difference between the predicted frame and the actual frame is recovered from the collected K-space samples of the current frame.

In Ref. [24], it was shown that the difference between the previous frame and the current frame is approximately sparse; thereby allowing for a CS based recovery. CS Theory says that other conditions remaining same (number of measurements and measurement basis), sparser the signal, better will be the reconstruction. In Ref. [30], the difference between the previous frame (already reconstructed) and the current frame (to be reconstructed) was being estimated using CS recovery. In the new hybrid model, the difference between the predicted frame and the current frame is estimated. Assuming that the prediction is good, the difference between the predicted and the current frame will be sparser than the difference between the previous and the current frame (as in Ref. [24]). Thus, one expects the hybrid method to yield better reconstruction results than Ref. [24]. The claim regarding superior sparsity is experimentally validated in Fig. 7 on a larynx sequence. It is shown that the difference between the previous and current frame (Fig. 7a) is less sparser than the difference between the predicted and current frame (Fig. 7b). The sorted

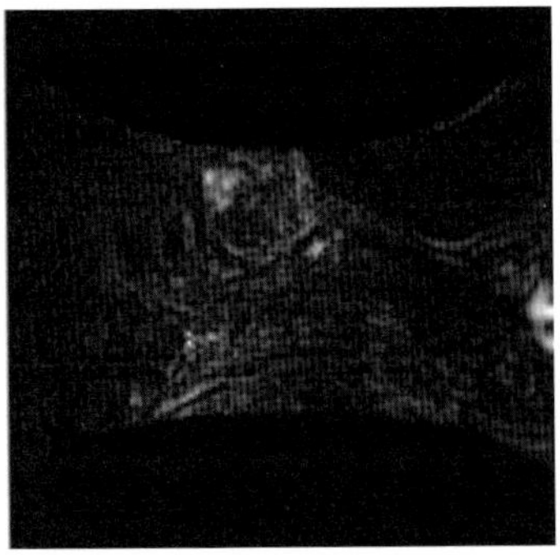

(a)

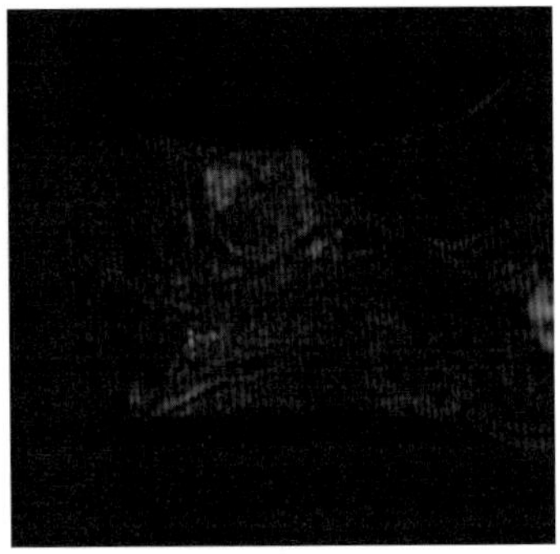

(b)

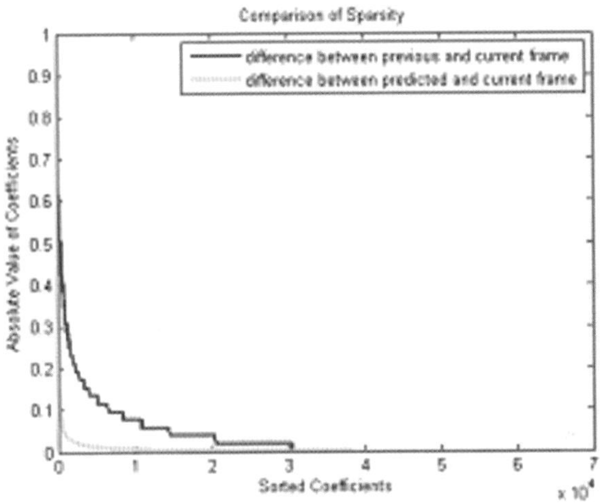

(c)

Fig. 7. 7a — Difference between previous and current frame; 7b — Difference between predicted and current frame; 7c — Sorted coefficients.

absolute values are shown in Fig. 7c; it can also be seen from Fig. 7c that the difference between the predicted and the current frame is sparser than the previous and current frame.

Once the prediction step is complete, the problem is to recover the difference between the predicted and the corrected frame (θ_t). This is the correction step.

$$x_t = \tilde{x}_t + \theta_t \tag{23}$$

It is expected that the difference will be sparse (as in Fig. 16). Hence, one can recover it by the solving the following problem,

$$\min_{\theta_t} \|y_t - RF\tilde{x}_t - RF\theta_t\|_2^2 + \lambda\|\theta_t\|_1 \tag{24}$$

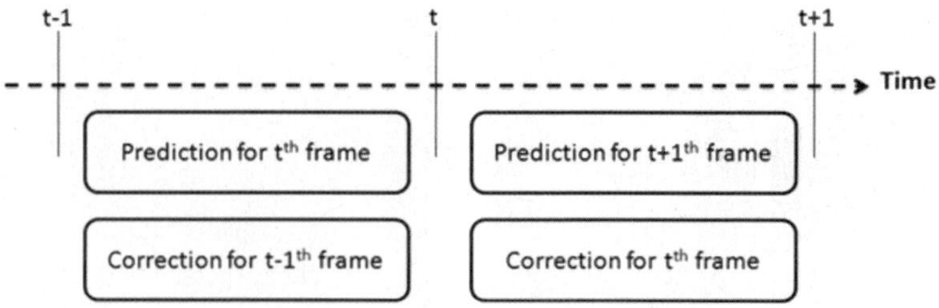

Fig. 8. Schematic Diagram for prediction and correction steps.

The prediction step of this hybrid method can be done while the K-space data for the current frame is being acquired since it is not dependent on acquired K-space data. However, the computational requirement for prediction step is negligible compared to the correction step. The major computational load arises from the solving (24). For real-time reconstruction, this step must be completed before the K-space data for the next frame is acquired. A schematic diagram explaining the sequence of prediction and correction steps is shown in Fig. 8.

The experimental data has been used previously to generate Fig. 3. The data consists of DCE MRI samples. Here the hybrid method is compared with the well-known (but naïve) sliding window technique, the Kalman Filter reconstruction method and the previous CS based reconstruction technique.[24] The ground-truth and the reconstructed images along with their difference images are shown in Fig. 9.

The quality of reconstruction is better assessed from the difference images (difference between ground-truth and reconstructed). The difference images corresponding to the SW and KF reconstruction are brighter, implying worse reconstruction. The difference images for CS reconstruction and the hybrid are darker meaning that the reconstruction is better compared to SW and KF. However, when looked closely one can see that hybrid method actually yields the best reconstruction.

For online reconstruction, one is also interested in the reconstruction times (or play-out rates) since the ultimate goal for online reconstruction is to achieve real-time speeds. By real-time, we mean that the reconstruction time for a frame is less than the time required to reconstruct it. The average reconstruction times for the different methods are shown in Table 1.

Both The SW method and the KF method has a constant reconstruction time. The reconstruction times for our proposed method and DiffCS varies by 10% around the mean. The table shows that SW has the fastest reconstruction times; it is about two times faster than KF. The reason is explained in Ref. [2].

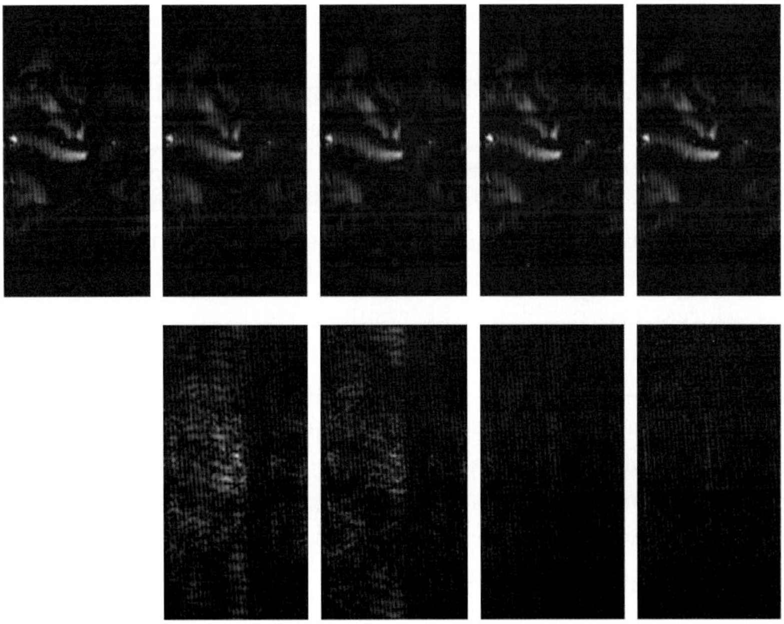

Fig. 9. Reconstructed (top) and Difference (bottom) Images. Left to Right: Ground-truth, Sliding Window, KF, DiffCS reconstruction,[24] Hybrid.

Table 1. Reconstruction Times (in seconds) for different methods.

Dataset	Sliding Window	KF	DiffCS	Hybrid
2D DCE 1	0.056	0.013	0.032	0.017
2D DCE 2	0.055	0.013	0.032	0.017
3D DEC	0.068	0.137	0.574	0.279

The reconstruction speed from our proposed methods is slightly slower than SW and KF and is about twice that of DiffCS.

4. Conclusion

In this chapter, we discuss about recent advances in online dynamic MRI reconstruction. This is the first comprehensive review on this topic. Broadly there are two classes of techniques to address this problem. First, the compressed sensing based methods — these presume that the difference image between consecutive frames are sparse and hence can be recovered. The second approach is to employ dynamical models like Kalman filtering. The major bottleneck with this approach is the computational bottleneck associated with it. The assumptions that reduce the computational overhead become too simplified for quality recovery. There is a final hybrid approach that combines the two. It predicts the frame based on a dynamical system; it then estimates the error between the prediction and the actual one by Compressed Sensing techniques.

Online dynamic MRI reconstruction will be of paramount importance in the future. It will enable image guided surgery and tracking applications amongst others. So far researchers have applied classical mathematical techniques to address this problem; the results have been modest. To push the limits of success, one cannot solely rely on mathematics — the trade-off is too predictable; we cannot improve results without increasing the computations. Mathematical algorithms, used so far are sequential in nature — they do not harness the power of recent advances in multi-core architectures. In the future, we need to focus on parallelizing algorithms so that they can run on multi-core systems; this would enable us to get speedy reconstruction even with sophisticated mathematical modeling.

References

1. M. Lustig, D.L Donoho and J.M Pauly, "Sparse MRI: The application of compressed sensing for rapid MR imaging," *Magn Reson Med*, **58**, 1182–1195 (2007).
2. U. Gamper, P. Boesiger, S. Kozerke, "Compressed sensing in dynamic MRI," *Magn Reson Med*, **59**, 365 (2008).
3. M. Lustig, J.M. Santos, D.L. Donoho, J.M Pauly, "k-t SPARSE: High frame rate dynamic MRI exploiting spatio-temporal sparsity," *International Symposium on Magnetic Resonance in Medicine* (2006).
4. H. Jung, J. C. Ye, E. Y. Kim, "Improved k-t BLAST and k-t SENSE using FOCUSS," *Phys Med Biol* **52**, 3201–3226 (2007).
5. H. Jung, J. Park, J. Yoo, and J. C. Ye, "Radial k-t FOCUSS for high-resolution cardiac cine MRI," *Magn Reson Med* **63**, 68–78 (2010).
6. H. Jung, J. Park, J. Yoo, and J. C. Ye, "k-t FOCUSS: A general compressed sensing framework for high resolution dynamic MRI," *Magn Reson Med* **61**, 103 (2009).
7. B.D. Rao and K. Kreutz-Delgado, "An affine scaling methodology for best basis selection," *IEEE Trans Signal Processing* **47**, 187 (1999).
8. L. Chen, M. C. Schabel and E. V. R. DiBella, "Reconstruction of dynamic contrast enhanced magnetic resonance imaging of the breast with temporal constraints," *Magn Reson Imaging* **28**, 637 (2010).
9. N. Todd, G. Adluru, A. Payne, E. V. R. DiBella and D. Parker, "Temporally constrained reconstruction applied to MRI temperature data," *Magn Reson Med* **62**, 406 (2009).
10. G. Adluru, S.P. Awate, T. Tasdizen, R.T. Whitaker and E.V.R. DiBella, "Temporally constrained reconstruction of dynamic cardiac perfusion MRI," *Magn Reson Med* **57**, 1027 (2007).

11. G. Adluru, C. McGann, P. Speier, E. G. Kholmovski, A. Shaaban and E. V. R. DiBella, "Acquisition and reconstruction of undersampled radial data for myocardial perfusion magnetic resonance imaging," *J Magn Reson Imaging* **29**, 466 (2009).
12. Z. Bo, J. P. Haldar, C. Brinegar and Z. P. Liang, "Low rank matrix recovery for real-time cardiac MRI," *IEEE Int Symposium Biomedical Imaging: From Nano to Macro* **996**, 999 (2010).
13. J. P. Haldar and Z. P. Liang, "Low-rank approximations for dynamic imaging," 2011 *IEEE Int Symposium Biomedical Imaging: From Nano to Macro* **1052** (2011).
14. S. Goud, Y. Hu, E. DiBella, M. Jacob, "Accelerated dynamic MRI exploiting sparsity and low-rank structure," *IEEE Trans Medical Imaging* **30**, 1042 (2011).
15. B. Zhao, J. P. Haldar, A. G. Christodoulou, Z.-P. Liang, "Image reconstruction from highly undersampled (k,t)-space data with joint partial separability and sparsity constraints," *IEEE Trans Med Imaging* **31**, 1809–1820 (2012).
16. A. Majumdar, R. K. Ward and T. Aboulnasr, "Non-convex algorithm for sparse and low-rank recovery: application to dynamic MRI reconstruction," *Magn Reson Imaging* **31**, 448 (2012).
17. A. Majumdar, "Improved dynamic MRI reconstruction by exploiting sparsity and rank-deficiency," *Magn Reson Imaging* **31**, 789 (2013).
18. S.G. Lingala and M. Jacob, "A blind compressive sensing frame work for accelerated dynamic MRI," *IEEE Int Symposium Biomedical Imaging*, 1060 (2012).
19. S. Goud, M. Jacob, "Blind compressed sensing dynamic MRI," *IEEE Trans Med Imaging* in press.
20. A. Majumdar, "Improved blind compressed sensing for dynamic MRI reconstruction," *International Symposium on Magn Reson Med* (2014).
21. N. Vaswani, "LS-CS-residual (LS-CS): Compressive sensing on the least squares residual," *IEEE Trans Signal Processing* **58**, 4108 (2010).
22. Y. Wiaux, G. Puy, R. Gruetter, J. P. Thiran, D. Van De Ville, D and P. Vandergheynst, "Spread spectrum for compressed sensing techniques in magnetic resonance imaging," *IEEE Int Symposium Biomedical Imaging* **756** (2010).
23. G. Puy, P. Vandergheynst, R. Gribonval and Y. Wiaux, "Universal and efficient compressed sensing by spread spectrum and application to realistic Fourier imaging techniques," *EURASIP J Adv Signal Processing* **6** (2012).
24. A. Majumdar, R. K. Ward and T. Aboulnasr, "Compressed sensing based near real-time online dynamic MRI reconstruction," *IEEE Trans Med Imaging* **31**, 2253 (2012).
25. A. Shukla, A. Majumdar and R. K. Ward, "Real-time dynamic MRI reconstruction: Accelerating compressed sensing on graphical processor unit," *IASTED Signal and Image Processing* (2013).
26. U. Sümbül, J. M. Santos and J. M. Pauly, "A practical acceleration algorithm for real-time imaging," *IEEE Trans Med Imaging* **28** (2009).
27. U. Sümbül, J. M. Santos and J. M. Pauly, "Improved time series reconstruction for dynamic magnetic resonance imaging," *IEEE Trans Med Imaging* **28** (2009).
28. X. Feng, M. Salerno, C. M. Kramer and C. H. Meyer, "Kalman filter techniques for accelerated Cartesian dynamic cardiac imaging," *Magn Reson Med* **69**, 1346 (2013).
29. A. Majumdar, "Motion predicted online dynamic MRI reconstruction from partially sampled k-space data," *Magn Reson Imaging* **31**, 1578 (2013).

Chapter 4

Using Prior Information To Enhance Sensitivity of Longitudinal Brain Change Computation

Evan Fletcher

IDeA Laboratory, Department of Neurology and Center for Neuroscience, University of California, Davis, California, USA
E-mail: emfletcher@ucdavis.edu

Longitudinal brain image registration is a technique that is crucial to investigate trajectories of brain change in normal aging and dementia. The goal of producing statistically robust profiles of change is challenging, confounded by image artifacts and algorithm bias. Tensor-based morphometry (TBM) computes deformation mappings between pairs of images of the same subject at different scan times, using log-determinants of the mapping jacobians to record localized change. These algorithms typically generate forces derived from image mismatch at edges to drive change computation, adding a penalty term to dampen spurious indications of change from bias and image artifacts. Mismatch and penalty terms necessitate a tradeoff between sensitivity and specificity.. Recent work has focused on techniques to minimize algorithm bias and ensure longitudinal consistency. Little has been done to improve the tradeoff using prior information, i.e. derived from the images themselves prior to matching. In the present chapter, we survey the recent literature and then propose an approach for enhancing specificity using prior information. Our experiments suggest that the resulting method has enhanced statistical power for discriminating between different trajectories of brain change over time.

1. Introduction

Computation of change in longitudinal MRI images is a crucial technique in the study of biological brain change over time, in order to identify differences between trajectories of normal aging and incipient dementia. It is vital for testing hypotheses about the succession of events in the unfolding of Alzheimer's Disease,[2–4] as well as determining patterns of individual change that distinguish cognitively normal from impaired subjects.[5] Such goals demand methods of longitudinal image registration that ideally should be free from bias (i.e. systematic spurious indication of change) and robust against noise (the interpretation of random image variability as change) while remaining sensitive to even small real biological changes and statistically powerful (requiring small samples to generate significant results). This goal is impossible to fulfill in practice. The existence of confounding factors — geometric distortion from MRI coils, intensity nonuniformities, random noise and head movement, as well as algorithmic bias — insures that no method can be robust with respect to artifacts and completely sensitive to real change at the same time.

A long-standing and necessary compromise is to optimize a matching functional consisting of an image intensity correspondence metric plus a penalty term. This is often also performed using smoothed images in which the contributions of random noise have been presumably dampened. In one line of research, the penalty functional is the "kinetic energy" — the integral of velocity magnitude squared — of the transformations from object to target along a path in the space of images. This penalty is used to guarantee that the deformation occurs via diffeomorphisms — smooth, one-to-one, invertible mappings — that push the image along a geodesic or minimal energy curve from object to target.[6,7] Diffeomorphisms preserve image topology, and forcing them to follow geodesic paths through image space guards against unwarranted complexity.[8]

In this chapter we shall be focused on tensor-based morphometry (TBM), which uses the log of the jacobian (i.e. 3×3 derivative matrix) determinants of the deformation fields to generate local maps of image change.[1,9,10] Recent work has shown that a penalty of a different sort than kinetic energy is necessary in TBM optimization because of inherent bias in the log-jacobian fields themselves, leading to overstated indications of change[9,11,12] even in image pairs where biological change does not exist, such as same-day scans. To redress this skewness of the log-jacobian field, a method has been proposed[9,12,13] that penalizes the Kullback-Liebler divergence[14] of the log-jacobian field from the identity distribution.

However, the Kullback-Liebler (KL) penalty term smoothes the log-jacobian fields and thus reduces their ability to record real change. This necessitates a tradeoff. We shall use the terminology of *sensitivity* and *specificity* in the statistical sense of accurately recording real change (sensitivity) while ignoring false indications of change due to artifacts or bias (specificity). Both are related to the concept of *localization*, the accurate representation of change only in regions where biological changes actually occur. Penalty functions such as KL are necessary to reduce false indications of change, thereby increasing specificity. But they have the inevitable effect of reducing sensitivity.

In a recent article,[15] we proposed to improve this tradeoff by combining estimates of edge location with the force driving the change calculation and the KL penalty. The rationale for introducing information about edge locations is that TBM algorithms compute optimal image matching by solving Euler-Lagrange equations, and these incorporate the intensity gradient of the target image.[16] The details will be elaborated in more detail in Section 2 below. Here, a qualitative description will help to make the intuition clearer. Intensity gradients are typically largest at tissue boundaries but they can also have non-trivial magnitudes elsewhere, due to noise artifacts or intensity inhomogeneities. When combined with apparent local intensity mismatches between the images, such instances may yield computations of change that do not correspond to biological difference. To counteract this, our recent proposal[15] used the distribution of gradient magnitudes to estimate the local probability of edge presence, *P(edge)*, which was inserted as a factor in the matching functional. We showed how *P(edge)* could be an enhancing or attenuating factor for the force driving the change computation, with 1 — *P(edge)* doing the same for the penalty function.

In sum, we locally attenuated the penalty while preserving change computation in places where observed change is more likely to be biological (at tissue boundaries), and conversely preserved the penalty while attenuating computation of change where it may more likely to be the result of artifacts (away from boundaries). The algorithm thus used *prior information* — known about the images prior to computing the deformation — in order to both improve the sensitivity and retain the robustness to noise of the change computations.

A survey of recent work suggests that a proposal to incorporate prior information in this way is relatively new in the literature of longitudinal image matching. Much of the recent effort to enhance robustness and accuracy has been devoted to reducing bias and ensuring consistency. The FreeSurfer approach has emphasized avoiding bias by complete symmetry of image preprocessing.[17] For two longitudinal images, this can be implemented by initial linear alignment of each to a "halfway" image[18] between them — thereby subjecting each image to the same amount of resampling, reducing bias resulting from the asymmetry in which one time point has sharper edges than the other. A related concept is to ensure inverse-consistent image matchings — at each iteration of the warping algorithm, the forward and backward deformations are each computed and constrained to be inverses of each other.[19–21] Several approaches have also proposed using a template to enforce registration consistency. The HAMMER approach[22,23] advocated simultaneous estimation of both the longitudinal subject correspondence and the relation of each subject with a template image. A refinement has sought to avoid potential bias from template selection by use of an "implicit template" combined with probabilistic spatio-temporal heuristics.[24]

Two recent techniques, however, have suggested adaptively changing the parameters of the diffeomorphic matching to adjust to image conditions. In this aspect, they are closer to our proposal. One method introduces prior knowledge about the images to be registered, generating a weighted multi-scale sum of smoothing kernels to capture features that have varying characteristic scales.[25] A second method directly addresses questions about the level of weighting given to the penalty term. Rather than use a fixed weight for all images, it evaluates image characteristics to estimate the level of noise and adjust the level of regularisation.[7]

Finally, recent work using generative and discriminative models in brain tissue segmentation is also relevant to our proposal for enhanced longitudinal image matching.[26,27] These articles have described how segmentation (tissue classification) can be improved by using *discriminative* models — local sampling of neighborhood characteristics including intensity, curvature, gradients and Haar measures — combined with *generative* models — adaptive estimates of structures guided by global image characteristics — to insure smoothness and structure coherence. The models consist of complex sums of various features, and necessitate the use of training sets and machine learning algorithms to estimate the optimal weights for combining them.

The relevance of these techniques for our approach to image matching is that a similar method, sampling an array of features, could be used to refine our original estimates of edge location likelihood. This might give greater certainty of edge estimation at locations where the intensity gradient magnitudes can typically be smaller than at the cortical boundaries. Examples of such locations include the hippocampus, the subcortical nuclei and certain sulci that are poorly defined in many MRI images because of small size or reduced tissue boundary contrast. Conversely, a refined probability estimate might also be more robust against false indications of "edges" resulting from artifacts, thereby leading to fewer errors and greater statistical power in groupwise studies of longitudinal change.

The rest of this chapter will describe one possible enhancement in detail (Section 2). We will then present experiments and their results for testing this model (Section 3) and conclude by a discussion (Section 4).

2. Incorporating Prior Information into Longitudinal Image Registration

In this section, we provide relevant details about the preprocessing sequence involved in longitudinal image registration, followed by an outline of the mathematical formalism of TBM and models of how prior information may be included in it.

2.1. *Image Preprocessing*

We start with two brain images of the same person, taken at different scan times. These images are processed to remove the skulls. Next, an affine alignment is performed to remove rotational and translational differences. To compensate for resampling asymmetry, which may generate spurious indications of change in the subsequent TBM registration as described above, we align each image to a point halfway between the two. Following Smith *et al.*[18] we compute halfway alignments. In order to treat both images as closely as possible alike, we resample the earlier time point to a lattice of isotropic voxels, introducing a slight interpolation blurring of edges. From the alignment of the later time point onto the resampled earlier point, an approximate square root matrix is created by halving each of the rotation and translation parameters, and the later time point is transformed by this matrix. Then the original earlier time point is aligned to this "halfway" point. This technique greatly reduces a systematic source of bias at prominent brain structure edges. It was not performed for the images used in our prevous article,[15] thereby adding extra edge bias to the results reported. Figure 1 illustrates the contrast between the "halfway" technique and the previous method of aligning the second time point onto

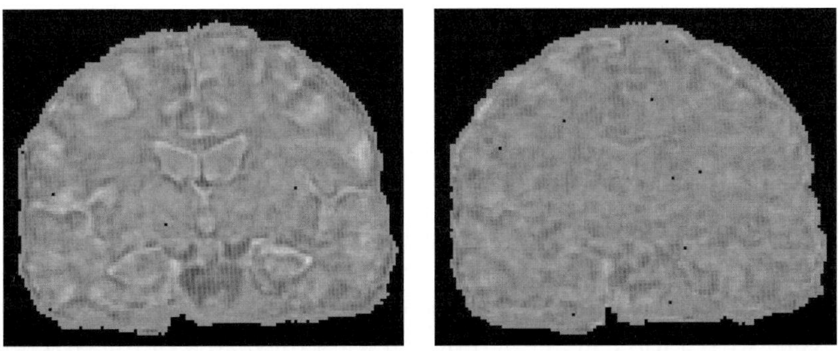

Fig. 1. Averaged difference images of 11 no-change subjects (two scans on the same day). Left: after aligning time 2 onto time 1. Right: after aligning each to halfway point.

the first. Each panel shows an average of 11 subtraction images (time 2 minus time 1) for individual subjects having two scans taken on the same day (therefore no biological change exists). The images were further nonlinearly deformed to a common template to enable voxelwise comparisons.

2.2. *Mathematical Formulation of TBM with Incorporated Prior Information*

2.2.1. *Formulation of the image matching problem*

Let Ω be a rectangular box in 3D Cartesian space. T_1 and T_2 are real-valued intensity functions on Ω representing our images at time 1 and time 2, respectively: the outcomes from affine-aligning time 1 and time 2 scans to the halfway point as described in the previous section. To compute a deformation of T_2 onto T_1, we compute an inverse-consistent deformation $\mathbf{g}$: $\Omega \to \Omega$ such that for each location $\mathbf{x}$ in Ω, $T_1(\mathbf{g}(\mathbf{x}))$ should equal $T_2(\mathbf{x})$. Let $\mathbf{u}$ be the displacement from a position in the deformed image back to its source in T_2. Then $\mathbf{g}(\mathbf{x}) = \mathbf{x} - \mathbf{u}(\mathbf{x})$. Matching T_1 and T_2 means finding an optimal $\mathbf{g}$ or equivalently an optimal $\mathbf{u}$ for the deformation between the images.

2.2.2. *Outline of the TBM algorithm*

The usual TBM algorithm optimizes an energy functional E to generate a matching $\mathbf{u}$ between the images. E has the format

$$E(T_1, T_2, \mathbf{u}) = M(T_1, T_2, \mathbf{u}) + \lambda R(\mathbf{u}), \tag{1}$$

where M is an image dissimilarity metric and R is a regularizing penalty term, both dependent on the deformation $\mathbf{u}$. The parameter λ governs the strength of the penalty term and is usually empirically tuned to give good results.

The algorithm solves the Euler-Lagrange equation $\partial_{\mathbf{u}} E = \mathbf{0}$, at least approximately, obtaining a $\boldsymbol{u}$ to optimize E. The variational derivative of the matching term M takes the form

$$\partial_{\mathbf{u}} M = m(T_1, T_2, \mathbf{u}) \nabla \mathbf{T}_1(\mathbf{g}(\mathbf{x})), \tag{2}$$

where m is a scalar function determined by the variational derivative and $\nabla \mathbf{T}_1(\mathbf{g}(\mathbf{x}))$ is the intensity gradient of T_1 at the location specified by $\mathbf{g}(\mathbf{x})$[16] (note that in our implementation T_1 is the target image).

The variational derivative of E is a force field $\partial_{\mathbf{u}} E = \mathbf{F}_1 + \lambda \mathbf{F}_2$, with $\mathbf{F}_1$ and $\mathbf{F}_2$ being the variational derivatives of the matching term and penalty term, respectively. $\mathbf{F}_1$ is a force generated by intensity mismatch of the two images at each voxel, driving the solution toward image matching. $\mathbf{F}_2$ is a force driving the solution to reduce the penalty term.

2.2.3. *The fluid-flow solution*

Instead of solving the Euler-Lagrange equation by gradient descent, *fluid flow* methods[28,29] solve for the flow velocity field $\mathbf{v}$, then use it to update the deformation $\mathbf{u}$ iteratively over small time interval increments Δt via Euler integration:

$$\mathbf{u}(\mathbf{x}, t + \Delta t) = \mathbf{u}(\mathbf{x}, t) + (\mathbf{v} - \mathbf{Du} * \mathbf{v})\Delta t \tag{3}$$

where Du is the 3×3 matrix jacobian derivative of u, here acting on the velocity v. This formula is based on a discrete approximation to the total time derivative of u.[28] The size of the time increment Δt is often varied so that a maximal u displacement is not exceeded at each iteration.

In our approach, the velocity $\mathbf{v}$ is derived by solving the Navier-Stokes partial differential equation[28]

$$\mu \nabla^2 \mathbf{v} + (\mu + \nu)\nabla(\nabla \cdot \mathbf{v}) = -\mathbf{F}(\mathbf{x}, \mathbf{u}) \tag{4}$$

where $\mathbf{F} = \mathbf{F}_1 + \lambda \mathbf{F}_2$ as described above.

Thus the fluid flow method consists of iterated steps, each step generating v from the current force field via (4), updating u via (3) and checking to see whether a termination condition — negligible improvement in E — is satisfied.

2.2.4. *The Kullback-Liebler penalty*

In our implementation, the penalty term will be the Kullback-Liebler penalty R_{KL} introduced by Yanovsky *et al.*,[8] based on the Kullback-Liebler divergence metric for log-jacobian distributions.[14] The metric is defined as:

$$R_{KL} = \int_\Omega \log |D\mathbf{g}(\mathbf{x})| d\mathbf{x} \tag{5}$$

where $|Dg|$ is the jacobian determinant of the 3×3 matrix derivative of g.

2.2.5. *Incorporating prior information into the energy functional*

Let $P(\mathbf{x})$ be an estimate of the likelihood that an intensity difference between $T_1(\mathbf{g}(\mathbf{x}))$ and $T_2(\mathbf{x})$ corresponds to an actual biological difference. Such an estimate, if available, could be a useful guide for modulating the mismatch force $\mathbf{F}_1$. Similarly, the complement of P — the likelihood that an intensity difference corresponds to an artifact and should be ignored — could be used to modulate the penalty force $\mathbf{F}_2$. A straightforward way of doing so would be to minimize a modified variational derivative of the form

$$P\mathbf{F}_1 + \lambda(1 - P)\mathbf{F}_2. \tag{6}$$

The intent of this formulation would be enhancement of both sensitivity and specificity and it is intuitively clear how the two summands with their probabilistic estimates would work to this end. At locations where image differences probably represent biological difference (with P close to 1), the force $\mathbf{F}_1$ derived from intensity mismatch would be preserved while the penalty force $\mathbf{F}_2$ would be attenuated. The opposite effect would occur at places where intensity differences are likely due to noise (with P close to 0).

Unfortunately, it is not guaranteed *a priori* that this formula is the variational derivative of any energy functional; thus it is not clear what sort of optimization problem would be "solved" by minimizing it. Furthermore, an ideal "likehood of real biological change" estimate is circular because it assumes knowledge of what we are trying to compute in the first place.

However, by making some simplifying assumptions, our recent article[15] proposed an approximation to the above formulation. We used for P a function that depended on T_2 alone (i.e. it was independent of the deformation mapping $\mathbf{g}$) and thus would be treated as a constant in the variational derivative of M. This enabled us to generate a force of the form (6) which was indeed the variational derivative of a valid matching functional, and we showed that minimizing this variational derivative led to matchings with increased sensitivity and specificity.

The "likelihood of biological change" function P was approximated by using likelihood of edges in T_2 as a proxy for "likelihood of change." We derived the likelihood of edges in T_2 from the cumulative distribution function (CDF) of its gradient magnitudes. Locations with large gradient magnitudes — having CDF value close to 1 — were considered as places where an edge occurrence was likely.

The reason for using edges as proxies for change can be seen from (2), where $\partial_{\mathbf{u}} M$ is a scalar function of intensity difference times the gradient of T_1. Thus intensity difference can only contribute to $\mathbf{F}_1$ at locations where $\nabla \mathbf{T}_1$ has appreciable magnitude. The gradient of T_1 is most strongly associated with tissue boundaries, and this leads to the association of edges with biological change. But $\nabla \mathbf{T}_1$ can also have nonzero magnitude at non-edge image artifacts, and we would like to dampen instances of the latter type, while preserving the former. This strengthens the rationale for associating edges with real change.

Basing P on edges in T_2 instead of T_1, however, may seem questionable. We found nonetheless that this approach at least partially achieves the intended consequences, because (1) in longitudinal registration the edges of T_1 and T_2 are usually not far apart, and their difference can be straddled by the smoothed gradient likelihood estimate; and (2) in places where $\nabla \mathbf{T}_1$ is large due to image artifacts rather than edges, it is a random occurrence that the corresponding location of T_2 also has a large gradient due to artifact. Thus when a T_2 edge is not present, it is likely that either the value of P or the gradient magnitude of T_1 will be low — and spurious computations of change force will be dampened.

2.2.6. *Refining the estimates of edge occurrence*

In our previous article, we used a simple formula equating the likelihood of an edge at a location with the proportion of all the gradients of the image having magnitudes less than the gradient at the current location, in other words, the CDF:

$$P_{old}(\mathbf{x}) = P(edge|\nabla \mathbf{T}_2(\mathbf{x})) = CDF(\|\nabla \mathbf{T}_2(\mathbf{x})\|) \tag{7}$$

However, this earlier choice of P has some drawbacks that might be improved. A main problem is that certain discrete brain structures like the hippocampi, small sulci and the subcortical nuclei have genuine edges but smaller-magnitude gradients than at the ventricles or brain boundary, leading to lower than desirable P values at the edges of these structures. The commonly seen indistinctness of gray-white tissue boundaries can create a similar problem. Secondly, T_2 may itself have nontrivial gradients elsewhere than at edges, so that the "random occurrence" of large T_1 and T_2 gradients, both due to artifacts, is still a possibility.

In this chapter, accordingly, we propose a refinement of P using both gradients and tissue segmentation in T_2. Tissue segmentation[30] is based on the assumption that intensity distribution in each tissue compartment of a noise-free image is close to homogeneous. Each brain voxel can be assigned an unambiguous label of the tissue class to which it most likely belongs. We can use the labels of the segmented image to further suppress spurious indications of change while enhancing edge delineations where biological change can occur.

We sample the $3 \times 3 \times 3$ voxel neighborhood of each location in the segmented image to generate a factor called $P(tissue)$. This depends on the tissue composition of the neighborhood. If all voxels are labeled the same tissue, we assign the value 0.1 (rather than 0, on the small possibility that the segmentation is incorrect). Otherwise, the neighborhood may straddle a tissue edge. If the proportion of one tissue is larger than 40%, we assume a strong edge presence is likely and assign the value of 1.0. Otherwise we assign a graduated scale of likelihoods, with 0.8 for a 30% proportion of one tissue, 0.4 for a 20% proportion of one tissue, and 0.2 for a 10% proportion.

We also wish to enhance edge strength for locations where gradient magnitudes are reduced but which are likely to be edges according to the brain segmentation. We do this by CDF "boosting." For voxels in which the neighborhood structure is close to 50% of one tissue according to the segmentation, we "boost" the gradient magnitude by a factor of 3.5 for gray-CSF boundaries and 2.0 for white-gray boundaries before inserting it into the gradient magnitude histogram. This has the effect of increasing the CDF value at this location, while causing little change in the CDF values of already strong gradients.

Our new model is now multiplicative in both probabilities:

$$P_{new}(\mathbf{x}) = P(edge|\nabla\mathbf{T}_2(\mathbf{x}), tissue) = CDF(\|\nabla\mathbf{T}_2(\mathbf{x})\|) \times P(tissue) \quad (8)$$

2.2.7. *Derivation of the variational derivatives incorporating prior information*

In this section, we will derive the formulas for the matching and penalty energy functionals and their variational derivatives enhanced by probability factors $P(\mathbf{x})$ as described above.

For the modified penalty functional based on R_{KL} define:

$$pR_{KL} = \int_{\Omega} (1 - P(\mathbf{x})) \log |D\mathbf{g}(\mathbf{x})| d\mathbf{x} \quad (9)$$

Then because $P(\boldsymbol{x})$ is independent of $\mathbf{g}$, we have:

$$\begin{aligned} \partial_{\mathbf{u}} pR_{KL} &= (1 - P(\mathbf{x}))\partial_{\mathbf{u}} \int_{\Omega} \log |D\mathbf{g}(\mathbf{x})| d\mathbf{x} \\ &= (1 - P(\mathbf{x}))\partial_{\mathbf{u}} R_{KL} \end{aligned} \quad (10)$$

For the modified image matching functional, we start with the cross-correlation (CC) metric. The variational derivative of CC can be found in Hermosillo *et al.*[16] In our approach, we compute a modified CC using terms weighted at each voxel by $P(\mathbf{x})$. Define the following terms:

$$v_1 = \int_{\Omega} P(\mathbf{x}) T_1^2(\mathbf{g}(\mathbf{x})) d\mathbf{x} \quad \text{(weighted variance of } \mathrm{T}_1) \quad (11)$$

$$v_2 = \int_{\Omega} T_2^2(\mathbf{x}) d\mathbf{x} \quad \text{(variance of } \mathrm{T}_2) \quad (12)$$

and

$$v_{12} = \int_{\Omega} P(\mathbf{x}) T_1(\mathbf{g}(\mathbf{x})) T_2(\mathbf{x}) d\mathbf{x} \quad \text{(weighted covariance } \mathrm{T}_1 \text{ and } \mathrm{T}_2). \quad (13)$$

Then our matching functional M is the modified cross-correlation:

$$M = v_{12}^2/(v_1 v_2)$$

Applying the rules of calculus to the variational derivative of M, and keeping in mind that $P(\mathbf{x})$ is independent of $\mathbf{g}$, we have the following:

$$\begin{aligned} \partial_{\mathbf{u}} M &= (2v_1 v_2 v_{12} \partial_{\mathbf{u}} v_{12} - v_{12}^2 v_2 \partial_{\mathbf{u}} v_1)/(v_1 v_2)^2 \\ &= 2P(\mathbf{x})(T_2(x) v_1 v_2 v_{12} - T_1(\mathbf{g}(\mathbf{x})) v_2 v_{12}^2)/(v_1 v_2)^2 \times \nabla\mathbf{T}_1(\mathbf{g}(\mathbf{x})) \end{aligned} \quad (14)$$

Examination of (14) shows that the variation of M is of the form $P(\mathbf{x}) \times \mathbf{F}_1$, where the $\mathbf{F}_1$ is a scalar function times the gradient of T_1. Similarly, (10) shows that the variation of our modified penalty is of the form $(1 - P(\mathbf{x})) \times \mathbf{F}_2$, where $\mathbf{F}_2$ is simply the variation of R_{KL}. Combining (10) and (14), we have obtained a variational vector field of the form given in (6).

3. Experiments and Results

We present experiments and their outcomes comparing the longitudinal brain change modeling computed by our earlier and new methods for incorporating prior information.

Data for our experiments were obtained from the Alzheimer's Disease Neuroimaging Initiative (ADNI) database (www.loni.usc.edu). The ADNI was launched in 2003 by the National Institute on Aging (NIA), the National Institute of Biomedical Imaging and Bioengineering (NIBIB), the Food and Drug Administration (FDA), private pharmaceutical companies and non-profit organizations, as a \$60 million, 5-year public-private partnership. The primary goal of ADNI has been to test whether serial magnetic resonance imaging (MRI), positron emission tomography (PET), other biological markers, and clinical and neuropsychological assessment can be combined to measure the progression of mild cognitive impairment (MCI) and early Alzheimer's disease (AD). ADNI is the result of efforts of many co-investigators from a broad range of academic institutions and private corporations, and subjects have been recruited from over 50 sites across the U.S. and Canada. The initial goal of ADNI was to recruit 800 adults, ages 55 to 90, to participate in the research — approximately 200 cognitively normal older individuals to be followed for three years, 400 people with MCI to be followed for three years, and 200 people with early AD to be followed for two years.

3.1. *Change vs. No-Change Images*

In order to test the statistical significance of change indications in each model, a first experiment computed change over two scans for a "no-change" (NC) group of 11 subjects having two scans on the same day, in which no biological change is expected, and 20 subjects with diagnosis of Alzheimer's Disease (AD), each subject's scans being close to one year apart. All group analyses were based upon log-Jacobian images of the longitudinal deformations. Group analyses required a further deformation of all subjects onto a "minimal deformation template" (MDT) constructed to be minimally distant from images in an

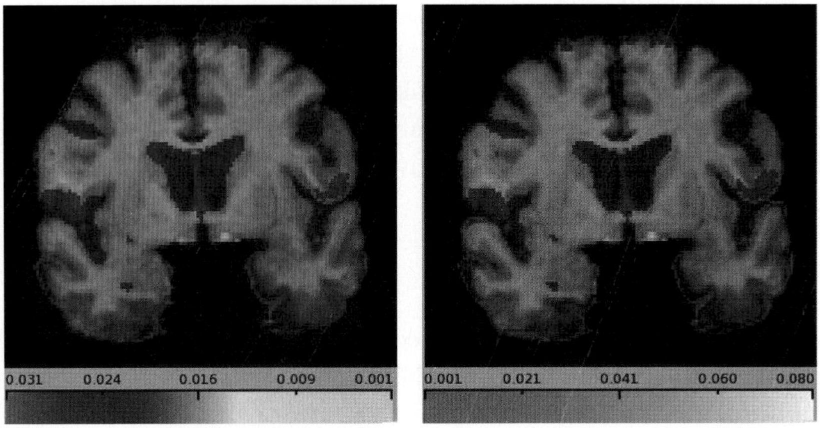

Fig. 2. Averaged log-jacobian values for old and new methods over group of 20 AD subjects with scan intervals of one year. Left: Old method. Right: New method. Color bars show values of log-jacobians: cool for negative values (tissue loss), warm for positive (expansion of fluid spaces). Color can be viewed in the e-book. In the present black and white version, the cool palette is under the left image while the warm palette is under the right image.

age-matched group.[31] We used an MDT made from 29 clinically normal individuals 60 years of age or older. Each subject T_2 image was warped to the MDT using a cubic B-spline warp,[32] and the deformation parameters were used to transform each native space jacobian image to template space.

Figure 2 shows color-coded average change values by method. The change values in each method are fairly similar, but with generally slightly larger magnitudes for our new method (right panel). Enhanced change computation of the new method is most visible in the medial temporal lobes.

To evaluate the indications of change for statistical significance, we compared the changes for each method with computed changes in the no-change group. We used groupwise t-tests to compare values at each voxel in the AD group with the same location in the NC group, after jacobian images from both groups were transformed to MDT space. A voxel t-value was the mean of the AD group minus the mean of the NC group at that voxel, the difference divided by the pooled standard deviation over both groups at the voxel. To assess statistical significance we performed non-parametric permutation testing.[33] In this technique the null hypothesis of no difference between the AD and NC groups is tested by randomly reconstituting the group memberships, swapping members from one to the other, and computing the range of t-values over all voxels with the new group composition. We performed 1000 iterations of this swapping, compiling histograms of maximum and minimum t-values generated at each iteration. At the end of the process, voxels with original t-values in the two-tailed top 5% (i.e. lower than 2.5% for the min t-values or larger than 97.5%

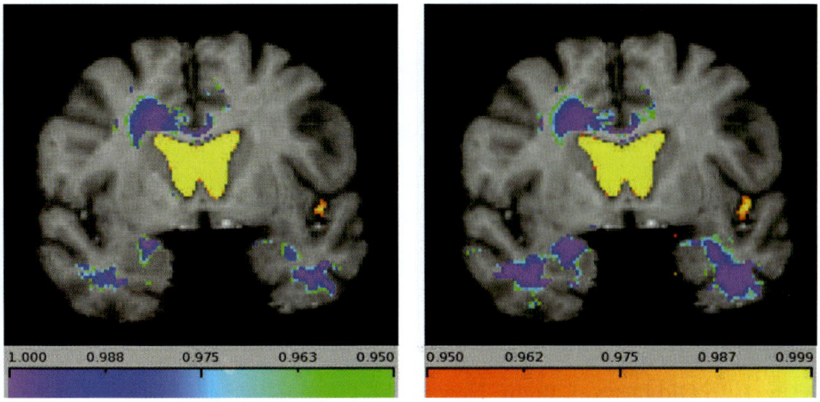

Fig. 3a. Statistically significant voxels for differences between AD and NC subjects, coronal view. This corresponds to the same slice as in Fig. 2. Left: Old method. Right: New method. Color bars show significances of t-values of log-jacobians: cool for negative values, warm for positive. Corrected p-values are $1 - \nu$ for ν shown in the color bar. Color bar also applies to Figs. 3b and 3c.

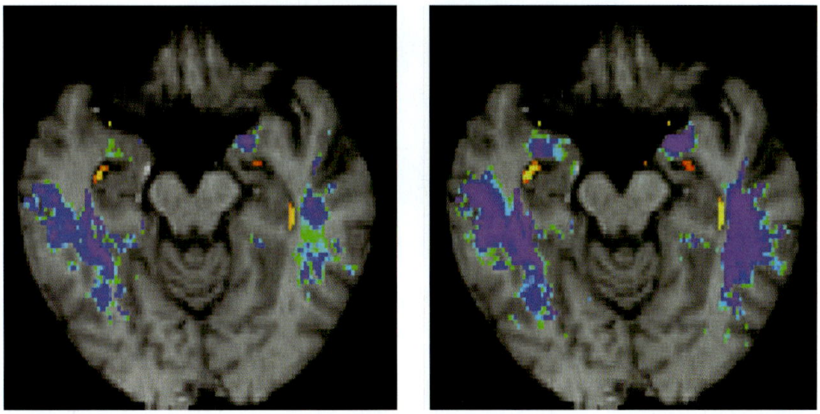

Fig. 3b. Statistically significant voxels for differences between AD and NC subjects, axial view. Color coding is the same as in Fig. 3a. Left: Old method. Right: New method.

for the max t-values) of all values in the histograms were considered to show significant differences between the groups at these locations.

Figure 3a shows comparisons of significant differences between AD and NC subjects in each method. Only statistically significant voxels are shown. Color bars indicate the ranges of statistical significance. Figure 3b gives an axial view also indicating more extensive temporal lobe change. Figure 3c shows a sagittal view indicating areas of signifcant change in the mid and posterior cingulate and the splenium.

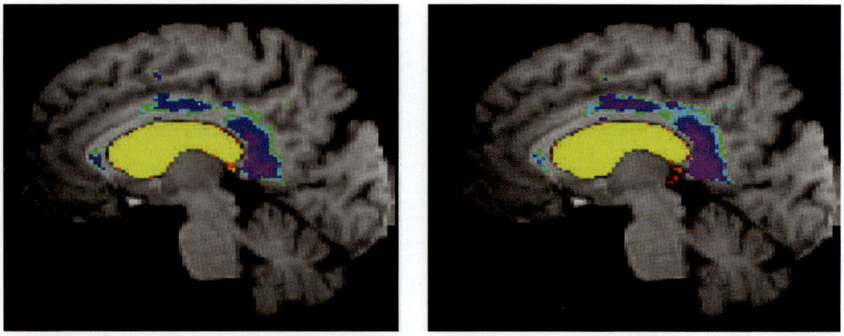

Fig. 3c. Statistically significant voxels for differences between AD and NC subjects, mid-sagittal view. Left: Old method. Right: New method. Color coding is the same as in Fig. 3a.

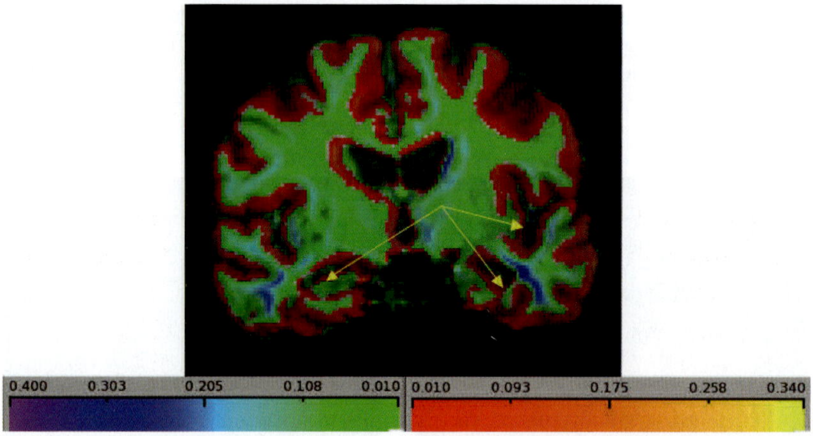

Fig. 4. Color coding of average $P_{new} - P_{old}$ values at each voxel: the difference between using CDF alone (old) and "boosted" CDF multiplied by neighborhood tissue information (new). Cold colors show decreases. Warm show increases. Arrows indicate sample edges of brain structures that were originally weak and are now enhanced: hippocampal boundaries and insular cortex. Other, stronger edges were often also enhanced.

3.2. *Examination of the Enhancements to Edge and Non-Edge Probabilities*

The gist of our approach is to associate likely brain change with the occurrence of tissue edges, accordingly enhancing the gradient magnitudes at likely edges via histogram "boosting" while suppressing them away from edges. Both of these operations make use of additional information when compared with our previous approach: the estimation of tissue class via segmentation.

Figure 4 illustrates changes to the P values of the new approach. It shows the average increment (positive or negative) over our 20 AD subjects after deformation to template space, when compared to our old P function. The image depicts $P_{new} - P_{old}$, i.e. formula (8) minus formula (7). We see increases in the P values at edges and decreases everywhere else. In homogeneous tissue areas away from edges, there are fairly uniform if small decreases in the P values. Yellow arrows in the figure point to the bilateral hippocampi (bottom arrows) and one of the insular cortices (right) — examples of structures whose gradient CDF values were formerly weak but are enhanced by the new method. The totality of changes in P resulted in enhanced computation of volume changes at or near edges and reduced intersubject variance of computed change at locations away from edges.

3.3. *Statistical Power of the Old and New Methods*

Our final experiment is a power analysis comparing the minimum sample size that each method would need to discern a 25% diminution of brain atrophy above normal aging levels, based on change computations for normal subjects (CN) and a second group of Alzheimer's (AD). For each method, we used *statistically defined ROIs* (statROIs)[34,35] over which to measure statistical power. The statROI for a TBM method is defined as a region in the template space where that method picks out significant differences between our original (in Section 3.1) AD and no-change (NC) groups. These ROIs were constructed by doing cluster-size permutation testing[33] to find significant ($p < 0.05$, corrected) clusters of voxels having t-values greater than 5 for the AD minus NC groups. To compute statistical power, we used a new set of AD subjects, not overlapping with the AD group of Section 1. This new set consisted of 25 AD subjects with scans close to 1 year apart. We also used a set of 24 CN subjects with scans at one-year intervals. The old and new methods each computed brain-change log-jacobians for each subject in each group. After warping to template space, the mean and standard deviation of each method over its own statROI was computed for each group. The statistical power of each method was estimated by the following formula[34]:

$$n80 = \frac{2\sigma_{AD}^2(z_{0.975} + z_{0.8})^2}{(0.25(\mu_{AD} - \mu_{CN}))^2} \tag{15}$$

where μ_{AD} and μ_{CN} denote the log-jacobian means of a method over AD and CN groups, σ_{AD} is the method standard deviation on the AD group and the z_b (for $b = 0.975$ or 0.8) are thresholds defined by $P(Z < z_b) < b$ in the standard normal distribution. Thus $n80$ is the minimum sample size needed to detect a 25% reduction in the atrophy rate beyond that of normal aging,[35] i.e. $\mu_{AD} - \mu_{CN}$, with 80% power at a significance level of 5%. Sample sizes with this approach will be larger than if they had been based on detecting 25% change in *total atrophy*, i.e. using μ_{AD} alone, but as pointed out by Holland *et al.*[35] this is a more realistic estimate for use in clinical trials where the concern is to detect effects of slowed atrophy beyond normal aging.

The *n*80 value of the old method was 144 subjects. For the new method, it was 130. Thus, our new method produced a gain in statistical power over the old.

4. Discussion

In this chapter, we have outlined a method for refining the calculation of longitudinal change. It has demonstrated increased ability to distinguish between AD and no-change subjects. Figures 2 and 3a–3c suggest that the new method outperforms the old one both in anatomical specificity and in capturing areas of significant change. Furthermore the new method has shown increased statistical power, reflected in decreased sample size needed to detect change beyond normal aging.

Thus, we believe this method has the potential to be useful in longitudinal image matching. Nonetheless we wish to discuss some of the limitations of the method. The first is that even though weak edge probabilities were enhanced (see Fig. 4), they did not appear to yield increased significance of change for structures associated with these edges. For example, it is well-known that the hippocampus is one of the first structures to undergo atrophy in AD, yet we did not find significant tissue loss in the hippocampus of the AD group as compared to the no-change images. One reason may stem from the difficulty of accurately deforming the hippocampi to the template during the B-spline transformation. The hippocampal topography varies greatly with amount of atrophy, creating difficulties for the B-spline deformations which match varying native subjects to the single hippocampal target in MDT. Inconsistency of cross-sectional deformation to the template introduces noise and reduces statistical power. Other brain structures (such as ventricles) show a more consistently successful matching. This observation may point to a problem inherent in cross-sectional analysis that cannot be addressed by metric enhancements of the TBM deformation, no matter how sophisticated. Inter-subject variation is always higher at tissue boundaries, and the issue is compounded in areas of imperfect registration during deformation to template space.

This leads to a second observation. Even though our new method shows slightly increased mean tissue losses at most edges, in fact almost no areas of significant brain differences in Figs. 3a–3c occur at edges. This means that the observed expansions of significant t-values for our new method depend crucially on the *reduced variation* caused by the multiplicative $P(tissue)$ term [see Eq. (8)], in regions away from edges, where segmentation estimates that the tissue neighborhood is homogeneous.

This scenario reflects a design feature intrinsic to the TBM algorithm. As explained in the introduction, TBM creates a model of brain change by generating forces at boundaries [see Eq. (2)], which drive movement of the deformation vectors. The movement is smoothed by coupling with a penalty function, thus spreading out indications of change. Our approach has been successful in improving TBM due to the adaptive P applied to $\mathbf{F_1}$ [Eq. (14)] which generates higher edge forces and stronger edge movements, and $1 - P$ applied to $\mathbf{F_2}$ [Eq. (10)] which allows them to propagate away from the edges, with reduced variation from noisy intensity fluctuations. Thus, our refinement takes advantage of and accentuates a characteristic already built into TBM.

It is important to note that "generating forces at edges and smoothing them" — the TBM model — is not the only approach to longitudinal change. Another model, the boundary shift integral (BSI),[36] quantifies changes only at tissue-CSF boundaries by counting the number of voxels that were brain tissue at baseline and converted to CSF at a later scan. To do so, it needs a "morphological operator" to estimate where the likely edges are, and an "intensity window" positioned to straddle intensity differences associated with boundary change, while excluding differences that lie outside the window. This observation highlights, again, the realization that change computation involves a tradeoff between localization and regularization. BSI implements these components using the morphological operator and the intensity window. By focusing on edges, we have incorporated an analog of the BSI morphological operator into TBM. The difference between the models is that TBM makes inferences about brain change in areas both near and far from edges, whereas BSI says nothing about change away from edges.

The question of whether tissue loss deep in the white matter is a real biological process might be answered by examining other MRI modalities such as DTI for evidence of white matter integrity decline. That question is beyond the scope of this chapter. In any case, the change computations enhanced by our proposed method are statistically powerful as discriminators between cognitive groups and as descriptors of differing brain trajectories in aging and disease.

References

1. C.R. Jack, D.S. Knopman, W.J. Jagust *et al.*, "Hypothetical model of dynamic biomarkers of the Alzheimer's pathological cascade," *Lancet Neurol* **9**, 119–128 (2010).

2. R.A. Sperling, P.S. Aisen, L.A. Beckett *et al.*, "Toward defining the preclinical stages of Alzheimer's disease: recommendations from the National Institute on Aging-Alzheimer's Association workgroups on diagnostic guidelines for Alzheimer's disease," *Alzheimers Dement* 7, 280–292 (2011).
3. C.R. Jack, D.M. Holtzman, "Biomarker modeling of alzheimer's disease," *Neuron* **80**, 1347–1358 (2013).
4. X. Hua, S. Lee, D.P. Hibar *et al.*, "Mapping Alzheimer's disease progression in 1309 MRI scans: Power estimates for different inter-scan intervals," *Neuroimage* **51**, 63–75. doi:10.1016/j.neuroimage.2010.01.104 (2010).
5. P. Dupuis, U. Grenander, M.I. Miller, "Variational problems in flows of diffeomorphisms for image matching," *Q J Appl Math.*
6. M.F. Beg, M.I. Miller, A. Trouvé *et al.*, "Computing large deformation metric mappings via geodesic flows of diffeomorphisms," *Int J Comput Vis* **61**, 139–157 (2005).
7. I.J. Simpson a, J. Schnabel a, A.R. Groves, J.L.R. Andersson, M.W. Woolrich, "Probabilistic inference of regularisation in non-rigid registration," *Neuroimage* **59**, 2438–2451 (2012).
8. I. Yanovsky, A.D. Leow, S. Lee, S.J. Osher, P.M. Thompson, "Comparing registration methods for mapping brain change using tensor-based morphometry," *Med Image Anal* **13**, 679–700 (2009).
9. X. Hua, A.D. Leow, N. Parikshak *et al.*, "Tensor-based morphometry as a neuroimaging biomarker for Alzheimer's disease: an MRI study of 676 AD, MCI, and normal subjects," *Neuroimage* **43**, 458–469 (2008).
10. X. Hua, B. Gutman, C.P. Boyle *et al.*, "Accurate measurement of brain changes in longitudinal MRI scans using tensor-based morphometry," *Neuroimage* **57**, 5–14 (2011).
11. A.D. Leow, I. Yanovsky, M.-C. Chiang *et al.*, "Statistical properties of jacobian maps and the realization of unbiased large-deformation nonlinear image registration," *IEEE Trans Med Imaging* **26**, 822–832 (2007).
12. I. Yanovsky, P.M. Thompson, S.J. Osher, A.D. Leow, "Topology preserving log-unbiased nonlinear image registration: theory and implementation," *IEEE Conference on Computer Vision and Pattern Recognition.* Minneapolois, MN; 1–8 (2007).
13. I. Yanovsky, "Unbiased nonlinear image registration," PhD Dissertation, UCLA (2008).
14. J. Shlens, "Notes on Kullback-Leibler Divergence and Likelihood Theory" (2007).
15. E. Fletcher, A. Knaack, B. Singh *et al.*, "Combining boundary-based methods with tensor-based morphometry in the measurement of longitudinal brain change," *IEEE Trans Med Imaging* **32**, 223–236 (2013).
16. G. Hermosillo, C.C. Hotel, O. Faugeras, I.S. Antipolis, C. Chefd'Hotel, "Variational methods for multimodal image matching," *Int J Comput Vis* **50**, 329–343 (2002).
17. M. Reuter, B. Fischl, "Avoiding asymmetry-induced bias in longitudinal image processing," *Neuroimage* **57**, 19–21 (2011).
18. S.M. Smith, N.D. De Stefano, M. Jenkinson, P. Matthews, "Normalized Accurate Measurement of Longitudinal Brain Change," *J Comput Assist Tomogr* **25**, 466–475 (2001).
19. G.E. Christensen, H.J. Johnson, "Consistent image registration," *IEEE Trans Med Imaging* **20**, 568–582 (2001).
20. W.K. Thompson, D. Holland, "Bias in tensor based morphometry Stat-ROI measures may result in unrealistic power estimates," *Neuroimage* **57**, 1–4 (2011).

21. X. Hua, D.P. Hibar, C.R.K. Ching *et al.*, "Unbiased tensor-based morphometry: improved robustness and sample size estimates for Alzheimer's disease clinical trials," *Neuroimage* **66**, 648–661 (2013).
22. D. Shen, C. Davatzikos, "HAMMER: hierarchical attribute matching mechanism for elastic registration," *IEEE Trans Med Imaging* **21**, 1421–1439 (2002).
23. D. Shen, C. Davatzikos, "Measuring temporal morphological changes robustly in brain MR images via 4-dimensional template warping," *Neuroimage* **21**, 1508–1517 (2004).
24. G. Wu, Q. Wang, D. Shen, "Registration of longitudinal brain image sequences with implicit template and spatial-temporal heuristics," *Neuroimage* **59**, 404–421 (2012).
25. L. Risser, F.-X. Vialard, R. Wolz, M. Murgasova, D.D. Holm, D. Rueckert, "Simultaneous multi-scale registration using large deformation diffeomorphic metric mapping," *IEEE Trans Med Imaging* **30**, 1746–1759 (2011).
26. C.-Y. Liu, J.E. Iglesias, Z. Tu, "Deformable templates guided discriminative models for robust 3D brain MRI segmentation," *Neuroinformatics* **11**, 447–468 (2013).
27. Z. Tu, K.L. Narr, P. Dollár, I. Dinov, P.M. Thompson, A.W. Toga, "Brain anatomical structure segmentation by hybrid discriminative/generative models," *IEEE Trans Med Imaging* **27**, 495–508 (2008).
28. G.E. Christensen, R.D. Rabbitt, M.I. Miller, "Deformable templates using large deformation kinematics," *IEEE Trans Image Process* **5**, 1435–1447 (1996).
29. E. D'Agostino, F. Maes, D. Vandermeulen, P. Suetens, "A viscous fluid model for multimodal non-rigid image registration using mutual information," *Med Image Anal* 7, 565–575 (2003).
30. E. Fletcher, B. Singh, D. Harvey *et al.*, "Adaptive image segmentation for robust measurement of longitudinal brain tissue change," *2012 Annu Int Conf IEEE Eng Med Biol Soc*, 5319–5322 (2012).
31. P. Kochunov, J.L. Lancaster, P. Thompson *et al.*, "Regional spatial normalization: toward and optimal target," *J Comput Assist Tomogr* **25**, 805–816 (2001).
32. D. Rueckert, P. Aljabar, R.A. Heckemann *et al.*, "Diffeomorphic registration using b-splines," *MICCAI 2006*. Vol 4191. Springer-Verlag 702–709 (2006).
33. T. Nichols, A.P. Holmes, "Nonparametric permutation tests for functional neuroimaging: a primer with examples," *Hum Brain Mapp* **15**, 1–25 (2001).
34. X. Hua, B. Gutman, C.P. Boyle *et al.*, "Accurate measurement of brain changes in longitudinal MRI scans using tensor-based morphometry," *Neuroimage* **57**, 5–14 (2011).
35. D. Holland, L.K. McEvoy, A.M. Dale, "Unbiased comparison of sample size estimates from longitudinal structural measures in ADNI," *Hum Brain Mapp*, 2586–2602 (2011).
36. P. Freeborough, N. Fox, "The boundary shift integral: an accurate and robust measure of cerebral volume change from registered repeat MRI," *IEEE Trans Med Imaging* **16**, 623–629.

Chapter 5

X-Ray Fluorescence Computed Tomography for Molecular Imaging

*Xia Li and Yu Kuang**

Medical Physics Program, University of Nevada Las Vegas,
Las Vegas, NV 89154 USA
**E-mail: yu.kuang@unlv.edu*

X-ray fluorescence computed tomography (XFCT) is a promising technique able to identify and quantify features in small samples of high-atomic-number (Z) elements such as iodine, gadolinium and gold. In this chapter, as a proof-of-concept, we investigated the feasibility of simultaneously imaging multiple elements (multiplexing) using XFCT. A polychromatic X-ray source was used to stimulate emission of X-ray fluorescence photons from multiple high-Z elements with low concentrations [2% (weight/volume) gold (Au), gadolinium (Gd) and barium (Ba)] embedded within a water phantom. The water phantom was used to mimic biological tissue targeted with high-Z nanoprobes. The emitted X-ray energy spectra from three elements were collected and then used to isolate the K shell X-ray fluorescence peaks and to generate sinograms for the three elements of interest. The tomographic distribution of the high Z elements within the phantom was reconstructed. A linear relationship between the X-ray fluorescence intensity of tested elements and their concentrations was observed, suggesting that XFCT is capable of quantitative molecular imaging.

1. Introduction

X-ray computed tomography (CT) imaging plays a critical role in the diagnosis, staging, treatment planning, and therapeutic assessment of cancer. CT is also indispensable in pre-clinical small animal studies, providing valuable anatomical information. However, while CT provides millimeter-resolved anatomical imaging, it lacks the ability to image multiple processes at the molecular level. It is difficult to use CT imaging to differentiate benign from cancerous nodules. This drawback also exists in sophisticated approaches such as dynamic contrast-enhanced CT (DCE-CT), which measures physiological properties.[1]

An intriguing alternative is X-ray fluorescence (XRF) CT (XFCT). XFCT detects characteristic X-ray emissions from high-atomic-number (Z) elements in patients exposed to an X-ray beam. Following photoelectric absorption, a vacancy in the K shell is subsequently filled by an electron from the L or M shells, and the energy difference between these shells is released as either an Auger electron or a characteristic K-shell X-ray (i.e., XRF).[2–4] In elements with an atomic number $Z \geq 47$ — such as gold (Au), gadolinium (Gd), iodine (I), and barium (Ba) — the L and M to K transitions are accompanied by characteristic K-shell X-rays $\geq 80\%$ of the time. Since the XRF energy spectrum is unique to a single element, this provides a way to quantitatively detect multiple elements, as well as exogenous molecular probes consisting of high-Z elements that are conjugated with antibodies or peptides that recognize disease specific biomarkers.

In this chapter, as a proof-of-concept, a XFCT system using polychromatic X-rays was developed. A water phantom, containing different high-Z elements, was used to mimic biological tissue targeted by nanoprobes. The results show that XFCT is a promising modality for multiplexed imaging of high atomic number probes.

2. Materials and Methods

2.1. *Phantom Preparation*

A water phantom containing Au, Gd and Ba insertions was shown in Fig. 1.[5] The insertions consisted of 2% (weight/volume) saline solutions of gold (Au), gadolinium (Gd) and barium (Ba) alone and a mixture of these three elements. The concentrations of these elements in saline solution were selected based on a previous animal study presenting achievable tumor-to-blood ratios with nanoparticles (NP).[6,7] After each solution was poured into an Eppendorf tube (0.7 ml), the tubes were sealed and inserted into a cylindrical water phantom measuring 3.5 cm (diameter) $\times$ 5 cm (height) as shown in Fig. 1. The centers of the four Eppendorf tubes were located 1 cm away from the center of the phantom.

2.2. *Experimental Setup*

2.2.1. *X-ray source*

A schematic example of experimental setup was shown in Fig. 2. The X-ray beam was generated by a Philips RT250 orthovoltage unit (Philips Medical System Inc., Shelton, CT) operating at 150 kV and a tube current of 20 mA. The X-ray beam was collimated by two led bricks ($10 \times 5 \times 5\ cm^3$ for each) separated by a 5 mm gap, and a lead block with a 5 mm-diameter cylindrical

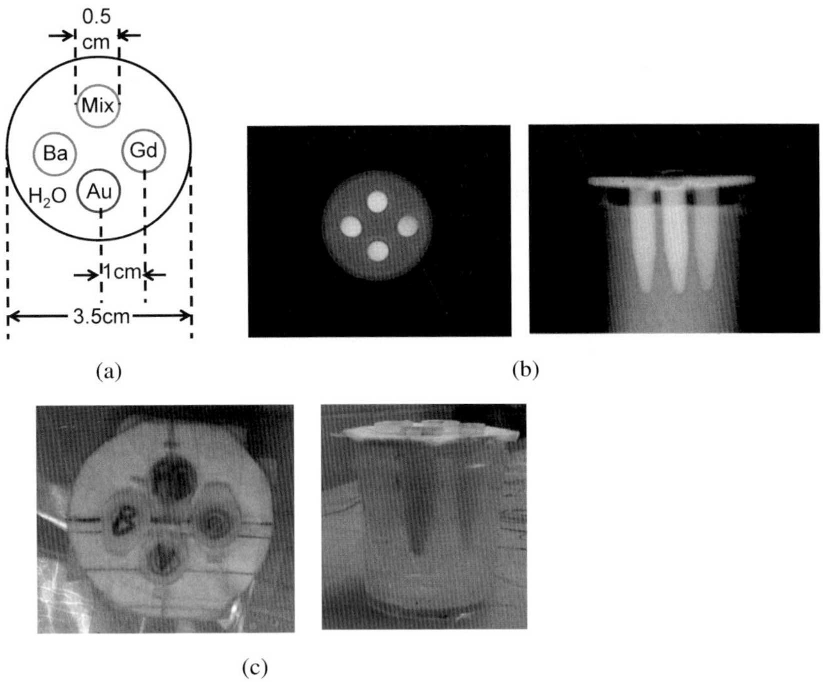

Fig. 1. (a) Schematic diagram of the cylindrical water phantom with four conical tube insertions. (b) X-ray transmission images of the water phantom scanned with a cone-beam CT system (40 kV, 0.64 mA): anterior to posterior projection (left) and left lateral projection (right). The measured Hounsfield Unit (HU) for each component was water 7 HU, Au 1107 HU, Ba 1882 HU, Gd 1025 HU and mixture 2768 HU. (c) Photographs of the cylindrical water phantom.

hole, to produce a pencil beam. To reduce the total dose deposited by X-ray photons with energies below the K-absorption edge for Au (80.7 keV), which is the highest K-edge among the three elements, a filter consisting of 1 mm Pb, 7.3 mm Al, and 1.4 mm Cu was placed at the exit of the collimator. The filter can be made of Pb, Sn, Cu, Al, and any combination of these elements. There were different kinds of polychromatic X-ray sources and filters for different XFCT systems.[8–10]

2.2.2. *XFCT acquisition scheme*

As a proof-of-concept, the XFCT acquisition was performed in a first generation CT geometry, acquiring a single line integral at a time. The water phantom was set to rotate and translate in precise steps using a computer-controlled motion stage (Velmex Inc., Bloomfield, NY), while the X-ray source and the detector were stationary. A single measurement slice was acquired by translating

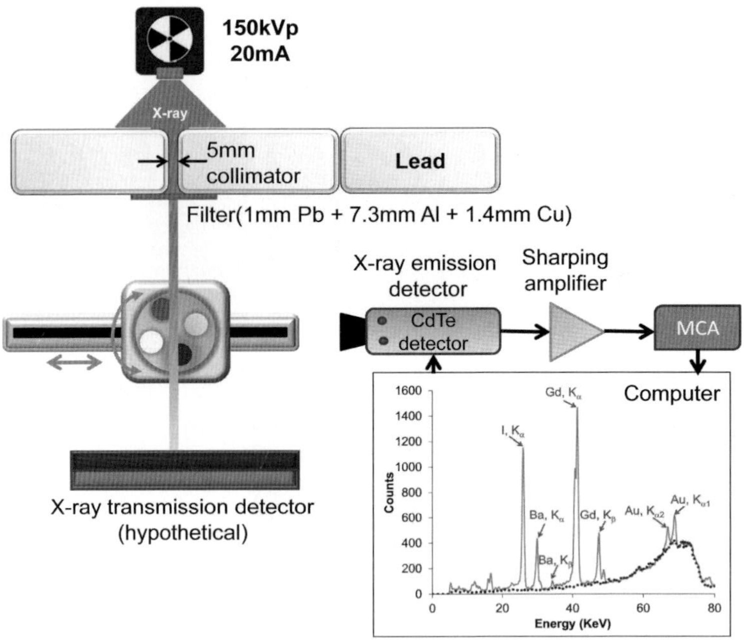

(a)

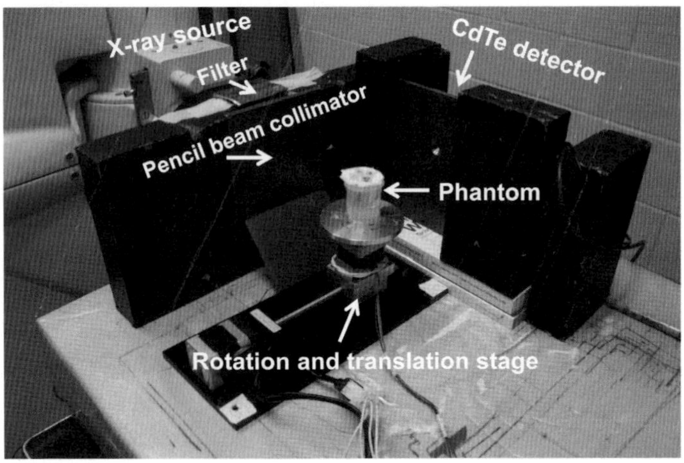

(b)

Fig. 2. Schematic of the experimental setup including the filtered X-ray source, the water phantom, and the CdTe detector. Multiplexing spectrum of Au, Gd, Ba and Iodine (I) is shown in the inset. The area under the dot line was the background photons derived from the Compton scatter.

the phantom 30 times in 1.5 mm increments, and rotating it 31 times to cover 360°. XRF photons, emitted from the narrow volume illuminated by the pencil beam, were collected using a thermoelectrically cooled cadmium telluride (CdTe) detector (X-123 CdTe, Amptek Inc., Bedford, MA). The detector and motion stage were controlled by motor-driving software. Data acquisition was paused during the movement of the stages to the next rotational or translational positions after the data collection for 18 s at each position. During the experiment, the collimated X-ray beam irradiated the phantom at a given view angle. After the completion of a scan at each position, the phantom was rotated by a small angular increment (30°) and the scanning process resumed again. This process was repeated until a full 360° rotation was completed. Subsequently, the scanning process continued while the phantom was translated by a 1.5 mm step over 4.5 cm along the axis normal to the beam direction, which covered the whole size of the phantom.

2.2.3. *X-ray fluorescence detector system*

The detector system was another important component in the experimental setup. It was used to capture the X-ray fluorescence signals from the sample containing elements at low concentration within the phantom. The X-ray detector module included a preamplifier with pile-up rejection, a digital pulse processor, and a multichannel analyzer (MCA) (PX4, Amptek Inc., Bedford, MA). The digital pulse processor and MCA were employed as interfaces between detector and personal computer for data acquisition, control and X-ray spectral data analysis. For any X-ray fluorescence measurement, there is a background count from Compton and elastically scattered X-rays and X-ray fluorescence from other elements in the sample. To minimize the number of unwanted scattered photons entering the detector, the detector system was placed at a 90° angle to the incident X-ray beam. To shield the X-ray detector from X-rays coming from outside the field of view, a conically shaped lead shield with a 5 mm-diameter opening end covered the sensitive element. Meanwhile, a second X-ray detector operating in the current mode could be placed behind the phantom along the beam direction to provide transmission measurements.

2.3. *Data Acquisition*

The raw data measured in an XFCT scan consists of a series of spectra, each spectrum corresponding to a beam position. The spectra included fluorescence peaks from elements of interest as well as background from scattered photons. Considering the low penetration of the L shell XRF, we only focused on

Table 1. Critical absorption and emission energies for photoelectric absorption and X-ray fluorescence emission.

Atomic number (Z)		Iodine (I) 53	Gadolinium (Gd) 64	Platinum (Pt) 78	Barium (Ba) 56	Gold (Au) 79
Critical absorption energies (keV)	K_{ab}	33.164	50.229	78.379	37.410	80.713
	L_{Iab}	5.190	8.393	13.873	5.995	14.353
	L_{IIab}	4.856	7.940	13.268	5.623	13.733
Emission energies from X-ray fluorescence (keV)[a]	L_{IIIab}	4.559	7.252	11.559	5.247	11.919
	$K_{\beta 2}$	33.016	49.961	77.866	37.255	80.165
	$K_{\beta 1}$	32.292	48.718	75.736	36.376	77.968
	$K_{\alpha 2}$	28.610	42.983	66.820	32.191	68.794
	$K_{\alpha 1}$	28.315	42.280	65.111	31.815	66.980
	$L_{\gamma 1}$	4.800	7.788	12.939	5.531	13.379
	$L_{\beta 2}$	4.507	7.102	11.249	5.156	11.582
	$L_{\beta 1}$	4.220	6.714	11.069	4.828	11.439
	$L_{\alpha 2}$	3.937	6.059	9.441	4.467	9.711
Peaks used for XRF imaging (keV)	$L_{\alpha 1}$	3.926	6.027	9.360	4.451	9.625
	$K_{\beta 2}$	32.42	48.87	—[b]	36.34	—[c]
	$K_{\beta 1}$					
	$K_{\alpha 2}$	29.00	43.13	66.89	32.42	68.46
	$K_{\alpha 1}$			65.59		66.63

[a]The emission energies are based on transition relations:

$$K_{\alpha 2} = K_{ab} - L_{IIab}, \quad K_{\alpha 1} = K_{ab} - L_{Iab}, \quad K_{\beta 1} = K_{ab} - M_{IIIab}, \text{ etc.}$$

[b,c]The K_β peaks of Pt (77.87 and 75.74 keV) and Au (77.97 and 80.1 keV) are only detectable in the high concentration of Pt and Au, and they are not clearly defined in the low concentration of Pt and Au. Thus, they are not used for data processing to relate fluorescence output to Pt and Au concentration within the phantom.

acquiring K shell XRF peaks (Table 1) to take advantage of the strong fluorescence yields as well as the deep tissue penetration of the emitted X-rays.

The incident X-ray photons with energies below Au K-absorption edge are not only useless, but also create unwanted scattering background counts during measurement. As shown in Table 1, X-ray photons above the Au K-edge energy (80.7 keV) can be used to excite the Au and other element XRF photons simultaneously. The undesired scattering can be easily reduced by placing a filter in the path of the incident beam. If the insertions of the phantom were changed to 2% (w/v) saline solutions of Pt, Gd, and I, X-ray photons above the Pt K-edge energy (78.4 keV) were applied to excite XRF photons.[5]

The number of fluorescence counts from the given element in tomography was obtained by the line integral of the concentration along the line traversed by the pencil beam. This integration process was accomplished by translating the detector and repeating the measurements described in Section 2.2.2 along the axis (parallel to the pencil beam direction), which covered the whole size of the phantom along the beam direction.

2.4. *Data Processing*

2.4.1. *Background subtraction*

The spectrum measured for each beam position includes the K-shell XRF peaks from different elements superimposed on a broad background of scattered photons. To estimate the concentrations of different elements from the spectral measurements, the scatter background in each energy window must be removed before XRF peaks can be isolated.

Energy windows are defined for the XRF peaks for the given elements as follows: Au: 65.1–67.7 and 67.8–70.1 keV; Gd: 40.3–45.0 and 47.3–49.9 keV; Ba: 30.1–33.7 and 34.8–38.2 keV. For insertions consisted of Pt, and I, the energy windows were defined as follows: Pt: 64.0–66.1 and 66.1–68.5 keV; I: 24.6–30.3 and 31.1–34.3 keV. A cubic spline function was used to fit the background counts for these energy windows. The net number of counts in the peaks was then calculated using

$$N_k = M_k - B_k \quad (1)$$

where k is the element of interest (e.g., Au, Gd, Ba, Pt, or I), M_k is the summation of the measured number of counts over the energy window for element k, and B_k is the fitted number of counts from the third-degree polynomial (fitted background counts) in energy window for element k.

The number of counts N_k corresponds to a line integral for a particular element along the beam. By processing spectra corresponding to different beam positions, a sinogram was generated for each of the elements present in the phantom using 30 radial positions and 31 angles.

2.4.2. *Image reconstruction*

The image formation process is similar to that of single photon emission computed tomography (SPECT) with parallel-hole collimators. The number of XRF photons detected at a given beam position is related to the line integral of the elemental distribution within the phantom. A rough attenuation correction was applied to the phantom sinogram to compensate for the exponential attenuations of the excitation X-ray beam and the emitted XRF signal. The excitation beam attenuation was modeled by an exponential fluence falloff using the total attenuation coefficient of water at 80 keV. Attenuation of the fluorescent emission was modeled in a similar fashion, by computing the distance traveled in water by the fluorescent photon. For the purpose of attenuation correction, it was assumed that measured fluorescent photons do not elastically scatter in the phantom. The distributions and concentrations of each individual element were reconstructed with 100 iterations of the maximum-likelihood expectation maximization (ML-EM) algorithm, which models the physical response of the imaging system.[11–16]

2.4.3. *Linearity*

The linearity between the XRF count value and concentration for each element (w/v) was also investigated. Serial dilutions were performed for each element and inserted into the water phantom. The phantom was placed in a 150 kV, 20 mA X-ray beam and imaged with a CdTe detector as described above. The peaks for each element were plotted as a function of the known elemental concentration.

2.5. *X-ray Dose From XFCT Imaging*

Micro LiF thermoluminescent dosimeters (TLDs) were used to measure the radiation dose of an XFCT imaging scan. The dimension of the TLD dosimeter is $1 \times 1 \times 1$ mm^3 (Harshaw TLD-100, Thermo Fisher Scientific Inc., Waltham, MA). Two sets of 3 TLD microcubes were used for the reference and the XFCT imaging dose measurements, respectively. For the reference dose measurement, an open-field TLD measurement was used, i.e. the TLDs were placed at the center of a water phantom and exposed to an unfiltered and non-collimated X-ray beam (open field, 150 keV, 20 mA). A dose conversion factor was determined by normalizing the open-field TLD reading to the absolute dose measured under the same condition with a calibrated Farmer ionization chamber (Model No. TN30006-0368, PTW, Freiburg, Germany). To measure the XFCT imaging dose, the TLDs were placed at the center of the water phantom (Fig. 2). The luminescent signals in TLDs were read out by an automatic dosimetry reader (Harshaw 5500 TLD reader, Solon, OH) after a 5-segment preheating process using a TLDO annealing oven (PTW, Freiburg, Germany). The imaging dose for the scan was computed by averaging three TLD readings and using the dose conversion factor.

3. Results

Figure 3 shows the spectra of the incident pencil beam after collimation and filtration measured by the CdTe detector along the X-ray beam direction.

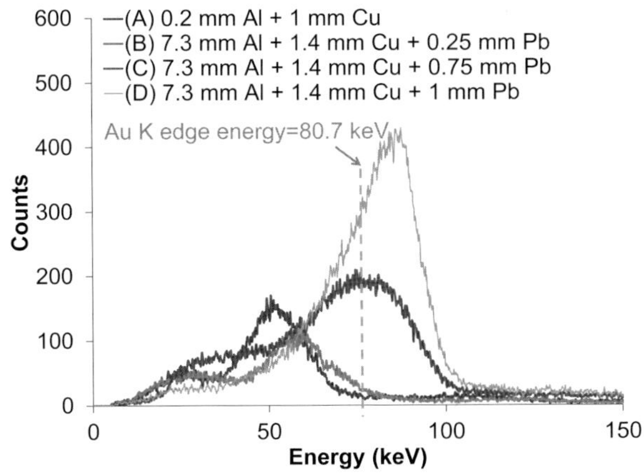

Fig. 3. A comparison of different filtered X-ray beams from the X-ray source operated at 150 keV, 20 mA. The Au K-edge energy is shown as a dotted line. Spectrum (D) was used for XFCT data acquisition.

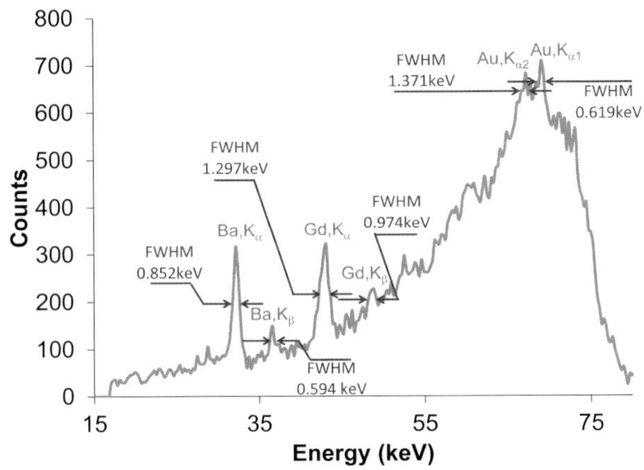

Fig. 4. A representative spectrum showing multiplexed detection in the water phantom containing a mixture of 2% Au, Gd, and Ba solutions.

Incident X-ray photons with energies below the K-absorption energies of the three elements (Table 1) not only create an unwanted scatter background, but also increase the dose deposited inside the phantom. As shown in Table 1, X-ray photons above the Au K-edge energy (80.7 keV) can be used to excite the Au, Gd and Ba XRF photons simultaneously. A filter with 1 mm thick Pb, 7.3 mm thick Al and 1.4 mm thick Cu was found to efficiently remove X-ray photons below the K-edge of Au while sustaining a sufficient X-ray fluence.

Figure 4 shows a representative XRF spectrum acquired using the line-by-line scan mode. The XRF spectrum showed sharp characteristic peaks for

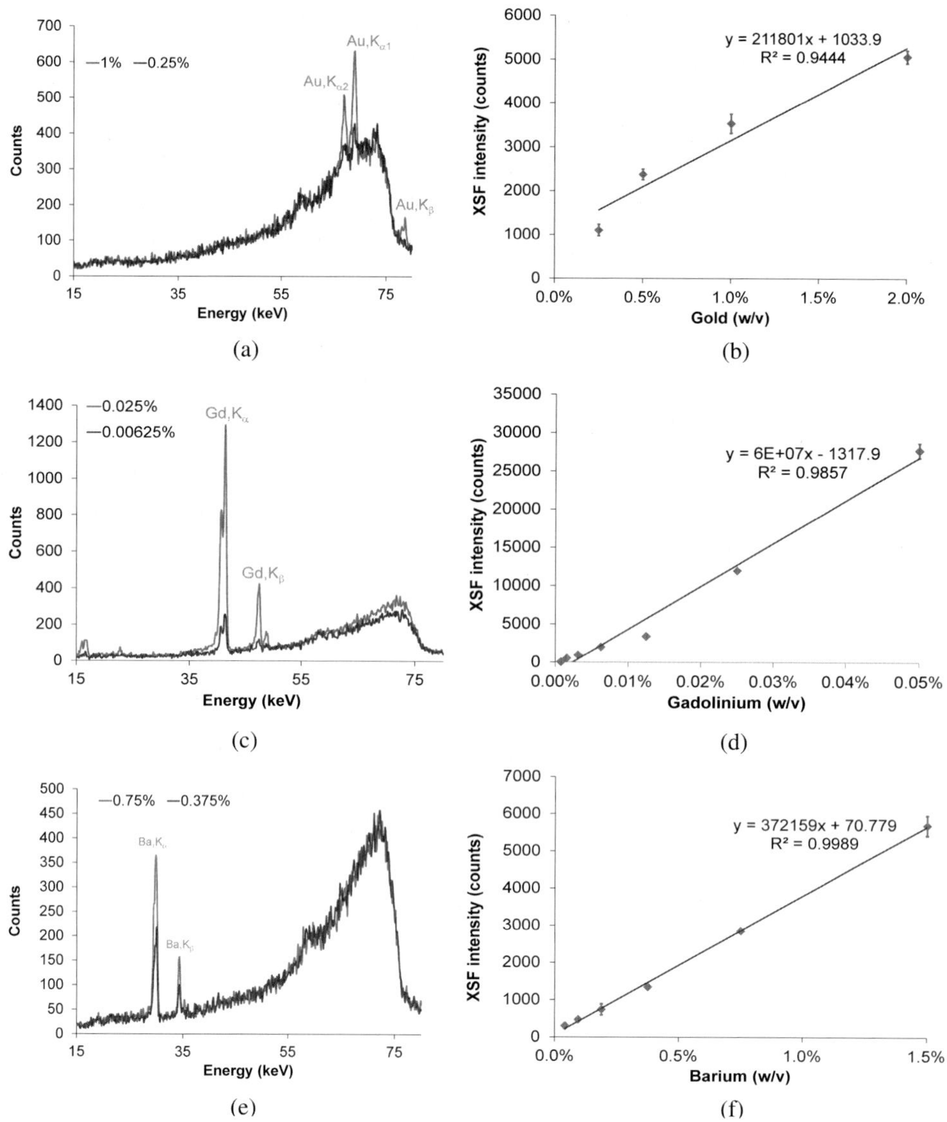

Fig. 5. Representative XRF spectra of three high-Z probes at two different concentrations: (a) Au (1% and 0.25%); (c) Gd (0.025% and 0.00625%); (e) Ba (0.75% and 0.375%). A linear relationship between the XRF intensity and the concentrations of the element solution was found.

Au, Gd, and Ba. The full width at half maximum (FWHM) for each peak was also measured in order to evaluate the capability of XFCT for multiplexed imaging of multiple elements (Fig. 4). The FWHM values of all these peaks were much smaller than the average peak-to-peak separation, suggesting that multiple elements can be used to probe different molecular processes *in vivo*.

Figure 5(a), (c), and (e) show the XRF spectra for different concentrations of Au, Gd and Ba solutions, respectively. The amplitudes of the Au $K_{\alpha 2}$ and $K_{\alpha 1}$ peaks [Fig. 5(a)], the Gd K_α and K_β peaks [Fig. 5(c)], as well as the Ba K_α and K_β peaks [Fig. 5(e)] were proportional to the concentration of Au, Gd and Ba saline solution, respectively. With the current experimental set-up, the minimum detectable concentrations were 0.25%, 0.00078% and 0.04% for Au, Gd and Ba respectively. The highly linear response of XFCT with respect to elemental concentrations ($R^2_{Pt} = 0.944$, $R^2_{Gd} = 0.986$, $R^2_I = 0.999$) suggests that XFCT is capable of quantitative imaging.

To evaluate the suitability of this technique for multiplexed imaging, a water phantom containing 2% (w/v) Au, Gd, and Ba insertions was imaged. The distribution of each element can be clearly identified in the reconstructed images (Fig. 6). Furthermore, all three elements were properly detected when mixed together. A cone-beam CT scan of the phantom is shown in Fig. 7. The X-ray dose from the entire XFCT imaging procedure was also measured with TLDs and found to be 77 cGy at the center of the phantom.

4. Discussion

An XFCT system built for multiplexed imaging of high Z elements was presented in this chapter. Nevertheless, the current technique was not yet practical for routine *in vivo* applications and requires further development. The ultimate feasibility of the current technique will depend on the successful resolution of a few technical issues, such as scanning time, X-ray dose, detection limit and image resolution. By filtering out most of the low-energy X-rays from the pencil beam with combined filter materials, the imaging dose was effectively reduced.

While the line-by-line acquisition used in this study was relatively slow, it provided flexibility in choosing sampling patterns if an XRF detector panel was used instead of a single pixel XRF detector.[17–19] Riviere *et al.* have demonstrated that the sampling pattern could be optimized to a full rotation half translation (FRHT) fashion in the 2D mode, i.e., rotate the object through a full 360°, but only the half of the object closest to the XRF detector panel side is scanned at each projection view. This scheme may result in both reduced imaging times and improved image quality.[20,21] Moreover, it was shown that there are advantages to adopting an interlaced sampling strategy in the 2D case, in which the sampling patterns at even and odd projection views are offset relative to one another. This technique provides two-fold more efficient sampling as compared to the conventional sampling pattern.[20] In the 3D helical scanning

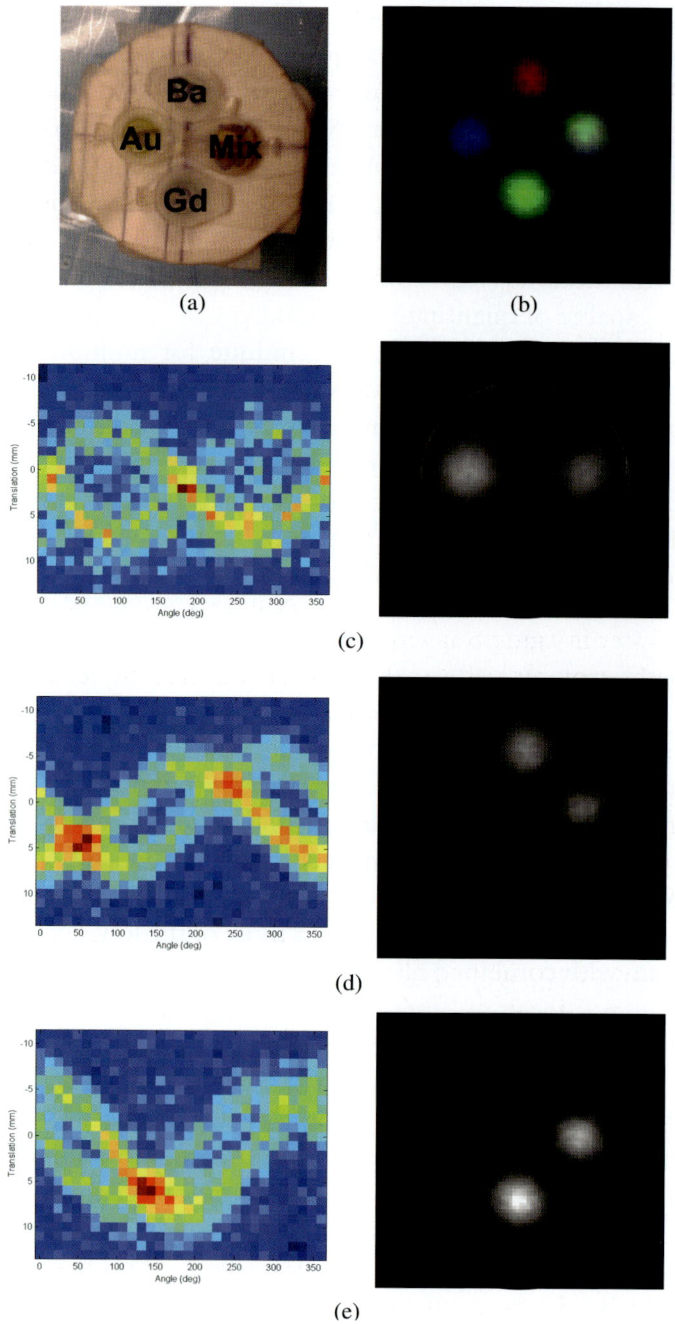

Fig. 6. Reconstructed XFCT multiplexed images of 2% (w/v) Au, Gd, and Ba solution embedded in a water phantom. (a) A photograph of the phantom, (b) Multicolor overlay of the reconstructed XFCT image (red: Ba; blue: Au; green: Gd). (c) to (e): For the three elements of interest [(c) Au; (d) Ba; (e) Gd], XRF peaks in the spectra were processed into a sinogram for each element (left column) and reconstructed with ML-EM (right column).

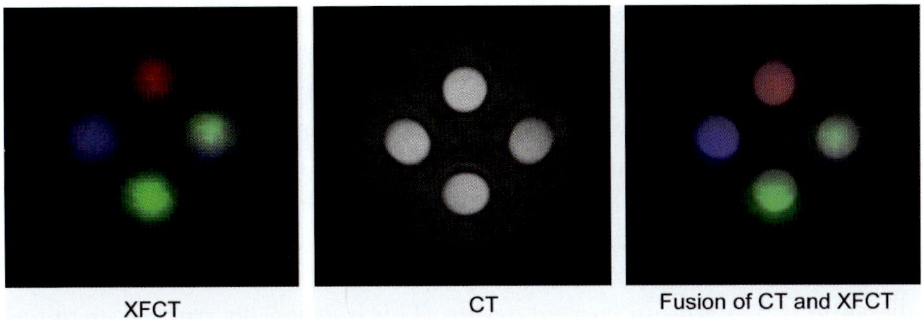

Fig. 7. Overlay of XFCT and X-ray transmission CT images of the phantom. Pseudo colors are used for different components in the XRF image: red for Ba; blue for Au; green for Gd.

mode (volumetric XFCT), FRHT sampling pattern coupled with a Fourier-based interpolation scheme could effectively improve longitudinal resolution.[20]

A ROI strategy could be employed to reduce dose and improve scan efficiency. This hybrid imaging scheme would provide high quality images of the ROIs with a faster imaging time and a limited radiation dose. Moreover, novel image reconstruction algorithms that can process incompletely sampled data could be helpful.[22] These algorithms allow for improved quantitative accuracy as well as for ROI imaging, which might lead to further reduction in data acquisition time and radiation dose.

In this study, we chose a single pixel photon counting detector and then pencil beam X-ray to excite the XRF signal. Alternatively, for faster acquisition, it is possible to use a wider excitation to stimulate XRF. For instance, a fan-beam can be used to illuminate a slide of the phantom with X-rays. Similarly, a cone beam can be applied to illuminate the entire phantom. However, these approaches require localization of the fluorescent emission at the detector side, because these fluorescent emissions may occur anywhere in the volume illuminated with X-ray (With a pencil beam, it is known that any fluorescent photon recorded was emitted within the narrow line formed by the beam). An array of photon-counting detectors coupled to a pinhole or parallel-hole collimator may be used in combination with a fan-beam or cone-beam to provide 2D or 3D localization of each fluorescent emission.

While fan-beam and cone-beam approaches offer the potential for shorter XFCT acquisitions, it should be noted that these approaches might dramatically increase the hardware complexity and cost due to the need for arrays of photon-counting detectors. Existing photon-counting arrays have worse energy resolution than off-the-shelf single-pixel detectors used in this study and require complex electronics to readout each detector pixel. An additional issue with cone-beam and fan-beam geometries is that those approaches may require higher imaging dose. With modern source technology, faster scanning with a pencil beam can also be achieved very quickly using a special scanning-beam X-ray source.[23,24] Collimation is not required in a pencil-beam geometry on the detector side because the fluorescent emissions are constrained to the narrow volume defined by the beam line. The trade-off between various geometries should be further investigated.

The interference between XRF photons and scatter photons poses a challenging issue with our current design. This is especially true for imaging of Au, because the Compton peak overlaps with the XRF signal thus affecting the lower detection limit. Scattering inside the sample and surrounding materials leads to a broad background (noise) in the XRF energy spectrum. This background reduces the signal to noise ratio of Au. To alleviate this problem, a plane-polarized X-ray beam could be used.[17–19] The plane-polarized X-rays can be produced by scattering an X-ray beam through 90 degree by a bi-layer polarizer (copper and silicon). The generated plane-polarized X-rays are not scattered isotropically. The differential scattering in one cross section of polarized X-rays is much lower than its orthogonal plane. If the XRF detectors are placed parallel to the plane of incident direction of lower scattering polarized X-rays, it will ensure minimum scattering of radiation into the detector,[19] thus improving the detection limit of Au.

In practice, quasi-monochromatic X-ray beams could be also used via a proper conversion from polychromatic X-ray beams.[25,26] The quasi-monochromatic X-ray beams would shift the X-ray energy with maximum intensity towards higher energy above the K-absorption energy of Au and reduce the background scattering X-rays beneath the Au peak, thus the detection limit of Au would be also improved.

It is noted that state-of-the-art clinical scanners have multiple detector rows (i.e. 64–320).[27] In this study, we only used a single pixel photon counting detector, resulting in longer scanning times. The use of an energy resolving XRF detector ring would also reduce the image time greatly, improve imaging performance and decrease the imaging radiation dose.

5. Conclusions

In this chapter, we have shown that the distributions of Au, Gd and Ba in the water phantom were clearly identifiable in the reconstructed XFCT images using a single scan. Our results also suggest that XFCT is capable of quantitative imaging. Additionally, with the proposed system, anatomical transmission CT and XFCT images can be acquired simultaneously. Further increase in imaging performance is expected when plane-polarized X-ray beams and quasi-monochromatic X-ray beams as well as an XRF detector ring are used for excitations.

Acknowledgements

This work was supported in part by an NIH/NIGMS grant (#1U54GM 104944-01A1) and a Lincy Endowed Assistant Professorship.

References

1. K.A. Miles, "Diagnostic imaging in undergraduate medical education: an expanding role," *Clin Radiol* **60**, 742–745 (2005).
2. S.K. Cheong, B.L. Jones, A.K. Siddiqi, F. Liu, N. Manohar, S.H. Cho, "X-ray fluorescence computed tomography (XFCT) imaging of gold nanoparticle-loaded objects using 110 kVp x-rays," *Phys Med Biol* **55**, 647–662 (2010).
3. B.L. Jones, S.H. Cho, "The feasibility of polychromatic cone-beam x-ray fluorescence computed tomography (XFCT) imaging of gold nanoparticle-loaded objects: a Monte Carlo study," *Phys Med Biol* **56**, 3719–3730 (2011).
4. M. Bazalova, Y. Kuang, G. Pratx, L. Xing, "Investigation of X-ray fluorescence computed tomography (XFCT) and K-edge imaging," *IEEE Trans Med Imaging* **31**, 1620–1627 (2012).
5. Y. Kuang, G. Pratx, M. Bazalova, B. Meng, J. Qian, L. Xing, "First demonstration of multiplexed X-ray fluorescence computed tomography (XFCT) imaging," *IEEE Trans Med Imaging* **32**, 262–267 (2013).
6. M. Almalki, S.A. Majid, P.H. Butler, L. Reinisch, "Gadolinium concentration analysis in brain phantom by X-ray fluorescence," *Australas Phys Eng Sci Med* **33**, 185–191 (2010).
7. C.M. Carpenter, C. Sun, G. Pratx, R. Rao, L. Xing, "Hybrid x-ray/optical luminescence imaging: characterization of experimental conditions," *Med Phys* **37**, 4011–4018 (2010).
8. S.H. Cho, B.L. Jones, S. Krishnan, "The dosimetric feasibility of gold nanoparticle-aided radiation therapy (GNRT) via brachytherapy using low-energy gamma-/x-ray sources," *Phys Med Biol* **54**, 4889–4905 (2009).
9. L. Ren, D. Wu, Y. Li, G. Wang, X. Wu, H. Liu, "Three-dimensional x-ray fluorescence mapping of a gold nanoparticle-loaded phantom," *Med Phys* **41**, 031902 (2014).
10. N.H. Manohar, "Effect of source X-ray energy spectra on the detection of fluorescence photons from gold nanoparticles," MS Thesis, Georgia Institute of Technology, 2011.
11. L.A. Shepp, Y. Vardi, "Maximum likelihood reconstruction for emission tomography," *IEEE Trans Med Imaging* **1**, 113–122 (1982).
12. P.P. Bruyant, "Analytic and iterative reconstruction algorithms in SPECT," *J Nucl Med* **43**, 1343–1358 (2002).
13. G. Pratx, C.M. Carpenter, C. Sun, L. Xing, "X-ray luminescence computed tomography via selective excitation: a feasibility study," *IEEE Trans Med Imaging* **29**, 1992–1999 (2010).

14. G. Pratx, C.M. Carpenter, C. Sun, R.P. Rao, L. Xing, "Tomographic molecular imaging of x-ray-excitable nanoparticles," *Opt Lett* **35**, 3345–3347 (2010).
15. K. Lange, R. Carson, "EM reconstruction algorithms for emission and transmission tomography," *J Comput Assist Tomogr* **8**, 306–316 (1984).
16. W. Cong, H. Shen, G. Wang, "Spectrally resolving and scattering-compensated x-ray luminescence/fluorescence computed tomography," *J Biomed Opt* **16**, 066014 (2011).
17. P.A. Ali, A.F. Al-Hussany, C.A. Bennett, D.A. Hancock, A.M. El-Sharkawi, "Plane polarized x-ray fluorescence system for the in vivo measurement of platinum in head and neck tumours," *Phys Med Biol* **43**, 2337–2345 (1998).
18. J. Borjesson, M. Alpsten, S. Huang, R. Jonson, S. Mattsson, C. Thornberg, "*In vivo* X-ray fluorescence analysis with applications to platinum, gold and mercury in man–experiments, improvements, and patient measurements," *Basic Life Sci* **60**, 275–280 (1993).
19. D.G. Lewis, "Optimization of a polarized source for *in vivo* x-ray fluorescence analysis of platinum and other heavy metals," *Phys Med Biol* **39**, 197–206 (1994).
20. P.V. P.J.L. Riviere, 2008 (unpublished).
21. P.V. P.J. La Riviere, M. Newville, S.R. Sutton, presented at the Nuclear Science Symposium Conference Record2007 (unpublished).
22. P.J. La Riviere, P.A. Vargas, "Monotonic penalized-likelihood image reconstruction for X-ray fluorescence computed tomography," *IEEE Trans Med Imaging* **25**, 1117–1129 (2006).
23. M.S.V.L. E.G. Solomon, R.E. Melen, J.W. Moorman, B. Skillicorn, "Low-exposure scanning-beam x-ray fluoroscopy system," *Proc. SPIE 2708, Medical Imaging 1996: Physics of Medical Imaging* (1996).
24. J. Zhang, G. Yang, Y. Cheng, B. Gao, Q. Qiu, Y.Z. Lee, J.P. Lu, O. Zhou, "Stationary scanning x-ray source based on carbon nanotube field emitters," *Appl Phys Lett* **86**, 184104 (2005).
25. G. Jost, T. Mensing, S. Golfier, R. Lawaczeck, H. Pietsch, J. Hutter, L. Cibik, M. Gerlach, M. Krumrey, D. Fratzscher, V. Arkadiev, R. Wedell, M. Haschke, N. Langhoff, P. Wust, L. Ludemann, "Photoelectric-enhanced radiation therapy with quasi-monochromatic computed tomography," *Med Phys* **36**, 2107–2117 (2009).
26. G.H. H.v. Busch, G. Martens, J.-P. Schlomka, B. Schweizer, 2005 (unpublished).
27. K.H. Schuleri, R.T. George, A.C. Lardo, "Applications of cardiac multidetector CT beyond coronary angiography," *Nat Rev Cardiol* **6**, 699–710 (2009).

Chapter 6

Dictionary Learning Based Low-Dose X-Ray CT Reconstruction

Qiong Xu[*,†], *Hengyong Yu*[‡], *Ge Wang*[§] *and Xuanqin Mou*[*,†,¶]

[*]*The Institute of Image Processing and Pattern Recognition, Xi'an Jiaotong University, Xi'an, Shaanxi, 710049 China*

[†]*Beijing Center for Mathematics and Information Interdisciplinary Sciences, Beijing, 10048 China*

[‡]*Biomedical Imaging Division, VT-WFU School of Biomedical Engineering and Sciences, Wake Forest University Health Sciences, Winston-Salem, NC 27157 USA*

[§]*Department of Biomedical Engineering, Rensselaer Polytechnic Institute, Troy, NY 12180 USA*

[¶]*E-mail: xqmou@mail.xjtu.edu.cn*

How to reduce radiation dose while maintaining the diagnostic performance is a major challenge in the computed tomography (CT) field. Inspired by the compressive sensing theory, the sparse constraint in terms of total variation (TV) minimization has already led to promising results for low-dose CT reconstruction. Compared to the discrete gradient transform used in the TV minimization method, dictionary learning is proven to be an effective way for sparse representation. On the other hand, it is important to consider the statistical property of projection data in low-dose CT cases. In this chapter, we present a dictionary learning based approach for low dose X-ray CT. In our method, the sparse constraint in terms of a redundant dictionary is incorporated into an objective function in a statistical iterative reconstruction framework. The dictionary can be either predetermined before an image reconstruction task or adaptively defined during the reconstruction process. An alternating minimization scheme is developed to minimize the objective function. Our approach is evaluated with low dose X-ray projections collected in an animal study. The results show that the proposed approach has potential to produce better images with lower noise and more detailed structural features.

1. Introduction

X-ray radiation is a kind of ionizing radiation, which may induce genetic, cancerous and other diseases to human health. The radiation risk has received more and more attention in X-ray based medical imaging field,[1] especially in X-ray CT which needs much more dosage compared to other imaging modalities such as radiography and so on. Therefore, the well-known ALARA (As Low As Reasonably Achievable) principle is applied to avoid excessive radiation dose in the CT field. In principle, there are two strategies for radiation dose reduction. The first one is to reduce the X-ray flux towards each detector element, which is usually implemented by adjusting the operating current, the operating potential and exposure time of an X-ray tube. Since X-ray imaging is a quantum accumulation process, the SNR (signal-to-noise ratio) depends on the X-ray dose quadratically. Given other conditions being identical, reducing the X-ray dose will lead to noisy projections, accordingly degrading image quality. The second one is to decrease the number of X-ray attenuation measurements across a whole object to be reconstructed. It necessarily produces insufficient projection data, suffering from few-view, limited-angle, interior scan, or other problems. This kind of insufficient data makes conventional reconstruction methods, such as FBP (Filtered Back-Projection), fail to reconstruct good images. These results are usually companied with some kinds of artifacts. How to reconstruct adequate images at a minimum dose level proposes a huge challenge to algorithm developments.

As the aforementioned, the low-dose CT data is usually noisy and incomplete. In order to reconstruct good images from this kind of data, the most natural idea is to preprocess the low-dose projection data before applying the conventional reconstruction methods. This kind of method is usually used in noisy situation. Therein, some kinds of filtering methods are proposed to denoise the projection data. Hsieh[2] proposed an adaptive filtering approach where the filter parameterization was adjusted according to the noise property. La Riviere[3] developed a penalized likelihood technique to smooth sinogram. Wang *et al.*[4] presented a penalized weighted least-squares approach to reduce sinogram noise. Different from these preprocessing methods, another class is to incorporate the available prior information and constraints into a reconstruction process. This kind of method is usually based on iterative reconstruction framework, especially on the SIR (statistical iterative reconstruction) framework. Since SIR optimizes the maximum-likelihood or penalized-likelihood function formulated according to the statistical characteristics of projection data, it intrinsically promises an optimal reconstruction quality from noisy projection data. Besides, due to the iterative reconstruction, it is more flexible for various incomplete data. Sidky and Pan[5] proposed an ADS-POCS method to solve the few-view and limited angle problem. Xu *et al.*[6] proposed an interior tomography method in SIR framework to address the few-view truncated noisy data reconstruction. As more prior information and constraints are incorporated appropriately, better reconstruction can be expected.

Now, we have a general impression about low-dose CT problem and its solution from the above background introduction. In the rest of this chapter, we will introduce a novel solution for low-dose CT based on SIR framework with dictionary learning and sparse representation constraints. We will concentrate on elaborating this method from the idea's origin to the specific formulations, experimental results and problem discussions.

2. Origin of Idea — From Total-Variation to Dictionary

In recent years, the compressive sensing (CS) theory has become more and more popular.[7,8] The CS theory allows a sparse signal to be accurately reconstructed from samples/measurements far less than what is usually required by the Shannon/Nyquist sampling theorem. The key for the success of CS is the sparsity property of signals under study. In general, a natural signal, such as natural image or vocality, has a sparse representation when it is applied for a sparsifying transform. One common sparsifying transform is the discrete gradient transform (DGT) whose coefficients can be summed up to form the so-called total variation (TV). Let μ be a 2D image, $D_j\mu = D_{m,n}\mu = \sqrt{(\mu_{m,n} - \mu_{m+1,n})^2 + (\mu_{m,n} - \mu_{m,n+1})^2}$, where the 1D index j has a one-one map to the 2D index (m, n). In mathematics, the TV can be simply expressed as $TV(\mu) = \|D\mu\|_1$ with $D\mu = (D_1\mu, \cdots, D_{N_J}\mu)^T$.

In the CT field, the CS theory has been known to be instrumental for image reconstruction from incomplete and noisy datasets. Most of these methods employed the TV minimization based algorithms to solve the few-view, limited angle, interior tomography, etc.[5,6] Although TV-based algorithms are successful in a number of cases, the power of the TV minimization constraint is still limited. The main reasons are two-folds. First, the TV constraint is a global requirement, which cannot directly reflect structures of an object. Second, the DGT operation cannot distinguish true structures and image noise. Consequently, images reconstructed with the TV constraint may lose some fine features and generate a blocky appearance in incomplete and noisy cases. Hence, it is necessary to investigate superior sparsifying methods for CS-inspired image reconstruction.

Very recently, the sparse representation in terms of a redundant dictionary has attracted increasing attention in image processing, imaging analysis and magnetic resonance imaging (MRI) fields.[9–13] Such a dictionary is an over-complete basis. The elements in this basis are called atoms, which are learned from application-specific training images. Then, an object image can be sparsely represented as a linear combination of these atoms. Usually, an object image is decomposed into small overlapped patches. The dictionary learning approach acts on these patches, and an average of the corresponding values in the overlapped patches is computed at a given location. Because the dictionary is learned from training images, it is expected to have a better sparsifying capability than any generic sparse transform. Also, the redundancy of the atoms facilitates a sparser representation. More importantly, the dictionary tends to capture local image features effectively because of the patch-based analysis and most importantly the structural self-similarity in many cases.

Therefore, our idea is to utilize the sparse constraint based on dictionary learning to achieve better performance with lower-dose in CT reconstruction.[14,15]

3. Background — Dictionary Learning based Sparse Representation

In this section, we will give some basic knowledge about dictionary learning and sparse representation for better understanding about our method presented in next section.

Let N and K be integers, and R be the real space. A dictionary is a matrix $\mathbf{D} \in \mathrm{R}^{N\times K}$ whose column $\mathbf{d}_k \in R^{N\times 1}$ $(k = 1,\dots, K)$ is a N dimensional vector, which is called an atom. Usually, the dictionary is redundant or over-complete; that is, $N \ll K$. An image patch of $\sqrt{N} \times \sqrt{N}$ pixels can be re-expressed as a N dimensional vector $\mathbf{x} \in \mathrm{R}^{N\times 1}$. Suppose that a patch $\mathbf{x}$ can be exactly or approximately represented as a sparse linear combination of the atoms in the dictionary $\mathbf{D}$; that is,

$$\|\mathbf{x} - \mathbf{D}\alpha\|_2^2 \leq \varepsilon, \tag{1}$$

where $\varepsilon \geq 0$ is a small error bound, and the representation vector $\boldsymbol{\alpha} \in R^{K\times 1}$ has few nonzero entries, $\|\boldsymbol{\alpha}\|_0 \ll N \ll K$ with $\|\cdot\|_0$ being the l_0-norm. The dictionary redundancy implies that the number of atoms is greater than the length of an atom.

Finding a sparse representation $\boldsymbol{\alpha} \in R^{K\times 1}$ of an image patch $\mathbf{x} \in R^{N\times 1}$ with respect to a given dictionary $\mathbf{D} \in R^{N\times K}$ is equivalent to solve the following optimization problem:

$$\min_{\boldsymbol{\alpha}} \|\boldsymbol{\alpha}\|_0 \quad s.t. \ \|\mathbf{x} - \mathbf{D}\boldsymbol{\alpha}\|_2^2 \leq \varepsilon. \tag{2}$$

By the Lagrange method, Eq. (2) can be rewritten in an unconstraint form

$$\min_{\boldsymbol{\alpha}} \|\mathbf{x} - \mathbf{D}\boldsymbol{\alpha}\|_2^2 + \nu\|\boldsymbol{\alpha}\|_0, \tag{3}$$

where ν is the Lagrange multiplier. It is pointed out that the above two problems are equivalent when a suitable ν is chosen. Since solving Eqs. (2) or (3) directly is NP-hard, an approximate alternative strategy is desirable. In this regard, there are several greedy algorithms available, such as matching pursuit (MP) and orthogonal matching pursuit (OMP) algorithms.[16,17] Also, the l_0-norm can be replaced by the l_1-norm to make the problem convex and manageable using a basis pursuit (BP) algorithm.[18]

Given a training set of S patches, the so-called dictionary learning is to seek a dictionary that makes each patch in the training set be sparsely represented by the atoms in this dictionary. Denote the given patch set as a matrix $\mathbf{X} \in R^{N\times S}$ with a patch $\mathbf{x}_s \in R^{N\times 1}$ $(s = 1, \ldots, S)$ being a column vector of $\mathbf{X}$, and the corresponding sparse representation vector as a matrix $\boldsymbol{\alpha} \in R^{K\times S}$ with the representation $\boldsymbol{\alpha}_s \in R^{K\times 1}$ of a patch being a column vector of $\boldsymbol{\alpha} \in R^{K\times S}$. Then, the dictionary learning is to solve

$$\min_{\mathbf{D},\boldsymbol{\alpha}} \sum_{s=1}^{S} (\|\mathbf{x}_s - \mathbf{D}\boldsymbol{\alpha}_s\|_2^2 + \nu_s\|\boldsymbol{\alpha}_s\|_0), \tag{4}$$

Equation (4) is basically equivalent to either of the following problems

$$\min_{\mathbf{D},\boldsymbol{\alpha}} \|\mathbf{X} - \mathbf{D}\boldsymbol{\alpha}\|_2^2 \quad s.t. \ \forall s, \quad \|\boldsymbol{\alpha}_s\|_0 \leq L_0, \tag{5}$$

$$\min_{\mathbf{D},\boldsymbol{\alpha}} \sum_{s=1}^{S} \|\boldsymbol{\alpha}_s\|_0 \quad s.t. \ \|\mathbf{X} - \mathbf{D}\boldsymbol{\alpha}\|_2^2 \leq \varepsilon, \tag{6}$$

where L_0 and ε are the sparsity and precision of the sparse representation, respectively. The l_0-norm in Eqs. (4)–(6) can be replaced by the l_1-norm to make them easier to solve. There are many algorithms available for dictionary learning, including the classical K-SVD method and the fast online learning technique.[19,20]

A successful application of the dictionary learning technique is image denoising.[9] Let a vector $\mathbf{z} \in R^{M\times 1}$ represent a noise image of $H \times W$ pixels and a vector $\mathbf{x} \in R^{M\times 1}$ denote its corresponding filtered version, $M = H \times W$. A set of small overlapping patches can be extracted from the image. With a sliding distance of one pixel, we will have $(H - \sqrt{N} + 1) \times (W - \sqrt{N} + 1)$ patches.

It is assumed that the patches extracted from the filtered image can be sparely represented in terms of a dictionary, and the filtered image should be close to the original noisy image. Hence, the denoising procedure is to minimize the following objective function:

$$\min_{\mathbf{x},\boldsymbol{\alpha},(\mathbf{D})} \|\mathbf{x}-\mathbf{z}\|_2^2 + \lambda \sum_{s=1}^{S} (\|\mathbf{E}_s\mathbf{x} - \mathbf{D}\boldsymbol{\alpha}_s\|_2^2 + \nu_s\|\boldsymbol{\alpha}_s\|_0), \tag{7}$$

where $\mathbf{E}_s \in R^{N\times M}$ is an operator to extract a patch from the filtered image $\mathbf{x}$, $S = (H - \sqrt{N} + 1) \times (W - \sqrt{N} + 1)$, and λ is a regularization parameter related to the noise level of $\mathbf{z}$. The dictionary $\mathbf{D}$ in Eq. (7) can be determined in two ways. One is to predetermine it from a training set, which should contain representative structures in the image to be filtered. The other is to construct the dictionary during the denoising procedure.

4. Dictionary Learning based CT Reconstruction

In this section, we will describe the proposed method in details from the following three aspects: algorithm framework, parameter selection and representative results and analysis.

4.1. *Reconstruction Framework*

4.1.1. *MAP based objective function*

Without loss of generality, we only assume a monochromatic source. Approximately, the measured data follows a Poisson distribution:

$$y_i \sim Poisson\{b_i e^{-l_i} + r_i\}, \quad i = 1, \ldots, I, \tag{8}$$

where y_i is the measurement along the ith X-ray path, and b_i is the blank scan factor, $l_i = \sum_{j=1}^{J} a_{ij}\mu_j = [\mathbf{A}\boldsymbol{\mu}]_i$ is the integral of the X-ray linear attenuation coefficients, $\mathbf{A} = \{a_{ij}\}$ is the system matrix, $\boldsymbol{\mu} = (\mu_1, \ldots, \mu_J)^T$ is a linear attenuation coefficient distribution, r_i accounts for read-out noise, I and J are the number of projections and pixels, respectively.

Assuming that the noise distributions along different paths are statistically independent, the Poisson log-likelihood function of the joint probability distribution can be written as

$$L(\mathbf{y}|\boldsymbol{\mu}) = \ln P(\mathbf{y}|\boldsymbol{\mu}) = \ln\left(\prod_{i=1}^{I}(e^{-\bar{y}_i}\bar{y}_i^{y_i}/y_i!)\right), \tag{9}$$

where $P(\cdot)$ is the probability function, and $\bar{y}_i = b_i e^{-l_i} + r_i$ is the expected value of y_i. Ignoring the constant terms, we obtain $L(\mathbf{y}|\boldsymbol{\mu}) = -\sum_{i=1}^{I}(\bar{y}_i - y_i \ln \bar{y}_i)$.

From the statistical perspective, an image can be reconstructed by maximizing *a posteriori* (MAP) of the function $P(\boldsymbol{\mu}|\mathbf{y})$. According to the Bayesian rule $P(\boldsymbol{\mu}|\mathbf{y}) = P(\mathbf{y}|\boldsymbol{\mu})P(\boldsymbol{\mu})/P(\mathbf{y})$ and the monotonic increment property of the natural logarithm, the reconstruction is equivalent to maximize the following objective function

$$\tilde{\Phi}(\boldsymbol{\mu}) = L(\mathbf{y}|\boldsymbol{\mu}) + \ln P(\boldsymbol{\mu}), \tag{10}$$

where $\ln P(\boldsymbol{\mu})$ is a regularization term based on the prior knowledge. Let $R(\boldsymbol{\mu}) = -\ln P(\boldsymbol{\mu})$, the task can be converted into minimizing the following objective function

$$\Phi(\boldsymbol{\mu}) = \sum_{i=1}^{I} ((b_i e^{-l_i} + r_i) - y_i \ln(b_i e^{-l_i} + r_i)) + R(\boldsymbol{\mu}), \tag{11}$$

Performing a second-order Taylor expansion of $g_i(l) = (b_i e^{-l} + r_i) - y_i \ln(b_i e^{-l} + r_i)$ with respect to an estimated line integral[21] $\hat{l}_i = \ln(b_i/(y_i - r_i))$, Eq. (11) becomes

$$\Phi(\boldsymbol{\mu}) = \sum_{i=1}^{I} \frac{w_i}{2}([\mathbf{A}\boldsymbol{\mu}]_i - \hat{l}_i)^2 + R(\boldsymbol{\mu}), \tag{12}$$

where $w_i = (y_i - r_i)^2/y_i$ is the statistical weight for each x-ray path.

While the simultaneous algebraic iterative technique (SART) also minimizes a least square function, statistical iterative reconstruction (SIR) deals with a statistically weighted least square function defined by Eq. (11). The statistical weight represents the confidence of the projection measurement along each path. The projection data through denser paths would have lower signal-to-noise-ratios (SNR). Although the measured realistic data may not fully satisfy the Poisson model[22] in practical applications, it is well-accepted in the CT field.[23]

4.1.2. *GDSIR and ADSIR*

The regularization term $R(\boldsymbol{\mu})$ in Eq. (12) represents prior information on reconstructed images. Various assumptions about the prior information lead to different reconstruction algorithms. For example, the assumption of smooth variation over adjacent pixels suggests a regularization in terms of quadratic differences between adjacent pixels.[21] The piecewise constant assumption supports a TV regularization.[5] A more general form of regularization is the q-generalized Gaussian Markov field (q-GGMRF) prior, which has two adjustable parameters.[24] The quadratic and TV regularization functions are special cases of q-GGMRF. Because all these regularization means are based on the relationship of adjacent pixels, it is difficult for them to distinguish weak structures and strong noise.

On the other hand, the dictionary learning and sparse representation techniques perform well in sensing structures and suppressing noise. So we propose to use the sparsity constraint in terms of a redundant dictionary as the regularization term of Eq. (12). In reference to Eq. (7), we have the following minimization problem:

$$\min_{\boldsymbol{\mu},\boldsymbol{\alpha},(\mathbf{D})} \sum_{i=1}^{I} \frac{w_i}{2}([\mathbf{A}\boldsymbol{\mu}]_i - \hat{l}_i)^2 + \lambda \left(\sum_s \|\mathbf{E}_s\boldsymbol{\mu} - \mathbf{D}\boldsymbol{\alpha}_s\|_2^2 + \sum_s \nu_s \|\boldsymbol{\alpha}_s\|_0 \right), \quad (13)$$

where $\mathbf{E}_s = \{e_{nj}^s\} \in R^{N\times J}$ is an operator to extract patches from an image.

Similar to the comments we made on Eq. (7), the dictionary $\mathbf{D}$ in Eq. (13) can be either predetermined or dynamically defined. According to these two options, we can perform either global dictionary based statistical iterative reconstruction (GDSIR) or adaptive dictionary based statistical iterative reconstruction (ADSIR). Because structures in various subjects are quite similar in a given application, a training set of patches for construction of a global dictionary can be extracted from images of similar objects. On the other hand, the training set of patches for construction of an adaptive dictionary can be extracted from an intermediate image and dynamically updated during the reconstruction process.

4.1.3. *Optimization via alternating minimization*

For GDSIR, the image reconstruction process is equivalent to solving the following optimization problem

$$\min_{\boldsymbol{\mu},\boldsymbol{\alpha}} \sum_{i=1}^{I} \frac{w_i}{2}([\mathbf{A}\boldsymbol{\mu}]_i - \hat{l}_i)^2 + \lambda \left(\sum_s \|\mathbf{E}_s\boldsymbol{\mu} - \mathbf{D}\boldsymbol{\alpha}_s\|_2^2 + \sum_s \nu_s \|\boldsymbol{\alpha}_s\|_0 \right), \quad (14)$$

where there are two variables $\boldsymbol{\mu}$ and $\boldsymbol{\alpha}$. An alternating minimization scheme can be used to optimize the two variables. First, an intermediate reconstructed image $\boldsymbol{\mu}$ with a fixed sparse representation $\tilde{\boldsymbol{\alpha}}$ is updated to reduce the data discrepancy. Thus, the objective function Eq. (14) becomes

$$\min_{\boldsymbol{\mu}} \sum_{i=1}^{I} \frac{w_i}{2}([\mathbf{A}\boldsymbol{\mu}]_i - \hat{l}_i)^2 + \lambda \sum_s \|\mathbf{E}_s\boldsymbol{\mu} - \mathbf{D}\tilde{\boldsymbol{\alpha}}_s\|_2^2. \quad (15)$$

By the separable paraboloid surrogate method, Eq. (15) can be iteratively solved as

$$\mu_j^t = \mu_j^{t-1} - \frac{\sum_{i=1}^{I} (a_{ij} w_i([\mathbf{A}\boldsymbol{\mu}^{t-1}]_i - \hat{l}_i)) + 2\lambda \sum_s \sum_{n=1}^{N} e_{nj}^s([\mathbf{E}_s\boldsymbol{\mu}^{t-1}]_n - [\mathbf{D}\tilde{\boldsymbol{\alpha}}_s]_n)}{\sum_{i=1}^{I}\left(a_{ij} w_i \sum_{k=1}^{J} a_{ik}\right) + 2\lambda \sum_s \sum_{n=1}^{N} e_{nj}^s \sum_{k=1}^{J} e_{nk}^s},$$

$$j = 1, \ldots, J, \tag{16}$$

where the superscript $t = 1, 2, \ldots, T$ is the iteration index. Second, the intermediate image $\boldsymbol{\mu}^t$ is re-expressed in terms of the dictionary for a better sparse representation. Thus, the objective function Eq. (13) becomes

$$\min_{\boldsymbol{\alpha}} \sum_s \|\mathbf{E}_s\boldsymbol{\mu}^t - \mathbf{D}\boldsymbol{\alpha}_s\|_2^2 + \sum_s \nu_s\|\boldsymbol{\alpha}_s\|_0, \tag{17}$$

which is a sparse representation problem. As an example, the OMP algorithm can be used to find the sparse representation of each patch. The above two steps are alternatingly performed until the stopping criteria are satisfied.

For ADSIR, the image reconstruction process is equivalent to solve the following optimization problem,

$$\min_{\boldsymbol{\mu},\mathbf{D},\boldsymbol{\alpha}} \sum_{i=1}^{I} \frac{w_i}{2}([\mathbf{A}\boldsymbol{\mu}]_i - \hat{l}_i)^2 + \lambda\left(\sum_s \|\mathbf{E}_s\boldsymbol{\mu} - \mathbf{D}\boldsymbol{\alpha}_s\|_2^2 + \sum_s \nu_s\|\boldsymbol{\alpha}_s\|_0\right), \tag{18}$$

where there are three variables $\boldsymbol{\mu}$, $\mathbf{D}$ and $\boldsymbol{\alpha}$. Similar to the GDSIR, an alternating minimization scheme is used to optimize the three variables. First, an intermediate reconstructed image $\boldsymbol{\mu}$ is updated to reduce the data discrepancy with a fixed sparse representation $\tilde{\boldsymbol{\alpha}}$ and a current dictionary $\tilde{\mathbf{D}}$. This step is exactly the same as that for the GDSIR expressed by Eq. (16). Second, keeping the intermediate image $\boldsymbol{\mu}^t$ unchanged, $\mathbf{D}$ and $\boldsymbol{\alpha}$ are estimated by

$$\min_{\mathbf{D},\boldsymbol{\alpha}} \sum_s \|\mathbf{E}_s\boldsymbol{\mu}^t - \mathbf{D}\boldsymbol{\alpha}_s\|_2^2 + \sum_s \nu_s\|\boldsymbol{\alpha}_s\|_0, \tag{19}$$

Equation (19) is the generic dictionary learning and sparse representation problem, which can be solved with respect to $\boldsymbol{\alpha}$ and $\mathbf{D}$ alternatingly using the classic K-SVD algorithm. For fast convergence, we can first use the fast online algorithm[25] to train a dictionary from the patches extracted from an intermediate image $\boldsymbol{\mu}^t$. Then, we fix the dictionary to update the sparse representation as in Eq. (17) using the OMP algorithm. The above procedures are alternatingly performed until the stopping criteria are satisfied.

4.2. *Parameter Selection*

Similar to other regularized iterative reconstruction algorithms, the regularization parameter λ is to balance the data fidelity and prior information terms. The final reconstruction depends on the parameter λ. It is an interesting problem on how to choose an optimal parameter. Usually, it is empirically selected in practice. For the GDSIR and ADSIR, we can also empirically select λ. Because the data fidelity term is proportional to the noise standard deviation in the projection domain, λ should be increased with the noise increment. Specifically, our parameter selection problem can be re-formulated as follows. After some variable exchanges and constant additions, we can rewrite Eq. (15) as

$$\min_{\boldsymbol{\mu}} \|\mathbf{B}\boldsymbol{\mu} - \mathbf{L}\|_2^2 + \lambda N \|\boldsymbol{\mu} - \tilde{\boldsymbol{\mu}}\|_2^2, \tag{20}$$

where $\mathbf{B} = \mathbf{w}\mathbf{A}$, $\mathbf{L} = \mathbf{w}\hat{\mathbf{l}}$, $\mathbf{w} = diag(\sqrt{w_i/2})$, $\hat{\mathbf{l}} = (\hat{l}_1, \ldots, \hat{l}_I)^T$, $\tilde{\boldsymbol{\mu}} = \{\frac{1}{N}\sum_{s\in\Omega j} \mathbf{F}_{sj}\mathbf{D}\tilde{\boldsymbol{\alpha}}_s\}$, N is the number of pixels in a patch, Ω_j denotes the set of patches covering a pixel j, and $\mathbf{F}_{sj} \in \mathbb{R}^{1\times N}$ extracts a pixel j from a patch s. Note that in Eq. (19) we can discard the pixels in margins and only consider the pixels in the intersection between the rows from $\sqrt{N}$ to $(H - \sqrt{N} + 1)$ and the columns from $\sqrt{N}$ to $(W - \sqrt{N} + 1)$ for an $H \times W$ image. Let $\boldsymbol{\xi} = \boldsymbol{\mu} - \tilde{\boldsymbol{\mu}}$ and $\tilde{\mathbf{L}} = \mathbf{L} - \mathbf{B}\tilde{\boldsymbol{\mu}}$. Then, Eq. (20) becomes

$$\min_{\boldsymbol{\mu}} \|\mathbf{B}\boldsymbol{\xi} - \tilde{\mathbf{L}}\|_2^2 + \lambda N \|\boldsymbol{\xi}\|_2^2. \tag{21}$$

Equation (21) is a classical regularization problem, which can be solved using existing methods, such as the Miller method and the generalized cross-validation method.[26–28] Nevertheless, λ is empirically selected in this feasibility study.

The dictionary redundancy improves the sparsity of representation. To ensure the redundancy, the number of atoms in a dictionary should be much greater than that of pixels in a patch, that means $K \gg N$. In the image processing field, $K = 4N$ is a conventional choice. Therefore, a larger patch size corresponds to a larger number of atoms in a dictionary, which would increase the computational cost. On the other hand, if the patch size is too small, it could not effectively catch features in an image. In Ref. [11], it was pointed out that there was no significant difference between the results with $N = 8 \times 8$, $K = 256$ and $N = 16 \times 16$, $K = 1024$, and a larger patch size may lead to an over-smoothed image. Hence, $N = 8 \times 8$, $K = 256$ are used in this chapter. In the dictionary learning process, we solve the optimization problem Eq. (5) by minimizing the representation error with a fixed sparse level L_0^D. The sparsity level is selected as $5 \sim 10$ atoms. The aforementioned parameter selection for N, K and L_0^D has been applied in many applications, and also worked well in our experiments to be described below.

Besides, there are two parameters in the sparse representation step of image reconstruction, which are the sparse level L_0^S and the precision level ε. The OMP process will stop when either $\|\boldsymbol{\alpha}_s\|_0 \geq L_0^S$ or $\|\mathbf{E}_s\boldsymbol{\mu} - \mathbf{D}\boldsymbol{\alpha}_s\|_2^2 \leq \varepsilon$. The sparse level L_0^S is the number of atoms involved in representing a patch, which is empirically determined according to the complexity of an image to be reconstructed and the property of the dictionary. Usually, L_0^S is greater than or equal to the L_0^D in dictionary learning, and smaller than $N/2$ for sparsity. The precision level ε represents the tolerance of the difference between the reconstructed and original images, which is determined by the image noise level and the property of the dictionary. The stronger the noise is, the greater ε is. We can estimate the image noise level over a flat region in a reconstructed image.

Based on the above discussions, the parameter selection guidelines are summarized as in Table 1.

4.3. *Representative Results — Sheep Lung Study*

4.3.1. *Data acquisition*

In a sheep lung perfusion study, an anesthetized sheep was scanned at normal and low doses respectively on a SIEMENS Somatom Sensation 64-slice CT scanner in a circular cone-beam scanning mode. A scan protocol was developed for low-dose studies with ECG gating: time point 1 for a normal X-ray dose

Table 1. Summary of the parameter selection guidelines.

No.	Variable	Meaning	Criterion/Range
1	λ	Parameter to balance the data fidelity and prior information terms	It should be increased with the noise level. It is usually empirically selected in practice.
2	K, N	Number of atoms and number of pixels in a patch	They are selected as $N = 64$ and $K = 256$ in the image processing field, and work well in our study.
3	L_0^D	Sparsity level L_0 for dictionary learning	It is usually set to 5~10 atoms.
4	L_0^S	Sparsity level L_0 for image reconstruction	It is determined by the complexity of an image and the power of a dictionary; $N/2 > L_0^S \geq L_0^D$.
5	ε	Tolerance of the difference between the reconstructed and original images	It is determined by the image noise and the dictionary capability, and normally comparable to the image noise level.

scan (100 kV/150 mAs) before a contrast agent injection, and time points 2–21 for low-dose scans (80 kV/17 mAs) after the contrast agent injection. All the sinograms of the central slice were extracted, which were in fan-beam geometry. The radius of the trajectory was 57 cm. Over a 360° range, 1160 projections were uniformly collected. For each projection, 672 detector elements were equi-angularly distributed defining a field of view (FOV) of 25.05 cm in radius. In this experiment, the reconstructed images were matrixes of 768×768 pixels covering a $43.63 \times 43.63\,\text{cm}^2$ region. The sparsity constraint was enforced on the entire lung region of 500×370 pixels.

4.3.2. *Global dictionary learning*

In this study, a baseline image was reconstructed from the normal-dose sinogram using the FBP algorithm to construct a global dictionary, and the performance of the proposed techniques were evaluated with other low-dose sinograms. Because of the discrepancy in the normal and low-dose X-ray kVp settings and injection of the contrast agent, the attenuation maps of the low-dose images were quite different from that of the baseline image. Also, the physiological motion of the sheep most likely introduced structural differences. As such, this group of sinograms actually offers a challenging case to evaluate the robustness of the GDSIR.

First, a set of overlapping patches were extracted from the lung region in the baseline image. The patch size was of 8×8 pixels. The patches with very small variance were removed from the extracted patch set. The direct current (DC) component was removed from each patch. Then, a global dictionary of 256 atoms was constructed using the online dictionary learning method with a fixed sparse level $L_0^D = 5$. The lung region and the final trained dictionary are shown in Fig. 1. Finally, a DC atom was added to the dictionary.

4.3.3. *Low-dose results*

For comparison, five reconstruction techniques were applied to the aforementioned low-dose sinograms. As the benchmark, low dose images were reconstructed using the FBP method. The corresponding reconstructions using the other four reconstruction techniques were described as follows.

First, the GDSIR algorithm with a pre-learned global dictionary (learned in Subsection 4.3.2) was employed to reconstruct low-dose images with the following empirical parameters: $\lambda = 0.04$, $\varepsilon = 2.5 \times 10^{-5}$, and $L_0^S = 25$. The initial image was from the FBP method. An ordered-subset strategy was used for acceleration. The number of subsets was 40. The iterative process was stopped after 50 iterations.

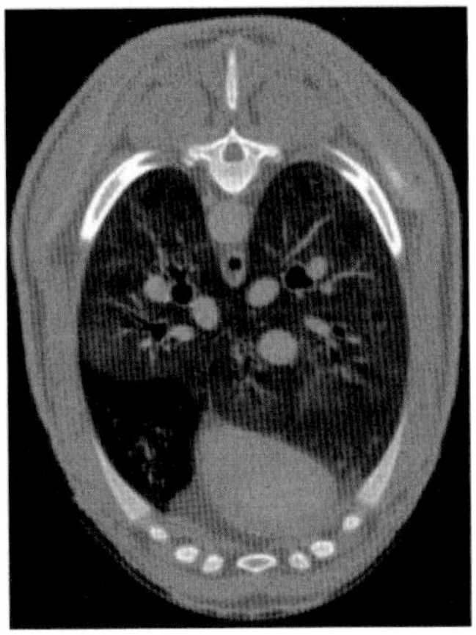

(a)

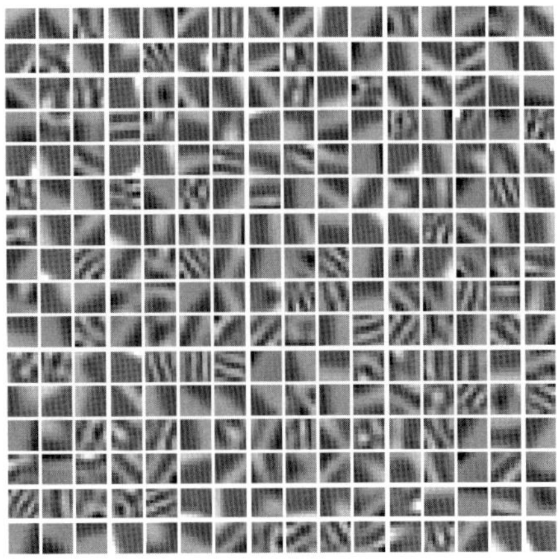

(b)

Fig. 1. Construction of a global dictionary. (a) is a sheep lung image with a display window [−700, 800] HU reconstructed from the normal-dose sinogram by the FBP method, which is used to extract the training patches. (b) is the learned dictionary consisting of 256 atoms. The attenuation coefficient of water was assumed as 0.018 to convert the reconstructed image (a) into HU and other images throughout this chapter.

Then, the ADSIR algorithm was tested with the same low-dose sinograms. In each iteration step, the dictionary was learned in real-time from the set of patches extracted from an intermediate image. The parameters for dictionary learning were the same as those in Subsection 4.3.2. Because there was strong noise in an intermediate image, the atoms in this dictionary are noisy. Therefore, the error control item ε for the ADSIR was made smaller than that for GDSIR in which the dictionary was learned from the normal-dose image. On the other hand, since the dictionary was learned from the reconstructed image itself, there was no need to use many atoms to capture the structures. The sparsity level parameter L_0^S was made much smaller than that for the GDSIR. Taking all these factors into account, the parameter were empirically chosen as $\lambda = 0.04$, $\varepsilon = 1 \times 10^{-5}$, and $L_0^S = 5$. The number of subsets was again 40. The iterative process was also stopped after 50 iterations.

Third, the popular TV regularization algorithm was included to demonstrate the merits of the proposed methods. For that purpose, the TV minimization constraint was used as the regularization term in Eq. (12), and enforced using the soft-threshold filtering based alternating minimization algorithm. We denote this method as TVSIR.

Fourth, to evaluate the effect of the statistical reconstruction technique in this dictionary learning based reconstruction framework, we replaced the log-likelihood term $\sum_{i=1}^{I} \frac{\omega_i}{2}([\mathbf{A}\boldsymbol{\mu}]_i - \hat{l}_i)^2$ in Eq. (13) with an un-weighted l_2-norm data fidelity term $\frac{1}{2}\|\mathbf{A}\boldsymbol{\mu} - \hat{\mathbf{I}}\|_2^2$. The global dictionary based algorithm was modified with this constant weighting scheme, which we denote as GDNSIR. The adaptive dictionary based algorithm can be modified in a similar way. The regularization parameter was empirically set to $\lambda = 0.35$ given the weight change of the data fidelity term in the objective function.

The results from a representative low-dose sinogram are in Fig. 2. It can be seen that there is strong noise in the FBP reconstruction, and streak artifacts along high attenuation structures, such as around bones. This kind of streak artifacts can be easily identified from the difference between the FBP image and the results with the SIR methods. The dictionary learning based algorithms generally performed well with low-dose data. While the GDSIR did better in preserving structures and suppressing noise, the ADSIR kept slightly more structures than the GDSIR (see the region indicated by the arrow "A"). The ADSIR generated a little less uniformity than the GDSIR in the whole image (see the region indicated by the arrow "B"), and some edges were obscurer than those with the GDSIR. The performance of the GDNSIR was not much different from that of the GDSIR. However, there were some streak artifacts with the GDNSIR as in the FBP reconstruction (see the difference from the FBP image), especially around the bone (see the region indicated by the arrow "C"). The image reconstructed by the TVSIR had much less noise than the FBP result, but it was a little blocky and had an inferior visibility compared to the dictionary learning based methods (see the regions indicated by the arrows "D" and "E"). Some bony structures in the TVSIR result were obscure or invisible (see the region indicated by the arrow "F").

4.3.4. *Few-view test*

Reducing the number of projection views is an important strategy to reduce image time and radiation dose, giving the few-view problem. To evaluate the proposed dictionary learning based algorithms for few-view tomography, the number of low-dose views was down-sampled from 1160 to 580, 290 and 116, respectively. The GDSIR and ADSIR methods were then applied. Also, the FBP and TVSIR methods were performed for comparison. The results are in Fig. 3.

It is seen that the FBP reconstruction results became worse and worse when the number of views was gradually decreased from 1160 to 116. The GDSIR, ADSIR and TVSIR results were much better than the FBP reconstruction. In the case of 580 views, the GDSIR and ADSIR results were almost as good as that reconstructed from 1160 views in Fig. 2. However, in the cases of 290 and 116 views, some details were lost. The TVSIR results always had more noise

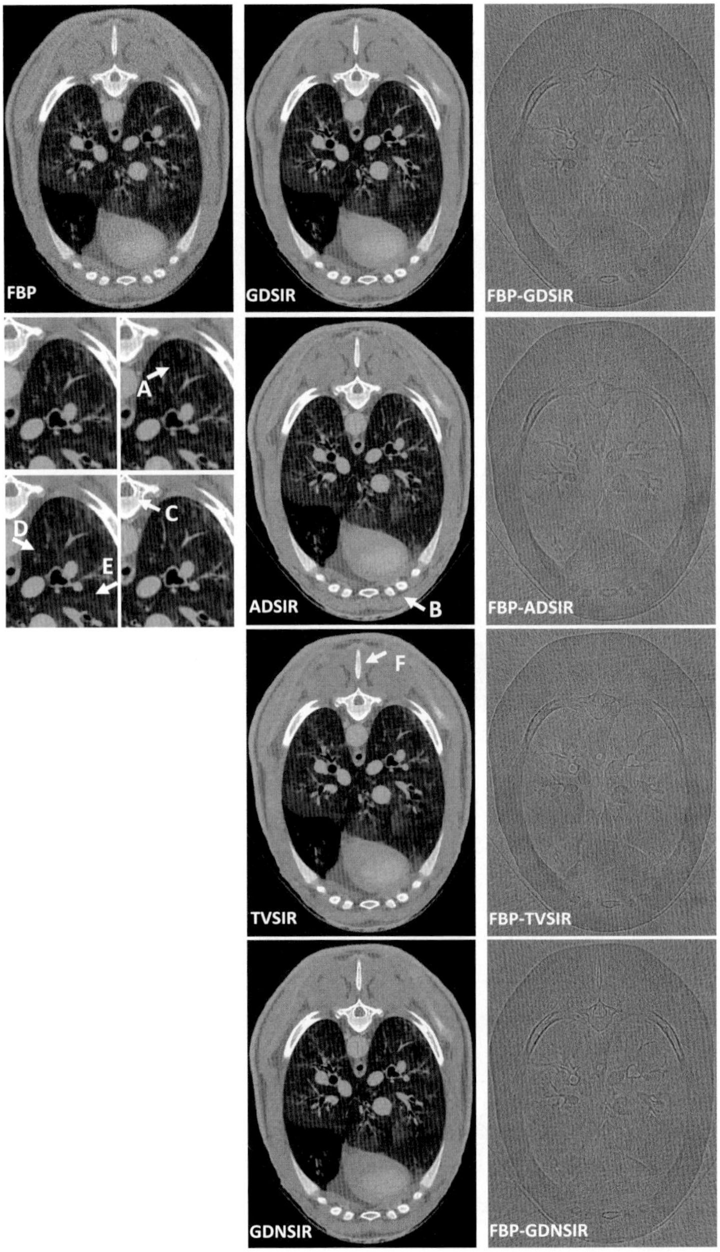

Fig. 2. Reconstructed images from a representative low-dose sinogram collected in the sheep lung CT perfusion study. The upper left image is reconstructed by the conventional FBP method. The middle column are the images reconstructed using the GDSIR, ADSIR, TVSIR and GDNSIR methods (from top to bottom), respectively. The magnified local regions of them are shown below the FBP results (upper left, upper right, lower left and lower right correspond to GDSIR, ADSIR, TVSIR and GDNSIR, respectively). The display window is $[-700, 800]$ HU. The right column are the difference images between the FBP image and the results by the GDSIR, ADSIR, TVSIR and GDNSIR with a display window $[-556, 556]$ HU.

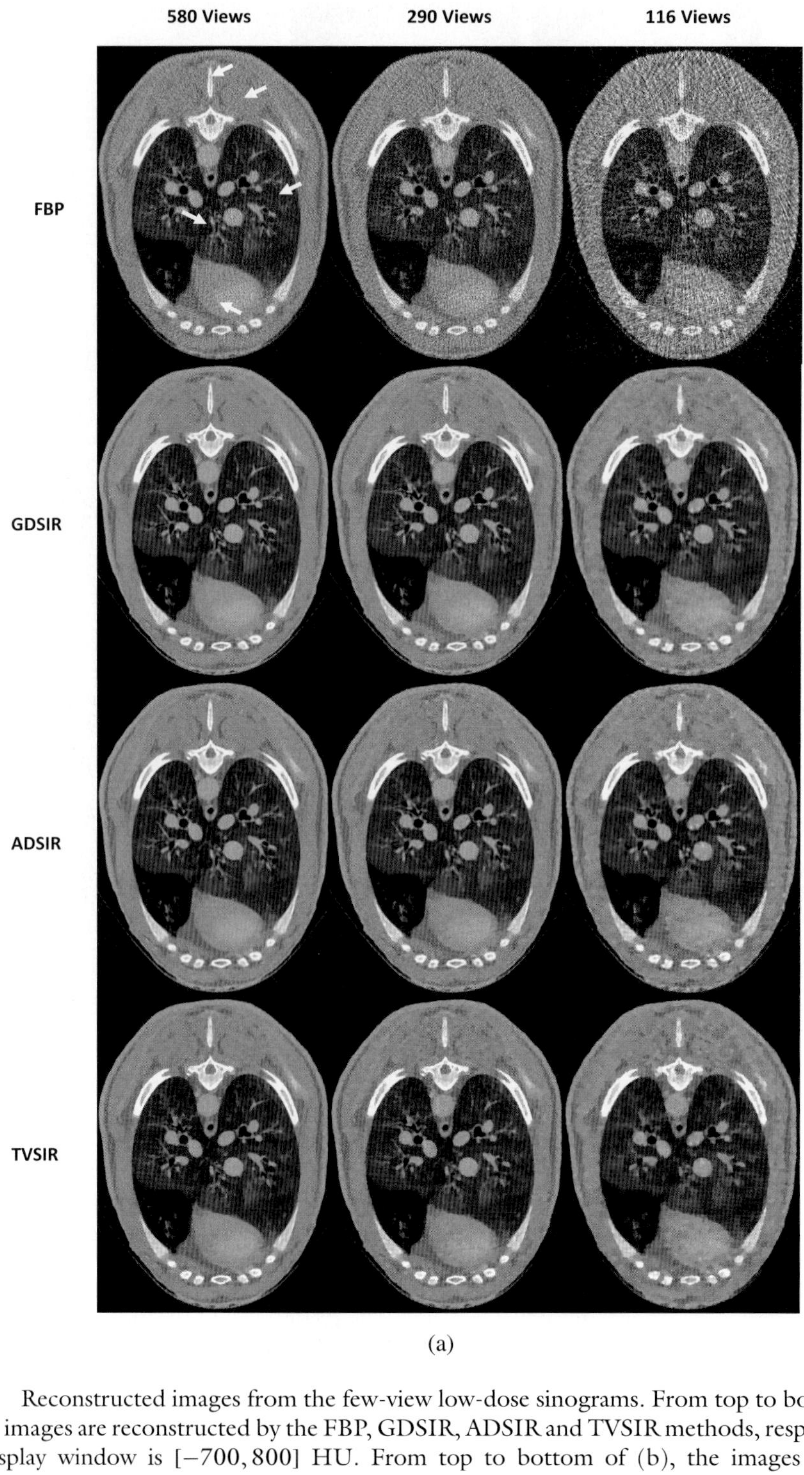

(a)

Fig. 3. Reconstructed images from the few-view low-dose sinograms. From top to bottom of (a), the images are reconstructed by the FBP, GDSIR, ADSIR and TVSIR methods, respectively. The display window is [−700, 800] HU. From top to bottom of (b), the images are the and fewer structures than the dictionary learning based reconstructions (see the regions indicated by the arrows).

4.3.5. *Plots of the terms in the objective function*

To monitor the convergence of the proposed dictionary learning based algorithms, we took the GDSIR as an example. Figure 4 plots the convergence

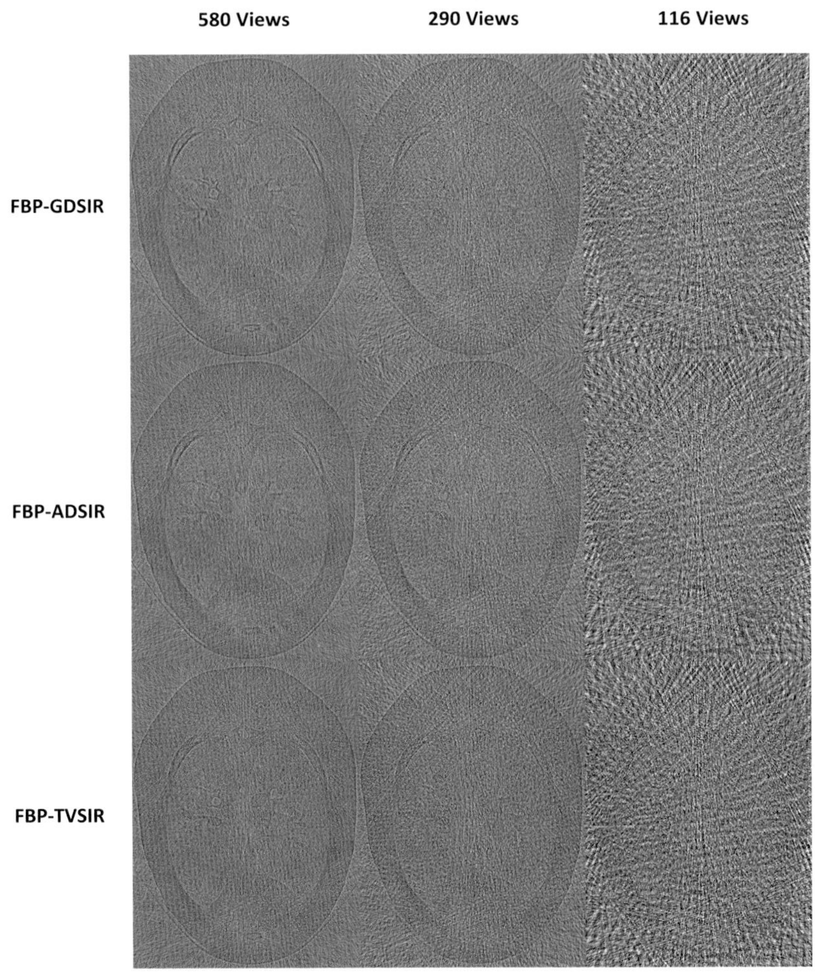

(b)

Fig. 3. (*Continued*)

differences between the FBP results and the corresponding results by the GDSIR, ADSIR and TVSIR methods, respectively. The display window is [−556, 556] HU. From left to right, the images are reconstructed from 580, 290, and 116 views, respectively.

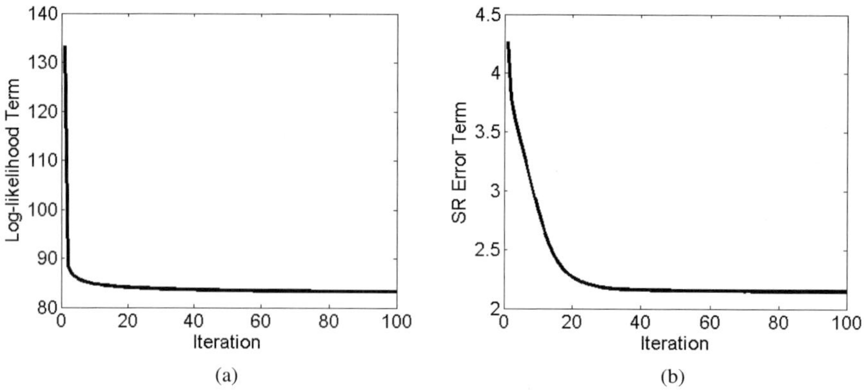

Fig. 4. Plots of objective functional terms associated with the GDSIR method applied to a representative low-dose sinogram. (a) and (b) are the curves for the log-likelihood and sparse representation errors, respectively.

curves of the log-likelihood term $\sum_{i=1}^{I} \frac{w_i}{2}([\mathbf{A}\boldsymbol{\mu}]_i - \hat{l}_i)^2$ and the sparse representation error term $\sum_s \|\mathbf{E}_s\boldsymbol{\mu} - \mathbf{D}\boldsymbol{\alpha}_s\|_2^2$ with respect to the iteration number. These curves show that both the log-likelihood term and the sparse representation error term would decrease monotonically. After ~40 iterations, both the two terms changed little with further iterations. Practically, the reconstruction process can be stopped after a fixed number of iterations when the log-likelihood term and sparse representation error term do not decrease significantly.

5. Discussion — TV or Dictionary?

Based on the CS theory, the TV regularization method was widely used for CT reconstruction, and produced good results from incomplete and noisy data. However, TV regularization method may produce blocky results in practical applications when there is too much noise. Moreover, the TV constraint uniformly penalizes the image gradient, and is not capable of distinguishing structural details from noise and artifacts. These problems dampen the enthusiasm for the clinical application of the TV regularization method.

Different from the TV regularization method, the dictionary learning approach aims at capturing localized structural information and suppressing image noise. The sparse representation in terms of a redundant dictionary is able to keep the atoms reflecting structural features and avoid the other atoms that may introduce artifacts. Use of the dictionary-based sparse representation as the regularization term for SIR is a new mechanism to improve image quality. Moreover, any missed structural information due to the enforcement of the sparsity constraint will be compensated for in the subsequent updating steps. The SIR is very effective to eliminate streak artifacts, and works well with a dictionary. In principle, the dictionary learning process should lead to a sparser representation of an underlying image in a specific application. The basic idea of the dictionary learning based approach is to find a best match to a true image from the dictionary-spanned image space. When the true image is outside the dictionary image space, the reconstructed image can be viewed as its projection on the dictionary image space with an unavoidable error. Therefore, some structures may be lost while artifacts may be introduced although the reconstructed results often have less noise and more structural information. A proper dictionary should represent the structural information of an object as much as possible. In this way, the reconstruction with a sparse representation in terms of the dictionary can perform well. With a global dictionary, the structural differences between its training images and a true image would affect the final reconstruction quality. Usually, it is not difficult to prepare an excellent training set with sufficiently many structural features and less noise for construction of a global dictionary. Since the GDSIR does not need to update the dictionary in each iteration step, it is much faster than the ADSIR. On the other hand, it is necessary to use an adaptive dictionary when a global dictionary does not match a specific application closely.

In fact, the CS theory is a general principle for image reconstruction and the key is to explore a sparsity constraint. In our opinion, practical sparsifying transforms have been developed in three generations. The first generation is the pixel-wise sparsity in the image domain, which includes the most popular DGT assuming a piecewise constant image model. The second generation is the pixel-wise sparsity in the transform domain, which includes Fourier transform, wavelet transform and other linear sparsifying transforms. The third generation is the structural sparsity, which includes the dictionary learning based sparse representation in this chapter as well as some low rank models for matrix completion. Due to the limitation of space, we only present some representative results from low-dose and/or few-view datasets. It can be expected that the dictionary learning based reconstruction methods will perform well for other CT applications, such as limited-angle, interior tomography, and so on.[15,29] Besides, more clinical applications are possible, such as ultra-low-dose lung cancer screening. Moreover, not only in the context of X-ray CT, our results could be extended to other tomographic modalities such as phase-contrast CT, PET and SPECT, etc.

Acknowledgments

This work was supported in part by National Natural Science Foundation of China (NSFC) (No. 61172163, 61302136), in part by the Research Fund for the Doctoral Program of Higher Education of China (No. 20110201110011), in part by China Postdoctoral Science Foundation (No. 2012M521775), in part by the National Science Foundation CAREER Award (CBET-1149679), in part by the National Institutes of Health/National Institute of Biomedical Imaging and Bioengineering (NIH/NIBIB) under Grant EB011785.

References

1. D. J. Brenner and E. J. Hall, "Computed tomography — an increasing source of radiation exposure," *New Eng J Med* **357**, 2277–2284 (2007).
2. J. Hsieh, "Adaptive streak artifact reduction in computed tomography resulting from excessive x-ray photon noise," *Med Phys* **25**, 2139–2147 (1998).
3. P. La Rivière, "Penalized-likelihood sinogram smoothing for low-dose CT," *Med Phys* **32**, 1676 (2005).
4. J. Wang, T. Li, H. Lu, and Z. Liang, "Penalized weighted least-squares approach to sinogram noise reduction and image reconstruction for low-dose X-ray computed tomography," *IEEE Trans Medical Imaging* **25**, 1272–1283 (2006).
5. E. Sidky and X. Pan, "Image reconstruction in circular cone-beam computed tomography by constrained, total-variation minimization," *Phys Med Biol* **53**, 4777–4807 (2008).
6. Q. Xu, X. Mou, G. Wang, J. Sieren, E. Hoffman, and H. Yu, "Statistical interior tomography," *IEEE Trans Medical Imaging* **30**, 1116–1128 (2011).
7. D. L. Donoho, "Compressed sensing," *IEEE Trans Infor Theory* **52**, 1289–1306 (2006).
8. E. J. Candes, J. Romberg, and T. Tao, "Robust uncertainty principles: Exact signal reconstruction from highly incomplete frequency information," *IEEE Trans Infor Theory* **52**, 489–509 (2006).
9. M. Elad and M. Aharon, "Image denoising via sparse and redundant representations over learned dictionaries," *IEEE Trans Image Process* **15**, 3736–3745 (2006).
10. J. Mairal, M. Elad, and G. Sapiro, "Sparse representation for color image restoration," *IEEE Trans Image Process* **17**, 53–69 (2007).
11. J. Mairal, G. Sapiro, and M. Elad, "Learning multiscale sparse representations for image and video restoration," *SIAM Multiscale Modeling Simulation* 7, 214–241 (2008).
12. Y. Chen, X. Ye, and F. Huang, "A novel method and fast algorithm for MR image reconstruction with significantly under-sampled data," *Inverse Problems Imaging* **4**, 223–240 (2010).
13. S. Ravishankar and Y. Bresler, "MR Image Reconstruction From Highly Undersampled k-space Data by Dictionary Learning," *IEEE Trans Medical Imaging* **30**, 1028–1041 (2011).
14. Q. Xu, H. Yu, X. Mou, and G. Wang, "Dictionary learning based low-dose X-ray CT reconstruction," *Proc. of the 11th International Meeting on Fully Three-Dimensional Image Reconstruction in Radiology and Nuclear Medicine*, 258–261, Potsdam, Germany (2011).

15. Q. Xu, H. Yu, X. Mou, L. Zhang, J. Hsieh, G. Wang, "Low-dose X-ray CT reconstruction via dictionary learning," *IEEE Trans Medical Imaging* **31**, 1682–1697 (2012).
16. S. G. Mallat and Z. Zhang, "Matching pursuits with time-frequency dictionaries," *IEEE Trans Signal Process* **41**, 3397–3415 (1993).
17. Y. C. Pati, R. Rezaiifar, and P. Krishnaprasad, "Orthogonal matching pursuit: Recursive function approximation with applications to wavelet decomposition," *Conf. Record of The Twenty-Seventh Asilomar Conference on Signals, Systems and Computers*, **1**, 40–44 (1993).
18. S. S. Chen, D. L. Donoho, and M. A. Saunders, "Atomic decomposition by basis pursuit," *SIAM J Scientific Computing* **20**, 33–61 (1999).
19. M. Aharon, M. Elad, and A. Bruckstein, "K-SVD: An Algorithm for Designing Overcomplete Dictionaries for Sparse Representation," *IEEE Trans Signal Process* **54**, 4311–4322 (2006).
20. J. Mairal, F. Bach, J. Ponce, and G. Sapiro, "Online learning for matrix factorization and sparse coding," *J Machine Learning Res* **11**, 19–60 (2010).
21. I. A. Elbakri and J. A. Fessler, "Statistical image reconstruction for polyenergetic X-ray computed tomography," *IEEE Trans Medical Imaging* **21**, 89–99 (2002).
22. B. R. Whiting, P. Massoumzadeh, O. A. Earl, J. A. O'Sullivan, D. L. Snyder, and J. F. Williamson, "Properties of preprocessed sinogram data in x-ray computed tomography," *Med Phys* **33**, 3290 (2006).
23. J. B. Thibault, K. D. Sauer, C. A. Bouman, and J. Hsieh, "A three-dimensional statistical approach to improved image quality for multislice helical CT," *Med Phys* **34**, 4526 (2007).
24. C. Bouman and K. Sauer, "A generalized Gaussian image model for edge-preserving MAP estimation," *IEEE Trans Image Process* **2**, 296–310 (1993).
25. http://www.di.ens.fr/willow/SPAMS/.
26. M. Bertero and P. Boccacci, *Introduction to Inverse Problems in Imaging*. Chapter 5.6: Taylor & Francis (1998).
27. K. Miller, "Least squares methods for ill-posed problems with a prescribed bound," *SIAM J Mathematical Analysis* **1**, 52 (1970).
28. G. H. Golub, M. Heath, and G. Wahba, "Generalized cross-validation as a method for choosing a good ridge parameter," *Technometrics* **21**, 215–223 (1979).
29. J. Wu, X. Mou, H. Yu, G. Wang, "Statistical interior tomography via dictionary learning without assuming anobject support," *Proc. of the 12th International Meeting on Fully Three-Dimensional Image Reconstruction in Radiology and Nuclear Medicine*, 440–443, California, USA (2013).

Chapter 7

Machine Learning Methods for Segmenting Psoriatic Lesions from 2D Images

Juan Lu,[*,§] *Ed Kazmierczak,*[*] *Jonathan H. Manton*[†] *and Rodney Sinclair*[‡]

[*]*Department of Computing and Information Systems, University of Melbourne*

[†]*Department of Electrical and Electronic Engineering, University of Melbourne*

[‡]*Department of Medicine (Dermatology), University of Melbourne*

[§]*E-mail: jualu@student.unimelb.edu.au*

Digital images combined with computer aided diagnosis techniques offer dermatologists a simple, robust, objective and portable means for assessing many kinds of dermatological conditions. Some of the conditions that are amenable to computer aided diagnosis include acne, psoriasis and rosacea. Computer aided diagnosis can act as an external reference point to verify clinicians' diagnoses or can act as another input to the diagnosis making process. In this chapter we examine machine-learning methods for the computer aided diagnosis of psoriasis severity by developing an algorithm for the analysis of psoriasis severity. Psoriatic lesions are analysed by first segmenting erythema, the inflamed red skin in lesions, and scaling, the flaky white skin in lesions. Erythema segmentation is achieved by decomposing the skin colour into its melanin and haemoglobin colour components, and a Support Vector Machine (SVM) is designed to identify erythema pixels. Scaling segmentation is done by first applying a contrast map to heighten the contrast between scaling and non-scaling pixels, and then using textures and neighbourhoods to identify the scaling pixels. Markov random fields (MRFs) are used in conjunction with SVMs to first identify candidate scaling pixels and then use the neighbourhood in which a pixel is located to determine its final classification. We demonstrate the effectiveness of the proposed segmentation and classification methods by testing them on a database of psoriasis images.

1. Introduction

Computer aided diagnosis using digital skin images is fast becoming an important tool in dermatology. Images can be acquired for analysis using a variety of different imaging modalities where each modality reveals different facets of a condition. Computer aided diagnosis in dermatology is often used to complement diagnoses by clinicians or is used to help achieve a correct diagnosis especially when the diagnosis is hard to make.[1]

The aim of this chapter is to describe algorithms for diagnosis of psoriasis severity using only 2D digital skin images. Two dimensional digital skin images are commonplace in dermatology practice and have been for a some time. A computer aided diagnosis system using just 2D digital skin images can not only analyse new images, but can also be used to analyse existing images.

The algorithm implements a processing pipeline that samples the image, applies filters to the image and transforms the image. In particular, machine learning and classification techniques are used to segment the key symptoms of psoriasis and then make a diagnosis of the psoriasis severity. The process for segmenting and diagnosing psoriasis severity is illustrated in Fig. 1. This type of processing pipeline is actually quite common and used in a number computer aided diagnosis systems.[2–4] The two key stages in the process are: (1) the segmentation of the symptoms in the image; and (2) the use of the symptoms to form a diagnosis or make a clinical decision. In the case of psoriasis the two steps become: (1) segmentation erythema and scaling; and (2) determining the severity of the erythema and scaling that, when combined with the area of lesion, allows the system to diagnose psoriasis severity. Note that this process of segmenting and diagnosing can be used with digital images of various modalities.

Segmenting the symptoms in a digital image and using the segmented image to make a diagnosis can both be implemented using statistical machine learning. Considering the digital image as a matrix of pixels allows us to treat both segmentation and diagnosis as classification problems. In the case of segmenting symptoms, the classification problem is to separate pixels that

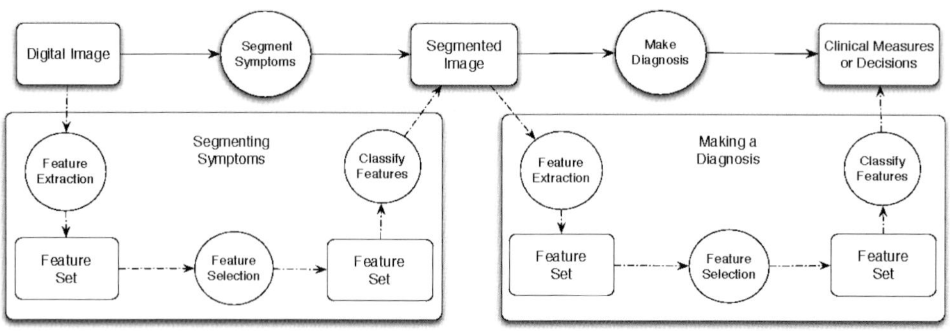

Fig. 1. A schematic for the design of our psoriasis diagnosis algorithm. In effect, the path through the dashed lines implements the path through the undashed lines.

are associated with a disease from those that are normal. In the diagnosis phase, where symptoms are associated with a region in the image, the classification problem is to differentiate between benign or malign symptoms, or to determine the severity of a symptom together with a description of the diagnosis.

There are three modules in a typical statistical machine learning system (see Fig. 1): feature extraction, feature selection and classification. In the case of digital images, features are typically numerical properties, or variables, that can be observed in the image. In most concrete problems, there are a number of different features that are observed and these features are grouped into *feature sets*. The feature set determined by the extraction module typically consists of the raw features extracted directly from images. The feature selection module determines a subset of the raw features that are better suited to the classification problem. Each pixel in the image will have a set of feature values associated with it and their feature values forms a feature space. The classifier then attempts to find boundaries between the classes of pixels based on pixels' feature values, for example, the pixels with feature vectors indicating erythema should all be in the same class.

This chapter will focus on developing machine learning methods for the segmentation of psoriasis. This is the preliminary step to diagnose psoriasis severity reliably and quantitatively.

2. Application of Machine Learning Methods for Psoriasis Segmentation

2.1. *Psoriasis*

Psoriasis is a chronic inflammatory skin disease and not much is known about the causes. There are around 125 million people worldwide suffering from this disease, and at present there is no known cure. The economic impact of psoriasis is also high. The overall annual cost of caring for individuals with clinically significant psoriasis has been estimated to as high as \$2 billion in the United States.[5] In Australia, individual expenditure on psoriasis treatment is estimated at around AUD \$2000 over a 2-year period.[6] The chronic nature of the disease often incurs a significant cost for patients over their lifetime.

The most common type of psoriasis is characterised by sharply demarcated scaly and erythematous plaques on the skin and can occur anywhere on the human body,[7] and individual psoriatic lesions vary greatly in appearance. Figure 2 shows some examples of psoriatic lesions.

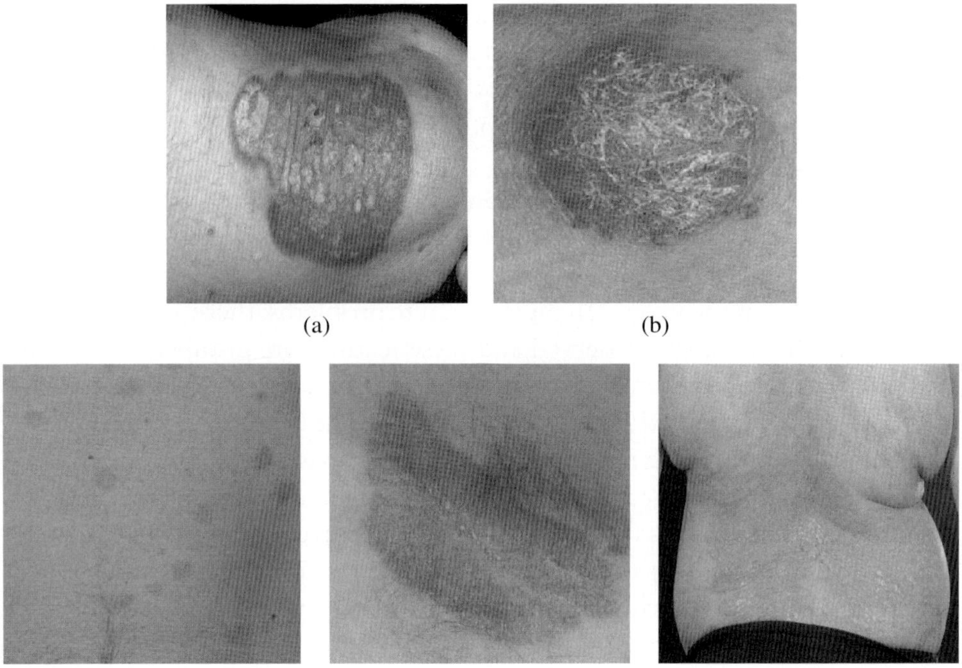

(a) (b) (c) (d) (e)

Fig. 2. Sample images of different types of psoriasis. (a) Plaque psoriasis; (b) Pustular psoriasis; (c) Guttate psoriasis; (d) Flexural psoriasis; (e) Erythrodermic psoriasis.

The problem for clinicians is to determine the efficacy of psoriasis treatment and to compare the efficacy of different psoriasis treatments. The current method for comparing treatments is to estimate a *severity index* from an individual's psoriasis lesions. A severity index is a single number derived from a variety of disease symptoms. One of the most common such indices is the PASI score.[8] PASI scores are derived by selecting a particular lesion and then visually estimating the area of selected lesions, the intensity of the erythema in the lesion, the degree of scaling in the region, and the thickness of the lesion. The four properties of a lesion are expressed as a numeric *severity index*. Despite training, intra- and inter- observer variances unavoidably occur in practice. An objective method of assessing psoriasis severity is in demand.

2.2. *Psoriasis Segmentation*

The first phase (see Fig. 1) in the computer aided diagnosis scheme is to segment the symptoms of the disease. In the case of psoriasis, this means segmenting erythema and scaling from normal skin. A body of work in segmenting psoriasis lesions exists but is focussed mostly on erythema and plaque psoriasis.

The methods for segmenting plaque psoriasis can be roughly divided into two types: pixel-based methods, and region-based methods. Pixel-based methods investigate color spaces and use only the color values of single pixels for segmentation. Region-based methods use color information and the information from neighbouring pixels to perform the segmentation and include methods like texture-based classification, watershed and region-based active contours.

A popular class of pixel-based methods for segmenting psoriasis are thresholding methods, for example, by thresholding G values in the normalised RGB color space[9] or by changing the thresholds based on assumptions about the distribution of normal skin and psoriasis lesions in the image.[10] In Refs. [11] and [12], the color space is changed to the CIE L*a*b* color space, where the hue and chroma color components are used to cluster pixels into psoriasis and normal skin classes. Delgado *et al.*[13] use a quadratic discriminant analysis that assumes that the difference between the G and B values in the RGB color space follows a Gaussian distribution. Nevertheless, problems with illumination and shadows remain unresolved with these thresholding methods.

Region-based segmentation of psoriasis have combined fuzzy texture spectrums with normalised RGB colors as features for a neuro-fuzzy classifier[14] and a multiresolution-decomposed signature subspace classifier.[15] The region-based segmentation offers better results in uneven illumination but has the drawback of missing small spot shaped psoriatic lesions. Another region-based approach to psoriasis segmentation is to use fractal features as in Refs. [16] and [17] that use the more complex textures in psoriasis to differentiate psoriasis from normal skin. Active contours work by initialising a seed region that grows outwards until a boundary between the psoriatic lesion and normal skin can be identified. This is done in Ref. [18] using color to seed the region and color change to detect the boundary. Region growing works well when the lesion exhibits erythema that almost completely surrounds the creamy white scaling. In the presence of scaling with no erythema, the technique can mis-classify scaling pixels as skin pixels.

Although plaque psoriasis is quite common, the segmentation methods listed above are not so successful with other types of psoriasis. The reason is that most algorithms rely on successfully segmenting erythema first, but the diversity of skin colors, psoriasis types and lighting conditions do not always make this possible. In this chapter we take a different strategy for segmentation which is to develop a pixel-based method to segment erythema, and a region-based method to segment scaling separately and then combine the results.

3. Segmenting Psoriasis Symptoms: Erythema

Erythema is the red inflamed skin that often, but not always, surrounds the creamy white scaling skin at the centre of psoriasis lesions. Erythema appears predominantly at the initial stages of psoriasis and some psoriatic lesions consist of erythema alone without any scaling. The redness of erythema when compared to normal skin makes it suitable to segment by developing a skin color model. Any segmentation algorithm for erythema based on skin color also needs to reject moles and other discolorations.

Our algorithm uses a skin color model and is composed of the following three steps:

(1) *Separating skin from background:* The skin is separated from the background using a histogram-based Bayesian classifier. Typical clinical images contain background objects such as clothes or wallpaper, that can confuse color based segmentation methods. Once the background is removed the algorithm can focus on segmenting psoriasis from normal skin without the need to deal further with background.
(2) *Determining the feature set by skin color decomposition:* The aim of this step is to extract features for classification by decomposing a skin color using a common model in which skin color is composed of melanin and hemoglobin color components. Melanin and hemoglobin are the features used by the classifier to segment erythema pixels from normal skin, moles and other skin discolorations. Independent Component Analysis (ICA) is used for the skin color decomposition.[19]
(3) *Segmenting erythema by using an SVM as the classifier:* The SVM classifies pixels in a feature space where the features are melanin and hemoglobin color components.[20]

3.1. *Separating Skin from Background*

The problem of separating skin from background has a long history,[21] for example, in human tracking,[22,23] gesture analysis,[24] and face recognition.[25,26] Skin segmentation is usually performed by using skin colors, because skin colors are robust information that is not affected by positions of the human body. Thresholding in a color-space, Bayesian classifiers and Gaussian classifiers are three of the most popular methods of skin segmentation.[27,28] Of these methods, color histogram based Bayesian classifiers perform the best on benchmark datasets,[27] because the color histogram is a stable representation of the skin colors unaffected by occlusion, while the explicit skin-color space thresholding is easily biased by illumination and the threshold values are hard to identify.[27] Additionally, the histogram-based Bayesian classifier is computationally faster than the Gaussian models.[27,29]

In this chapter we use the YCbCr color space combined with a Bayesian classifier and a color based histogram. The reason for choosing the YCbCr color space is that skin color is known to be compactly clustered in the YCbCr color space.[20,26]

Bayesian modelling separates skin pixels from non-skin pixels by using a Bayesian maximum likelihood estimation.[30] Given a color value x in the YCbCr color space, the likelihood of being skin $P(\text{skin}|x)$ and non-skin $P(-\text{skin}|x)$ is defined as:

$$P(\text{skin}|x) = \frac{P(x|\text{skin})P(\text{skin})}{P(x|\text{skin})P(\text{skin}) + P(x|-\text{skin})P(-\text{skin})}$$

$$P(-\text{skin}|x) = \frac{P(x|-\text{skin})P(-\text{skin})}{P(x|\text{skin})P(\text{skin}) + P(x|-\text{skin})P(-\text{skin})} \tag{1}$$

where $P(x|\text{skin})$ and $P(x|-\text{skin})$ are the conditional probabilities of a pixel color x given that we are dealing with a skin class and a non-skin class respectively, which are obtained through histograms of skin pixels and non-skin pixels, and $P(-\text{skin})$ and $P(\text{skin})$ are prior probabilities of being skin and non-skin respectively, which are case dependent.

A comparison of likelihoods $P(\text{skin}|x)$ and $P(-\text{skin}|x)$ can be performed through the ratio of $P(\text{skin}|x)$ to $P(-\text{skin}|x)$:

$$\frac{P(\text{skin}|x)}{P(-\text{skin}|x)} = \frac{P(x|\text{skin})\text{P}(\text{skin})}{P(x|-\text{skin})P(-\text{skin})} \tag{2}$$

If a pixel color x is such that

$$\frac{P_{\text{skin}}(x|\text{skin})}{P_{-\text{skin}}(x|-\text{skin})} \geq t_{\text{skin}} \tag{3}$$

exceeding the threshold t_{skin}, then x is labeled as a potential skin pixel. The threshold t_{skin} is a function of $P(\text{skin})$ and $P(-\text{skin})$ as follows:

$$t_{\text{skin}} = \frac{c_p P(-\text{skin})}{c_n P(\text{skin})} \tag{4}$$

where c_p is the introduced cost of a false positive, and c_n is the introduced cost of a false negative. In this way, a comparison of the likelihoods is converted to a comparison of the conditional probabilities.

The Cb and Cr components of the YCbCr color space are used to build the histograms, and the luminance component Y is discarded to reduce the disturbance from uneven illumination, for example, highlights and shadows.

Trading off between correct detection of skin and false positives, we set t_{skin} to be 0.2 and 0.1 for the Bayesian classifiers built with Cb and Cr components respectively. This gives the sets of pixels

$$X_{\text{skin}}^{\text{Cb}} = \left\{ x_{\text{Cb}} | \frac{P_{\text{skin}}(x_{\text{Cb}}|\text{skin})}{P_{\text{skin}}(x_{\text{Cb}}|-\text{skin})} \geq 0.2 \right\}$$
$$X_{\text{skin}}^{\text{Cr}} = \left\{ x_{\text{Cr}} | \frac{P_{\text{skin}}(x_{\text{Cr}}|\text{skin})}{P_{\text{skin}}(x_{\text{Cr}}|-\text{skin})} \geq 0.1 \right\} \tag{5}$$

with the result that the skin pixels are given by the set $A_{\text{skin}} = X_{\text{skin}}^{\text{Cb}} \bigcap X_{\text{skin}}^{\text{Cr}}$.

3.2. *Feature Extraction: Decomposing Skin Color into Melanin and Hemoglobin Components*

Once the skin has been separated from background we can look for features that can be used to distinguish erythema from normal skin. Figure 3 shows a dichromatic reflection model of skin. Human skin is a turbid media with a multi-layered structure. Melanin occurs in the epidermal layer and causes the skin to present as brown or black in color. Hemoglobin occurs in the dermal layer and causes the reddish color in the skin.

After identification of the skin region, the skin color is decomposed into melanin and hemoglobin components. These two components correlate directly with skin coloring and can be used to distinguish between erythema and other non-inflamed skin such as normal skin and moles. The quantities of these two pigments vary between individuals which in turn causes the variation in skin color that we see. In the case of erythema and its accompanying inflammation, there is an increase in hemoglobin causing the abnormal redness on the surface

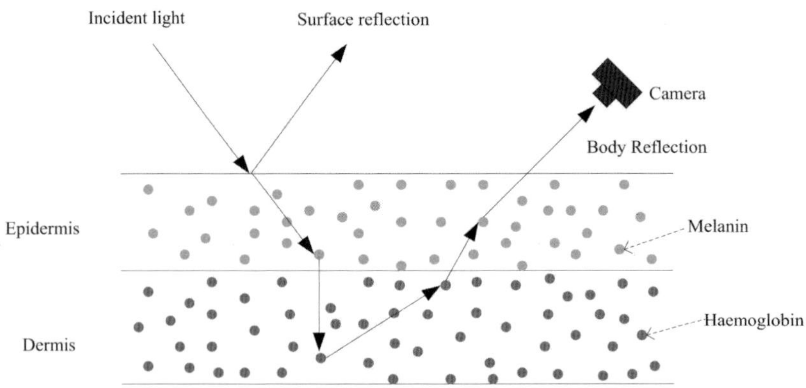

Fig. 3. Dichromatic reflection model of skin.

of the skin. In contrast, normal skin maintains a more balanced mixture of the hemoglobin and melanin pigments.

If we assume that skin color is a direct result of the melanin and hemoglobin pigments in the skin then we can attribute a *melanin* component and a *hemoglobin* component to skin color. Further if we assume that these two components of skin color are orthogonal then we can use ICA to decompose a skin color into melanin and hemoglobin components which then become our *features* for the classification step. This is an extension of the method proposed in[19] that synthesises skin color based on the ICA decomposition.

There are four steps in the skin color decomposition algorithm:

(1) A skin color model can be defined in a three dimensional optical density domain,[19] such that the skin color density can be linearly represented by melanin and hemoglobin components. We have:

$$\begin{aligned}\mathbf{l}_{x,y} &= \mathbf{c}^m q^m_{x,y} + \mathbf{c}^h q^h_{x,y} + \Delta \\ &= C\mathbf{q}_{x,y} + \Delta \end{aligned} \tag{6}$$

where $\mathbf{l}_{x,y}$ is the color intensity in the optical density domain, $\mathbf{c}^m$ and $\mathbf{c}^h$ are the melanin and hemoglobin components, $q^m_{x,y}$ and $q^h_{x,y}$ are relative quantities of the melanin and hemoglobin components respectively, and Δ is a spatially stationary vector modelling the other pigments and skin structure.

$$\mathbf{l}_{x,y} = [-\log(r_{x,y}), -\log(g_{x,y}), -\log(b_{x,y})]^t \tag{7}$$

In Eq. (7) $r_{x,y}, g_{x,y}$ and $b_{x,y}$ are the normalised color densities of a pixel at coordinate (x, y) with RGB values r, g and b respectively. Equation (6) can be rewritten using a pure density matrix $C = [\mathbf{c}^m, \mathbf{c}^h]$ and quantity vector $\mathbf{q}_{x,y} = [q^m_{x,y}, q^h_{x,y}]$.

(2) Principle Component Analysis (PCA)[31] is a technique for reducing dimensionality while preserving information. PCA is used here to reduce the three dimensional optical densities to two dimensions while preserving the major skin color information and discarding any redundant information from other pigments in the process. The resulting two dimensional color intensity vector $\mathbf{w}_{x,y}$ is given below:

$$\begin{aligned}\mathbf{w}_{x,y} &= \tilde{P}^t \mathbf{l}_{x,y} \\ &= \tilde{P}^t (C\mathbf{q}_{x,y} + \Delta) \\ &= \tilde{P}^t C\mathbf{q}'_{x,y} \end{aligned} \tag{8}$$

where $\mathbf{q}'_{x,y} = \mathbf{q}_{x,y} + (\tilde{P}^t C)^{-1} \tilde{P}^t \Delta$, and $\tilde{P} = [\mathbf{p}(1), \mathbf{p}(2)]$ is composed of two principle components $\mathbf{p}(1)$ and $\mathbf{p}(2)$ corresponding to the first two largest eigenvalues, $\lambda(1)$ and $\lambda(2)$ in the PCA analysis.[31]

(3) Starting now with the two dimensional space, ICA is used to estimate the melanin and hemoglobin components from the two dimensional density vectors. To simplify the ICA computation the vectors $\mathbf{w}_{x,y}$ are *whitened* to have zero mean and unit variance.[32] The whitened value $\mathbf{e}_{x,y}$ is given by:

$$\begin{aligned}\mathbf{e}_{x,y} &= \tilde{\Lambda}^{-\frac{1}{2}}[\mathbf{w}_{x,y} - \bar{\mathbf{w}}] \\ &= \tilde{\Lambda}^{-\frac{1}{2}}\tilde{P}^t C[\mathbf{q}'_{x,y} - (\tilde{P}^t C)^{-1}\bar{\mathbf{w}}] \\ &= H\mathbf{s}_{x,y} \end{aligned} \tag{9}$$

where $\tilde{\Lambda} = \mathrm{diag}[\lambda(1), \lambda(2)]$ and $\bar{\mathbf{w}}$ is the mean vector of $\mathbf{w}_{x,y}$ taken over all the coordinates in the image. $H = \tilde{\Lambda}^{-\frac{1}{2}}\tilde{P}^t C$ is a separation matrix, and $\mathbf{s}_{x,y} = [s_{x,y}(1), s_{x,y}(2)]^t = \mathbf{q}'_{x,y} - (\tilde{P}^t C)^{-1}\bar{\mathbf{w}}$, where $s_{x,y}(1)$ and $s_{x,y}(2)$ are independent of each other and represent the source *signal* $\mathbf{w}_{x,y}$.
What we want now is an estimate of the synthesised skin color $\tilde{I}_{x,y}$ from the independent melanin and hemoglobin components $\tilde{C} = [c^{\mathrm{m}}, c^{\mathrm{h}}]$. We use the separation matrix H and the source signals $\mathbf{s}_{x,y}$ to estimate $\tilde{C}$ and consequently $\tilde{I}_{x,y}$: The pure density matrix $\tilde{C}$ can be estimated from the separation matrix $H = \tilde{\Lambda}^{-\frac{1}{2}}\tilde{P}^t C$ as $\tilde{C} = (\tilde{\Lambda}^{-\frac{1}{2}}\tilde{P}^t)^{-1}H$. The quantities of pigments from Eq. (6) can now be estimated as $\tilde{\mathbf{q}}_{x,y} = \tilde{C}^{-1}\mathbf{l}_{x,y} - \mathbf{d}$ where $\mathbf{d}$ is given by $\tilde{C}^{-1}\Delta$. Our problem however, is that Δ is unknown but assuming that the smallest value of $\tilde{\mathbf{q}}_{x,y}$ is zero, which we can do because of the whitening process performed earlier, we have $\mathbf{d} = \min_{x,y}(\tilde{C}^{-1}\mathbf{l}_{x,y})$.

(4) The melanin and hemoglobin quantities of a skin color can now be derived by using the skin color model below:

$$\tilde{\mathbf{l}}_{x,y} = \tilde{C}(K\tilde{\mathbf{q}}^t_{x,y} + j\mathbf{d}) + j\Delta \tag{10}$$

where $\tilde{\mathbf{l}}_{x,y}$ is the *synthesised skin color* based on the melanin and hemoglobin components. K and j are introduced synthesis parameters. The spatial effect can be removed by setting $j = 0$ and setting $K = \mathrm{diag}[1, 0]$ the color intensity $\tilde{\mathbf{l}}^m_{x,y}$ of the melanin component is obtained and setting $K = \mathrm{diag}[0, 1]$ the color intensity $\tilde{\mathbf{l}}^h_{x,y}$ of the hemoglobin component is obtained. Transforming $\tilde{\mathbf{l}}^m_{x,y}$ and $\tilde{\mathbf{l}}^h_{x,y}$ from the optical density domain back into the RGB color space, we have:

$$\tilde{I}^m_{x,y} = \exp(-\tilde{\mathbf{l}}^m_{x,y}) \quad \tilde{I}^h_{x,y} = \exp(-\tilde{\mathbf{l}}^h_{x,y}) \tag{11}$$

where $\tilde{I}^m_{x,y}$ and $\tilde{I}^h_{x,y}$ are the estimated color intensities of the melanin component and the hemoglobin component in the RGB color space respectively.

3.3. *Erythema Pixel Extraction*

After decomposing skin color into independent components, erythema pixels can be separated from non-erythema pixels by using the hemoglobin and melanin component color intensities. Thus, we have a binary classification problem for which we use an SVM.

In this section, an SVM is used to perform the classification. The reason for using an SVM classifier is that its performance is shown to be quite promising.[33–35] SVMs are attractive because they are able to linearise non-linear classification problems through the use of the kernel trick[36] where data points are embedded into a high dimensional space where the decision rule can be linearised. SVMs classify by deriving a hyperplane in feature space that separates the data points into separate classes. An optimum hyperplane is the one with the largest distance between the hyperplane and the closet data points on each side of the hyperplane in feature space.

Suppose that we have a training set $\mathcal{T}$:

$$\mathcal{T} = \{(\mathbf{v}_1, \alpha_1), \ldots (\mathbf{v}_i, \alpha_i), \ldots (\mathbf{v}_n, \alpha_n)\}, \quad \mathbf{v}_i \in \Re^6, \alpha_i \in \{-1, 1\} \tag{12}$$

where if $\alpha_i = -1$, $\mathbf{v}_i$ is the feature vector for an erythema pixel, and if $\alpha_i = 1$, $\mathbf{v}_i$ is the feature vector of a non-erythema pixel. Let n is the number of training samples.

The objective function of the SVM determines a hyperplane with the equation $h(\mathbf{v}) = \boldsymbol{\omega}^t \mathbf{v} + b = 0$, intercept b and normal vector $\boldsymbol{\omega}$ such that b and $\boldsymbol{\omega}$ can be determined from the training samples by solving a minimisation problem:

$$\begin{aligned} \text{minimise} \quad & \frac{1}{2}\boldsymbol{\omega}^t \boldsymbol{\omega} + c\sum_{i=1}^{n} \xi_i \\ \text{subject to} \quad & \alpha_i(\boldsymbol{\omega}^t \phi(\mathbf{v}_i) + b) \geq 1 - \xi_i, \quad i = 1, 2, \ldots, n \\ & \xi_i \geq 0, \quad i = 1, 2, \ldots, n \end{aligned} \tag{13}$$

The variables ξ_i are slack variables that allow some data points to be misclassified by the hyperplane, c is an error tolerance constant that controls the tolerance of the slack variables, and $\phi(\cdot)$ is a *mapping function* that maps training samples to a higher dimensional space. A Gaussian radial basis function[30] is used in our algorithm because of its simplicity and its computational efficiency:

$$K(F_{x',y'}, F_{x,y}) = \exp\{-\gamma \| F_{x',y'} - F_{x,y} \|^2\} \tag{14}$$

where $\gamma > 0$, σ is the variance and $\gamma = \frac{1}{2\sigma^2}$.

4. Segmenting Psoriasis Symptoms: Scaling

The appearance of scaling varies with different psoriatic lesions. It typically appears as white or creamy colored scales on regions of red and inflamed skin (erythema), but can also appear in isolation without the accompanying erythema. When psoriasis appears without the accompanying erythema, it appears as discernibly white or creamy flakes on normal skin. Scaling can present as small spots or as patches scattered within erythema. Moreover, the color of scaling may be very similar to that of normal skin, especially if the skin is fair, making it difficult to differentiate between scaling and normal skin using color alone. However, the rough textured surface of scaling is markedly different from normal skin.

The algorithm presented in this chapter uses a feature space derived from both color and texture to identify scaling pixels. There are two stages in the algorithm: (1) the algorithm first analyses skin color and skin texture using the L*a*b* color space and a bank of Gabor filters to create a feature space for the image; (2) the algorithm next removes erythema pixels from consideration and resamples the image to collect training samples for the classification process. The segmentation is achieved by using a combination of an MRF and the hyperplane derived from an SVM.[37]

4.1. *Developing the Feature Space for the Detection of Scaling*

4.1.1. *Scaling contrast map for enhancing the contrast between scaling and surrounding erythema*

A scaling contrast map is developed to enhance the contrast between scaling and erythema, especially in situations where scaling is scattered in erythema and is hard to discern visually. The L*a*b* color space is used to develop a pair of multi-scale centre-surround filters that increases the contrast between scaling and normal skin.

In the L*a*b* color space, the color distance is linearised for the perception of color difference. The L^* dimension specifies lightness where an L^* value of 0 is black and an L^* value of 100 is a diffuse white. The a^* dimension is the red-green dimension, where a positive value of a^* is red and a negative value is green, and the b^* dimension is the blue-yellow dimension, where a positive value of b^* is blue and a negative value is yellow.

The color of scaling correlates well with higher values of L^* and erythema with positive values of a^*. With this in mind a **scaling contrast map** S is defined as the result of multi-scale centre-surround filtering in the L^* and a^*

components:

$$S_{x,y} = J(L^*_{x,y}) + J(\text{inv}(a^*_{x,y})) \tag{15}$$

where $S_{x,y}$ is the value of scaling contrast map S at the image coordinate (x, y), $J(\cdot)$ is a multi-scale centre-surround filter that detects contrast in the specific color component, and $\text{inv}(a^*_{x,y})$ inverts the image in the a^* dimension, which is defined by $\text{inv}(a^*_{x,y}) = \max_{i,j}(a^*_{i,j}) - a^*_{x,y}$, where (i, j) runs through all the coordinates in the image. By inverting the color intensity values of the erythema, the a^* values become lower and the contrast between scaling and any surrounding erythema is enhanced.

The multi-scale centre-surround filter $J(\cdot)$ is now defined by:

$$J(X_{x,y}) = \sum_{s=1}^{3} \left(X_{x,y} - \frac{1}{N} \sum_{\substack{x-w(s)\leq m\leq x+w(s)\\ y-w(s)\leq n\leq y+w(s)}} X_{m,n} \right) \tag{16}$$

where $X_{x,y}$ is the color intensity of the current pixel with coordinate (x, y) and s is the scale. The subtracted term is the average intensity value of the surrounding area with pixel number N. The size of the surrounding area is determined by scale s, $w(s) = \frac{d}{2^s}$, where d is the larger value between the image width and the image height, and the scale s is set to be $s \in \{1, 2, 3\}$.[38]

4.1.2. *Texture analysis with Gabor filters for differentiating rough scaling from normal skin*

The scaling contrast map S behaves well when segmenting scaling from erythema but is not sufficient for segmenting scaling from normal skin, especially when the color difference between the two is small. However, scaling presents as a rough textured surface that distinguishes it from the more smoothly textured normal skin. The rough texture of scaling combined with the scaling contrast map can provide a good combination of features for segmenting scaling.

Gabor filters are used to differentiate rough scaling from smooth normal skin. A 2D Gabor filter is defined as:

$$g(x, y; \gamma, \sigma, \lambda, \psi) = \exp\left(-\frac{x'^2 + \gamma^2 y'^2}{2\sigma^2}\right) \exp\left(i\left(2\pi\frac{x'}{\lambda} + \psi\right)\right)$$
$$x' = x\cos\theta + y\sin\theta$$
$$y' = -x\sin\theta + y\cos\theta \tag{17}$$

where the Gaussian distribution function $\exp(-(x'^2+\gamma^2 y'^2)/2\sigma^2)$ with standard deviation σ and spatial aspect ratio γ is called the envelop, the complex

Table 1. Parameters defining the bank of Gabor filters used for scaling texture analysis.

Spatial frequencies	$1/\lambda$	23, 31, 47 cycles per image
Rotation angles	θ	$0, \frac{\pi}{8}, \frac{\pi}{4}, \frac{3\pi}{8}, \frac{\pi}{2}, \frac{5\pi}{8}, \frac{3\pi}{4}, \frac{7\pi}{8}, \pi$
Phase shift	ψ	0
Spatial aspect ratio	γ	0.5

sinusoidal $\exp(i(2\pi x'/\lambda + \psi))$ with spatial frequency $1/\lambda$ and phase shift ψ is called the carrier, and θ is the rotation angle.

We have the Gabor energy $E_{x,y}$:

$$E_{x,y}^2 = \mathrm{Re}(r_{x,y})^2 + \mathrm{Img}(r_{x,y})^2 \tag{18}$$

Where $r_{x,y}$ is the response of a Gabor filter. We use the square of the Gabor energy, because it is better in accentuating the differences between scaling and normal skin than the more commonly used Gabor energy. Since the variations in the textures of scaling and normal skin in different lesions and people make the choice of one single Gabor filter unlikely, the algorithm uses a bank of 24 Gabor filters designed to respond well in a variety of skin and scaling texture conditions. Parameters for the Gabor filters are shown in Table 1.

A Gabor texture image is constructed with the purpose of covering the responses of the Gabor filters whose spatial frequencies and rotation angles are between the selected ones in Table 1. The technique given in Ref. [39] is applied, that filters the square of Gabor energy image using hyperbolic tangent and mean filters subsequently, and sums the flittering outputs over all of the rotation angles and frequencies of the Gabor filters.

4.2. *Semi-supervised Scaling Segmentation*

The second stage of the algorithm segments scaling from 2D skin images through a semi-supervised algorithm to ensure the invariance of segmentation to scaling and skin changes from different patients. This part of the algorithm implements a three step process: (1) the scaling contrast map is applied to threshold out all dark pixels representing darker pigments in the skin and including erythema, hair, moles and other blemishes; (2) a training set for the scaling classifier is extracted from the image, and is composed of pixels that are highly likely to be scaling and pixels that are highly likely to be normal skin; (3) the pixels are classified using an SVM defined by the training set and the resulting image smoothed using an MRF.

4.2.1. *Removing erythema and other dark pixels*

The first step is to threshold out the dark pixels representing erythema, hair, moles and other blemishes in the scaling contrast map S. Scaling and normal skin pixels remain in consideration after the application of the contrast map because they result in a significantly high value of S. We define a binary image M by:

$$M_{x,y} = \begin{cases} 1 & \text{if } S_{x,y} \geq t_s \\ 0 & \text{otherwise} \end{cases} \tag{19}$$

where t_s is the threshold value. Pixels labelled with 1 including scaling and normal skin are retained for further analysis. Pixels labelled with 0 denote darker pigments. Besides erythema, hair, moles and other blemishes are removed from further consideration by the thresholding. This step changed the scaling segmentation problem into a binary classification problem. In the following steps, a classifier is designed to differentiate scaling from normal skin.

4.2.2. *Collecting training samples for segmenting scaling from normal skin*

Since there is a great deal of variation in skin colors and psoriasis lesions, a generic set of training data is unlikely to yield good classification results. Our algorithm gathers the training data needed from the image being analysed. Training data is collected by identifying the regions of scaling and normal skin using the position of erythema, which is often found between scaling and normal skin. Collecting training data proceeds with three steps:

(1) First, the erythema location is approximately localised based on the scaling contrast map. A rough segmentation of erythema, but one that serves our purposes, can be obtained through a threshold method:

$$X_{x,y} = \begin{cases} 1 & \text{if } S_{x,y} \leq 0.2 \min_{i,j} S_{i,j} \\ 0 & \text{otherwise} \end{cases} \tag{20}$$

where X is a binary image, which indicates location of erythema with value '1' and other objects with value '0'. The threshold value is determined empirically, based on the fact that erythema would show negative values in the scaling contrast map, and the values would still be lower than darkened normal skin. It is noted that not all the erythema can be identified, but normal skin and scaling are not included in the identified erythema locations.

Algorithm 1 An algorithm to extract a sample of scaling pixels and a sample of normal skin pixels from an image.

Input: The initial location of the erythema X and image M.

Output: Regions of candidate scaling L_{scaling} pixels and regions of candidate skin L_{skin} pixels.

$n \leftarrow 0$
repeat
    $X \leftarrow X \oplus U$
    $n \leftarrow n + 1$
    if an enclosed region is formed in X **then**
        $X \leftarrow \text{FloodFill}(X)$
    end if
until no more enclosed regions are formed
$L_{\text{Scaling}} \leftarrow M_{x,y} \cap X_{x,y} \ominus nU$
$L_{\text{Skin}} \leftarrow M_{x,y} \cap X^{C}_{x,y}$
return: L_{Scaling}, L_{Skin}

(2) Second, using the location of erythema, areas of potential scaling and normal skin pixel samples are identified with a series of morphological operations. The algorithm given in Algorithm 1 describes the process. The input is a binary image X, that is given by Eq. (20). The algorithm returns two sets of pixels, the set of possible scaling pixels L_{scaling} and the set of possible skin pixels L_{skin}.

(3) Third, a soft-constrained k-means clustering is used to identify candidate training regions of scaling and normal skin from the potential samples L_{scaling} and L_{skin}. The soft-constrained k-means adapted the traditional k-means by putting weights in the clustering process, that are related with the probabilities of a pixel belonging to scaling and normal skin classes. It is assumed that pixels in the potential scaling location have a higher probability of being scaling than normal skin. A similar assumption holds for pixels in the potential skin locations. A cluster of scaling pixels C_1 and a cluster of skin pixels C_2 are formed by using the soft-constrained k-means clustering, and then within each of these clusters the pixels with the greater likelihood of being scaling and normal skin are chosen.

Let $F_{x,y}$ be an element of the scaling feature set F_{scaling}, that is composed of a scaling contrast map and Gabor texture, at location (x, y). The objective function for the soft-constrained k-means is defined as the sum of the weighted distances of a sample to each of the cluster centroids:

$$h(\mathcal{C},\mathcal{O}) = \sum_{i=1}^{2} \sum_{(x,y)\in C_i} W(L_{x,y}, C_i)\|F_{x,y} - \mathcal{O}_i\|^2 \tag{21}$$

where $\mathcal{O} = (\mathcal{O}_1, \mathcal{O}_2)$ is the pair of centroids for the clusters $\mathcal{C} = (C_1, C_2)$, and $\|\cdot\|$ is the Euclidean norm. The weight $W(L_{x,y}, C_i) = P(L_{x,y}, C_i)^{-1}$, where $P(L_{x,y}, C_i)$ is the probability that a pixel with location $L_{x,y}$ is in the class C_i. If $L_{x,y}$ is in a region that indicates the same class as C_i, the probability is assigned a higher value, and otherwise is assigned a lower value. Note that the equality $P(L_{x,y}, C_1) + P(L_{x,y}, C_2) = 1$ must hold.
The objective function $h(\mathcal{C}, \mathcal{O})$ is minimised. The centroid for each of the two clusters can be obtained by setting the first-order partial derivative with respect to the centroid to be zero. The centroid is given by:

$$\mathcal{O}_i = \frac{\sum_{(x,y)\in C_i} W(L_{x,y}, C_i) F_{x,y}}{\sum_{(x,y)\in C_i} W(L_{x,y}, C_i)} \tag{22}$$

A partitioning of the feature set into those that are closer to $\mathcal{O}_1$ and those that are closer to $\mathcal{O}_2$ with respect to the weighted distance now occurs. The minimum of the objective function $h(\mathcal{C},\mathcal{O})$ is achieved by iteration of Eq. (22) and the partitioning of the feature set until the clusters converge. The training set T_i for the class C_i is taken to be those samples $F_{x,y}$ in the image such that:

$$\frac{W(L_{x,y}, C_i)\|F_{x,y} - \mathcal{O}_i\|^2}{W(L_{x,y}, C_j)\|F_{x,y} - \mathcal{O}_j\|^2} \leq t_h \tag{23}$$

where $j = 2$ if $i = 1$ and $j = 1$ if $i = 2$. The threshold $t_h = 0.1$ ensures that training samples have a high likelihood of being within their respective classes.

4.2.3. *Identifying scaling pixels*

After the training sets for scaling and normal skin are identified, we again have a classification problem for which an SVM is well-suited. The problem however, is that a purely pixel-based classification method does not perform well when scaling is directly adjacent to normal skin. In such cases, the classification of a pixel more often depends on the neighbourhood of the pixel than on clear distinctions in feature space. MRFs are formulated with precisely this kind of problem in mind.[40] Our strategy for identifying scaling is to define an MRF where the probability of a pixel being scaling or normal skin depends on the distance from the hyperplane of an SVM of the pixels in its neighbourhood.

An MRF[40] is an undirected graph $(\mathcal{S}, \mathcal{E})$ that models joint probability distributions. Each site $(x, y) \in \mathcal{S}$ is associated with a random variable and each edge models conditional dependencies. The *neighbourhood* $N_{x,y}$ of a site $(x, y) \in \mathcal{S}$ is the set of nodes adjacent to (x, y) in the graph.

Now let $A = \{A_{x,y}|M_{x,y} = 1\}$ be the set of scaling features for all pixels classified as non-erythema pixels using Eq. (19). Each $A_{x,y} \in A$ is a vector consisting the values of the scaling contrast map and Gabor textures at the coordinate (x, y). Further, let $\omega = \{\omega_{x,y}|(x, y) \in S\}$ be a labelling of the pixels in S using the features in A where each $\omega_{x,y} \in$ {scaling, skin}. The labelling ω is a segmentation and can also be considered as an MRF.

In the context of an MRF, we would like to know the probability of a labelling ω given the features in A, that is, $P(\omega|A)$. According to the Bayesian interpretation

$$P(\omega|A) = \frac{P(A|\omega)P(\omega)}{P(A)} \tag{24}$$

Maximum a posteriori (MAP) estimation theory[30] is the mathematical tool most commonly used to estimate ω with maximum likelihood. To this end, we wish to maximise the objective function:

$$\omega = \text{argmax} P(A|\omega)P(\omega) \tag{25}$$

where we assume that the feature variables are conditionally independent of the class labels. Now, $P(A|\omega)$ can be expressed in terms of the individual pixels:

$$P(A|\omega) = \prod_{x,y} P(A_{x,y}|\omega_{x,y}) \tag{26}$$

The usual assumption in image processing is that the individual terms of the likelihood $P(A_{x,y}|\omega_{x,y})$ have a Gaussian distribution. However, in our case this is a strong assumption. Instead, we first classify the pixels using an SVM and then use the distance between a pixel and the separating hyperplane to derive a likelihood function for the MRF. Thus, pixels that are a long way from the hyperplane are assigned a high probability of being either skin pixels or scaling pixels. Pixels that are close to the SVM hyperplane, such as those where scaling and normal skin are directly adjacent are assigned a much lower probability [see Eq. (27)]. Pixels that are close to the hyperplane are classified according to the neighbourhood in which they are located using a MRF.

We define the probability of a single pixel $P(A_{x,y}|\omega_{x,y})$ to be:

$$P(A_{x,y}|\omega_{x,y}) = \begin{cases} \dfrac{1}{1+\exp(-d(A_{x,y}))} & \text{if } a_{x,y} = \omega_{x,y} \\ \dfrac{\exp(-d(A_{x,y}))}{1+\exp(-d(A_{x,y}))} & \text{otherwise} \end{cases} \quad (27)$$

where $a_{x,y}$ is the classification result from the SVM (either skin or scaling), and $d(A_{x,y})$ measures the distance of the feature $A_{x,y}$ to the hyperplane of the classifying SVM. The distance $d(A_{x,y})$ is given by:

$$\begin{aligned} d(A_{x,y}) &= |\mathbf{w} \cdot \phi(A_{x,y}) + b| \\ &= \left| \sum_{x',y'} a_{x',y'} \lambda_{x',y'} K(F_{x',y'}, A_{x,y}) + b \right| \end{aligned} \quad (28)$$

where $\lambda_{x',y'}$ is a Lagrange multiplier,[30] and $K(\cdot,\cdot)$ is the kernel function. The SVM used in the initial scaling segmentation is similar to that used in Section 3 with the same radial basis function.

We also need to calculate the prior $P(\omega)$. The prior is assumed to be an MRF where the underlying graph of the field is a regular grid. The probability of a labelling ω can be expressed in terms of an energy function over cliques in the underlying graph.[41] We wish to capture homogeneous regions in the image which is achieved here by using pairs of connected vertices. The prior is then given:

$$P(\omega) = \frac{1}{Z} \exp\left(-\sum_{x,y} \sum_{x',y' \in N_{x,y}} V(\omega_{x,y}, \omega_{x',y'}) \right) \quad (29)$$

where $N_{x,y}$ is an 8-connected neighbourhood, and (x', y') is the coordinate of a pixel in the neighbourhood $N_{x,y}$. In particular, the energy function $V(\omega_{x,y}, \omega_{x',y'})$ is defined between pairs of pixels that are adjacent in $N_{x,y}$. The energy function $V(\omega_{x,y}, \omega_{x',y'})$ is here given by:

$$V(\omega_{x,y}, \omega_{x',y'}) = \begin{cases} k \cdot \exp(\|A_{x,y} - A_{x',y'}\|) & \text{if } \omega_{x,y} \neq \omega_{x',y'} \\ 0 & \text{otherwise} \end{cases} \quad (30)$$

where k is a penalty constant and is experimentally chosen to be 4. $V(\omega_{x,y}, \omega_{x',y'})$ gives the probability of observing the features of the pixel $A_{x,y}$ given the features at a neighbouring pixel $A_{x',y'}$. The probability is higher for homogeneous regions and lower for heterogenous regions. Furthermore, higher penalty values are assigned if neighbouring pixels with different labels show a larger difference of the feature values.

5. Experimental Results

5.1. *Erythema Segmentation*

The performance of the SVM-based classifier is tested on 100 images. The set included images with a variety of skin colors, different severities of erythema and scaling and various lighting conditions. The image set was divided into a 40-image training set, where 150000 erythema pixels and 170000 non-erythema pixels are extracted, and a testing set consisting of the remaining 60 images. The LIBSVM library is used to build the SVM classifier.[42] The error tolerance is set to $c = 1000$ and the parameter of the Radial Basis Function kernel $\sigma^2 = 5$ in this research. The parameters σ and c is determined through a "grid-search" with cross-validation.[42]

The performance of the SVM-based method is compared with a nearest neighbour classification method. In Ref. [43], the nearest neighbour classification is used to segment vitiligo, a skin depigmented disorder due to a lack of melanin, from normal skin by building on the decomposition of skin into the melanin and hemoglobin components. The method used in Ref. [43] is amended by calculating the Euclidean distance of color vectors in hemoglobin skin images to separate erythema from healthy skin, since erythema is accompanied by an increase of hemoglobin pigment.

Figure 4 shows the experimental results of a subset of images. Observe that the SVM-based method is able to segment more erythema pixels with minor severity degree than the nearest neighbour classification method.

Table 2 shows the sensitivity and specificity of our proposed algorithm together with the nearest neighbour classification method used in Ref. [43]. Even though the nearest neighbour classification method has a higher specificity value, the SVM-based method shows a higher sensitivity value. In dermatology, the requirement is to have a higher sensitivity than other metrics, so that the progress of a treatment an be presented clearly. The lower specificity of our algorithm is mainly due to shade on the skin or gradually darkening skin. Some moles are misclassified as erythema with both our algorithm and the method in Ref. [43]. This misclassification is because red pigments sometimes appear around moles as shown in the second column of Fig. 4.

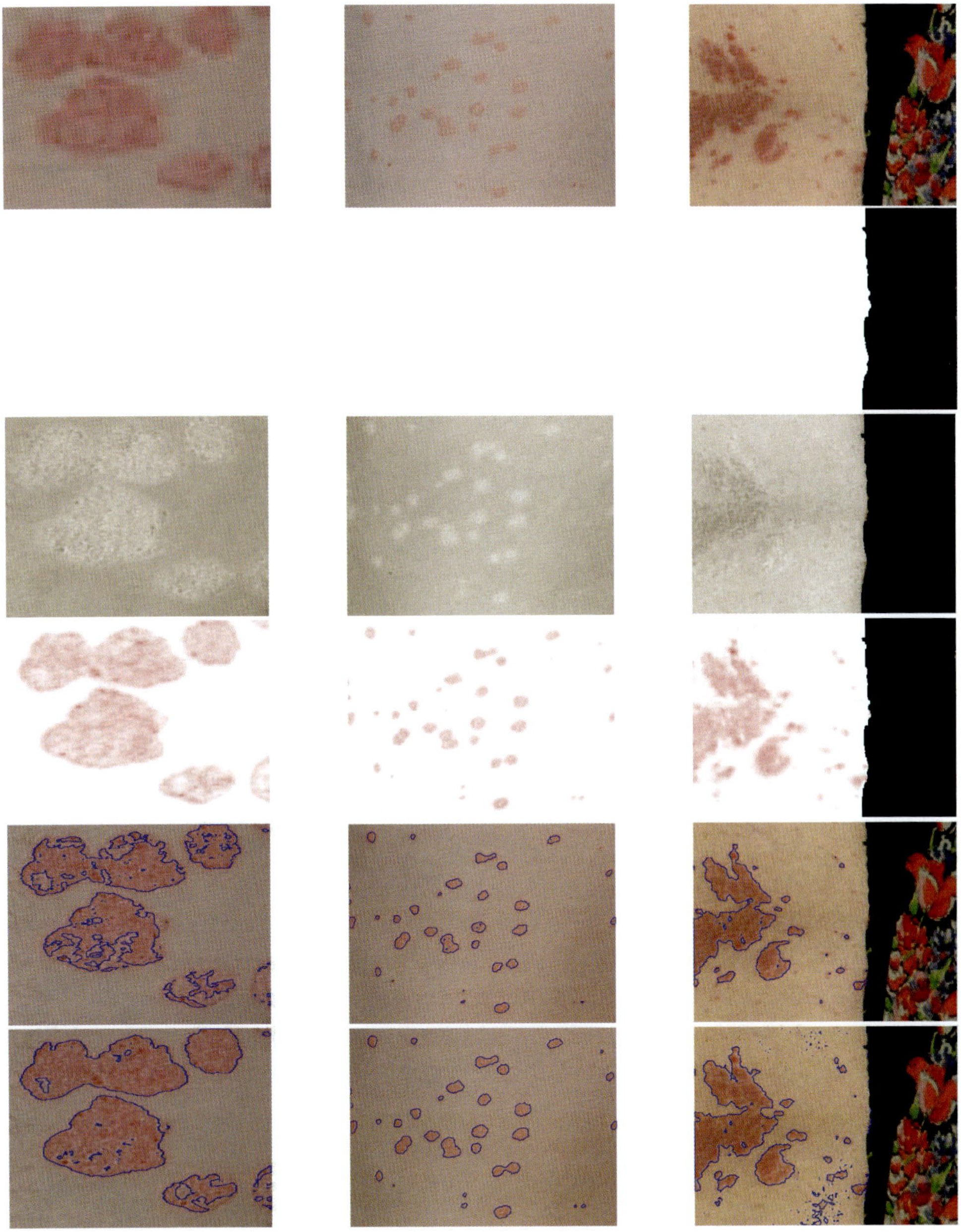

Fig. 4. Examples of the erythema segmentation result. From top to bottom: original image, skin segmentation result, melanin component image, hemoglobin component image, segmentation result with method in Ref. [43] and our segmentation result.

Table 2. Performance of algorithms.

Methods	Sensitivity	Specificity
Methods in[43]	89.41%	85.34%
Our methods with the SVM	95.32%	75.01%

Table 3. Parameters in the soft-constrained k-means procedure.

Parameter	Value
$P\{L_{x,y} \in L_{\text{scaling}}, C_1\}$	0.67
$P\{L_{x,y} \in L_{\text{scaling}}, C_2\}$	0.33
$P\{L_{x,y} \in L_{\text{skin}}, C_1\}$	0.20
$P\{L_{x,y} \in L_{\text{skin}}, C_2\}$	0.80

5.2. *Scaling Segmentation*

The scaling segmentation algorithm has been tested on a set of 103 images, which are collected from a dataset containing 722 psoriasis scaling images. The images were chosen so that there was a good distribution of images taken under different lighting conditions and at different angles, images with shadows, images with wrinkles, and images with hair. The images in each category were randomly selected.

We set the threshold $t_s = 0.004$ for the scaling contrast map in the definition of $M_{x,y}$ [see Eq. (19)] as a balance between removing erythema and retaining scaling. Note that even potential regions of scaling are highly likely to contain areas of normal skin and so the parameter values are chosen to reflect this fact. The parameters used in the soft-constrained k-means procedure are given in Table 3.

We compare the performance of the proposed scaling classifier with a stand alone SVM classifier and a standard MRF as in Ref. [40]. In Ref. [40], the MRF is constructed with the likelihood term of a Gaussian Distribution and with the smoothing term $V(\omega_{x,y}, \omega_{x',y'})$ defined by a Gibbs distribution.

Some examples of the segmentation of scaling are shown in Fig. 5. Observe that our segmentation results are better than the SVM and the MRF for differentiating normal skin from scaling when normal skin is adjacent to psoriatic lesions.

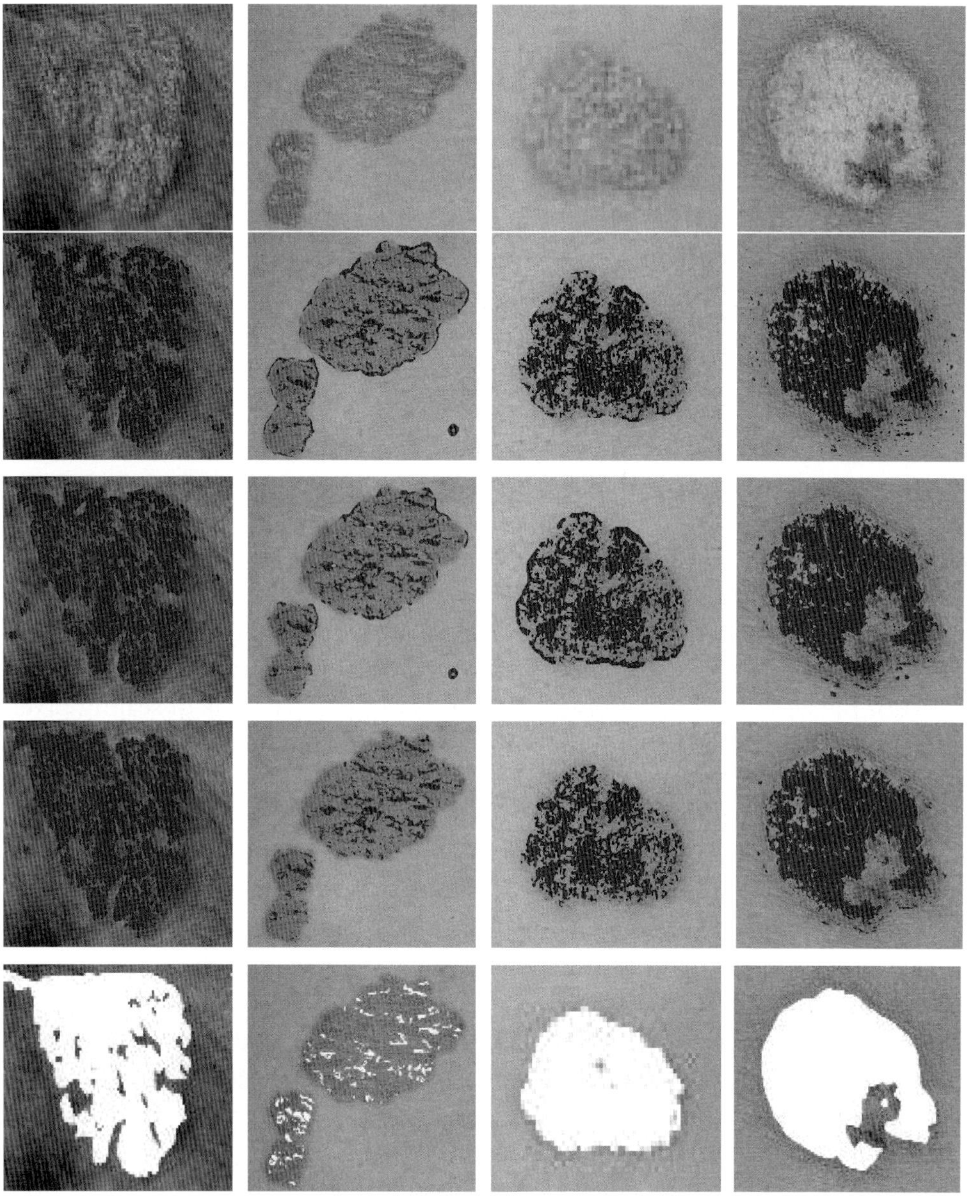

Fig. 5. From top to bottom: original image, SVM segmentation result, MRF segmentation result, our segmentation result, and Ground truth.

Table 4. A comparison of scaling segmentation results with training sets from the soft-constrained k-means.

	Sensitivity	Specificity	Dice
SVM	0.7303	0.8764	0.3817
MRF	0.7638	0.8677	0.3642
Proposed method	0.7229	0.8946	0.4249

Table 4 shows the sensitivity, specificity, and Dice's coefficient of the proposed segmentation method compared with the SVM and a standard MRF. The sensitivity of our proposed method is less clear cut in Table 4 and the sensitivity of our method is very similar to that given by the SVM. The oversegmentation of the MRF method with the Gaussian likelihood function, where some normal skin is also classified as scaling, causes the sensitivity to be the highest in both cases. The differences are in the specificity results. The specificity is higher for our classifier than either SVM or MRF alone, indicating fewer false non-scaling pixels classified as scaling pixels. Moreover, Dice's coefficient is much higher for the combined classifier than either the SVM or the MRF indicating higher similarity between the sets of scaling pixels and non-scaling pixels as found by the combined classifier and the "ground truth."

The robustness of our algorithm is tested against 16 images with wrinkled skin, 29 images with hair, 19 images with shadows, 11 images where the imaging direction has been changed, and 11 image where the illumination is changed. Some examples of the results are shown in Fig. 6.

The evaluation of the 16 images is summarised in Table 5. Dice's coefficient for our method is always higher than the other two classifiers where manually selected training sets are used. In all cases, either sensitivity or specificity for our method is highest as well. The use of the contrast map enables our algorithm to differentiate scaling from shadows, images captured in high illumination and images captured in low illumination. The changes of imaging direction do not affect the segmentation results, even though the lighting condition changes in this situation. In addition, our algorithm shows robustness to wrinkles and skin with short hair. This is the contribution of the Gabor features. The bank of Gabor filters is good at characterising the difference between scaling and wrinkles as well as short hair, due to the use of multiple scales and orientations. However, when the hair is long and clear in the image, our Gabor features fail to suppress the disturbance.

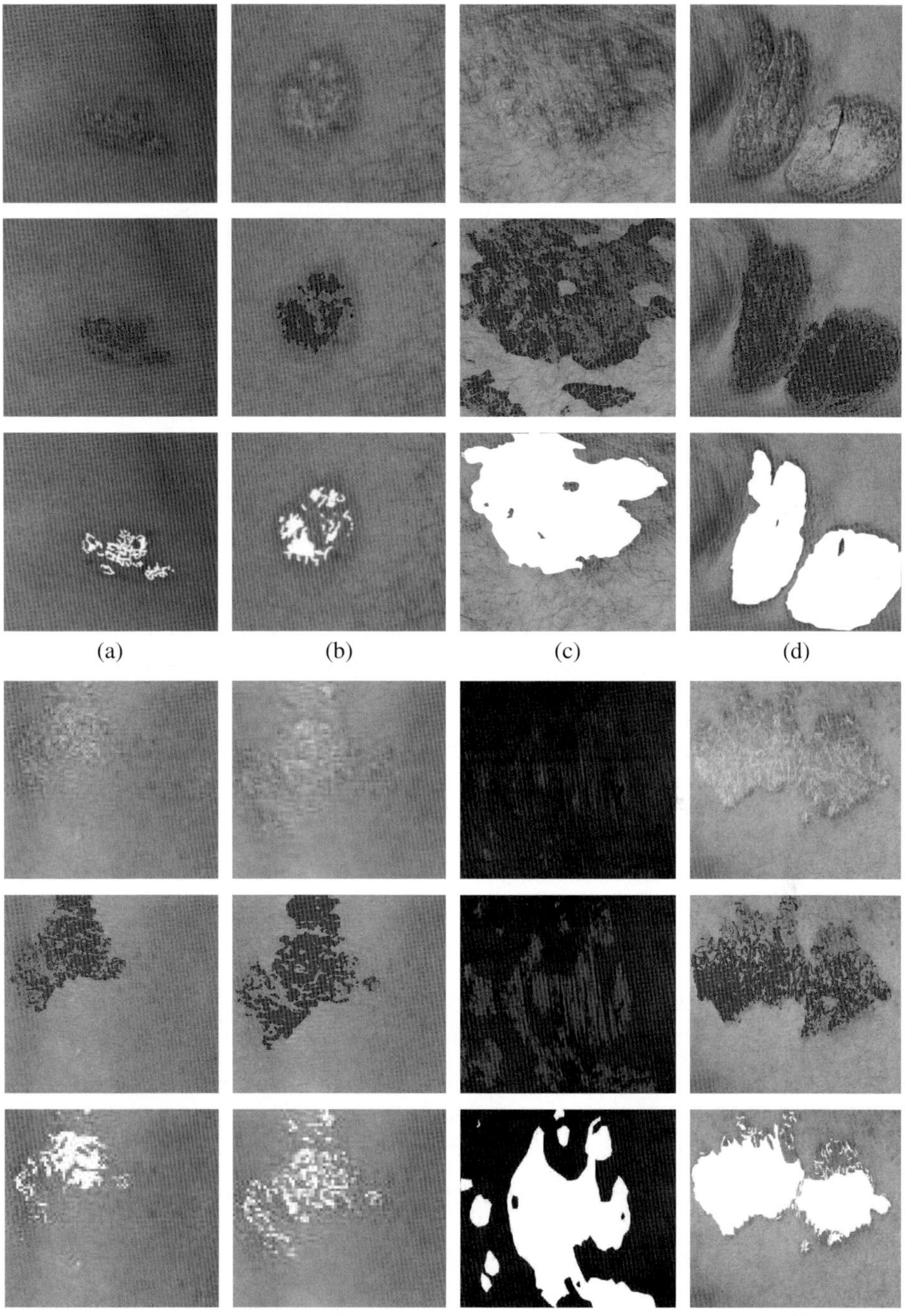

Fig. 6. Segmentation results for a variety of scaling images. The first row in each group is the original image; the second row in each group is our segmentation result; the third row in each group is the ground truth. (a) Image with shadow; (b) Image with short hair; (c) Image with long hair; (d) Image with wrinkled skin; (e) Image captured from a certain angle; (f) Image captured with a different angle from the image in (e); (g) Image with a low illumination; (h) Image with a high illuminance.

Table 5. A comparison of scaling segmentation results for images under a variety of different conditions.

	Sensitivity	Specificity	Dice
Images with shadows			
SVM	0.8048	0.8734	0.4265
MRF	0.8334	0.8502	0.3995
Proposed method	0.8179	0.8707	0.4505
Images with wrinkles			
SVM	0.7303	0.8347	0.5180
MRF	0.7653	0.8019	0.5010
Proposed method	0.7278	0.8849	0.5503
Images with hair			
SVM	0.7334	0.9009	0.4427
MRF	0.7273	0.8426	0.3954
Proposed method	0.7591	0.8769	0.4737
Images about changes of imaging direction			
SVM	0.8264	0.8255	0.3747
MRF	0.7176	0.6444	0.2351
Proposed method	0.8035	0.8855	0.4398
Images about changes of illuminance			
SVM	0.7948	0.8225	0.3291
MRF	0.7370	0.8271	0.2739
Proposed method	0.7830	0.9112	0.4001

6. Discussions and Conclusion

This chapter works on different color spaces to perform the segmentation of psoriasis. This is because of the different properties of segmentation objects. We use the YCbCr color space to separate skin from the background, since the YCbCr color space reduces color redundancy in a RGB color space, and the skin color is compactly clustered in the YCbCr color space. The L*a*b* color space is used in the scaling segmentation. The reason is that the color distance in the L*a*b* color space is linearised for the perception of color difference. The L*a*b* color space is thus good at the description of color difference between scaling and erythema.

In this chapter, we proposed methods for the segmentation of a general psoriatic lesion by separately segmenting erythema and scaling from a psoriasis skin image. We researched on SVM and MRF building on feature analysis of erythema and scaling. The advantage of our proposed method for erythema segmentation is shown by comparing with a nearest neighbour classification method. Our erythema segmentation method is more sensitive to mild erythema. The proposed scaling segmentation method is superior to the SVM alone and the MRF alone, and is good at the segmentation of scaling under different imaging conditions and with different skin types. In the future, more psoriasis images will be collected to validate the performance of the algorithm, and other feature analysis and classification methods will be investigated to improve the segmentation results.

Acknowledgement

We would like to appreciate the Skin & Cancer Foundation, Victoria and St. Vincent Hospital for providing the psoriasis image data set and the assistance in the research.

References

1. K. Doi, "Computer-aided diagnosis in medical imaging: Historical review, current status and future potential," *Comp Med Imaging Graphics* **31**, 198–211 (2007).
2. K. Suzuki, "A review of computer-aided diagnosis in thoracic and colonic imaging," *Quantitative Imaging In Medicine And Surgery* **2**, 163–176 (2012).
3. Q. Abbas, M. Emre Celebi, and I. Fondón, "Computer-aided pattern classification system for dermoscopy images," *Skin Res Techn* **18**, 278–289 (2012).
4. H. Masmoudi, S. Hewitt, N. Petrick, K. Myers, and M. Gavrielides, "Automated quantitative assessment of HER-2/neu immunohistochemical expression in breast cancer," *Medical Imaging, IEEE Trans* **28**, 916–925 (2009).
5. H. S. Javitz, M. M. Ward, E. Farber, L. Nail, and S. G. Vallw, "The direct cost of care for psoriasis and psoriatic arthritis in the united states," *J Am Acad Dermatology* **46**, 850–860 (2002).
6. N. Jenner, J. Campbell, A. Plunkett, and R. Marks, "Cost of psoriasis: A study on the morbidity and financial effects of having psoriasis in Australia," *Aust J Dermatology* **43**, 255–261 (2002).
7. J. F. Fowler, M. S. Duh, L. Rovba, S. Buteau, L. Pinheiro, F. Lobo, J. Sung, J. J. Doyle, A. Swensen, D. A. mallett, and G. Kosicki, "The impact of psoriasis on health care costs and patient work loss," *J Am Acad Dermatology* **59**, 772–780 (2008).
8. E. Puzenat, V. Bronsard, S. Prey, P. Gourraud, S. Aractingi, M. Bagot, B. Cribier, P. Joly, D. Jullien, M. Le Maitre, C. Paul, M. Richard-Lallemand, J. Ortonne, and F. Aubin, "What are the best outcome measures for assessing plaque psoriasis severity? a systematic review of the literature," *J Eur Acad Dermatology Venereology* **2**, 10–16 (2010).
9. L. Savolainen, J. Kontinen, J. Röning, and A. Oikarinen, "Application of machine vision to assess involved surface in patients with psoriasis," *Brit J Dermatology* **137**, 395–400 (1997).

10. J. Röing, R. Jacques, and J. Kontinen, "Area assessment of psoriatic lesions based on variable thresholding and subimage classification," *Vision Interface '99*, (Trois-Riviéres, Canda), 303–311, 19–21 (1999).
11. D. Ihtatho, M. Fadzil, A. Affandi, and S. Hussein, "Area assessment of psoriasis lesion for PASI scoring," *Engineering in Medicine and Biology Society, 2007. EMBS 2007. 29th Annual International Conference of the IEEE* 3446–3449 (2007).
12. D. Ihtatho, M. Ahmad Fadzil, A. Mohd Affandi, and S. Hussein, "Automatic PASI area scoring," *Intelligent and Advanced Systems, 2007. ICIAS 2007. International Conference on* 819–822 (2007).
13. D. Delgado, B. Ersboll, and J. M. Carstensen, "An image based system to automatically and objectively score the degree of redness and scaling in psoriasis lesions," *13th Danish Conference on Image Analysis and Pattern Recognition* 130–137 (2004).
14. J. Taur, "Neuro-fuzzy approach to the segmentation of psoriasis images," *J VLSI Signal Processing* **35**, 19–27 (2003).
15. J. Taur, G. Lee, C. Tao, C. Chen, and C. Yang, "Segmentation of psoriasis vulgaris images using multiresolution-based orthogonal subspace techniques," *Systems, Man, and Cybernetics, Part B: Cybernetics, IEEE Trans* **36**, 390–402 (2006).
16. A. Caliman and M. Ivanovici, "Psoriasis image analysis using color lacunarity," *Optimization of Electrical and Electronic Equipment (OPTIM), 2012 13th International Conference on* 1401–1406 (2012).
17. A. Caliman, M. Ivanovici, and N. Richard, "Fractal feature-based color image segmentation for a healthcare application in dermatology," *E-Health and Bioengineering Conference (EHB) 2011* 1–4 (2011).
18. F. Bogo, M. Samory, A. Fortina, S. Piaserico, and E. Peserico, "Psoriasis segmentation through chromatic regions and geometric active contours," *Engineering in Medicine and Biology Society (EMBC), 2012 Annual International Conference of the IEEE* 5388–5391 (2012).
19. N. Tsumura, H. Haneishi, and Y. Miyake, "Independent compnent analysis of skin color image," *J Optical Soc Am A* **16**, 2169–2176 (1999).
20. J. Lu, J. Manton, E. Kazmierczak, and R. Sinclair, "Erythema detection in digital skin images," *Image Processing (ICIP), 2010 17th IEEE International Conference on* 2545–2548 (2010).
21. R. Chellappa, C. Wilson, and S. Sirohey, "Human and machine recognition of faces: A survey," *Proc IEEE* **83**, 705–741 (1995).
22. M. Yeasin, E. Polat, and R. Sharma, "A multiobject tracking framework for interactive multimedia applications," *Multimedia, IEEE Trans* **6**, 398–405 (2004).
23. S. Kawato and J. Ohya, "Automatic skin-color distribution extraction for face detection and tracking," *Signal Processing Proceedings, 2000. WCCC-ICSP 2000. 5th International Conference on* **2**, 1415–1418 (2000).
24. J. Han, G. Awad, and A. Sutherland, "Automatic skin segmentation and tracking in sign language recognition," *Computer Vision, IET* **3**, 24–35 (2009).
25. L. H. Xuan and S. Nitsuwat, "Face recognition in video, a combination of eigenface and adaptive skin-color model," *Intelligent and Advanced Systems, 2007. ICIAS 2007. International Conference on* 742–747 (2007).
26. R.-L. Hsu, M. Abdel-Mottaleb, and A. Jain, "Face detection in color images," *Pattern Analysis and Machine Intelligence, IEEE Trans* **24**, 696–706 (2002).

27. P. Kakumanu, S. Makrogiannis, and N. Bourbakis, "A survey of skin-color modeling and detection methods," *Pattern Recognition* **40**, 1106–1122 (2007).
28. W.-H. Lai and C.-T. Li, "Skin colour-based face detection in colour images," *Video and Signal Based Surveillance, 2006. AVSS '06. IEEE International Conference on* 56–61 (2006).
29. M. J. Jones and J. M. Rehg, "Statistical color models with application to skin detection," *Int J Comp Vision* **46**, 81–96 (2002).
30. T. Sergios and K. Koutroumbas, *Pattern Recognition*. Academic Press, 4th edition ed. (2009).
31. J. Shlens, "A tutorial on principal component analysis," (2009).
32. A. Hyvärinen and E. Oja, "Independent component analysis: Algorithms and applications," *Neural Networks* **13**, 411–430 (2000).
33. M. E. Mavroforakis, H. V. Georgiou, N. Dimitropoulos, D. Cavouras, and S. Theodoridis, "Mammographic masses characterization based on localized texture and dataset fractal analysis using linear, neural and support vector machine classifiers," *Artificial Intelligence Med* **37**, 145–162 (2006).
34. K. Chan, T.-W. Lee, P. Sample, M. Goldbaum, R. Weinreb, and T. Sejnowski, "Comparison of machine learning and traditional classifiers in glaucoma diagnosis," *Biomed Eng, IEEE Trans* **49**, 963–974 (2002).
35. J. Maroco, D. Silva, A. Rodrigues, M. Guerreiro, I. Santana, and A. de Mendonca, "Data mining methods in the prediction of dementia: a real-data comparison of the accuracy, sensitivity and specificity of linear discriminant analysis, logistic regression, neural networks, support vector machines, classification trees and random forests," *BMC Res Notes* **4**, 299–312 (2011).
36. B. E. Boser, I. M. Guyon, and V. N. Vapnik, "A training algorithm for optimal margin classifiers," *Proceedings of the 5th Annual ACM Workshop on Computational Learning Theory* 144–152 (1992).
37. J. Lu, E. Kazmierczak, J. Manton, and R. Sinclair, "Automatic segmentation of scaling in 2-d psoriasis skin images," *Med Imaging, IEEE Trans* **32**, 719–730 (2013).
38. R. Achanta, F. Estrada, P. Wils, and S. Susstrunk, "Salient region detection and segmentation," *Lecture Notes in Computer Science*, (5008), 66–78 (2008).
39. A. K. Jain and F. Farrokhnia, "Unsupervised texture segmentation using gabor filters," *Pattern Recognition* **24**, 1167–1186 (1991).
40. Z. Kato and T. chuen Pong, "A Markov random field image segmentation model for color textured images," *Image and Vision Computing* **24**, 1103–1114 (2006).
41. S. Li, *Markov Random Field Models in Computer Vision*. Springer-Verlag (1995).
42. C. Chang and C. Lin, *LIBSVM: A library for support vector machines*, 2001. Software available at http://www.csie.ntu.edu.tw/ cjlin/libsvm (2001).
43. M. Ahmad Fadzil, H. Nugroho, S. Norashikin, and H. H. Suraiya, "Assessment of therapeutic response in skin pigment disorder treatment," *Information Technology, 2008. ITSim 2008. International Symposium on* **1**, 1–8 (2008).

Part 2
Image Processing in Medical Imaging

Chapter 8

Classification on Brain Functional Magnetic Resonance Imaging: Dimensionality, Sample Size, Subject Variability and Noise

Jean Honorio

CSAIL, MIT
Cambridge, MA 02139, USA
Email: jhonorio@csail.mit.edu

Our aim in this chapter is to study the conditions for the reasonably good performance of classifiers on brain functional magnetic resonance imaging. We propose a synthetic model for the systematic study of aspects such as dimensionality, sample size, subject variability and noise. Our simulations highlight the key factors that affect generalization accuracy.

1. Introduction

Functional magnetic resonance imaging (fMRI) has become one of the methods of choice for looking at human brain activity. Neural activity is followed by an increase in blood flow and oxygenation in the local vasculature. This phenomenon is called *hemodynamic response* and it is used by fMRI in order to indirectly measure neural activity.

Classification on brain fMRI faces various challenges. fMRI data is three-dimensional and thus, datasets are very highly dimensional. Typical datasets contain tens of thousands of voxels. Due to the cost and time needed in order to capture fMRI along with other imaging modalities and clinical data, the number of available subjects is small. Usually, datasets have only a few tens of subjects. Many datasets also show high subject variability, depending on the nature of the neuropsychological process and task. Additionally, it is well-known that fMRI signal is noisy.

Classification has been used on brain fMRI for two goals: the *prediction of cognitive states* and *group classification*. In the *prediction of cognitive states*,[1–15] the goal is to infer the experimental condition (e.g. calculation vs. reading) that a given subject was undergoing at a given time. In *group classification*,[16–23] the goal is to infer the group membership (e.g. cocaine addicted vs. control) of a given subject.

Besides using all voxels as features,[5,8,10,14] classifiers are also trained with features extracted from the original data. Feature extraction methods can be categorized into two groups. Some of the methods extract features that are a weighted combination from all the available voxels by using different schemes, such as principal component analysis,[6,13,20,21] independent component analysis[16,17,19] and a coarse resolution of the original image.[3] The remaining methods select a subset of voxels by following different criteria, such as most discriminative voxels,[12] most active voxels,[1,2,9,12,15,17,18] searchlight accuracy,[24] mutual information,[11] threshold-split region[22,23] and recursive feature elimination.[4,7]

Several classifiers commonly encountered in the machine learning literature have been proposed for brain fMRI data, such as Gaussian naïve Bayes,[12] k-nearest neighbors,[15] Fisher linear discriminant,[18–20] logistic regression,[14] linear support vector machines,[1,2,4,5,7,8,11–13,15,21] Gaussian support vector machines,[3,6,9] Adaboost,[10] random forests,[16] neural networks[17] and majority voting.[22,23]

Some of the proposed classification frameworks use a predefined set of regions of interest (ROIs).[2,5,10,15,17,19] As noted Ref. [23], a possible drawback in these frameworks is that the practitioner needs either prior knowledge of the underlying neuropsychological process or an additional independent dataset in order to find the set of ROIs. If one selects the set of ROIs from the same dataset (*double dipping*), the significance of the cross-validation results is compromised.[25]

Our goal in this chapter is to study the conditions for the reasonably good performance of linear support vector machines (SVMs) on brain fMRI data. To this end, we propose a synthetic model for the systematic study of aspects such as dimensionality, sample size, subject variability and noise. We believe this study is a first step in understanding the key factors that affect generalization accuracy in brain fMRI data.

We chose to focus on linear SVMs since it has been largely used for group classification as well as the prediction of cognitive states.[1,2,4,5,7,8,11–13,15,21] Other linear classifiers such as the Fisher linear discriminant and logistic regression have also been proposed in the literature.[14,18–20] Besides using all voxels as features,[5,8,10,14] we chose a method that extracts features that are a weighted combination from all the available voxels, namely principal component analysis.[6,13,20,21] We also chose to evaluate a feature extraction method that selects a subset of voxels, namely the most discriminative voxels.[12]

2. Materials and Methods

In this section, we present our synthetic model, its parameters and the procedure for data generation. We also describe the feature extraction methods used in our experiments, as well as the techniques used for estimating the generalization accuracy of the classifiers.

Our synthetic model is based on a number of Gaussian-distributed regions with Gaussian spatially-correlated noise. Despite our simplifying assumptions, we believe our model introduces many intuitions from neuroscience. First, we assume that a number of brain regions are involved in a specific activity, such that their activation level differs between two classes. (Class refers to a group in *group classification* or a experimental condition in the *prediction of cognitive states.*) Second, it is well-known that brain fMRI data contains spatially-correlated noise and that there is high subject variability, and thus we introduce these elements to our model. Finally, our experimental setting assumes high dimensionality of the feature vector and a small number of samples.

For simplicity of presentation, we consider a *one-dimensional* brain. Note that most classification algorithms (including linear SVMs) do not take into account the three-dimensional structure of the data. In fact, voxels are treated as one-dimensional. Our synthetic model has the following parameters:

- the number of original features: F,
- the number of samples per class: S,
- the number of involved brain regions: R,
- the distance between the means of the classes: μ_{signal},
- the variance per class: σ^2_{signal} (both parameters μ_{signal} and σ^2_{signal} allow for modeling subject variability),
- the radius of the involved brain regions: r_{signal},
- the noise variance: σ^2_{noise} and
- the radius of the spatially-correlated noise: r_{noise}.

We generate a complete synthetic dataset with F features and $2S$ samples (each class contains S samples) by using the following procedure:

(1) We select R features from $\{1, \ldots, F\}$ uniformly at random.
(2) For each of the S samples in class $\in \{-1, +1\}$:

   (a) We create an F-dimensional "signal vector" as follows: Each of the R selected features is independently sampled from a Gaussian distribution with mean $+\mu_{\text{signal}}/2$ for class $+1$ ($-\mu_{\text{signal}}/2$ for class -1) and variance σ^2_{signal}. The remaining $F - R$ unselected features are set to zero. After this vector has been created, we smooth it with a Gaussian filter of radius r_{signal} and standard deviation $r_{\text{signal}}/2$. (We normalize the Gaussian filter so that its center has weight 1 and thus, each of the R selected features in the signal vector retains its variance.)

(b) We create an F-dimensional "noise vector" as follows: Each of the F features is independently sampled from a Gaussian distribution with mean zero and variance σ^2_{noise}. After this vector has been created, we smooth it with a Gaussian filter of radius r_{noise} and standard deviation $r_{\text{noise}}/2$. (We normalize the Gaussian filter so that it has unit ℓ_2-norm and thus, each of the F features in the noise vector retains its variance.)

(c) The generated sample is the summation of the "signal vector" from step (2a) the "noise vector" from step (2b).

We used LIBLINEAR[26] in order to train linear SVMs with ℓ_2^2-regularization, hinge loss and soft-margin parameter $C = 1$. Additionally, we use the following feature extraction methods:

- *Original features.* We use the F generated features from the above-described procedure.
- *Principal component analysis (PCA) features.*[6,13,20,21] We perform singular value decomposition of the F original features and use all available components.
- *Most discriminative features.*[12] We first rank each of the F original features independently with a Gaussian classifier and then select the top 100 performing features.

In order to estimate the generalization accuracy of the classifiers, we rely on three different methods:

- *k-fold cross-validation.* We hold out S/k samples in turn while training on the other $S(k-1)/k$ samples. The held out samples are used for measuring the classification accuracy. (We chose $k = 5$.)
- *.632 Bootstrapping.* For each of B independent repetitions, we perform the following procedure. From the S samples in the dataset, we pick S random samples with replacement as training set. (The training set has approximately $0.632\,S$ unique samples.) After training, we measure the classification accuracy for the samples not in the training set. The final estimator is an average between the above quantity and the classification accuracy by using the whole dataset of S samples for training and testing. We refer the interested reader to Ref. [27]. (We chose $B = 5$.)

- *Independent set.* After training in the whole dataset of S samples, we measure the classification accuracy in an independent set of 1000 samples per class.

The latter method is an unbiased estimator which we use only for assessing the quality of the former two biased methods, which are used in practice. Indeed, the independent-set-of-samples method is impractical for most brain fMRI problems.

3. Results

We perform several synthetic experiments in order to analyze the different aspects of brain fMRI data. For each experiment, we change one parameter while keeping the rest of the parameters fixed to a default value. In order to obtain a measure of confidence of the results, we perform 20 repetitions and report error bars at 90% significance level. Next, we show the set of values for each parameter (the default values are in parentheses): $F \in \{500, 1000, 2000, 5000, 10000, 20000, (50000)\}$, $S \in \{10, (20), 50, 100, 200, 500, 1000\}$, $R \in \{1, 2, 3, (4), 5, 6, 7\}$, $\mu_{\text{signal}} \in \{0.5, 1, 1.5, (2), 2.5, 3, 3.5\}$, $\sigma^2_{\text{signal}} \in \{0.05, 0.1, 0.2, 0.5, (1), 2, 5\}$, $r_{\text{signal}} \in \{1, 2, 3, 4, 5, (6), 7\}$, $\sigma^2_{\text{noise}} \in \{0.05, 0.1, 0.2, 0.5, (1), 2, 5\}$ and $r_{\text{noise}} \in \{1, (2), 3, 4, 5, 6, 7\}$. We believe that some of these default values are typically encountered in brain fMRI problems, specifically the number of original features (F), the number of samples per class (S) and the signal-to-noise ratio $\sigma^2_{\text{signal}}/\sigma^2_{\text{noise}}$.

We report the generalization accuracy of linear SVMs with the original features in Fig. 1, with PCA features in Fig. 2 and with the most discriminative features in Fig. 3. Note that k-fold cross-validation is a better estimator than .632 bootstrapping, since it is always closer to the unbiased independent-set-of-samples method. For the three feature extraction methods, generalization accuracy is increasing with respect to the number of samples per class (S), the number of involved brain regions (R), the distance between means of the classes (μ_{signal}) and the radius of the involved brain regions (r_{signal}). Generalization accuracy is also decreasing with respect to the number of original features (F), the variance per class (σ^2_{signal}), the noise variance (σ^2_{noise}) and the radius of the spatially correlated noise (r_{noise}). Although, for the original features as well as PCA features, generalization accuracy does not significantly change with respect to the variance per class (σ^2_{signal}). The behavior with the most discriminative voxels is more pronounced than with the other two feature extraction methods.

Figure 4 shows a comparison of the three feature extraction methods: the original features, PCA features and the most discriminative features. The results with the original features and PCA features are almost equal. In general, the

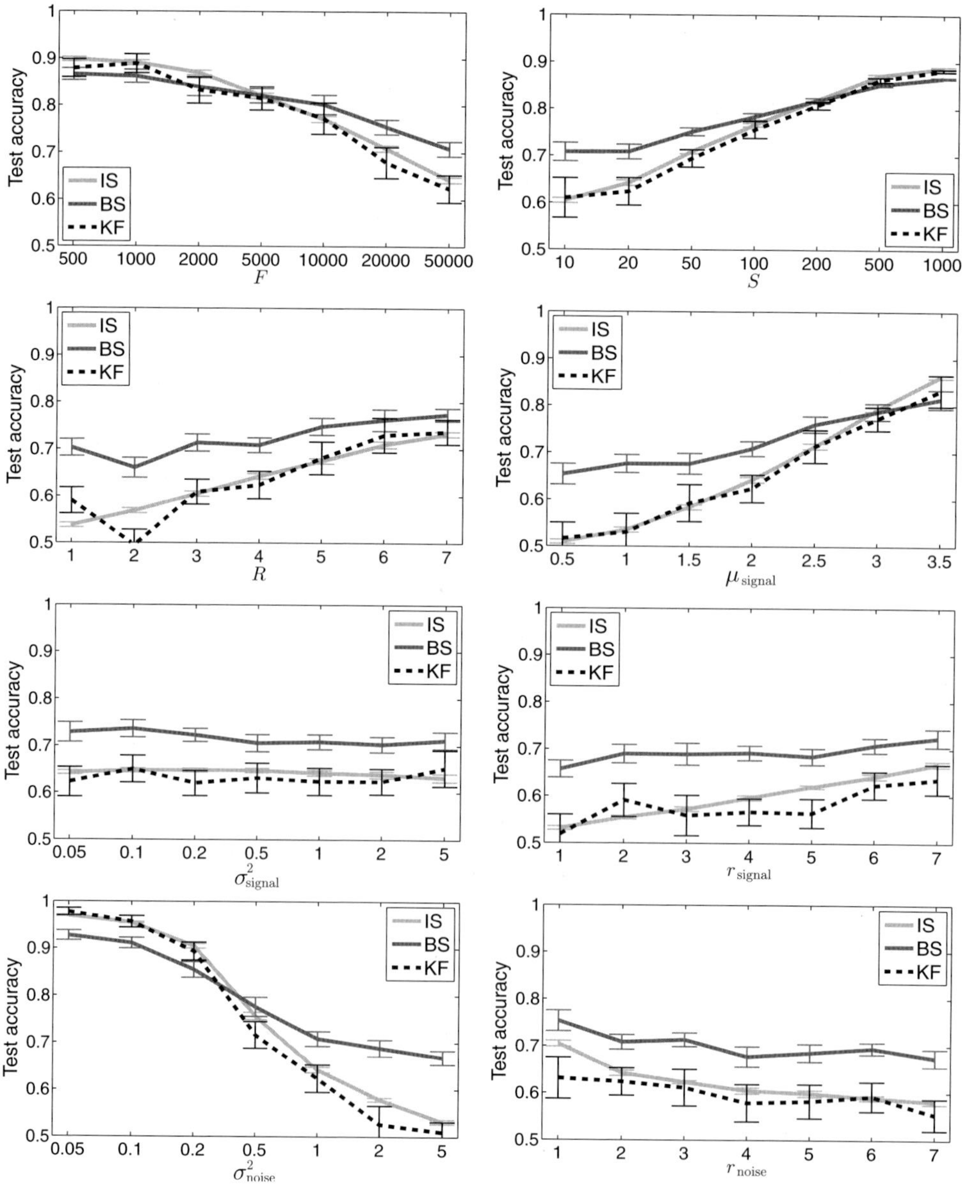

Fig. 1. Generalization accuracy for linear SVMs with the original features, for a different: number of original features (F), number of samples per class (S), number of involved brain regions (R), distance between means of the classes (μ_{signal}), variance per class (σ^2_{signal}), radius of the involved brain regions (r_{signal}), noise variance (σ^2_{noise}) and radius of the spatially correlated noise (r_{noise}). Default values were set to $F = 50000$, $S = 20$, $R = 4$, $\mu_{\text{signal}} = 2$, $\sigma^2_{\text{signal}} = 1$, $r_{\text{signal}} = 6$, $\sigma^2_{\text{noise}} = 1$ and $r_{\text{noise}} = 2$. We also include error bars at 90% significance level. Note that k-fold cross-validation (KS) is a better estimator than .632 bootstrapping (BS), since it is always closer to the unbiased independent-set-of-samples method (IS). Note that generalization accuracy is increasing with respect to S, R, μ_{signal} and r_{signal}. It is also decreasing with respect to F, σ^2_{noise} and r_{noise}. Generalization accuracy does not significantly change with respect to σ^2_{signal}.

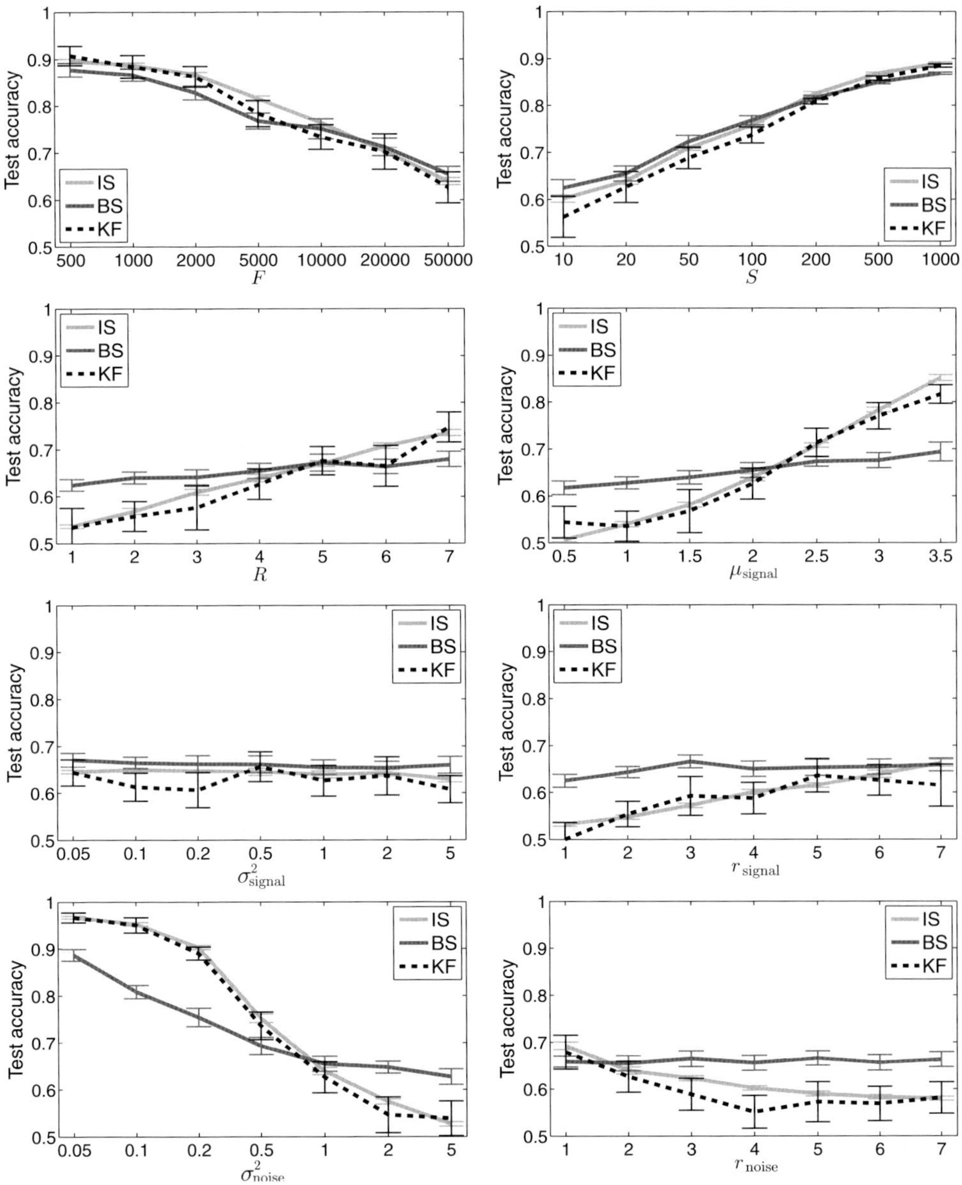

Fig. 2. Generalization accuracy for linear SVMs with PCA features, for a different: number of original features (F), number of samples per class (S), number of involved brain regions (R), distance between means of the classes (μ_{signal}), variance per class (σ^2_{signal}), radius of the involved brain regions (r_{signal}), noise variance (σ^2_{noise}) and radius of the spatially correlated noise (r_{noise}). Default values were set to $F = 50000$, $S = 20$, $R = 4$, $\mu_{\text{signal}} = 2$, $\sigma^2_{\text{signal}} = 1$, $r_{\text{signal}} = 6$, $\sigma^2_{\text{noise}} = 1$ and $r_{\text{noise}} = 2$. We also include error bars at 90% significance level. Note that k-fold cross-validation (KS) is a better estimator than .632 bootstrapping (BS), since it is always closer to the unbiased independent-set-of-samples method (IS). Note that generalization accuracy is increasing with respect to S, R, μ_{signal} and r_{signal}. It is also decreasing with respect to F, σ^2_{noise} and r_{noise}. Generalization accuracy does not significantly change with respect to σ^2_{signal}.

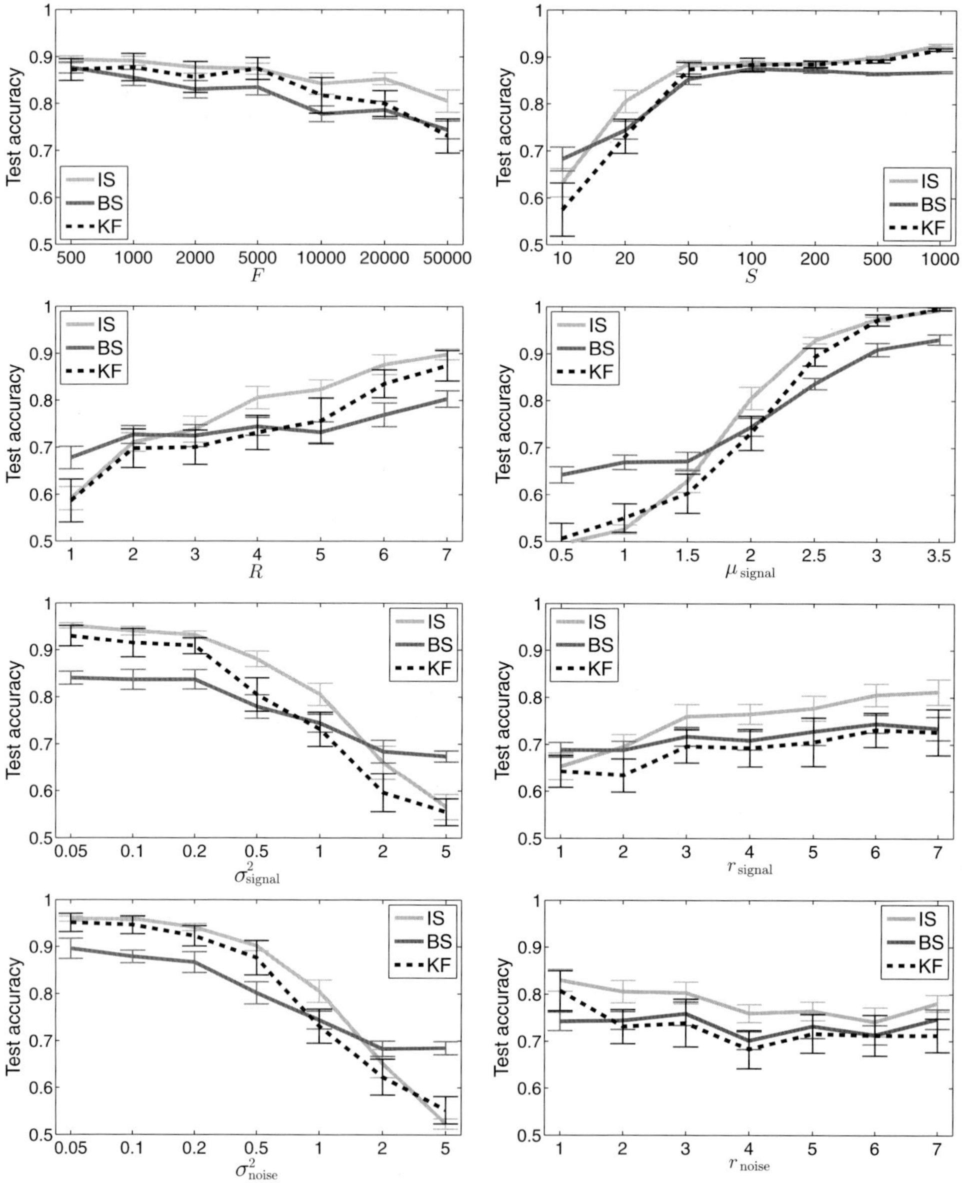

Fig. 3. Generalization accuracy for linear SVMs with the most discriminative features, for a different: number of original features (F), number of samples per class (S), number of involved brain regions (R), distance between means of the classes (μ_{signal}), variance per class (σ^2_{signal}), radius of the involved brain regions (r_{signal}), noise variance (σ^2_{noise}) and radius of the spatially correlated noise (r_{noise}). Default values were set to $F = 50000$, $S = 20$, $R = 4$, $\mu_{\text{signal}} = 2$, $\sigma^2_{\text{signal}} = 1$, $r_{\text{signal}} = 6$, $\sigma^2_{\text{noise}} = 1$ and $r_{\text{noise}} = 2$. We also include error bars at 90% significance level. Note that k-fold cross-validation (KS) is a better estimator than .632 bootstrapping (BS), since it is always closer to the unbiased independent-set-of-samples method (IS). Note that generalization accuracy is increasing with respect to S, R, μ_{signal} and r_{signal}. It is also decreasing with respect to F, σ^2_{signal}, σ^2_{noise} and r_{noise}.

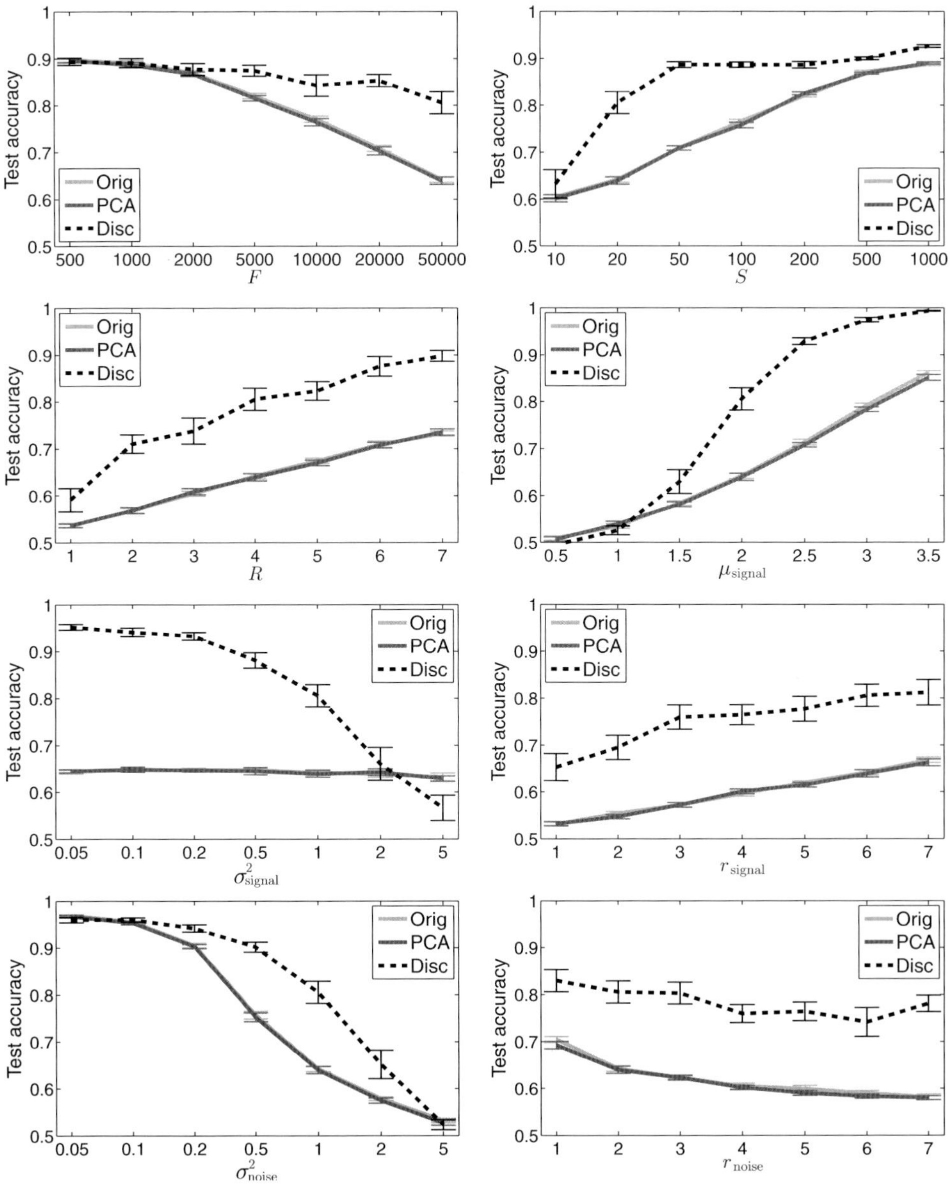

Fig. 4. Generalization accuracy for linear SVMs with the most discriminative features, for a different: number of original features (F), number of samples per class (S), number of involved brain regions (R), distance between means of the classes (μ_{signal}), variance per class (σ^2_{signal}), radius of the involved brain regions (r_{signal}), noise variance (σ^2_{noise}) and radius of the spatially correlated noise (r_{noise}). Default values were set to $F = 50000$, $S = 20$, $R = 4$, $\mu_{\text{signal}} = 2$, $\sigma^2_{\text{signal}} = 1$, $r_{\text{signal}} = 6$, $\sigma^2_{\text{noise}} = 1$ and $r_{\text{noise}} = 2$. We report the unbiased independent-set-of-samples method. We also include error bars at 90% significance level. The results with the original features (Orig) and PCA features (PCA) are almost equal. In general, the results with the most discriminative features (Disc) are significantly better than Orig and PCA.

results with the most discriminative features are significantly better than the other two methods.

4. Discussion

As in many classification tasks, having a small number of discriminative features allows for obtaining good generalization accuracy. Thus, the goal of a practitioner is to decrease the number of features while retaining discriminability. In brain fMRI, we recommend to use methods such as the most discriminative voxels,[12] which obtained significantly better results than using all voxels as features[5,8,10,14] or PCA features.[6,13,20,21] Note that the latter fact is not surprising since the objective of PCA is not to find discriminative features but to best explain the variance in the whole dataset.

In what follows, our observations are mainly with respect to the best performing feature extraction method, i.e. the most discriminative features.

Our experiments suggest that it is recommendable to collect data from at least $S = 50$ samples per class, which allows for obtaining good classification accuracy ($\sim$ 90%). Having more than $S = 50$ samples per class seems to increase generalization accuracy only marginally.

Some aspects of brain fMRI data cannot be controlled since they depend on the nature of the neuropsychological process and task. Among these aspects, we have the number and radius of the involved brain regions (R and r_{signal}) and the subject variability parameters (μ_{signal} and σ^2_{signal}). When there are few involved brain regions or when the brain regions are small, we obtain poor classification accuracies (60–65%). When there are several involved brain regions or when the brain regions are large, we obtain good classification accuracies (80–90%). Additionally, in a regime of *low subject variability*, when the distance between means of the classes (μ_{signal}) is large or when the variance per class (σ^2_{signal}) is small, we obtain almost perfect classification (96–100%). In a regime of *high subject variability*, when the distance between means of the classes (μ_{signal}) is small or when the variance per class (σ^2_{signal}) is high, we obtain very poor classification accuracies (50–56%).

Other aspects of brain fMRI data can be controlled up to some extent. Controlling for the noise variance (σ^2_{noise}) seems far more important than controlling for the amount of spatial-correlatedness of the noise (r_{noise}). Indeed, when the noise variance is small, all the feature extraction methods obtained remarkably good generalization accuracy ($\sim$96%). In this sense, we recommend to take into account the reduction of noise variance when designing neuropsychological tasks as well as when devising proper signal processing methods for the captured data.

5. Concluding Remarks

We chose a reasonable model based on a number of Gaussian-distributed regions with Gaussian spatially-correlated noise, although other more complex synthetic models could have been chosen. Note that it is not possible to know the *true* probabilistic model that generated real-world data, unless we work under the unsatisfiable assumption of having access to infinite data. In practice, only a finite number of samples is available and *objectively* assessing the *level of realism* of a model is not possible. Despite the simplifying assumptions made in our model, we believe it introduces many intuitions from neuroscience. Having said that, we believe that more complex synthetic models that better introduce other neuropsychological aspects will be very beneficial.

We did not include the *leave-one-out* method, where we hold out each of the samples in turn while training on the other $S - 1$ samples. The main reason for excluding this method is that our experimental setting includes training sets of up to $S = 1000$ samples, where leave-one-out is computationally demanding. We preferred to include k-fold cross-validation, since this includes leave-one-out as a specific instance ($k = S$). Moreover, in our experiments, k-fold cross-validation was a good estimator of the generalization accuracy, since it was always close to the unbiased (but impractical) independent-set-of-samples method. Experiments with leave-one-out cross-validation will be of importance, given its use in many studies.

Note that in most experimental settings, the parameters (e.g. number of PCA components, number of most discriminative features, soft-margin parameter C) are selected for each training set by using either a validation set or a nested cross-validation procedure. We chose to keep the parameters fixed for computational reasons. The experimental study of parameter selection will be also beneficial.

While we focused exclusively on generalization accuracy, it is also important to analyze other aspects of feature selection and classification. For instance, it would be interesting to analyze whether the most discriminative features include the R ground-truth involved brain regions, or whether linear SVMs with the original features produce higher weights for the R ground-truth involved brain regions.

References

1. S. Balci, M. Sabuncu, J. Yoo, S. Ghosh, S. Whitfield-Gabrieli, J. Gabrieli, and P. Golland, "Prediction of successful memory encoding from fMRI data," *MICCAI Workshop on Analysis of Functional Medical Images*, 97–104 (2008).

2. D. Cox and R. Savoy, "Functional magnetic resonance imaging (fMRI) "brain reading": Detecting and classifying distributed patterns of fMRI activity in human visual cortex," *NeuroImage* **19**, 261–270 (2003).
3. C. Davatzikos, K. Ruparel, Y. Fan, D. Shen, M. Acharyya, J. Loughead, R. Gur, and D. Langlebenb, "Classifying spatial patterns of brain activity with machine learning methods: Application to lie detection," *NeuroImage* **28**, 663–668 (2005).
4. F. De Martino, G. Valente, N. Staeren, J. Ashburner, R. Goebel, and E. Formisano, "Combining multivariate voxel selection and support vector machines for mapping and classification of fMRI spatial patterns," *NeuroImage* **43**, 44–58 (2008).
5. J. Etzel, V. Gazzola, and C. Keysers, "An introduction to anatomical ROI-based fMRI classification analysis," *Brain Res* **1282**, 114–125 (2009).
6. Y. Fan, D. Shen, and C. Davatzikos, "Detecting cognitive states from fMRI images by machine learning and multivariate classification," *IEEE CVPR Workshop on Mathematical Methods in Biomedical Image Analysis* (2006).
7. S. Hanson and Y. Halchenko, "Brain reading using full brain support vector machines for object recognition: There is no 'face' identification area," *Neural Comput* **20**, 486–503 (2008).
8. S. La Conte, S. Strother, V. Cherkassky, J. Anderson, and X. Hu, "Support vector machines for temporal classification of block design fMRI data," *NeuroImage* **26**, 317–329 (2005).
9. J. Lee, M. Marzelli, F. Jolesz, and S. Yoo, "Automated classification of fMRI data employing trial-based imagery tasks," *Med Image Anal* **13**, 392–404 (2009).
10. M. Martínez-Ramón, V. Koltchinskii, G. Heileman, and S. Posse, "fMRI pattern classification using neuroanatomically constrained boosting," *NeuroImage* **31**, 1129–1141 (2006).
11. V. Michel, C. Damon, and B. Thirion, "Mutual information-based feature selection enhances fMRI brain activity classification," *IEEE International Symposium on Biomedical Imaging*, 592–595 (2008).
12. T. Mitchell, R. Hutchinson, R. Niculescu, F. Pereira, X. Wang, M. Just, and S. Newman, "Learning to decode cognitive states from brain images," *Machine Learning* **57**, 145–175 (2004).
13. J. Mourão-Miranda, A. Bokde, C. Born, H. Hampel, and M. Stetter, "Classifying brain states and determining the discriminating activation patterns: Support vector machine on functional MRI data," *NeuroImage* **28**, 980–995 (2005).
14. S. Ryali, K. Supekar, D. Abrams, and V. Menon, "Sparse logistic regression for whole-brain classification of fMRI data," *NeuroImage* **51**, 752–764 (2010).
15. X. Wang, R. Hutchinson, and T. Mitchell, "Training fMRI classifiers to discriminate cognitive states across multiple subjects," *Neural Inf Process Syst* **16**, 709–716 (2003).
16. A. Anderson, I. Dinov, J. Sherin, J. Quintana, A. Yuille, and M. Cohen, "Classification of spatially unaligned fMRI scans," *NeuroImage* **49**, 2509–2519 (2010).
17. J. Arribas, V. Calhoun, and T. Adali, "Automatic Bayesian classification of healthy controls, bipolar disorder and schizophrenia using intrinsic connectivity maps from fMRI data," *IEEE Transactions on Biomedical Engineering* **57**, 2850–2860 (2010).
18. C. Damon, P. Pinel, M. Perrot, V. Michel, E. Duchesnay, J. Poline, and B. Thirion, "Discriminating between populations of subjects based on fMRI data using sparse feature selection and SRDA classifier," *MICCAI Workshop on Analysis of Functional Medical Images*, 25–32 (2008).

19. O. Demirci, V. Clark, and V. Calhoun, "A projection pursuit algorithm to classify individuals using fMRI data: Application to Schizophrenia," *NeuroImage* **39**, 1774–1782 (2008).
20. J. Ford, H. Farid, F. Makedon, L. Flashman, T. Mc Allister, V. Megalooikonomou, and A. Saykin, "Patient classification of fMRI activation maps," *Med Image Comput Computer Assisted Intervention* **2879**, 58–65 (2003).
21. C. Fu, J. Mourão-Miranda, S. Costafreda, A. Khanna, A. Marquand, S. Williams, and M. Brammer, "Pattern classification of sad facial processing: Toward the development of neurobiological markers in depression," *Biol Psychiatry* **63**, 656–662 (2008).
22. J. Honorio, D. Samaras, D. Tomasi, and R. Goldstein, "Simple fully automated group classification on brain fMRI," *IEEE International Symposium on Biomedical Imaging*, 1145–1148 (2010).
23. J. Honorio, D. Tomasi, R. Goldstein, H.C. Leung, and D. Samaras, "Can a single brain region predict a disorder?" *IEEE Transactions on Medical Imaging* **31**, 2062–2072 (2012).
24. F. Pereira, T. Mitchell, and M. Botvinick, "Machine learning classifiers and fMRI: A tutorial overview," *NeuroImage* **45**, S199–S209 (2009).
25. N. Kriegeskorte, W. Simmons, P. Bellgowan, and C. Baker, "Circular analysis in systems neuroscience: The dangers of double dipping," *Nat Neurosci* **12**, 535–540 (2009).
26. R. Fan, K. Chang, C. Hsieh, X. Wang, and C. Lin, "LIBLINEAR: A library for large linear classification," *J Machine Learning Res* **9**, 1871–1874 (2008).
27. T. Hastie, R. Tibshirani, and J. Friedman, *The Elements of Statistical Learning*, Springer (2001).

Chapter 9

Regression Mixture Modeling for fMRI Data Analysis

V. P. Oikonomou and K. Blekas†*

**School of Business and Economics,
Department of Business Administration,
TEI of Ionian Islands, 31100 Lefkada, Greece
E-mail:viknmu@gmail.com*

*†Department of Computer Science & Engineering,
University of Ioannina,
45110 Ioannina, Greece
E-mail: kblekas@cs.uoi.gr*

Functional magnetic resonance imaging (fMRI) has become a novel technique for studying the human brain and obtaining maps of neuronal activity. An important goal in fMRI studies is to decompose the observed series of brain images in order either to detect activation when a stimulus is presented to the subject, or to identify and characterize underlying brain functional networks when the subject is at rest. In this chapter, a model class is presented for addressing this issue that consists of finite mixture of generalized linear regression models. The main building block of the method is the general linear model which constitutes a standard statistical framework for investigating relationships between variables of fMRI data. We extend this into a finite mixture framework that exploits enhanced modeling capabilities by incorporating some innovative *sparse* and *spatial* properties. In addition, a weighted multi-kernel scheme is employed dealing with the selection problem of kernel parameters where the weights are estimated during training. The proposed regression mixture model is trained using the maximum *a posteriori* approach, where the Expectation-Maximization (EM) algorithm is applied for constructing update equations for the model parameters. We provide comparative experimental results in both activation-based and resting state applications that illustrate the ability of the proposed method to produce improved performance and discrimination capabilities.

1. Introduction

Human brain represents the most complex system in the nature. It is the center of the nervous system. This organ of 1.5 kg and a volume around of 1200 cm^3 is responsible for almost every complex task of a human being.

Millions of elementary components, called neurons, are interconnected to each other creating a complex information processing network. The activity of this network is associated with the mind and gives rise to consciousness. Despite the rapid scientific progress of the last few decades, how the brain works remains a mystery. While the brain is protected by the bones of the skull, it is still vulnerable to damage and disease. Also it is susceptible to degenerative disorders, such as Parkinson's disease, multiple sclerosis, and Alzheimer's disease. Understanding the human brain is one of the greatest scientific challenges of the years to come.[1,2]

Brain imaging uses various techniques to produce images of the brain. Electroencephalography (EEG) is the oldest technique for brain imaging and it produces images of the brain by recording the electrical activity along the scalp. Another neuroimaging technique is the Magnetoencephalography (MEG) which records the magnetic fields produced by the electric currents of the brain. While both techniques present excellent temporal resolution, their spatial resolution is a major drawback since they cannot describe the anatomical structures of the brain. Hence, the use of them has decreased after the introduction of anatomical imaging techniques with high spatial resolution such as Magnetic Resonance Imaging (MRI). Positron Emission Tomography (PET) is a functional neuroimaging technique used to examine various tissues of human body. This technique presents very good spatial resolution. However, the time resolution is very bad and this affects the experimental design since only blocked design experiments can be performed. PET is an invasive technique since a radiotracer is injected into the human body.

Today, the most popular technique for functional neuroimaging is the fMRI. It is a noninvasive technique which presents very good spatial resolution while its time resolution is better compared to other similar techniques such as PET, that offers the opportunity to perform more complicated experimental designs. The fMRI analysis is based mostly on the Blood Oxygenation Level Dependent (BOLD) effect, firstly reported in Ref. [3]. When a stimulus is applied to a subject, regions of the brain involved in the process are becoming active. As a result the rate of blood flow is increased and more oxygenated blood arrives. Furthermore, the blood contains iron which is a paramagnetic material. In the above metabolic procedure, oxygenated and deoxygenated blood are taking part. However, the deoxygenated blood is more paramagnetic than oxygenated. This difference on the magnetic properties between oxygenated and deoxygenated blood is exploited by MRI technology to produce brain images. The increase in blood flow is known as the *hemodynamic response*. For the statistical analysis of the fMRI data, two properties of the hemodynamic response are important. First, the hemodynamic response is slow compared to the neuronal activity. Second, it can be treated (or approximated) as a linear time invariant system. The linearity property together with the mathematical operation of convolution constitute the basic tools to construct statistical models and environments such as the SPM[4] and the FSL,[5] for studying fMRI applications.

Image acquisition of fMRI constructs a 4D dataset consisting of 3D brain volumes that evolve in time. The basic element is called *voxel* and represents a value on a grid in 3D. By taking the values of voxels over time we create a set of *time-series*, i.e. sequential type of data measured in successive time instances at uniform intervals. The fMRI data contains various important properties and a careful analysis of them is needed for the subsequent analysis. Temporal correlations between the samples are found due to physiological properties and experimental conditions. This phenomenon depends mostly on how frequently we acquire the images in conjunction with the duration of BOLD effect. Also, spatial correlation can be observed in the data. This is derived from physiological properties, such as the activated brain areas and the connectivity between brain areas, as well as technical considerations, such as the smallest size of brain location in space that we can obtain. In addition, what affects the quality of fMRI data is the presence of noise that is observed in the data. There are two main sources of noise: noise due to the imaging process and noise due to the human subject.

The types of fMRI experiments can be divided into two large groups according to the desired target. In the *activation-based* fMRI experiments the human subject is exposed to a series of stimulated events according to the experimental design, which provides a binary vector (stimulus is either present, or not). This vector is combined with the hemodynamic response function, through the convolution operator, to give the BOLD regressor which is very important for the statistical analysis of our data. The second group is the *resting state* type of fMRI experiments where we try to find connections between various brain areas when the human subject is at rest, i.e. no stimulus is present. Figure 1 illustrates briefly the overall procedure of the fMRI data analysis process in a flow diagram design.

2. An Overview of fMRI Data Analysis

The objective of fMRI data analysis is to detect the weak BOLD signal from the noisy data and determine the activated areas of the brain. It usually consists of two stages: preprocessing and statistical analysis. The first stage

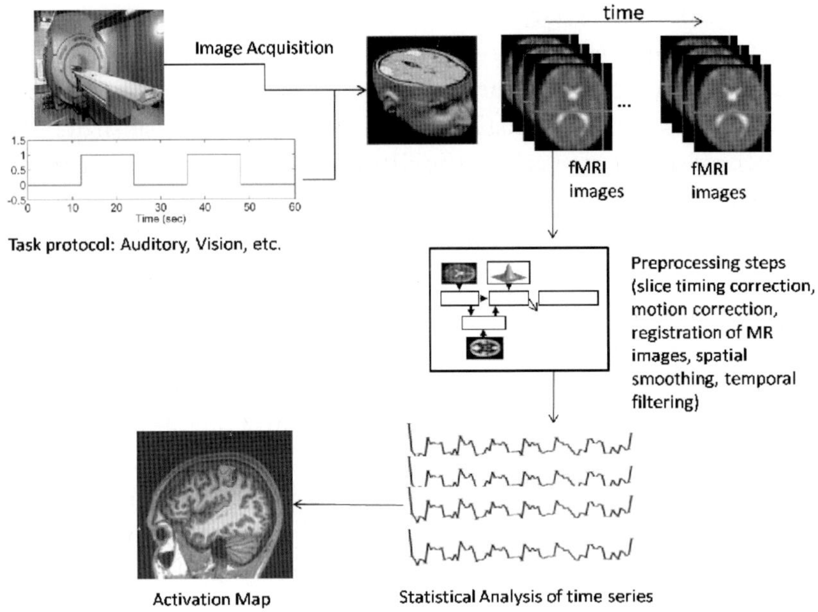

Fig. 1. Overall scheme in fMRI analysis.

contains various techniques that could be made in order to remove artifacts, validate the assumptions of the model and standardize the brain regions across subjects.[6,7] Among them, the most common preprocessing schemes are: slice timing correction, realignment, coregistration of images, normalization, spatial smoothing and temporal filtering.

In literature, there are many methodologies that have been proposed for the analysis of fMRI data. They can be divided into two major categories: the *model-based* and the *data driven* (or model-free). The term "model" is referred to the process of modeling the hemodynamic response. The model-based approaches are used only for activation-based fMRI studies, and are mainly based on the general linear regression model (GLM)[8] and its extensions.[9,10] At the end of the learning process the statistical activation map is drawn based on t- or F-statistics displaying the activation areas and the importance of each voxel.[8] On the other hand, the data driven methods are applied on both resting state and activation-based studies and include the principal component analysis (PCA),[11] independent component analysis (ICA)[12,13] and clustering algorithms.[11,13–15]

A significant drawback of the GLM is that spatial and temporal properties of fMRI data are not taken into account in its basic scheme. More specifically, autoregressive modeling of noise have been proposed in Refs. [9, 10] so as to incorporate temporal correlations, while non-stationary models of noise have been presented in Refs. [16, 17] for the analysis of fMRI time series. Moreover, spatial properties of data are included by usually performing a smoothing with a fixed Gaussian kernel as a preprocessing step.[9,18] Other approaches have also been proposed with elaborate denoising techniques, see Refs. [9, 19] for example. Under the Bayesian framework, spatial dependencies have been modeled through Markov Random Field (MRF) priors applied either to temporal and spatial components of the signal, or to the noise process.[20] Also, Gaussian spatial priors have been placed over the regression coefficients, as well as on autoregressive coefficients of the noise process.[9]

An important feature of the GLM is the type of the design matrix used which may affect significantly the subsequent statistical analysis. Some typical examples are the Vandermonde or B-splines matrix (dealing with polynomial or spline regression models), while others use some predefined dictionaries (basis functions) derived from transformations, such as Fourier, Wavelets, or Discrete Cosine Transform.[10] Other more advanced techniques apply kernel design matrix constructing from an appropriate parametric kernel function.[21,22] Alternatively, for the activation-based fMRI studies, the design matrix could contain information about the experimental paradigm.[8] Also, regressors related to head motion can be included since remnants from head motion noise could be present in the time series.[10] Finally, following the Bayesian framework, sparse priors over regression coefficients could be introduced so as to determine automatically the design matrix.[21–23]

Another family of methods for the fMRI data analysis with special advantages is through clustering techniques. Clustering is the procedure of dividing a set of unlabeled data into a number of groups (clusters), in such a way that similar in nature samples belong to the same cluster, while dissimilar samples become members of different clusters.[24] Cluster analysis of fMRI data constitutes a very interesting application that has been successfully applied during last years. The target is to create a partition into distinct regions, where each region consists of voxels with similar temporal behavior. Most popular clustering methods use partitioning methodologies such as k-means, fuzzy clustering and hierarchical clustering. They are applied to either entire raw data, or feature sets which are extracted from the fMRI signals.[14,15,25–31]

Recently, more advanced approaches have been introduced in order to meet spatial correlation properties of data. In Ref. [32] a spatially constrained mixture model has been adopted for capturing the Hemodynamic Response Function (HRF), while in Ref. [33] the fuzzy c-means algorithm in cooperation with a spatial MRF was proposed to cluster the fMRI data. Furthermore, a mixture model framework with spatial MRFs applied on statistical maps was described in Refs. [19, 34]. However, in the above works the clustering procedure was performed indirectly, either through careful construction of the regression model, or using features extracted from the fMRI time series. Also, temporal patterns of clusters have not been taken into account. A solution to this is to perform the clustering directly to fMRI time series, as for example in Ref. [35], where a mixture of GLMs was presented using a spatial prior based on the Euclidean distances between the positions of time series and cluster centers in a 3D space head model. An alternative solution was given in Ref. [36], where spatial correlations among the time series is achieved through Potts models over the hidden variables of the mixture model.

In this chapter, we present an advanced regression mixture modeling approach for clustering fMRI time series[22] that incorporates very attractive features to facilitate the analysis of fMRI data. The main contribution of the method lies on three aspects:

- Firstly, it achieves a sparse representation of every regression model (cluster) through the use of an appropriate sparse prior over the regression coefficients.[37] Enforcing sparsity is a fundamental machine learning regularization principle[24,37] and has been used in fMRI data analysis.[9,17,23]
- Secondly, spatial constraints of fMRI data have been incorporated directly to the body of mixture model using a Markov random field (MRF) prior over the voxel's labels,[21] so as to create smoother activation regions.
- Finally, a kernel estimation procedure is established through a multi-kernel scheme over the design matrix of the regression models. In this way, we can manage to improve the quality of data fitting and to design more compact clusters.

Training of the proposed regression mixture model is performed by setting a Maximum A Posteriori (MAP) estimation framework and employing the Expectation-Maximization (EM) algorithm.[38,39] Numerous experiments have been conducted using both artificial and real fMRI datasets where we have considered applications on activation-based, as well as on resting state fMRI data. Comparison has been made using a regression mixture model with only spatial properties and the known k-means clustering algorithm. As experiments have shown, the proposed method offers very promising results with an excellent behavior in difficult and noisy environments.

This chapter is structured as follows. At first we present the basic regression mixture model and then we show how it can be adapted in order to fit the fMRI data and their properties. This is split into descriptions of the priors, the general construction and the MAP likelihood, where we show how the EM algorithm can be used for estimating the model parameters. The experiments section presents several results from functional activation studies of auditory and event-related (foot movement) experiments, as well as from resting state fMRI studies. Comparison has been also made with standard approaches. The chapter finishes with some concluding remarks.

3. Finite Mixture of Regression Models

3.1. *Mixture Models*

Mixture models provides a powerful probabilistic modeling tool for data analysis. It has been used in many scientific areas including machine learning, pattern recognition, signal and image analysis and computer vision.[24,39] That makes mixture models so popular and suitable as they are parametric models of an elegant way, yet they are very flexible and easily extensible in estimating any general and complex density and finally, they are capable of accounting for unobserved heterogeneity.

A mixture model of order K is a linear combination of K probability density parametric functions $p(y|\boldsymbol{\theta}_j)$ of different sources and it is formulated as:

$$p(y|\Theta) = \sum_{j=1}^{K} \pi_j p(y|\boldsymbol{\theta}_j). \tag{1}$$

The parameters π_j are the mixing weights satisfying the constraints:

$$0 \leq \pi_j \leq 1 \quad \text{and} \quad \sum_{j=1}^{K} \pi_j = 1, \tag{2}$$

while $\Theta = \{\pi_j, \theta_j\}_{j=1}^{K}$ is the set of model parameters which are unknown and must be estimated. According to this model, each observation is generated by first selecting a source j based on the probabilities $\{\pi_j\}$ and then by performing sampling based on the corresponding distribution with parameters θ_j. Having found the parameters Θ, the posterior probabilities that an observation $\boldsymbol{y}$ belongs to the j-th component can be calculated:

$$P(j|\boldsymbol{y}) = \frac{\pi_j p(\boldsymbol{y}|\theta_j)}{\sum_{k=1}^{K} \pi_k p(\boldsymbol{y}|\theta_k)} \tag{3}$$

Then, an observation belongs to the component j^* with the largest posterior value, i.e. $P(j^*|y) > P(j|y)\ \forall j \neq j^*$.

Let us assume that we have a data set of N samples $Y = \{y_1, \dots, y_N\}$ which are independent. The estimation of the mixture model parameters Θ can be made by maximizing the log-likelihood function:

$$l(\Theta) = \log p(Y|\Theta) = \sum_{n=1}^{N} \log p(y_n|\Theta) = \sum_{n=1}^{N} \log \left\{ \sum_{j=1}^{K} \pi_j p(y_n|\boldsymbol{\theta}_j) \right\}. \quad (4)$$

The Expectation-Maximization (EM)[38] algorithm provides a useful framework for solving likelihood estimation problems. It uses a data augmentation scheme and is a general estimation method in the presence of missing data. In the case of finite mixture models, the component memberships play the role of missing data. EM iteratively performs two main steps. During the *E-step*, the expectation of hidden variables are calculated based on the current estimation of the model parameters:

$$z_{nj} = P(j|y_n) = \frac{\pi_j p(y_n|\theta_j)}{\sum_{k=1}^{K} \pi_k p(y_n|\theta_k)}. \quad (5)$$

At the *M-step*, the maximization of the complete data log-likelihood function (Q-function) is performed:

$$Q(\Theta|\Theta^{(t)}) = \sum_{n=1}^{N} \sum_{j=1}^{K} z_{nj} \{\log \pi_j + \log p(y_n|\theta_j)\} \quad (6)$$

This leads to obtaining new estimates of the mixture weights:

$$\pi_j = \frac{\sum_{n=1}^{N} z_{nj}}{N}, \quad (7)$$

as well as of the model components parameters $\theta_j^{(t+1)}$. The received update rules depend on the type of component density functions. In the case of multivariate Gaussian mixture models for example, i.e. $p(y|\theta_j) = N(y; \mu_j, \Sigma_j)$, these rules become[24,39]:

$$\boldsymbol{\mu}_j = \frac{\sum_{n=1}^{N} z_{nj} y_n}{\sum_{n=1}^{N} z_{nj}} \quad (8)$$

$$\boldsymbol{\Sigma}_j = \frac{\sum_{n=1}^{N} z_{nj} (y_n - \boldsymbol{\mu}_j)(y_n - \boldsymbol{\mu}_j)^T}{\sum_{n=1}^{N} z_{nj}} \quad (9)$$

The E- and M-steps are alternated repeatedly until some specified convergence criterion is achieved.

3.2. *Regression Mixture Modeling*

In the case of fMRI data analysis, we are dealing with *time-series* type of data which are sequences of values measured at T successive time instances x_l, i.e. $\boldsymbol{y}_n = \{y_{nl}\}_{l=1}^{T}$. Linear regression modeling constitutes an elegant functional description framework for analyzing sequential data. It is described with the following form:

$$\boldsymbol{y} = \boldsymbol{X}\boldsymbol{w} + \boldsymbol{e}_n, \tag{10}$$

where $\boldsymbol{w}$ is the vector of M (unknown) linear regression coefficients. The $\boldsymbol{e}_n$ is an additive error term (T dimensional vector) that is assumed to be zero mean Gaussian with a spherical covariance $\boldsymbol{e}_n \sim \mathcal{N}(0, \sigma^2 I)$, i.e. errors are not correlated.

For constructing the design matrix $\boldsymbol{X}$ several approaches can be employed. A common choice is to use Vandermonde or B-splines matrix in cases where we assume polynomial or splines regression models, respectively. Another option is to assume a kernel design matrix using an appropriate kernel basis function over time instances $\{x_l\}_{l=1}^{T}$, with the RBF kernel function to be the most commonly used:

$$[X]_{lk} = K(x_l, x_k; \lambda) = \exp\left(-\frac{(x_l - x_k)^2}{2\lambda}\right),$$

where λ is a scalar parameter. Specifying the proper value for this parameter is an important issue that may affect drastically the quality of the fitting procedure. In general, its choice depends on the amount of local variations of data which must be taken into account. In addition, the design matrix may contain information about the experimental paradigm of fMRI experiment.

Following Eq. (10) it is obvious that, given the set of regression model parameters $\theta = \{\boldsymbol{w}, \sigma^2\}$, the conditional probability density of time-series $\boldsymbol{y}_n$ is also Gaussian, i.e.

$$p(\boldsymbol{y}_n|\theta) = \mathcal{N}(\boldsymbol{X}\boldsymbol{w}, \sigma^2 I).$$

Regression mixture models[39] provides a natural framework for fitting a given set of sequential data $\Upsilon = \{\boldsymbol{y}_1, \ldots, \boldsymbol{y}_n\}$. They allow for simultaneously modeling heterogeneous regression functions by training a mixture of distinct distributions where each one corresponds to a latent class. Obviously, this is equivalent to the task of time-series clustering, i.e. the division of the set Υ into K clusters, in such a way that each cluster contains similar in nature elements. Therefore each cluster has its own regression generative mechanism, as given by a conditional density with parameters $\theta_j = \{\boldsymbol{w}_j, \sigma_j^2\}, j = 1, \ldots, K$.

The EM algorithm can be then applied in order to train regression mixture models. That differs from the basic scheme described previously — the expected complete log-likelihood Q-function which takes the following form:

$$Q(\Theta|\Theta^{(t)}) = \sum_{n=1}^{N}\sum_{j=1}^{K} z_{nj}\left\{\log \pi_j - \frac{T}{2}\log 2\pi - T\log\sigma_j - \frac{\|\boldsymbol{y}_n - \boldsymbol{X}\boldsymbol{w}_j\|^2}{2\sigma_j^2}\right\}, \tag{11}$$

as well as the update rules of the regression component parameters θ_j which are

$$\boldsymbol{w}_j = \left(\sum_{n=1}^{N} z_{nj}\boldsymbol{X}^T\boldsymbol{X}\right)^{-1}\boldsymbol{X}^T\sum_{n=1}^{N}(z_{nj}\boldsymbol{y}_n), \tag{12}$$

$$\sigma_j^2 = \frac{\sum_{n=1}^{N} z_{nj}\|\boldsymbol{y}_n - \boldsymbol{X}\boldsymbol{w}_j\|^2}{T\sum_{n=1}^{N} z_{nj}}. \tag{13}$$

After the convergence of the EM algorithm, each sequence $\boldsymbol{y}_n$ is assigned to the cluster with the maximum posterior probability $P(j|\boldsymbol{y}_n)$ [similar to Eq. (3)].

4. Regression Mixture Analysis of fMRI Time-Series

The application of the basic ML-based scheme of regression mixture models to the task of fMRI data analysis has some limitations due to its weakness to capture some important features arisen from the nature of these observations. In particular, the fMRI data are structures that involve spatial properties, where adjacent voxels tend to have similar activity behavior.[40] Furthermore, there are temporal correlations which are derived from neural, physiological and physical sources.[10] These are physical constraints that must be incorporated to the model.

4.1. *General Construction*

A significant advantage of Bayesian estimation is its flexibility of incorporating appropriate priors and its full characterization of the posterior. Bayesian modeling also enable us to model the uncertainty of the hyperparameters so that the final performance is more robust. In such a way, we can eliminate the phenomenon of data overfitting found in the ML case. These are the main building blocks for constructing a maximum a-posteriori (MAP) approach which offers a more advanced solution: *sparseness, spatial, and multi-kernel.*

4.1.1. *Sparse modeling*

An important issue when using a regression model is how to estimate its order M, i.e. the size of linear regression coefficients $\boldsymbol{w}_j$. Estimating the proper value of M depends on the shape of data to be fitted, where models of small order may lead to underfitting, while large values of M may become responsible for data overfitting. This may deteriorate significantly the clustering performance. Bayesian regularization framework provides an elegant solution to this problem.[24,37] It initially assumes a large value of order M. Then, a heavy tailed prior distribution $p(\boldsymbol{w}_j)$ is imposed upon the regression coefficients that will enforce most of the coefficients to be zero out after training. This has been successfully employed in the Relevance Vector Machine model.[37]

More specifically, the prior is defined in an hierarchical way by considering first a zero-mean Gaussian distribution over the regression coefficients:

$$p(\boldsymbol{w}_j|\boldsymbol{\alpha}_j) = \mathcal{N}(\boldsymbol{w}_j|0, A_j^{-1}) = \prod_{l=1}^{M} \mathcal{N}(w_{jl}|0, \alpha_{jl}^{-1}), \tag{14}$$

where A_j is a diagonal matrix containing the M components of the precision (inverse variance) vector $\boldsymbol{\alpha}_j = (a_{j1}, \ldots, a_{jM})$. At a second level, precision can be seen as hyperparameters that follow a Gamma prior distribution:

$$p(\alpha_j) = \prod_{l=1}^{M} \Gamma(\alpha_{jl}|b, c) \propto \prod_{l=1}^{M} \alpha_{jl}^{b-1} \exp^{-c\alpha_{jl}}. \tag{15}$$

Note that both Gamma parameters b and c are *a priori* set to zero so as to achieve uninformative priors. The above two-stage hierarchical sparse prior is actually the student's t-distribution enforcing most of the values α_{jl} to be large and thus eliminating the effect of the corresponding coefficients w_{jl} by setting to zero. In such a way, the regression model order for every cluster is automatically selected and overfitting is avoided.

4.1.2. *Spatial regularization*

A common approach to achieve spatial correlations between voxels is to apply a spatial Gaussian filter to smooth the signal prior to statistical analysis. This is used for instance in Statistical Parametric Mapping (SPM).[4] However, this can lead to overlay blurred results, where effects with small spatial extend can be lost and detected regions may extend beyond their actual boundaries. A more advanced approach to spatial regularization is through the use of Markov Random Field (MRF) prior[41] which models the conditional dependence of the signals in neighboring voxels.

MRFs have been successfully applied to computer vision applications.[41,42] Conventional use of MRFs requires the set of sites of the random field as the image voxels, with the neighborhood structure given by a regular lattice. More specifically, we can treat the probabilities (voxel labels) π_{nj} of each fMRI sequence $\boldsymbol{y}_n$ belongs to the j-th cluster (mixture component) as random variables, which also satisfy the constraints $\pi_{nj} \geq 0$ and $\sum_{j=1}^{K} \pi_{nj} = 1$. We assume that the set of voxel labels $\Pi = \{\boldsymbol{\pi}_n\}_{n=1}^{N}$ follows the Gibbs prior distribution with density[41]

$$p(\Pi) = \frac{1}{Z} \exp\left\{ -\sum_{n=1}^{N} V_{N_n}(\Pi) \right\}. \tag{16}$$

The function $V_{N_n}(\Pi)$ denotes the clique potential function around the neighborhood N_n of the n-th voxel taking the following form:

$$V_{N_n}(\Pi) = \sum_{m \in N_n} \sum_{j=1}^{K} \beta_j (\pi_{nj} - \pi_{mj})^2. \tag{17}$$

In our case we consider neighbourhood consisted of eight (8) voxels which are horizontally, diagonally and vertically adjacent. We also assume that every cluster has its own regularization parameter β_j. This has the ability to increase the flexibility of model, since it allows different degree of smoothness at each cluster. It is interesting to note here that in this framework, the regularization parameters β_j belong to the set of the unknown parameters and thus can be estimated during the learning process. Finally, the term Z of Eq. (16) is the normalizing factor that is analogous to $Z \propto \prod_{j=1}^{K} \beta_j^{-N}$.

An alternative methodology on using a capable MRF prior to leverage spatial correlations in brain maps is through a recent non-parametric scheme shown in Ref. [43]. In particular, an appropriate class-specific Gibbs potential function has been proposed of the following form:

$$\vartheta_{nj} = \sum_{m \in N_n} z_{nj} z_{mj}, \tag{18}$$

that gives the influence of the neighborhood to the decision process. This function acts as a smooth filter to the estimated posteriors and it works like a voting system, where the majority cluster-label among its closest neighbors is assigned to every sequence. Then, probabilities of voxels' labels are given according to a *softmax* function:

$$\pi_{nj} \propto \frac{e^{\vartheta_{nj}}}{\sum_{k=1}^{K} e^{\vartheta_{nk}}}. \tag{19}$$

4.1.3. *Multi-kernel scheme*

As mentioned before, the construction of the design matrix $\boldsymbol{X}$ is a crucial part of the regression model and may be significantly affected by the parameter value of the desired kernel function. This problem can be solved by adopting a multi-kernel scheme.[44,45] In particular, we assume a pool of S kernel matrices $\{\boldsymbol{\Phi}_s\}_{s=1}^S$, each one having its own scalar parameter value λ_s. Thus, the composite kernel matrix $\boldsymbol{X}_j$ for the $j-th$ cluster can be written as a linear combination of S kernel matrices Φ_s:

$$\boldsymbol{X}_j = \sum_{s=1}^{S} u_{js}\boldsymbol{\Phi}_s, \tag{20}$$

where u_{js} are the coefficients of the multi-kernel scheme which are unknown and satisfy the constraints $u_{js} \geq 0$ and $\sum_{s=1}^{S} u_{js} = 1$. These parameters should be estimated during learning in order to construct the kernel design matrix that better suits to every cluster. As experiments have shown, the use of the proposed multi-kernel scheme has the ability to significantly improve the performance and the quality of the data fitting procedure.

4.2. *Estimation of Model Parameters*

After defining the sparse and sparse priors together with the multi-kernel scheme, we are now ready to describe the estimation process of the model parameters. The incorporation of the above properties leads to a modification of the regression mixture model which is written as:

$$f(\boldsymbol{y}_n|\Theta) = \sum_{j=1}^{K} \pi_{nj} p(\boldsymbol{y}_n|\theta_j), \tag{21}$$

where $\Theta = \{\{\pi_{nj}\}_{n=1}^N, \theta_j = (\boldsymbol{w}_j, \boldsymbol{\alpha}_j, \sigma_j^2, \boldsymbol{u}_j, \beta_j)\}_{j=1}^K$ is the set of mixture model parameters. The clustering procedure becomes now a Maximum-A-Posteriori (MAP) estimation problem, where the MAP log-likelihood function is given by

$$\begin{aligned} l_{MAP}(\Theta) &= \log p(\Upsilon|\Theta) + \log p(\Theta) \\ &= \sum_{n=1}^{N} \log f(\boldsymbol{y}_n|\Theta) + \log p(\Pi) + \sum_{j=1}^{K}\{\log p(\boldsymbol{w}_j|\boldsymbol{\alpha}_j) + \log p(\boldsymbol{\alpha}_j)\}. \end{aligned} \tag{22}$$

The EM algorithm can then be applied for MAP-estimating the model parameters. Likewise, it requires at each iteration the conditional expectation values z_{nj} of the hidden variables to be computed first (E-step):

$$z_{nj} = P(j|\boldsymbol{y}_n, \Theta) = \frac{\pi_{nj} p(\boldsymbol{y}_n|\theta_j)}{f(\boldsymbol{y}_n|\Theta)}. \tag{23}$$

During the M-step the maximization of the complete data MAP log-likelihood expectation is performed:

$$\begin{aligned} Q(\Theta|\Theta^{(t)}) = &\sum_{n=1}^{N}\sum_{j=1}^{K} z_{nj} \left\{ \log \pi_{nj} - \frac{T}{2}\log 2\pi - T\log\sigma_j - \frac{\|\boldsymbol{y}_n - \boldsymbol{X}_j\boldsymbol{w}_j\|^2}{2\sigma_j^2} \right\} \\ &- \sum_{j=1}^{K} \left\{ -N\log\beta_j + \beta_j \sum_{n=1}^{N}\sum_{m\in N_n} (\pi_{nj} - \pi_{mj})^2 + \frac{1}{2}\boldsymbol{w}_j^T A_j \boldsymbol{w}_j \right. \\ &\left. - \sum_{l=1}^{M} [(b-1)\log\alpha_{jl} - c\alpha_{jl}] \right\}. \end{aligned} \tag{24}$$

By setting the partial derivatives of the above Q function with respect to all model parameters, we can obtain the update rules. For the regression model parameters $\{\boldsymbol{w}_j, \sigma_j^2, \boldsymbol{\alpha}_j, \beta_j\}$ we can easily obtain the next equations:

$$\boldsymbol{w}_j = \left[\left(\sum_{n=1}^{N} z_{nj} \right) \frac{1}{\sigma_j^2} \boldsymbol{X}_j^T \boldsymbol{X}_j + A_j \right]^{-1} \cdot \frac{1}{\sigma_j^2} \boldsymbol{X}_j^T \left(\sum_{n=1}^{N} z_{nj} \boldsymbol{y}_n \right), \tag{25}$$

$$\sigma_j^2 = \frac{\sum_{n=1}^{N} z_{nj} \|\boldsymbol{y}_n - \boldsymbol{X}_j \boldsymbol{w}_j\|^2}{T\sum_{n=1}^{N} z_{nj}}, \tag{26}$$

$$\alpha_{jl} = \frac{1+2c}{w_{jl}^2 + 2b}, \tag{27}$$

$$\beta_j = \frac{N}{\sum_{n=1}^{N}\sum_{m\in N_n} (\pi_{nj} - \pi_{mj})^2}. \tag{28}$$

In the case of the label parameters π_{nj} we obtain the following quadratic equation:

$$\pi_{nj}^2 - <\pi_{nj}> \pi_{nj} - \frac{1}{2\beta_j |N_n|} z_{nj} = 0\ , \tag{29}$$

where $|N_n|$ is the cardinality of the neighborhood N_n and $\langle \pi_{nj} \rangle$ is the mean value of the j-th cluster's probabilities of the spatial neighbors of the n-th voxel, i.e. $\langle \pi_{nj} \rangle = \frac{1}{|N_n|} \sum_{m\in N_n} \pi_{mj}$. The above quadratic expression has two roots, where we select only the one with the positive sign since it yields $\pi_{nj} \geq 0$:

$$\pi_{nj} = \frac{\langle \pi_{nj} \rangle + \sqrt{\langle \pi_{nj} \rangle^2 + \frac{2}{\beta_j |N_n|} z_{nj}}}{2}. \tag{30}$$

Note that in the above update rule the neighborhood N_n may contain label parameters π_{mj} that have been either already updated or not. However, these values do not satisfy the constraints $0 \leq \pi_{nj} \leq 1$ and $\sum_{j=1}^{K} \pi_{nj} = 1$, and there is a need to project them on their constraint convex hull. For this purpose, we apply an efficient convex quadratic programming approach presented in Ref. [42], that is based on the active-set theory.[46]

Finally, the weights u_{js} of the multi-kernel scheme are adjusted by solving the following minimization problem, where we have considered only the part of likelihood function that involves $\boldsymbol{u}_j$:

$$\begin{aligned} \min_{\boldsymbol{u}_j} \sum_{n=1}^{N} z_{nj} \parallel \boldsymbol{y}_n - \sum_{s=1}^{S} u_{js} \boldsymbol{\Phi}_s \boldsymbol{w}_j \parallel^2 &= \min_{\boldsymbol{u}_j} \sum_{n=1}^{N} z_{nj} \parallel \boldsymbol{y}_n - \mathcal{X}_j \boldsymbol{u}_j \parallel^2 \\ &= \min_{\boldsymbol{u}_j} \left\{ \boldsymbol{u}_j^T \mathcal{X}_j^T \mathcal{X}_j \boldsymbol{u}_j - 2 \boldsymbol{u}_j^T \mathcal{X}_j^T \frac{\sum_{n=1}^{N} z_{nj} \boldsymbol{y}_n}{\sum_{n=1}^{N} z_{nj}} \right\}, \\ \text{s.t.} \sum_{s=1}^{S} u_{js} = 1 \quad &\text{and} \quad u_{js} \geq 0. \end{aligned} \tag{31}$$

In the above formulation, the matrix $\mathcal{X}_j$ has S columns calculated by $\boldsymbol{\Phi}_s \boldsymbol{w}_j$, i.e. $\mathcal{X}_j = [\boldsymbol{\Phi}_1 \boldsymbol{w}_j \; \boldsymbol{\Phi}_2 \boldsymbol{w}_j \; \cdots \; \boldsymbol{\Phi}_S \boldsymbol{w}_j]$. The minimization problem described in Eq. (31) is a typical constrained linear least-squared problem that can be solved again with the active-set theory.[46]

At the end of the learning process, the *activation map* of the brain is constructed with the following manner: Initially, we select the cluster h that best match with the BOLD signal $\boldsymbol{\xi}$ (which is known before the data analysis) among the K mixture components. This is done according to the Pearson correlation measurement (cosine similarity) between the estimated mean curve $\boldsymbol{\mu}_j = \boldsymbol{X}_j \boldsymbol{w}_j$ of each cluster with the BOLD signal $\boldsymbol{\xi}$, i.e.

$$h = \arg \max_{j=1}^{K} \frac{\boldsymbol{\mu}_j^T \boldsymbol{\xi}}{|\boldsymbol{\mu}_j||\boldsymbol{\xi}|}. \tag{32}$$

Then, the voxels that belong to cluster h determine the brain activation region, while the rest voxels (that belong to all other $K - 1$ clusters) correspond to the non-activation region. In this way, we create a binary image with activated and non-activated pixels.

A drawback of the EM algorithm is its sensitivity to the initialization of the model parameters due to its local nature. Improper initialization may lead to poor local maxima of the log-likelihood that sequentially affects the quality of the clustering solution. A common practice is to initialize mixture model parameters by randomly selecting K input time-series and to perform only a few EM steps. Several trials of such procedure can be made and finally the solution with the maximum log-likelihood value can be selected for the initialization.

A more advanced approach has been proposed in Ref. [22] that follows an incremental strategy for building the regression mixture model. Starting with a mixture model with one regression component, the learning methodology adds a new component to the mixture based on a *component splitting* procedure. In activation-based fMRI data analysis, this is done by selecting a cluster for splitting based on their similarity with the BOLD signal. A detailed description can be found in Ref. [22]. It must be noted that an obvious advantage of the incremental learning scheme is that of simultaneously offering solutions for the intermediate models with $k = \{1, \dots, K\}$ components. This can be seen as very convenient for introducing model order selection criteria and terminating the evolution of learning: stop training when the insertion of a new component does not offer any significant improvement of the (penalized) likelihood function.

5. Experiments

The proposed regression mixture model (called as SSRM) has been evaluated using a variety of artificial datasets and real fMRI data. In all experiments for constructing the multi-kernel scheme, we calculated first the total variance of samples, λ. Next, we used a set of $S = 10$ RBF kernel functions, where each one had a scalar parameter $\lambda_s = k_s\lambda$, where $k_s = [0.1, 0.2, \dots, 1.0]$ (level of percentage). It must be noted that during the activation-based experiments another column has been added to the design matrix which describes the BOLD signal. Note that the time instances x_l were normalized before to $[0, 1]$. Finally, the linear weights of the multi-kernel scheme were in all cases initialized equally to $u_{js} = 1/S$. Comparison has been made using the SRM method which is a regression mixture model with only spatial properties (and without sparse properties), and the k-means which is a well-known vector-based clustering approach. An extended experimental study can be found in Refs. [22, 43], that present additional comparative results with the standard GLM model[8] and various types of noise.

5.1. *Activation-based fMRI Experiments*

The goal of this series of experiments is to discover the brain activation areas when the human subject is exposed to a stimulus. At first we have studied the performance of the proposed method using synthetic data, where the ground truth of activation is known. Additional experiments were made using real fMRI datasets taken from block design auditory and event-related foot movement studies.

5.1.1. *Experiments with artificial datasets*

During the experiments with simulated fMRI data, we have created 3D set of time series using linear regression models with known design matrix and regression coefficients. We have also added white Gaussian noise of various SNR levels according to the formula: $SNR = 10\log_{10}(\frac{s^T s}{N\sigma^2})$, where σ^2 is the noise variance and s is the BOLD signal. The spatial correlation among time series is achieved through the regression coefficients. Figure 2(a) represents the spatial patterns used, while the BOLD signal used to model the neural activity is shown in Fig. 2(b). Also, in these time series we have added a slow varying component to model the drift in the fMRI time series. This is done by using a linear regression model where the regressors are the first ten basis vector of DCT basis and the regression coefficients are sampled by the standard normal distribution $\mathcal{N}(0, 1)$. The size of the obtained dataset was $80 \times 80 \times 84$. Finally, for each SNR level we studied the performance of the comparative methods by executing 50 Monte Carlo simulations, where we took the statistics of the depicted results (mean and variance). To measure the quality of each clustering approach, we have used two evaluation criteria: the accuracy performance (percentage of correct classifying data) and the Normalized Mutual Information (NMI).[22]

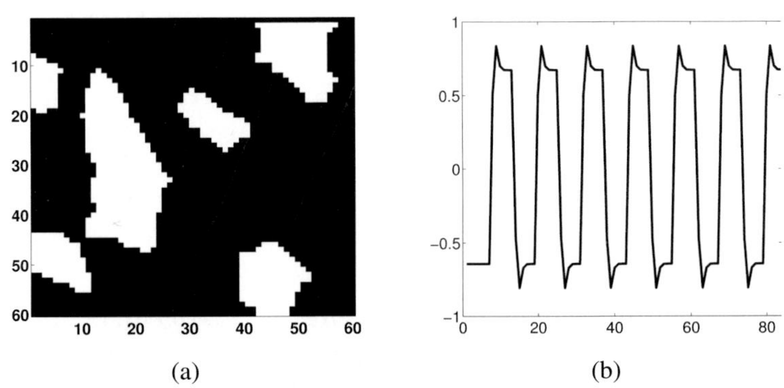

Fig. 2. (a) Spatial patterns and (b) the BOLD signal used in experiments with simulated data.

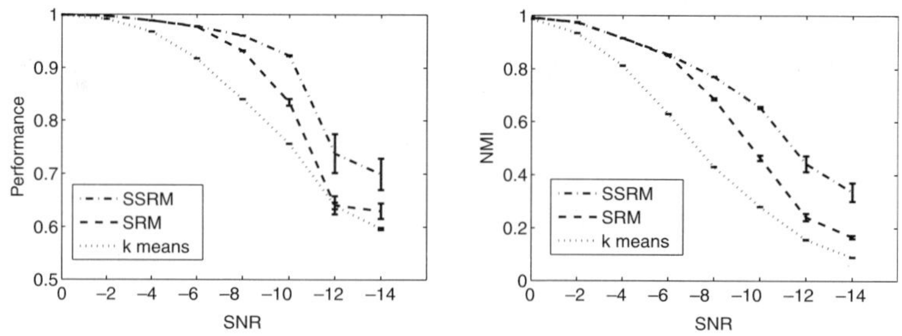

Fig. 3. Comparative results for our dataset of Fig. 2. Error bars for the two evaluation criteria are shown in terms of several SNR values.

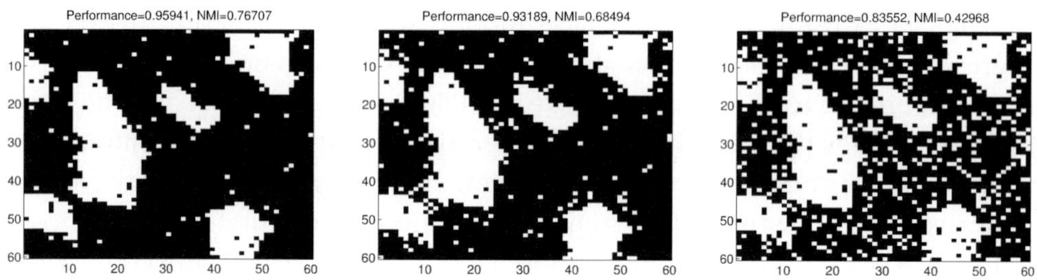

(a) SSRM (b) SRM (c) k-means

Fig. 4. Spatial patterns as estimated by all methods in the case of −8 dB.

Figure 3 shows the comparative results for our simulated dataset of Fig. 2. The superiority of the SSRM is obvious based on two evaluation criteria, especially in small SNR values (noisy data). Comparison with the SRM method that holds only the spatial properties, has shown a significant improvement in terms of both evaluation criteria. This proves the usefulness of the sparse term to modeling procedure. An example of the activation maps as estimated by each method is shown in Figs. 4 in the case of $SNR = -8$ dB. Clearly, our method had better discrimination ability and achieved to discover more accurately the original spatial pattern, while at the same time reduced significantly the false negative activation cases. A more comprehensive experimental analysis can be found on Ref. [22].

5.1.2. *Experiments using real fMRI data*

We have made additional experiments using real fMRI data. In our study, we have selected a dataset with a block-designed auditory paradigm. In this experiment, we have followed the standard preprocessing steps of the SPM package. The BOLD signals for the experiment is shown in Fig. 2(b). This

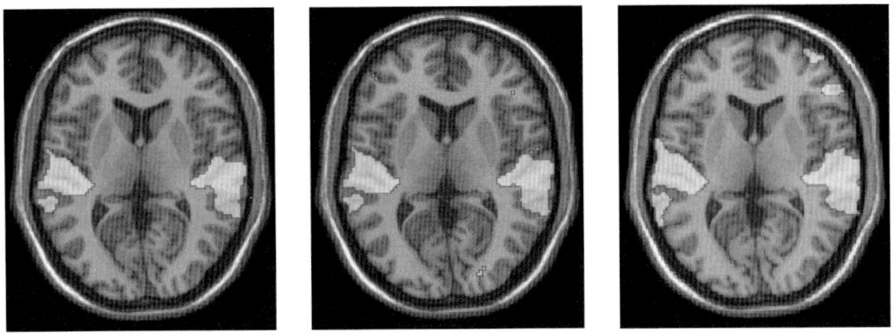

Fig. 5. The binary activation map as estimated by each method in the case of the auditory experiment.

dataset was downloaded from the SPM webpage[a] and it was based on an auditory processing task as executed by a healthy volunteer. Its functional images consisted of $\mathcal{M} = 68$ slices ($79 \times 95 \times 68$, $2\,\text{mm} \times 2\,\text{mm} \times 2\,\text{mm}$ voxels). Experiments were made with the slice 29 of this dataset, which contains a number of $N = 5118$ time series. In this series of experiments, we have employed the incremental learning strategy of the proposed method SSRM[22] which provided us with the proper number of clusters. We have found a number of $K = 5$ cluster and then we have used this value in order to run the other two approaches, SRM and k-means. Figure 5 represents the comparative results of all clustering methods giving the resulting position of the activation area inside the brain. Note that the activated areas are overlaid on grayscale T1 weighted anatomical images. All methods have detected the auditory cortex as the brain activation area. However, the SSRM methods have clearly detected only three distinct areas of activation, while the remaining two approaches have additionally detected other small activated islands that may bring difficulties in the decision making process.

Furthermore, we have studied the capability of our method to construct the 3D activation model. In particular we have applied our method independently to all available slices (68) of the auditory experiment. The resulting activation maps are fed to the 3D Slicer toolkit[47] that sequentially produces the 3D head model with the activation areas. Figure 6 illustrates the resulting 3D models of our method and the standard GLM approach.[8] Obviously, both methods have detected a significant activation on the temporal lobe. However, our method has detected an extra activated region into the frontal lobe which is expected in auditory experiments.

[a]http://www.fil.ion.ucl.ac.uk/spm/

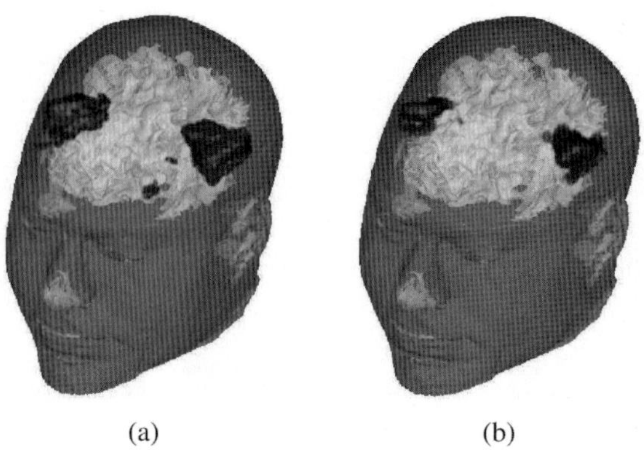

Fig. 6. The 3D head activation maps as estimated by (a) the proposed method SSRM and (b) the standard GLM.

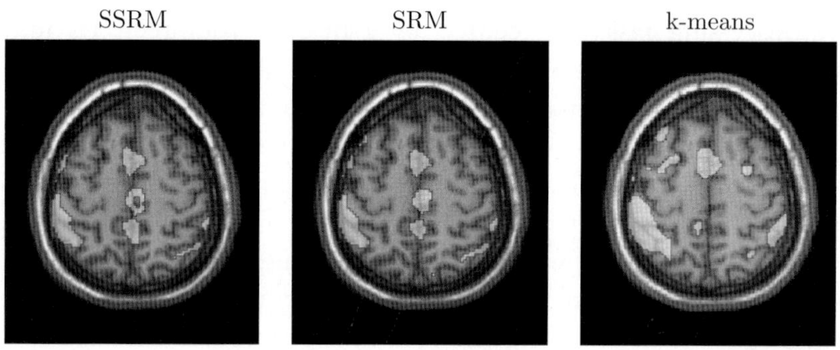

Fig. 7. Estimated motor activated areas of comparative methods in white overlaid on greyscale T1 weighted anatomical images.

In the event-related foot-movement experiment, we analyzed fMRI data consisted of images acquired from the University Hospital of Ioannina, Greece.[48] Details about the protocol that was followed for constructing the fMRI data can be found in Ref. [22]. Experiments were made with the slice 54 of this dataset, which contains a number of $N = 2644$ time series. Figure 7 presents the comparative results in this dataset overlaid on greyscale T1 weighted anatomical images. As expected, all methods have detected the primary and the supplementary motor areas of the brain as the activation cluster. Although there is no ground truth for the fMRI data on individual cases, the motor system in general is well-studied and described in literature. The proposed regression mixture model gives more activated areas closer to the established motor circuitry and therefore the results are more reasonable (at least in this case).

5.2. *Resting State fMRI Experiments*

We have also made experiments with resting state fMRI data obtained from the Neuroimaging Informatics Tools and Resources Clearinghouse (NITRC)[b] under the project name: NYU CSC TestRetest. A detailed description of the dataset can be found in Ref. [49]. In our experiments we have selected a subject from this dataset, where we have used the slice 34 (of 52). Two versions of the proposed SSRM method were studied that differ on the spatial prior: (a) SSRM with the exponential potential function of Eqs. (16), (17) and (b) SSRM with the softmax MRF prior of Eqs. (18), (19). The task in these series of experiments was to estimate the Default Mode Network (DMN), which is a resting state network that consists of precuneus, medial frontal, inferior parietal cortical regions and medial temporal lobe. The DMN is expected to be presented in almost every fMRI experiment.

The depicted brain images are shown in Fig. 8 that illustrate the DMN cluster as estimated by each clustering approach. What is interesting to observe is that, although all methods are able to properly identify the DMN, the other two methods, SRM and k-means, tend to overestimate it and construct small islands (almost uniformly the brain) not belonging to DMN. Clearly, the proposed SSRM method seems to have better discrimination ability to discover more accurately the network. Both versions do not show any significant difference, with the second version (b) to appear to be more consistent producing slightly smoother regions. However, a more systematic comparative study is required to evaluate their effectiveness.

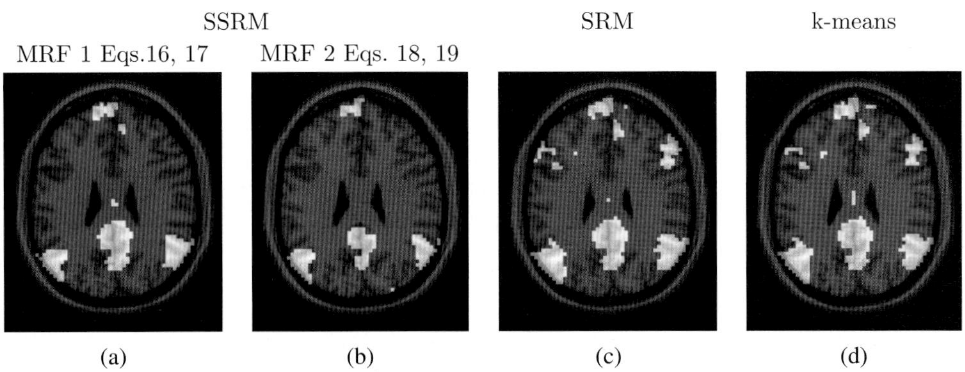

Fig. 8. Default Mode Network estimation from resting state fMRI data using two versions of SSMR (a) and (b) that differ in the type of MRF-based spatial prior, (c) the SRM and (d) the k-means approaches.

[b] http://www.nitrc.org

6. Conclusions

In this chapter, we have presented a regression mixture modeling framework for the analysis of fMRI data. This model class is very flexible and can embody prior knowledge of the nature of data. The key aspect of the proposed technique lies on the superior sparse regression performance to model data of latent classes, as well as the ability to evoke responses which are spatially homogeneous and locally contiguous. It also includes a multi-kernel scheme for composing the kernel matrix of each component that offers better fitting capabilities. Therefore, the proposed method manages to incorporate significant physiological properties of human brain and to tackle important issues that they are possible to deteriorate the performance of fMRI data analysis. As compared to standard approaches, the sparse and spatial regularization procedures of the method have been shown to increase the robustness of detection and to result in inferences with higher sensitivity.

Further extensions of the finite mixtures are possible for the regression case. Instead of using GLMs as component specific models, generalized additive models can be used which allow to relax some assumptions we have made. Another future research direction is to examine the possibility of applying alternative sparse priors, as well as to assume Student's-t type of distribution for modeling the noise (instead of Gaussian) so as to achieve more robust inference and handle outlying observations.[24] Finally, another possibility is to extend our model to 3D cases and to group analysis applications.

References

1. Human brain project. https://www.humanbrainproject.eu/ (2012).
2. Brain initiative. http://www.nih.gov/science/brain/ (2013).
3. S. Ogawa, T. Lee, A. Kay, and D. Tank, "Brain magnetic resonance imaging with contrast dependent on blood oxygenation," *Proc Nat Acad Sci USA* **87**, 9868–9872 (1990).
4. K. Friston, Statistical parametric mapping. http://www.fil.ion.ucl.ac.uk/spm/ (2009).
5. M. Jenkinson, C. Beckmann, T. Behrens, M. Woolrich, and S. Smith, "FSL," *NeuroImage* **62**, 782–790 (2012).
6. N. A. Lazar, *The Statistical Analysis of Functional MRI data*. Springer (2008).
7. R. A. Poldrack, J. A. Mumford, and T. E. Nichols, *Handbook of Functional MRI Data Analysis*. Campridge University Press (2011).
8. K. J. Friston, "Analysis of fMRI time series revisited," *Neuroimage* **2**, 45–53 (1995).
9. G. Flandin and W. Penny, "Bayesian fMRI data analysis with sparse spatial basis function priors," *NeuroImage* **34**, 1108–1125 (2007).
10. W. Penny, N. Trujillo-Barreto, and K. Friston, "Bayesian fMRI time series analysis with spatial priors," *NeuroImage* **24**, 350–362 (2005).

11. R. Baumgartner, L. Ryner, W. Richter, R. Summers, M. Jarmasz, and R. Somorjai, "Comparison of two exploratory data analysis methods for fMRI: fuzzy clustering vs. principal component analysis," *Magn Res Imaging* **18**, 89–94 (2000).
12. M. J. Mckeown, S. Makeig, G. G. Brown, T. P. Jung, S. S. Kindermann, A. J. Bell, and T. J. Sejnowski, "Analysis of fMRI data by blind separation into independent spatial components," *Hum Brain Mapp* **6**, 160–188 (1998).
13. A. Meyer-Baese, A. Wismueller, and O. Lange, "Comparison of two exploratory data analysis methods for fMRI: Unsupervised clustering versus independent component analysis," *IEEE Trans Inf Technol Biomed* **8**, 387–398 (2004).
14. A. Meyer-Base, A. Saalbach, O. Lange, and A. Wismller, "Unsupervised clustering of fMRI and MRI time series," *Biomed Signal Process Control* **2**, 295–310 (2007).
15. C. G. Laberge, A. Adler, I. Cameron, T. Nguyen, and M. Hogan, "A bayesian hierarchical correlation model for fMRI cluster analysis," *IEEE Trans Biomed Eng* **57**, 1967–1976 (2011).
16. H. Luo and S. Puthusserypady, "fMRI data analysis with nonstationary noise models: A bayesian approach," *IEEE Trans Biomed Eng* **54**, 1621–1630 (2007).
17. V. Oikonomou, E. Tripoliti, and D. Fotiadis, "Bayesian methods for fMRI time-series analysis using a nonstationary model for the noise," *IEEE Trans Inf Technol Biomed* **14**, 664–674 (2010).
18. R. Frackowiak, J. Ashburner, W. Penny, S. Zeki, K. Friston, C. Frith, R. Dolan, and C. Price, *Human Brain Function, Second Edition*. Elsevier Science, USA (2004).
19. N. Hartvig and J. Jensen, "Spatial mixture modeling of fMRI data," *Human Brain Mapping* **11**, 233–248 (2000).
20. M. Woolrich, M. Jenkinson, J. Brady, and S. Smith, "Fully bayesian spatio-temporal modeling of fMRI data," *IEEE Trans Med Imaging* **23**, 213–231 (2004).
21. V. Oikonomou, K. Blekas, and L. Astrakas, "A sparse and spatially constrained generative regression model for fMRI data analysis," *IEEE Trans Biomed Eng* **59**, 58–67 (2012).
22. V. P. Oikonomou and K. Blekas, "An adaptive regression mixture model for fMRI cluster analysis," *IEEE Trans Med Imaging* **32**, 649–660 (2013).
23. H. Luo and S. Puthusserypady, "A sparse Bayesian method for determination of flexible design matrix for fMRI data analysis," *IEEE Trans Circuits Syst I Reg Papers* **52**, 2699–2706 (2005).
24. C. M. Bishop, *Pattern Recognition and Machine Learning*. Springer (2006).
25. R. Baumgartner, C. Windischberger, and E. Moser, "Quantification in functional magnetic resonance imaging: Fuzzy clustering vs. correlation analysis," *Magn Reson Imaging* **16**, 115–125 (1998).
26. C. Goutte, P. Toft, E. Rostrup, F. ï. Nielsen, and L. K. Hansen, "On clustering fMRI time series," *NeuroImage* **9**, 298–310 (1999).
27. A. Wismüller, O. Lange, D. R. Dersch, G. L. Leinsinger, K. Hahn, B. Pütz, and D. Auer, "Cluster analysis of biomedical image time-series," *Int J Comput Vision* **46**, 103–128 (2002).
28. F. G. Meyer and J. Chinrungrueng, "Spatiotemporal clustering of fMRI time series in the spectral domain," *Med Image Anal* **9**, 51–68 (2005).
29. A. Mezer, Y. Yovel, O. Pasternak, T. Gorfine, and Y. Assaf, "Cluster analysis of resting-state fMRI time series," *NeuroImage* **45**, 1117–1125 (2009).

30. C. Windischberger, M. Barth, C. Lamm, L. Schroeder, H. Bauer, R. C. Gur, and E. Moser, "Fuzzy cluster analysis of high-field functional MRI data," *Artif Intel Med* **29**, 203–223 (2003).
31. A. Wismüller, A. Meyer-Base, O. Lange, D. Auer, M. F. Reiser, and D. Sumners, "Model-free functional MRI analysis based on unsupervised clustering," *J Biomed Inform* **37**, 10–18 (2004).
32. T. Vincent, L. Risser, and P. Ciuciu, "Spatially adaptive mixture modeling for analysis of FMRI time series," *IEEE Trans Med Imaging* **29**, 1059–1074 (2010).
33. L. He and I. R. Greenshields, "An MRF spatial fuzzy clustering method for fMRI SPMs," *Biomed Signal Process Control* **3**, 327–333 (2008).
34. M. Woolrich, T. Behrens, C. Beckmann, and S. Smith, "Mixture models with adaptive spatial regularization for segmentation with an application to FMRI data," *IEEE Trans Med Imaging* **24**, 1–11 (2005).
35. W. Penny and K. Friston, "Mixtures of general linear models for functional neuroimaging," *IEEE Trans Med Imaging* **22**, 504–514 (2003).
36. J. Xia, F. Liang, and Y. M. Wang, "On clustering fMRI using potts and mixture regression models," *Proc Conf IEEE Eng Med Biol Soc* 4795–4798 (2009).
37. M. E. Tipping, "Sparse bayesian learning and the relevance vector machine," *J Mach Learn Res* **1**, 211–244 (2001).
38. A. Dempster, L. A., and R. D., "Maximum likelihood from incomplete data via the EM algorithm," *J Royal Stat Soc B* **39**, 1–38 (1977).
39. G. M. McLachlan and D. Peel, *Finite Mixture Models*. New York: Wiley (2001).
40. L. Harrison, W. Penny, J. Daunizeau, and K. Friston, "Diffusion-based spatial priors for functional magnetic resonance images," *NeuroImage* **41**, 408–423 (2008).
41. S. Geman and D. Geman, "Stochastic relaxation, Gibbs distributions, and the Bayesian restoration of images," *IEEE Trans Pattern Anal Mach Intell* **6**, 721–741 (1984).
42. K. Blekas, A. Likas, N. P. Galatsanos, and I. E. Lagaris, "A Spatially-Constrained Mixture Model for Image Segmentation," *IEEE Trans Neural Netw* **16**, 494–498 (2005).
43. V. Oikonomou, K. Blekas, and L. Astrakas, "Resting state fmri analysis using a spatial regression mixture model," *Bioinformatics and Bioengineering (BIBE), 2013 IEEE 13th International Conference on* 1–4 (2013).
44. S. Gunn and J. Kandola, "Structural modelling with sparse kernels," *Mach Learning* **48**, 137–163 (2002).
45. M. Girolami and S. Rogers, "Hierarchic Bayesian models for kernel learning," *ICML '05: Proceedings of the 22nd Intern Conf on Mach Learning*, (New York, NY, USA), 241–248, ACM (2005).
46. J. Nocedal and S. J. Wright, *Numerical Optimization*. Springer-Verlag New York, Inc. (1999).
47. S. Pieper, M. Halle, and R. Kikinis, "3D SLICER," *IEEE Int Symp Biomed Imaging ISBI 2004* 632–635 (2004).
48. L. Astrakas, S. Konitsiotis, P. Margariti, S. Tsouli, L. Tzarouhi, and M. I. Argyropoulou, "T2 relaxometry and fMRI of the brain in lateonset restless legs syndrome," *Neurology* **71**, 911–916 (2008).
49. Z. Shehzad, A. M. C. Kelly, P. T. Reiss, D. G. Gee, K. Gotimer, L. Q. Uddin, S. H. Lee, D. S. Margulies, A. K. Roy, B. B. Biswal, E. Petkova, F. X. Castellanos, and M. P. Milham, "The resting brain: Unconstrained yet reliable," *Cerebral Cortex* **19**, 2209–2229 (2009).

Chapter 10

Tree Structure for Modeling Skin Lesion Growth

Tim K. Lee,[*,†,‡,§] *Sina Khakabi,*[‡] *Paul Wighton,*[#] *Harvey Lui,*[*,†] *David I. McLean*[†] *and M. Stella Atkins*[†,‡]

[*] *Departments of Cancer Control Research and Integrative Oncology, BC Cancer Agency, Vancouver, Canada*

[†] *Photomedicine Institute, Department of Dermatology and Skin Science, University of British Columbia and Vancouver Coastal Health Research Institute, Vancouver, Canada*

[‡] *School of Computing Science, Simon Fraser University, Burnaby, Canada*

[#] *Martinos Center for Biomedical Imaging, Harvard Medical School, Boston, USA*

[§] *Email: tlee@bccrc.ca*

Cutaneous malignant melanoma is one of the most frequent types of cancer in the world; but if the malignancy is detected and treated early, it can be cured. Many dermatologists promote dermoscopy as an early detection tool; however, dermoscopy requires formal training with a steep learning curve. In this chapter, we introduce a novel tree-based framework to automate the melanoma detection from dermoscopic images. Inspired by the radial and vertical growth pattern of skin lesions, we designed a flexible and powerful framework by decomposing dermoscopic images recursively. Pixels are repeatedly clustered into sub-images according to the color information and spatial constraints. This framework allows us to extract features by examining the tree from a graphical aspect, or from a textural/geometrical aspect on the nodes. In order to demonstrate the effectiveness of the proposed framework, we applied the technique, in completely different manners, to two common tasks of a computer-aided diagnostic system: segmentation and classification. The former task achieved a per-pixel sensitivity and specificity of 0.89 and 0.90 respectively on a challenging data set of 116 pigmented skin lesions. The latter task was tested on a public data set of 112 malignant and 298 benign lesions. We obtained 0.86 and 0.85 for precision and recall, respectively, along with an F-measure of 0.83 using a 3-layer perceptron. These experiments testified the versatility and the power of the tree-structure framework for dermoscopic analyses.

1. Introduction

Malignant melanoma of the skin, a life-threatening disease, has been increasing rapidly and steadily among fair-skinned populations over last few decades. In British Columbia, Canada, a low sun country of the world, the incidence rate has been tripled since 1970's.[1] South of Canada, the USA recorded a 3.1% average annual increase.[2] In Australia, melanoma has surpassed lung cancer as the third most common cancer for both men and women and the most common cancer for men between the age of 15 and 44.[3] Overall, the disease has become a major health problem for the countries with a large white population.

Malignant melanoma is very treatable if it is detected early. The five-year survival rate is greater than 90%. However, the prognosis is poor for many patients with advanced or late staged disease. For these patients, the 5-year survival rate can reduce dramatically to only 15% after their initial diagnosis.[4] Thus, early detection is essential for a successful treatment of the disease.

Early melanoma detection is, however, challenging because the malignancy often resembles benign lesions such as melanocytic nevi and seborrheic keratoses.[5,6] Diagnosis with naked eyes often results in false negatives or false positives.[5,7,8] In order to improve the diagnostic accuracy, many experts have been advocating the use of a non-invasive hand-held device, dermoscopy, which provides a magnified view of the skin internal structure.[9] Applying either polarized light or oil immersion to render the outermost layer of the skin, epidermis to be translucent, physicians who have specially trained for the technique can examine the morphology of the skin lesion at the dermal-epidermal junction and render a diagnosis. (Figure 1 shows two examples of dermoscopic images.) Studies showed that this non-invasive technique improved the diagnostic accuracy only for the trained physicians. Untrained doctors, even dermatologists, are often confused by the complex and unfamiliar visual patterns, thereby reducing their diagnostic capability.[9] Recently, many research groups have been developing automated computer algorithms to assist physicians in analyzing the complex dermoscopic patterns in the hope to neutralize the steep learning curve of the technique. The common approach is to detect and analyze various dermoscopic structures such as pigment networks, streaks and blood vessels.[10–14] This approach achieves various degrees of success.

In this chapter, we introduce a new framework for automatic analysis of dermoscopic images. It is a novel approach inspired by the analysis of the growth pattern of skin lesions. In this approach, a dermoscopic image is decomposed using a simple growth model estimated using a single image; then a tree-structure is constructed to represent the growth model.

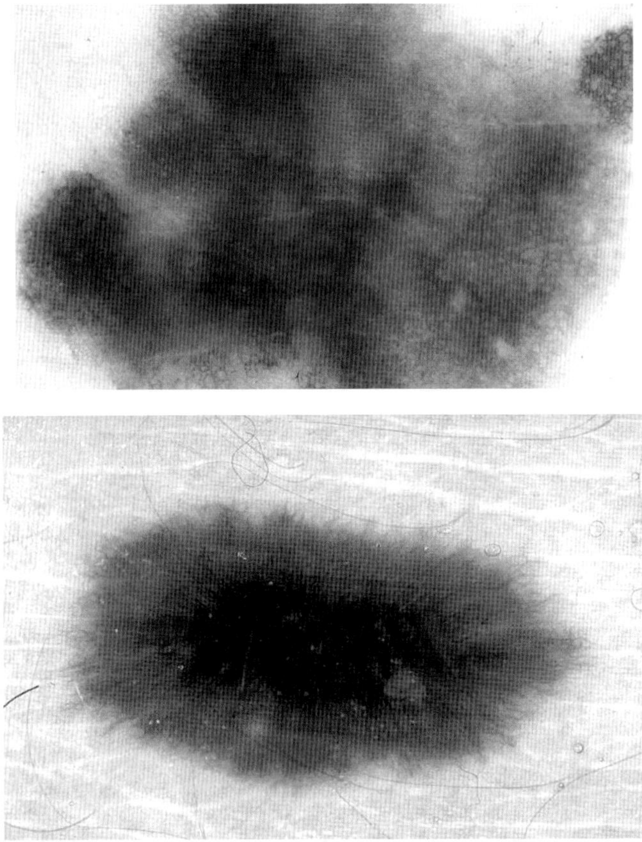

Fig. 1. Samples of dermoscopic images. The top lesion has an irregular shape, while the bottom figure has a regular oval shape.

The remaining of the paper is organized as follows: the next section reviews the lesion growing model and previous works on decomposition. Section 3 describes the construction of the tree-based framework, a very flexible structure allowing it to adopt for various scenarios and needs. Sections 4 and 5 demonstrate the flexibility of the technique by applying it to two common tasks of a computer-aided diagnostic system: lesion segmentation and classification. Finally, a short conclusion is presented in Section 6.

2. Background and Previous Work

2.1. *Lesion Growth Model*

Cuteneous malignant melanomas are often identified with two growth phases: radial and vertical.[15] Both malignant and benign pigmented skin lesions usually

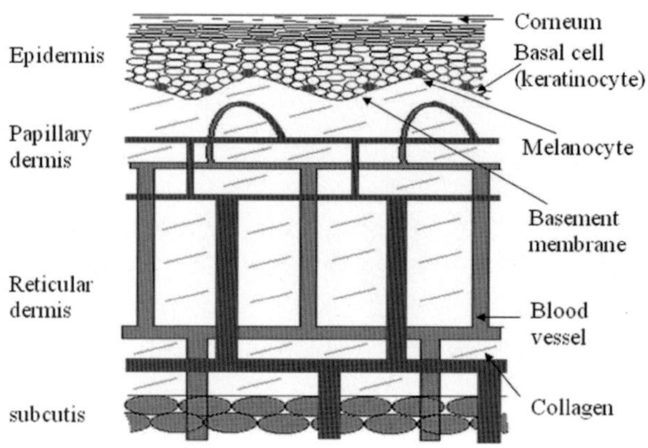

Fig. 2. Schematic of the epidermis and dermis strcutures.

begin with a radial growth. In this phase, a pigmented lesion is formed by nests of melanocytes, which synthesize a brown pigmentation called melanin. This phase commences at the dermal-epidermal junction and the entire horizontal growth phase is confined in epidermis, the outer layer of the skin. The vertical growth phase is marked by the penetration of the basement membrane of the outer skin into the dermis. (Figure 2 depicts the structure of the epidermis and dermis.) During the growth of a lesion, the width and depth of the lesion extend out from the initial melanocytic nest of the lesion. Due to the natural history of normal and abnormal cells, benign skin lesions tend to grow evenly, often in a regular oval shape, while abnormal lesions often result in an irregular shape. (Figure 1 illustrates two lesions, one with an irregular shape and another one with a regular oval shape.)

Using a single dermoscopic image, the growth pattern of a pigmented lesion can be postulated because the center the lesion is often the initial melanocytic nest. Zhou *et al.* utilized this hypothesis[16] and observed that most dermatologists placed the center of the lesion in the middle of a dermoscopic image frame, and constrained a segmentation algorithm spatially by assuming the middle of the image frame as the initial growing point of the lesion. We further observed that the periphery of a skin lesion often has a lighter brown color than the interior of the lesion. This phenomenon could be explained by the fact that the center of the lesion is usually thicker with more layers of melanocytes than the newly grown areas near the periphery. Because melanin absorbs light, the central area tends to have less reflected light and, hence, darker than the periphery. Thus, we modified Zhou *et al.*'s growth model in the following way: the center of a skin lesion is determined by the dark-color portion of the skin lesion. Based on this extended growth model, we decompose the skin image into a tree structure.

2.2. *Decomposition*

Shape and image decomposition can be categorized into boundary-based or area-based approaches. The former method has been successfully used to analyze border irregularity of a lesion by decomposing a lesion border into a series of indentation and protrusion segments.[17] However, in order to analyze the growth pattern of a lesion, an area-based method is required to analyze the image texture. There are many successful ways to perform area-based decomposition, such as morphological shape decomposition and skeleton decomposition.[18] Unfortunately, a pigmented skin lesion may manifest one or more of the following patterns: reticular, globular, cobblestone, starburst, parallel and homogeneous. In addition, the spatial relationship between any texture patterns is unknown. Hence, it is a nontrivial task to design an optimal structural element for the morphological operations. On the other hand, skeleton decomposition is the complement problem of boundary decomposition; both depend strongly on the border shape and may not reflect the internal texture patterns. In this chapter, a new decomposition method by clustering is proposed. The method represents the growth pattern of the lesion.

3. Decomposing Skin Images into Tree Structures

Unlike Zhou *et al.*'s approach,[16] our goal is to represent the growth pattern of a skin lesion by creating a tree structure. this chapter assumes that the center of the lesion (or part of a lesion in the middle of the recursion) is defined by the center of the dark pixels of the lesion. The central point is used to constraint the clustering the image pixels into dark and light regions. The identification of the central point and clustering are performed recursively in order to decompose a skin region into two sub-regions, which are also marked as the node of a tree. Thus the tree-building process can be divided into three subtasks: identifying the central point, clustering the image pixels and constructing the tree.

3.1. *Extraction of the Central Point*

Let us denote a pixel p of a color skin lesion image by its image coordinate (x, y). A set of connected pixels CP can be divided into dark and light pixels according to their luminance intensities $I(x, y)$, normalized by the maximum luminance intensity I_m. Thus, the coordinates of the dark pixels, denoted by the set $\{(DX, DY)\}$, is defined as:

$$\{(DX, DY)\} = \left\{ (x, y) \left| \frac{I(x, y)}{I_m} \leq I_d \right. \right\}, \tag{1}$$

for all $p \in CP$. I_d is the pre-defined cut-off threshold for the dark pixels.

The central point (x_c, y_c) of CP is defined by the centroid of the dark pixels only. For n connected dark pixels as determined by Eq. (1), the centroid of CP is defined as:

$$(x_c, y_c) = \left(1/n \sum_{i=1}^{n} x_i,\ 1/n \sum_{i=1}^{n} y_i \right), \quad x_i \in DX, \quad y_i \in DY. \tag{2}$$

Note that the detection of dark pixels in Eq. (1) is only for the determination of the central point. We hypothesize that a lesion expands from the central point (x_c, y_c), the centroid of the dark pixels, as it grows. Thus, an ideal normal skin lesion will have concentric circles or ellipses for the dark and light pixels as shown in Fig. 3. However, real lesions often show a complex shape, especially, for melanomas which consist of unstable malignant cells and produces irregular growth rate in different directions. Sometimes, the dark or light pixels may not form a connected component. Nevertheless, the scheme in the following section decomposes a skin lesion into a tree structure according to the distance from the central point (x_c, y_c), along with the color information of the lesion.

Fig. 3. The growth pattern of an ideal skin lesion, as shown in dark and light pixels. For this paper, the center point of the lesion is defined by the centroid of the dark pixels only.

3.2. *Clustering Decomposition*

A set of connected pixels *CP* is decomposed into two regions using the well-known k-means clustering algorithm, which minimizes the sum of squares of the distance between the feature (variable) associated with the pixels of the region and the region centroids.[19,20] For the dark and light regions, i.e. $k = 2$, the k-means clustering is formulated as:

$$\arg\min_{S} \sum_{i=1}^{2} \sum_{f_j \in S_i} \frac{1}{w_i} \|f_j - \mu_i\|^2, \tag{3}$$

where f_j is the j feature (variable) of the region, and μ_i is the centroid of the region S_i. For our task, one spatial feature and two chromatic features are applied in the clustering algorithm: the radial distance D and the blue and green intensity channels of the RGB color image. The red channel is eliminated in order to reduce the effect of the blood vessels. The radial distance D of a pixel (x, y) is defined as the Euclidean distance between the pixel and the central point of the original connected pixels *CP*, which is computed by Eq. (2). The features are weighted by w_i. Such a weight is especially important for the radial distance D because too strong a weight on D places the emphasis on the spatial feature over the chromatic features and results artificially rounded regions. After clustering, the parent region formed by *CP* is divided into two disjoint sibling regions CP_1 and CP_2.

3.3. *Tree Construction*

The root node of the tree structure is initialized to the cluster of all pixels of the skin lesion image. Then the nodes for the subsequent depth is built recursively by clustering the pixels of the parent's node into the two disjoint sibling regions (CP_1 and CP_2), using 2-means clustering, according to the distances to the centroid of the parent nodes and the red and blue intensity values. The termination condition varies according to the analysis need. As demonstrated in the following sections, a tree with a fixed depth is used in the segmentation task, while a tree with variable length is constructed for lesion diagnosis.

The resultant tree structure has two important properties:

(1) Summation of the pixel counts at every level of the tree is equal to the number of pixels in the original image, and
(2) Every pixel belongs to exactly one cluster at every level of the tree.

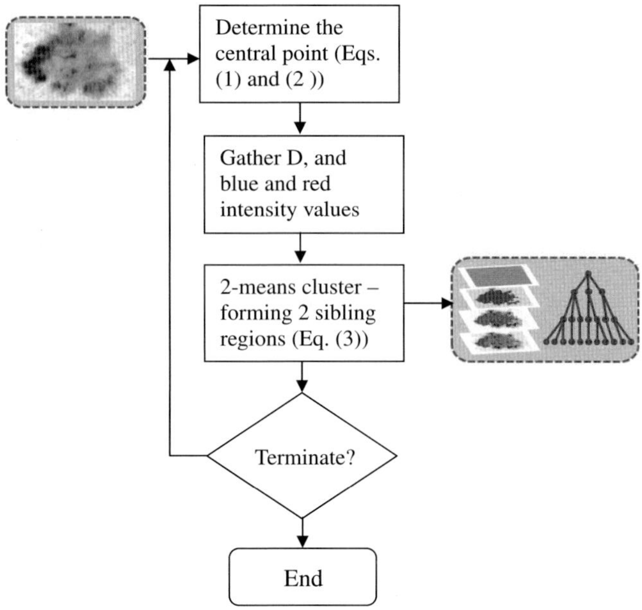

Fig. 4. Flowchart of the image decomposition process.

These two properties along with the flexibility of the termination condition during the tree construction provide a rich representation over which many salient features of the color skin lesion can be extracted.

The flowchart of the decomposition process and tree construction is shown in Fig. 4, outlining the entire process from an input image to the final tree structure.

4. Skin Lesion Segmentation

The usefulness of the tree representation is first demonstrated in a skin lesion segmentation application. The tree is constructed with the following parameters. The cut-off intensity I_d in Eq. (1) was set to 0.25, and the weights w_j in Eq. (2) were set to 2 for the radial distance D, and to 1 for both blue and green channels. In addition, the depth of the tree was set to 4. In other words, after decomposing a color skin image, the root level places all image pixels into one cluster, and other level decomposes the pixels into different clusters according to the procedure described in Section 3. Because a RGB color image consists of 3 intensity channels, the tree decomposition method generates 12 intensity images (3 color channels and 4 depth levels) as shown

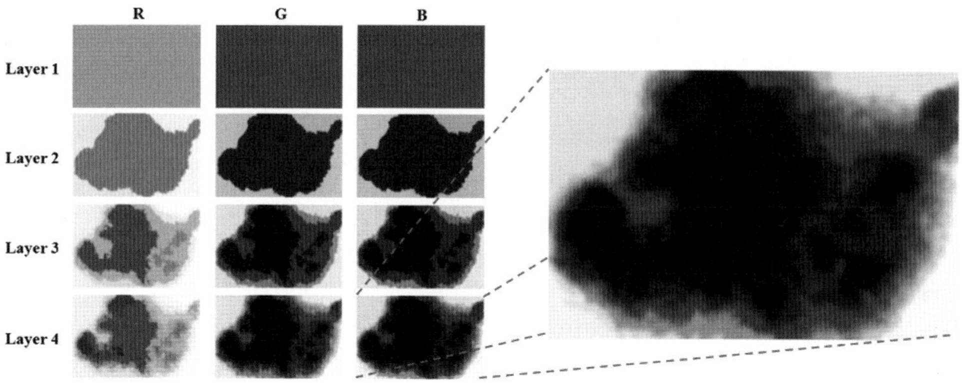

Fig. 5. Decompose the top figure of Fig. 1 for segmentation. The tree has 4 levels and 3 channels in each level.

in Fig. 5. The intensity value in each cluster is first assigned to the mean cluster intensity value. Then each intensity image was smoothed by a 15×15 Gaussian filters with $\sigma = 5$.

A feature vector of 13 elements was extracted for each pixel using the above data representation. The feature elements were the 12 intensity values in all levels and color channels, along with a spatial feature, the Euclidean distance between the pixel and the center of the lesion (x_c, y_c) of the root level. The feature vector was applied to a MAP estimation based on supervised learning model for automated skin lesion analysis.[21] The label set for the segmentation task in this model was $L = \{\text{'}lesion\text{'}; \text{'}background\text{'}\}$.

The first stage in the supervised learning model was the training stage in which parameters for the multivariate Gaussian distribution were estimated for the labeling phase. The posterior probabilities $P(p_j|l_i)$ (i.e. probability of a pixel p given the label l_i in the label set L) were modeled as multivariate Gaussian distribution. In the second stage which was the labeling stage, labels l^* were assigned to the pixels of previously unseen images using maximum likelihood estimation in the following way:

$$l^* = \arg\max_{l_i \in L}(\log P(p|l_i) + \log P(l_i)). \tag{4}$$

As in this case there were two classes $l_1 = lesion$ and $l_2 = background$, the following constraint was considered:

$$P(l_1) + P(l_2) = 1. \tag{5}$$

The ROC curve was obtained by varying the values of $P(l_1)$ and $P(l_2)$ according to constraint in equation above. Equivalently, the ROC curve could be generated using a simple threshold method over the pixel probability map obtained using the following equation:

$$l_i(p) = \frac{P(p|l_i)}{P(p|l_2) + P(p|l_2)}, \tag{6}$$

where $l_i(p)$ is the likelihood of each label.[21]

The segmentation method was tested in a dataset, which has been used in several segmentation algorithms. The dataset contained 116 images of which 100 were considered challenging from a dermoscopic atlas.[22] An image is considered challenging if at least one of the following conditions are true[21]:

(1) the contrast between skin and lesion is low,
(2) there is significant occlusion by oil or hair,
(3) the entire lesion is not visible (partial lesion),
(4) the lesion contains variegated colors, or
(5) the lesion border is not clearly defined.

In addition, each image was segmented by a dermatologist to provide the ground truth, and pixels were labeled from the set L = {'*lesion*'; '*background*'}. Ten-fold cross-validation was used to validate the method.

Examples of five segmentation results from our method are provided in Fig. 6, where the first row is an easy image to segment and the remaining rows are the challenging cases containing lesions occluded with hair, partial lesions and low contrast borders of the lesions. No pre-processing of removing hairs or noise is applied to this segmentation test of the data representation.

The segmentation results are tabulated in Table 1 along with six other state-of-the-art skin lesion segmentation techniques: G-LoG/LDA,[21] KPP,[16] JSEG,[23] DTEA,[24] SRM,[25] and FSN.[26] The dataset was tested using the authors' implementation of their methods. Similar to G-LoG/LDA,[21] the output of the current method is a probability map of the pixels. Consequently, by changing the threshold of the segmentation over this probability map, the ROC curves were obtained (see Fig. 7). The output of the five other methods is binary segmentation of lesions; therefore, the nearest point on the ROC curve was compared with the sensitivity/specificity pairs. Table 1 lists ΔSens and ΔSpec, which show the difference between the sensitivity/specificity of methods with the closest pair on ROC curve of the current method. The area under the curve is only used to compare the current method with G-LoG/LDA in the column AUC. The sensitivity/specicity reported in the table for the current method and for G-LoG/LDA is the closest point to (0; 1), the optimal performance, on the ROC curve.

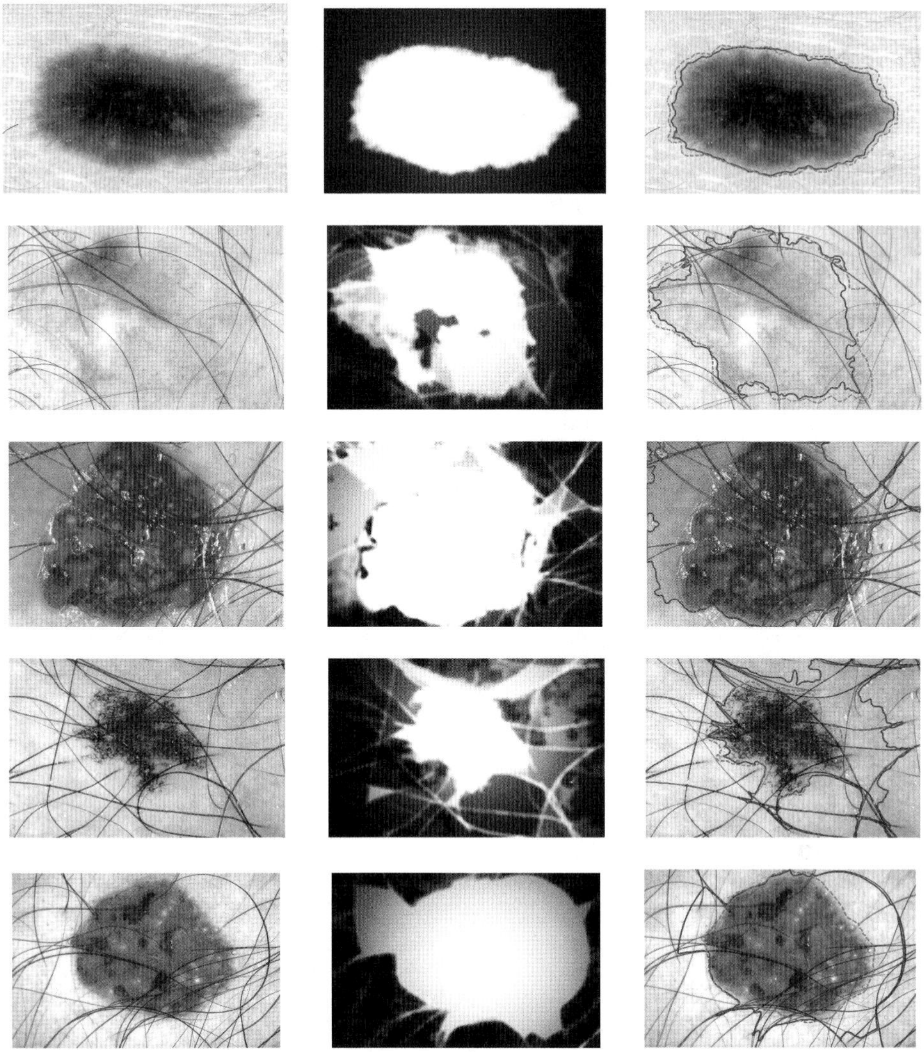

Fig. 6. Examples for the segmentation model. Examples of easy (first row) and challenging (second to the fifth rows) images are shown. The first column shows the original dermoscopic images. The second column demonstrates resulting probability maps obtained using the learning model. Our segmentation results and the ground-truth are depicted as blue and red dashed line, respectively, in the third column. Note: hair or noise removal pre-processing was not applied in this experiment.

The current method with tree decomposition achieved excellent AUC, sensitivity and specificity of 0.96, 0.89 and 0.90, respectively. These indicators showed that the technique outperformed G-LoG/LDA. The tree-based approach also outperformed KPP, DTEA, SRM, and FSN, and was comparable to JSEG's performance according to ΔSens and ΔSpec.

Table 1. Comparison of results of our segmentation method with six other methods.

Method	AUC	Sens.	Spec.	ΔAUC	ΔSens.	ΔSpec.
Our method	0.954	0.881	0.903	N/A	N/A	N/A
G-LoG/LDA	0.948	0.880	0.887	0.006	0.001	0.016
KPP	N/A	0.717	0.790	N/A	0.164	0.025
DTEA	N/A	0.641	0.987	N/A	0.035	−0.001
SRM	N/A	0.770	0.946	N/A	0.002	0.024
JSEG	N/A	0.678	0.986	N/A	−0.002	−0.001
FSN	N/A	0.812	0.935	N/A	0.012	0.017

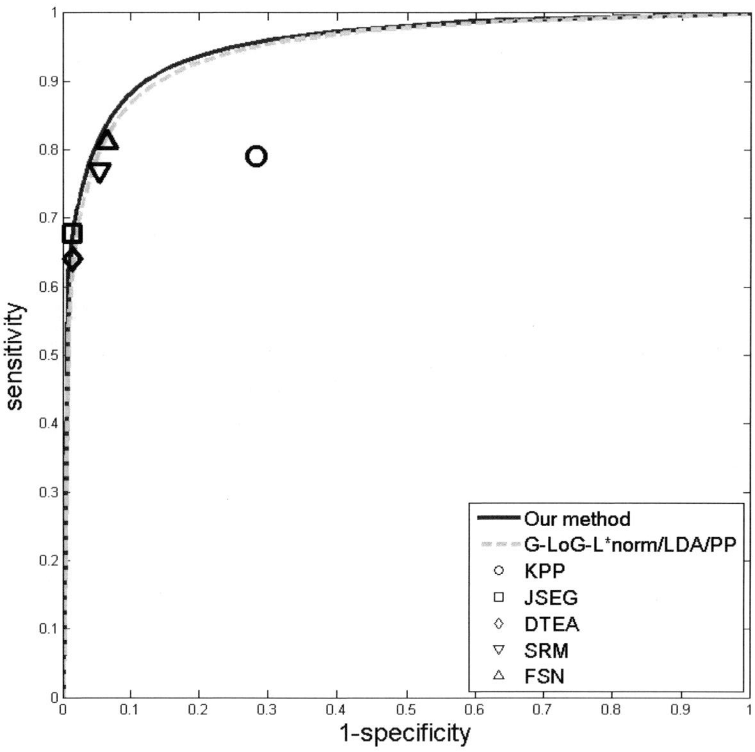

Fig. 7. Comparing the ROC curves for our method and six other methods, G-LoG/LDA,[21] KPP,[16] JSEG,[23] DTEA,[24] SRM,[25] and FSN.[26]

5. Skin Lesion Diagnosis

In the second experiment, we demonstrated the flexibility of the framework by modifying the decomposition process for a lesion diagnosis problem. The cut-off intensity I_d in Eq. (1) and the weights w_j for spatial parameter D and chromatic channels in Eq. (2) were kept to 0.25, 1, and 2, respectively, similar to the skin lesion segmentation experiment. However, instead of using the RGB color channels, hue, saturation, and intensity of HSI color space were used in the k-means clustering procedure described in Section 3.2. There were two other major modifications for building the data structure: a tree structure with a variable depth is constructed and a cluster and shrink procedure is deployed for pruning one of the regions. During the tree construction, the lighter regions obtained from the k-means were pruned. Only the darker regions were kept and decomposed again. In additional, the following four conditions were set for the termination of the tree construction:

(1) A dark region was too small in size;
(2) A dark region consisted of similar colors;
(3) The decomposed dark region had not significantly changed in comparison to its parent; and
(4) The depth of the constructed tree reached a predefined limit.

When one of the above conditions was met, the decomposition terminated. Figure 8 depicts the resultant tree structure for a benign and an abnormal lesion.

Features used for analysing lesion condition were also changed. Observing the new tree structures in Fig. 8 for a typical benign and a malignant lesion, we realized that the tree itself (graphical aspect) could be used to differentiate the disease condition. Thus the following feature vector was selected: the number of nodes and leaves of the tree, the depth of the tree and the average compactness index for each level of the tree. Compactness index CI was defined as

$$CI = \frac{PE}{4\pi A}, \tag{7}$$

where PE and A denoted the perimeter and the corresponding area, respectively, of the darker region. The CI was calculated for all the nodes in the tree; then, the mean value of the all CIs over each depth of the tree was calculated and stored in the feature vector. Because the root region was rectangular, the CI for this node was ignored. Thus, the number of CIs was one less than the maximum possible depth of the tree which was defined in the termination condition.

The tree representation and the feature vector were tested in a two-class classification (malignant vs. benign) experiment, using a data set of 410 pigmented skin images randomly selected from Interactive Atlas of Dermoscopy.[27] In this dataset, there were 112 malignant lesion images (containing melanoma and pigmented basal cell carcinomas), and 298 benign lesion images (consisting

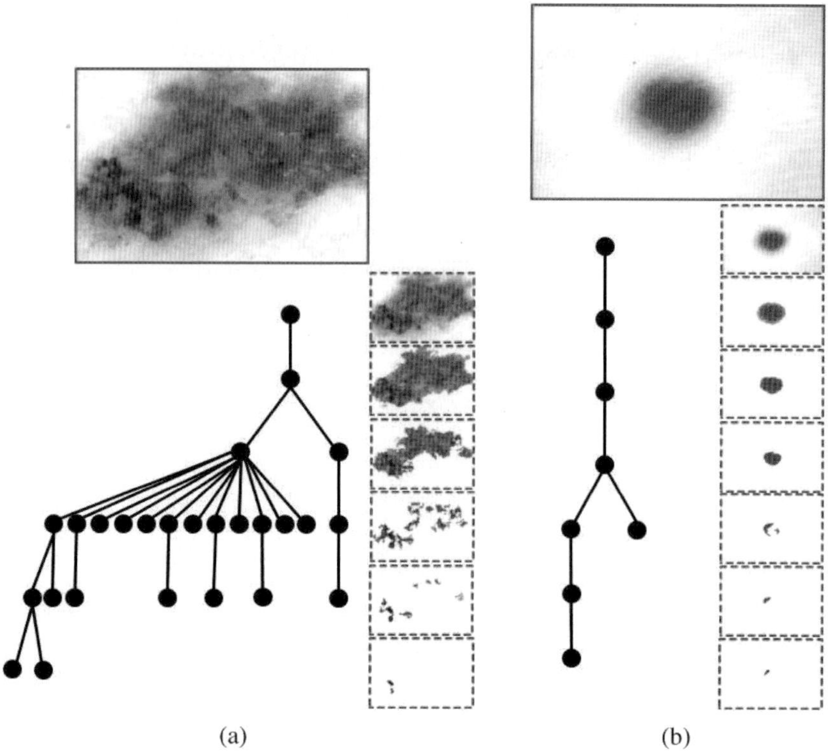

Fig. 8. The variable tree structures with the lighter region pruned for (a) a melanoma and (b) a benign lesion.

Table 2. Classification results for the two-class classification, benign and malignant, using a data set of 410 lesion images.

Feature set	Classifier	Precision	Recall	F-Measure	AUC of ROC
All features	3-layer perceptron	0.855	0.849	0.834	0.786
Graphical features	3-layer perceptron	0.848	0.841	0.824	0.787
CI1 to CI3	3-layer perceptron	0.639	0.712	0.641	0.617
CI4 to CI9	3-layer perceptron	0.713	0.729	0.622	0.494
All features	AdaBoost	0.829	0.832	0.817	0.745
Graphical Features	AdaBoost	0.835	0.837	0.823	0.776
CI1 to CI3	AdaBoost	0.692	0.732	0.685	0.637
CI4 to CI9	AdaBoost	0.596	0.722	0.614	0.490

of atypical, congenital, compound, dermal, Spitz, and blue nevi; seborrheic keratosis; and dermatofibroma). The ground truth was provided by the atlas.

Publicly available machine learning tools, a 3-layer perceptron and AdaBoost of WEKA[28] were used to classify the 410 images into malignant and benign. The parameters for the perceptron were set as follows: learning rate was set to 0.3, momentum was set to 0.2, training time was set to 500 and validation threshold was set to 20. The parameters of AdaBoost were set as follows: the number of iterations was set to 10, the seed was randomly generated and the weight threshold was set to 100.

The data set was tested in four different ways. In the first approach, all twelve features were gathered in a 12-dimensional feature set [number of nodes, number of leaves, depth, and 9 compactness index (*CI*) components] and the resulting set was fed into the two classifiers separately. The second evaluation was done by just using the graphical feature set (number of nodes, number of leaves, depth). In the third and fourth approaches, *CI1* to *CI3* and *CI4* to *CI9* were evaluated respectively to validate the discriminative power of different layers in the tree in our method. In all these approaches, the validation method was set to a ten-fold cross validation. The malignant and benign images were randomly chosen from separate classes and uniformly merged and distributed over the folds. Table 2 provides the classification results between the malignant and benign classes for our dataset using two classifiers and four approaches. Figure 9 shows the ROC curves from the 3-layer perceptron and AdaBoost classifiers.

Table 2 shows that using all features, both classifiers returned very good results in precision, recall and F-Measure. The 3-layer perceptron achieved 0.86, 0.85 and 0.83 for precision, recall and F-measure, respectively. The results for AdaBoost were slightly lower, but were above 0.8 for precision and recall. Interestingly, the graphical features alone were performing so well. They achieved similar performance as all features under the perceptron classifier, and they surpassed the all features results under the AdaBoost classifier. This illustrated the strength of the tree structure over the other methods that were only based on textural/geometrical features. These results also explained that the *CI1* to *CI3* feature set, the top three layers, had more discriminative power than the *CI4* to *CI9* feature set, the lower layer set.

The ROC curves in this study are obtained using WEKA machine learning software.[28] The reason behind the more jagged ROC curve for AdaBoost was likely due to the low density of the grid search over the parameters of the classifier. The denser grid for the 3-layer perceptron classifier results in the smoother curves.

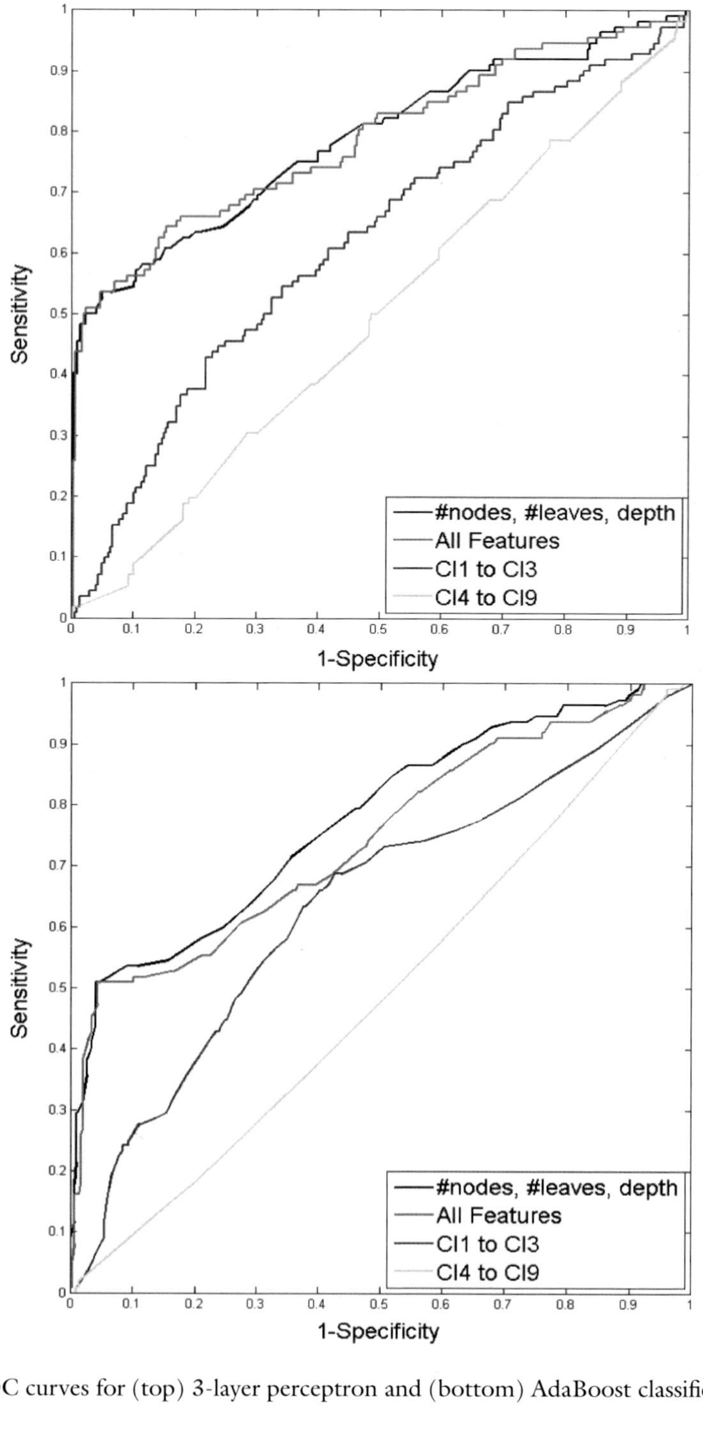

Fig. 9. ROC curves for (top) 3-layer perceptron and (bottom) AdaBoost classifiers for lesion diagnosis.

6. Conclusions

In this chapter, we introduce a novel tree structure-based framework for dermoscopic image analysis. Inspired by skin lesion growth patterns, we designed a flexible and powerful framework, which decomposes a skin image into a mutli-level tree structure. All pixels are represented uniquely in each level; hence, task-specific salient features can be extracted. In order to demonstrate the flexibility and the power of the framework, it was tested in two common skin image analysis tasks of segmentation and diagnosis. Both segmentation and diagnosis programs returns good and promising results. However, the configurations and the parameters for these two programs are not the emphasis of this chapter because we believe one can extract new features to future improve the results. The main focus is the tree structure framework itself, which can be applied to other skin image analysis tasks.

Acknowledgments

This work was supported in part by the Natural Sciences and Engineering Research Council of Canada (NSERC) and the Canadian Institute of Health Research (CIHR), and by a scholarship from the CIHR Skin Research Training Centre.

References

1. D. I. McLean, N. Phillips, Y. Zhou, R. Gallagher and T. K. Lee, "40-Year Trends in Skin Cancer in British Columbia, Canada, 1973 to 2003," *J Cutaneous Med Surg* **16**, 83–91 (2012).
2. E. Linos, S. M. Swetter, M. G. Cockburn, G. A. Colditz and C. A. Clarke, "Increasing burden of melanoma in the United States," *J Invest Dermatol* **129**, 1666–1674 (2009).
3. Australian Institute of Health and Welfare, "Cancer incidence projections Australia 2002 to 2011," Cat. no. CAN 25, Canberra, 166 (2005).
4. C. M. Balch, J. E. Gershenwald, S. J. Soong, J. F. Thompson, M. B. Atkins, D. R. Byrd, A. C. Buzaid, A. J. Cochran *et al.*, "Final version of 2009 AJCC melanoma staging and classification," *J Clin Oncol* **27**, 6199–6206 (2009).
5. D. D. Witheiler and C. J. Cockerell, "Sensitivity of diagnosis of malignant melanoma: A clinicopathologic study with a critical assessment of biopsy techniques," *Exp Dermatol* **1**, 170–175 (1992).
6. L. Izikson, A. J. Sober, M. C. Mihm, Jr. and A. Zembowicz, "Prevalence of melanoma clinically resembling seborrheic keratosis: Analysis of 9204 cases," *Arch Dermatol* **138**, 1562–1566 (2002).
7. C. M. Grin, A. Kopf, B. Welkovich, R. Bart and M. Levenstein, "Accuracy in the clinical diagnosis of malignant melanoma," *Arc Dermatol* **126**, 763–766 (1990).

8. J. Mayer, "Systematic review of the diagnostic accuracy of dermatoscopy in detecting malignant melanoma," *Med J Aust* **167**, 206–210 (1997).
9. M. Binder, M. Schwarz, A. Winkler, A. Steiner, A. Kaider, K. Wolff and H. Pehamberger, "Epiluminescence microscopy: A useful tool for the diagnosis of pigmented skin lesions for formally trained dermatologists," *Arch Dermatol* **131**, 286–291 (1995).
10. M. Sadeghi, T. K. Lee, D. McLean, H. Lui and M. S. Atkins, "Global pattern analysis and classification of dermoscopic images using textons," In D. R. O. S. Haynor, editor, *Medical Imaging 2012: Image Processing* (2012).
11. M. Sadeghi, T. K. Lee, D. McLean, H. Lui and M. S. Atkins, "Detection and analysis of irregular streaks in dermoscopic images of skin lesions," *Ieee T Med Imaging* **32**, 849–861 (2013).
12. M. Sadeghi, M. Razmara, T. K. Lee and M. S. Atkins, "A novel method for detection of pigment network in dermoscopic images using graphs," *Comput Med Imaging Graph* **35**, 137–143 (2011).
13. H. Mirzaalian, T. K. Lee and G. Hamarneh, "Learning features for streak detection in dermoscopic color images using localized radial flux of principal intensity curvature", *IEEE Workshop on Mathematical Methods in Biomedical Image 2012*, Jan. 9–10, 2012, Breckenridge, Colorado, USA (2012).
14. P. Kharazmi and T. K. Lee, "Automatic segmentation of vascular patterns in dermoscopy images", *The 37th Canadian Medical and Biological Engineering Conference*, May 20–23, 2014, Vancouver, Canada (2014).
15. W. H. Clark, Jr., A. M. Ainsworth, E. A. Bernardino, C. H. Yang, C. M. Mihm, Jr. and R. J. Reed, "The developmental biology of primary human malignant melanomas," *Semin Oncol* **2**, 83–103 (1975).
16. H. Zhou, M. Chen, L. Zou, R. Gass, L. Ferris, L. Drogowski and J. M. Rehg, "Spatially constrained segmentation of dermoscopy images," *I S Biomed Imaging*, 800–803 (2008).
17. T. K. Lee, D. I. McLean and M. S. Atkins, "Irregularity index: A new border irregularity measure for cutaneous melanocytic lesions," *Medical Image Analysis* 7, 47–64 (2003).
18. D. N. Vizireanu, "Generalizations of binary morphological shape decomposition," *J Electronic Imaging* **16**, 013002 (2007).
19. G. A. F. Seber, *Multivariate Observations*, John Wiley & Sons, Inc., Hoboken, New Jersey, (1984).
20. H. Spath, *The Cluster Dissection and Analysis Theory FORTRAN Programs Examples*, Prentice-Hall Inc., Upper Saddle River, New Jersey, (1985).
21. P. Wighton, T. K. Lee, H. Lui, D. I. McLean and M. S. Atkins, "Generalizing Common Tasks in Automated Skin Lesion Diagnosis," *IEEE Trans Information Techn Biomed* **15**, 622–629 (2011).
22. G. Argenziano, H. P. Soyer, S. Chimenti, R. Talamini, R. Corona, F. Sera, M. Binder, L. Cerroni *et al.*, "Dermoscopy of pigmented skin lesions: Results of a consensus meeting via the Internet," *J Am Acad Dermatol* **48**, 679–693 (2003).
23. M. E. Celebi, Y. A. Aslandogan, W. V. Stoecker, H. Iyatomi, H. Oka and X. H. Chen, "Unsupervised border detection in dermoscopy images," *Skin Res Techn* **13**, 454–462 (2007).

24. H. Iyatomi, H. Oka, M. Celebi, M. Hashimoto, M. Hagiwara, M. Tanaka and K. Ogawa, "An improved internet-based melanoma screening system with dermatologist-like tumor area extraction algorithm," *Comp Medical Imaging Graphics* **32**, 566–579 (2008).
25. M. Celebi, H. Kingravi, H. Iyatomi, Y. Aslandogan, W. Stoecker, R. Moss, J. Malters, J. Grichnik *et al.*, "Border detection in dermoscopy images using statistical region merging," *Skin Res Tech* **14**, 347–353 (2008).
26. M. Celebi, S. Hwang, H. Iyatomi and G. Schaefer, "Robust border detection in dermoscopy images using threshold fusion," *17th IEEE International Conference on Image Processing (ICIP)*, 2541–2544 (2010).
27. G. Argenziano, H. P. Soyer, V. D. Giorgio, D. Piccolo, P. Carli, M. Delfino, A. Ferrari, R. Hofmann-Wellenhof *et al.*, *Interactive Atlas of Dermoscopy*, Edra Medical Publishing and New Media, Milan, Italy (2000).
28. M. Hall, E. Frank, G. Holmes, B. Pfahringer, P. Reutemann and I. H. Witten, "The WEKA data mining software: an update," *SIGKDD Explorations* **11** (2009).

Chapter 11

Automatic Detection of Retinal Structures Based on Mathematical Morphology

Sandra Morales, Valery Naranjo and Mariano Alcañiz*

Instituto Interuniversitario de Investigación en Bioingeniería y Tecnología Orientada al Ser Humano
Universitat Politècnica de València, I3BH/LabHuman
Camino de Vera s/n, 46022 Valencia, Spain
**E-mail: smorales@labhuman.i3bh.es*

The retinal vascular network and optic disc are two of the most important anatomical structures of the fundus. Two methods to detect them have been included in this chapter. Their goal is to form part of some disease screening system since the segmentation of these structures can be a key process to assist clinicians in different pathology diagnosis. For example, both of them can be used as reference to detect several retinal lesions or other ocular structures in addition to identifying some fundus features. This chapter presents an in-depth study about the use of mathematical morphology to locate these main retinal structures. In particular, the proposed methods are characterized by combining several morphological operators and by making use of a variant of the watershed transformation, the stochastic watershed. This transformation avoids sub-segmentation problems related to the classical watershed. The methods have been validated in several public databases by improving the results of other state-of-the-art algorithms. Therefore, it has been demonstrated that the performance of the stochastic watershed allows us to apply it for clinical purposes.

1. Introduction

Retinal vasculature is able to indicate the status of other vessels of the human body. Indeed, the retina is the only location where blood vessels can be directly visualised non-invasively *in vivo*.[1] That is the reason why its study is usually included in the standard screening of any patient with diseases in which the vessels may be altered. In many instances preclinical signs are not easily recognized and often appear as signs or symptoms that are not specific for a particular disease, but the retina and its blood vessel characteristics have been shown to be a window into several disease processes.[2]

Retinal imaging is, nowadays, a mainstay of the clinical care and management of patients with retinal as well as systemic diseases. Many important diseases manifest themselves in the retina and originate either in the eye, the brain or the cardiovascular system. In particular, the most prevalent diseases that can be studied via eye imaging and image analysis are: diabetes, diabetic retinopathy, age-related macular degeneration, glaucoma and cardiovascular disease.[3] Screening campaigns are usually considered effective if the disease in question is identified at an early, preferably preclinical, stage and if it is amenable to treatment.[2] In the main, the best approach for risk population assessment seems to be a direct, regular and complete ophthalmologic examination.[4] However, population growth, ageing, physical inactivity and rising levels of obesity are contributing factors to increase retinopathies, so that the number of ophthalmologists for the assessment by direct examination of the population risk is high.[5] Moreover, it must be stressed that this type of retinal disease identification, that is based on manual observation, is highly subjective.[6] So, for those reasons, automatic screening systems are increasingly important. They are able to relieve physicians of repetitive work, increase efficiency and provide remarkable cost-savings in addition to be accessible in rural and remote areas where there is a lack of eye specialists.[7]

Retinal segmentation is a fundamental component of most automatic retinal disease screening systems.[8] It is usually a prerequisite before systems achieve more complex tasks as identifying different pathologies. In general, several anatomical structures are segmented through fundus image processing and then some features are extracted from them to characterize each pathology. The most important anatomical structures of the fundus are the vascular network, that is the retinal blood vessels, and the optic disc (OD). Both of them can be used as reference to detect other anatomical ocular structures or several retinal lesions and to identify some fundus features. For example, among their multiples uses, the following can be stressed. Morphological attributes of retinal blood vessels, such as length, width, tortuosity and/or branching pattern and angles are utilized for diagnosis, screening, treatment, and evaluation of various cardiovascular and ophthalmologic diseases.[9] The relation between the size of the optic disc and the cup (cup-disc-ratio) is widely used for glaucoma diagnosis.[10] The relatively constant distance between the optic disc and the fovea is useful for estimating the location of the macula, area of the retina related to fine vision.[11]

This chapter presents an in-depth study about the use of mathematical morphology in order to detect the main retinal structures. The methods that will be presented are characterized by combining several morphological operators, basic ones and other more complex, and by making use of a variant of the watershed transformation, the stochastic watershed, which avoids sub-segmentation problems related to the classical watershed.

Numerous segmentation methods of retinal structures have been reported in literature. Nevertheless, this chapter is only focused on detection methods of the vascular tree and the optic disc. Moreover, it must be emphasized that the method proposed for vascular tree detection obtains directly the retinal network skeleton avoiding a complete vessel segmentation stage. This approach is different than most of literature about this topic where a skeletonization is usually performed on the vessels previously detected. However, it should be taken into account that the major drawback of this strategy is the dependence of the different stages on the previous ones in addition to computational cost. So, presenting a method which obtains the retinal tree centerline without the necessity of vessel segmenting can reduce the number of necessary steps in fundus image processing and at the same time the dependency of previous stages can also be reduced.

Referring to vessel extraction techniques, they can be mainly divided into four categories: edge detectors, matched filters, pattern recognition techniques and morphological approaches. A more extensive classification can be found in Ref. [8]. Most edge detection algorithms assess changes between pixels values by calculating image gradient magnitude and then it is thresholded to create a binary edge image.[12,13] Matched filters are filters rotated in different directions in order to identify the cross section of blood vessels.[14,15] Pattern recognition techniques can be divided into supervised and unsupervised approaches. Supervised methods, such as artificial neural networks[16] or support vector machines,[17,18] exploit some prior labelling information to decide whether a pixel belongs to a vessel or not, while unsupervised algorithms[19] perform the vessel segmentation without any prior labelling knowledge. Morphological processing is based on vessels characteristics known *a priori* (line connected segments) and combines morphological operators to achieve the segmentation.[20,21] Although most state-of-the-art methods look for detecting all vessel pixels of the vascular tree, there are also some attempts based on finding the vessel skeleton, or in other words, the vessel centerline. The work of Chen *et al.* is based on shortest path connection,[22] Sofka and Stewart on the use of matched filters,[23] Wu and Derwent on ridge descriptors[24] and Walter and Klein and Bessaid *et al.* on the application of watershed transformation[25,26] but none of them is based on the use of stochastic watershed.

Regarding the OD-boundary detectors, the presented techniques can mainly be grouped into template-based methods, deformable models, and morphological algorithms. Different approaches have been proposed according to template-based methods: edge detection techniques followed by the Circular Hough Transform;[27,28] pyramidal decomposition and Hausdorff-based template matching;[29] colour decorralated templates;[30] or a kNN-regressor along with a circular template.[11] Concerning deformable models, GVF-snake,[31] ASM,[32] and modified active contours, which exploit specific features of the optic disc anatomy[33] or incorpore knowledge-based clustering and updating,[34] have also been used to this purpose. As for algorithms based on mathematical morphology, most of them detect the OD by means of watershed transformation, generally through marker-controlled watershed,[35–37] although each author chooses different markers. The centroid of the largest and brightest object of the image is considered as an approximation for the locus of the OD and it is used as internal marker.[35] The extended minima transformation[38] is applied to select the internal markers and external markers are calculated as an effectively partition of the image into regions, so that each region contains single internal marker and part of the background.[36] A list of pixels belonging to the main vessels arcade in the vicinity of an internal OD point previously detected are also used.[37] On the other hand, some authors propose combining various algorithms to get a better approximation of the OD-boundary.[39,40]

The rest of the chapter is organized as follows: in Section 2 a basic theoretical background about morphological operators and the stochastic watershed transformation is included. Sections 3 and 4 describe two methods based on mathematical morphology to detect the main retinal structures. Section 5 shows the experimental results of the methods explained above and they are compared with other state-of-the-art algorithms. Finally, Section 6 provides conclusions.

2. Theoretical Background

2.1. *Morphological Operators*

Mathematical morphology is a non-linear image processing methodology based on minimum and maximum operations whose aim is to extract relevant structures of an image.[41]

Let f be a grey-scale image which is defined as $f(\mathbf{x}): E \rightarrow T$ where $\mathbf{x}$ is the pixel position. In the case of discrete valued images, $T = \{t_{min}, t_{min} + 1, \ldots, t_{max}\}$ is an ordered set of gray-levels. Typically, in digital 8-bit images $t_{min} = 0$ and $t_{max} = 255$. Furthermore, let $B(\mathbf{x})$ be a sub-set of Z^2 called structuring element (shape probe) centred at point $\mathbf{x}$, whose shape is usually chosen according to some *a priori* knowledge about the geometry of the relevant and irrelevant image structures. The two basic morphological operators are:

$$\begin{aligned} \textit{Dilation}: [\delta_B(f)](\mathbf{x}) &= \max_{b \in B(\mathbf{x})} f(\mathbf{x}+\mathbf{b}) \\ \textit{Erosion}: [\varepsilon_B(f)](\mathbf{x}) &= \min_{b \in B(\mathbf{x})} f(\mathbf{x}+\mathbf{b}). \end{aligned} \tag{1}$$

Their purpose is to expand light or dark regions, respectively, according to the size and shape of the structuring element. Those elementary operations can be combined to obtain a new set of operators or basic filters given by:

$$\begin{aligned} \textit{Opening}: \gamma_B(f) &= \delta_B(\varepsilon_B(f)) \\ \textit{Closing}: \varphi_B(f) &= \varepsilon_B(\delta_B(f)). \end{aligned} \tag{2}$$

Light or dark structures are respectively filtered out from the image by these operators regarding the structuring element chosen.

Other morphological operators that complement the previous ones are geodesic transformations. The *geodesic dilation* is the iterative unitary dilation of an image f (marker) which is contained within an image g (reference),

$$\delta_g^{(n)}(f) = \delta_g^{(1)}\delta_g^{(n-1)}(f), \text{ being } \delta_g^{(1)}(f) = \delta_B(f) \wedge g. \tag{3}$$

The *reconstruction by dilation* is the successive geodesic dilation of f regarding g up to idempotence,

$$\gamma^{rec}(g,f) = \delta_g^{(i)}(f), \quad \text{so that } \delta_g^{(i)}(f) = \delta_g^{(i+1)}(f). \tag{4}$$

Using the *geodesic reconstruction*, a *close-hole operator* can also be defined. For a grey-scale image, it is considered a hole any set of connected points surrounded by connected components of value strictly greater than the hole values. This operator fills all holes in an image f that do not touch the image boundary f_∂ (used as marker):

$$\psi^{ch}(f) = [\gamma^{rec}(f^c, f_\partial)]^c, \tag{5}$$

where f^c is the complement image (i.e., the negative).

2.2. *Stochastic Watershed Transformation*

Watershed transformation is a segmentation technique for gray-scale images.[42] This algorithm is a powerful segmentation tool whenever the minima of the image represent the objects of interest and the maxima are the separation boundaries between objects. Due to this fact, the input image of this method is usually a gradient image. In mathematical morphology, the gradient $\varrho(f)(\mathbf{x})$

of an image $f(\mathbf{x})$ can be obtained as the pointwise difference between a unitary dilation and a unitary erosion, i.e.,

$$\varrho(f)(\mathbf{x}) = \delta_B(f)(\mathbf{x}) - \varepsilon_B(f)(\mathbf{x}). \quad (6)$$

In the case of a gradient image is considered as input image, the watershed transformation produces a segmentation which can be viewed as: a set of closed contours of segmented regions which will be noted by $WS(\varrho(f))$, or a partition of the space E in a set of classes named $\Pi(WS(\varrho(f)))$.

However, one problem of this technique is the over-segmentation, which is caused by the existence of numerous local minima in the image normally due to the presence of noise. One solution to this problem is using marker-controlled watershed, $WS(\varrho)_{f_{mrk}}$, in which the markers f_{mrk} artificially indicate the minima of the image. Nevertheless the controversial issue consists in determining f_{mrk} for each region of interest,

$$f_{mrk}(\mathbf{x}) = \begin{cases} 0 & \text{if } \mathbf{x} \in \mathit{marker} \\ 255 & \mathit{Otherwise}. \end{cases} \quad (7)$$

Note that the use of few markers along with the existence of borders within the structure to be segmented can also cause some parts of it to not be detected (sub-segmentation). So, the choice of correct markers is crucial for the effectiveness and robustness of the algorithm.

A watershed transformation variant is used to solve this conflict, the stochastic watershed.[43] In this transformation, a given number M of marker-controlled-watershed realizations are performed selecting N random markers in order to estimate a probability density function (pdf) of image contours and filter out non significant fluctuations. Let $\{f_{mrk\,i}\}_{i=1}^{M}$ be M sets of N uniform random markers and $WS_i = WS(\varrho)_{f_{mrk\,i}}$ the ith output image of the marker-controlled watershed imposed by $f_{mrk\,i}$. The pdf of image contours is computed by Parzen window method[44] as follows

$$pdf(\mathbf{x}) = \frac{1}{M}\sum_{i=1}^{M}(WS_i(\mathbf{x}) * G(\mathbf{x}; s)), \quad (8)$$

where $G(\mathbf{x}; s)$ represents a Gaussian kernel of variance σ^2 and mean μ ($\mu = 0$)

$$G(\mathbf{x}; s) = \frac{1}{2\pi\sigma^2} e^{-\left(\frac{\|\mathbf{x}\|^2}{2\sigma^2}\right)}. \quad (9)$$

Afterwards, it is necessary to perform a last marker-controlled watershed on the pdf obtained.

This type of watershed works better than other marker-based watershed transformations used previously in literature. In the next section, two different applications of the stochastic watershed will be explained in detail.

2.3. *Image Enhancement*

Non-uniform illumination and low contrast are typical and inherent problems to the image capture technique. Moreover, in the case of retinal images, both problems are especially pronounced due to the fact that the retina is a spherical structure and it is necessary for the use of a spotlight to capture the image. So, they should be corrected prior to the image processing. For instance, in this chapter, next local transformation for shade correction is proposed

$$\Gamma(f)(t) = \begin{cases} \dfrac{\frac{1}{2}(u_{max} - u_{min})}{(\mu_f - t_{min})^r}(t - t_{min})^r + u_{min} & \text{if } t \leq \mu_f \\ \dfrac{-\frac{1}{2}(u_{max} - u_{min})}{(\mu_f - t_{max})^r}(t - t_{max})^r + u_{max} & \text{if } t > \mu_f. \end{cases} \tag{10}$$

where t_{min} and t_{max} are the minimum and maximum grey level of the image respectively, u_{min} and u_{max} are the target levels (typically 0 and 255 respectively), μ_f is the mean value of the image for all pixels within a window centred at the current pixel $\mathbf{x}$ of the fixed size, and the parameter r is used to control the contrast increasing (experimentally $r = 2$).

3. Retinal Vessel Centerline Extraction

This section is focused on obtaining directly the skeleton of the retinal vascular tree by means of mathematical morphology and curvature evaluation. Its goal is to reduce the number of necessary steps in fundus image processing at the same time that the dependency of previous stages is reduced in comparison with methods that perform a complete segmentation of retinal vessels. Specifically, it involves two main steps: in the first step, the principal curvature is calculated on the retinal image. In the second step, the stochastic watershed is applied to extract the vascular skeleton.

Although fundus images are RGB format [Fig. 2(a)], the present work is drawn on monochrome images obtained from the green component extraction because this band provides improved visibility of the blood vessels [Fig. 2(b)]. Moreover, this grey image is enhanced with the algorithm of Section 2.3. Then, a small opening, using a disc of radius 1 as SE (B_1), is performed on the enhanced green component image to fill in any gaps in vessels that could provoke subsequent errors, for example due to brighter zone within arteries. Next, a dual top-hat, with a SE larger than the widest vessel (B_2), is applied with the goal of extracting all of them and eliminating structures with high gradient that are not vessels, as occurs with the optic disc border [Fig. 2(c)]. Afterwards, with the aim of highlighting the vessels on the background, principal curvature, f_κ, is calculated as the maximum eigenvalue of the Hessian matrix[12] resulting the image shown in Fig. 2(d). Finally, stochastic watershed is applied to the curvature image.

This transformation uses random markers to build a probability density function (*pdf*) of contours [Fig. 2(e)], which is then segmented by a last marker-controlled watershed. Thereby, the vascular skeleton is part of the frontiers of the resultant regions [Fig. 2(f)]. In addition to the random markers some controlled markers are also included. It is forced that there is at least one marker in the area delimited by the crossing of two vessels. These areas are determined by means of the residue of the close-hole operator on f_κ. This methodology avoids the fact that some vessels are not detected by the watershed transformation (see Fig. 1).

In order to discriminate which frontiers are significant and which ones are not and should be filtered out, the frontiers are multiplied by f_κ and then are thresholded [Fig. 2(g)] using a fixed threshold, experimentally $t = 0.05$. Once the skeleton is obtained, a pruning process is applied to remove possible spurs giving rise to the final result of the method [Fig. 2(h) and 2(i)]. The implemented pruning process is characterized by removing spur branches but without altering the main branches. Only the branches whose size is less than an threshold are removed while the others are remained intact.

Next, the algorithm and figure summarizes the steps of the vessel centerline extraction method which has been explained.

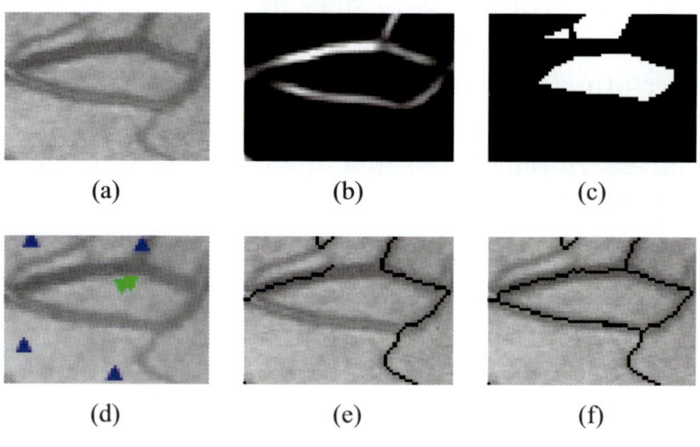

Fig. 1. Stochastic watershed on the crossing of two vessels: (a) Enhanced green component, (b) Principal curvature (f_κ), (c) Residue of close-hole operator, (d) Random (blue ▲) and controlled (green ▼) markers, (e) Result of the stochastic watershed using only the random markers shown in blue and (f) Result of the stochastic watershed combining random and controlled markers (blue and green).

Algorithm 1: Vessel centerline extraction

Data: Original RGB fundus image $\mathbf{f} = (f_R, f_G, f_B)$
Result: Vessel centerline, f_{out}

initialization: B_1, B_2 ;
$f_{in} \leftarrow f_G$ Green component selection ;
$f_{enh} \leftarrow \Gamma(f_{in})$ Image Enhancement ;
$f_{op} \leftarrow \gamma_{B_1}(f_{enh})$ Opening ;
$f_{dth} \leftarrow \rho_{B_2}(f_{op})$ Dual top-hat ;
$f_{\kappa} \leftarrow max[eig(H(f_{dth}))]$ Principal curvature ;
$f_{ws} \leftarrow WS(f_{\kappa})_{f_{mrk}}$ Stochastic Watershed ;
$f_{th} \leftarrow (f_{\kappa} \times f_{ws}) < t$ Thresholding ;
$f_{out} \leftarrow \Upsilon(f_{th})$ Pruning ;

4. Optic Disc Segmentation

The automatic OD-segmentation method proposed in this section is focused on using different operations based on mathematical morphology on a fundus image to obtain the OD-contour. Previously, a pre-processing of the original RGB image is required. The first step of the pre-processing consists in applying PCA to transform the input image to grey scale. This technique combines the most significant information of the three components RGB in a single image so that it is a more appropriate input to the segmentation method. After segmentation, a post-processing is also performed to fit the final region contour by a circumference. In Fig. 3, the main steps of the segmentation process are depicted. Note that the whole image is processed although only a region of interest is shown for better visualisation. A detailed explanation of the method can be found in Ref. [45].

4.1. *Pre-processing*

Generally, an initial gray-scale image is necessary to carry out most of the segmentation algorithms of the literature. However, in the case of OD segmentation, each author considers appropriate a different intensity image, such as a band of the original RGB image[11,35] or a component of other color spaces.[31,33] In this work, the use of a new grey-scale image is proposed. Specifically, it is calculated by means of principal component analysis (PCA)[46] because this type of analysis maximizes the separation of the different objects that compose a image so that the structures of the retina are better appreciated.

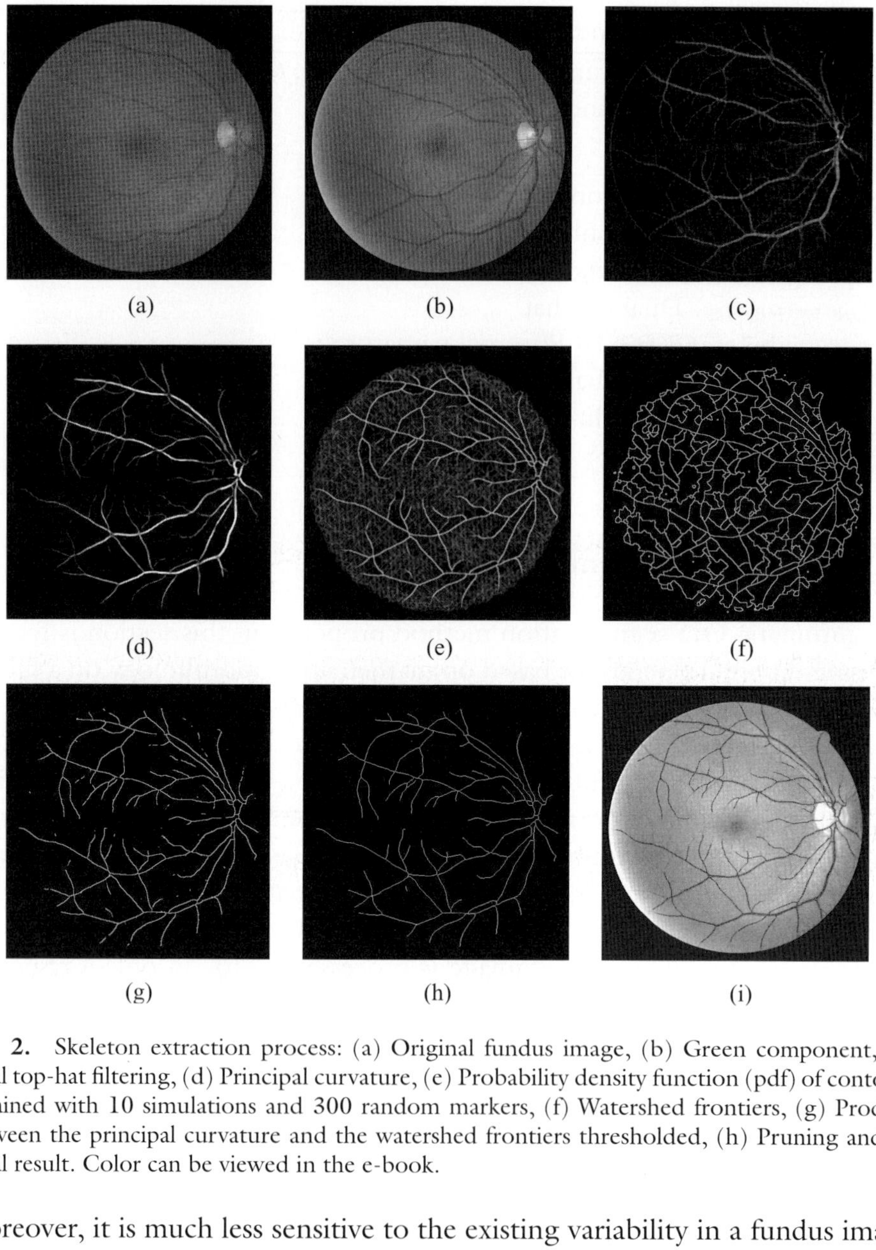

Fig. 2. Skeleton extraction process: (a) Original fundus image, (b) Green component, (c) Dual top-hat filtering, (d) Principal curvature, (e) Probability density function (pdf) of contours obtained with 10 simulations and 300 random markers, (f) Watershed frontiers, (g) Product between the principal curvature and the watershed frontiers thresholded, (h) Pruning and (i) Final result. Color can be viewed in the e-book.

Moreover, it is much less sensitive to the existing variability in a fundus image regarding color, intensity, etc. The first principal component retains most of the variations present in all of the original components, so that it is chosen as the input image of the method. Afterwards, this image is enhanced through the algorithm explained in Section 2.3.

Retinal vessels are originated from the OD, therefore there are numerous vessels crossing its border which makes its discrimination difficult. Vessel

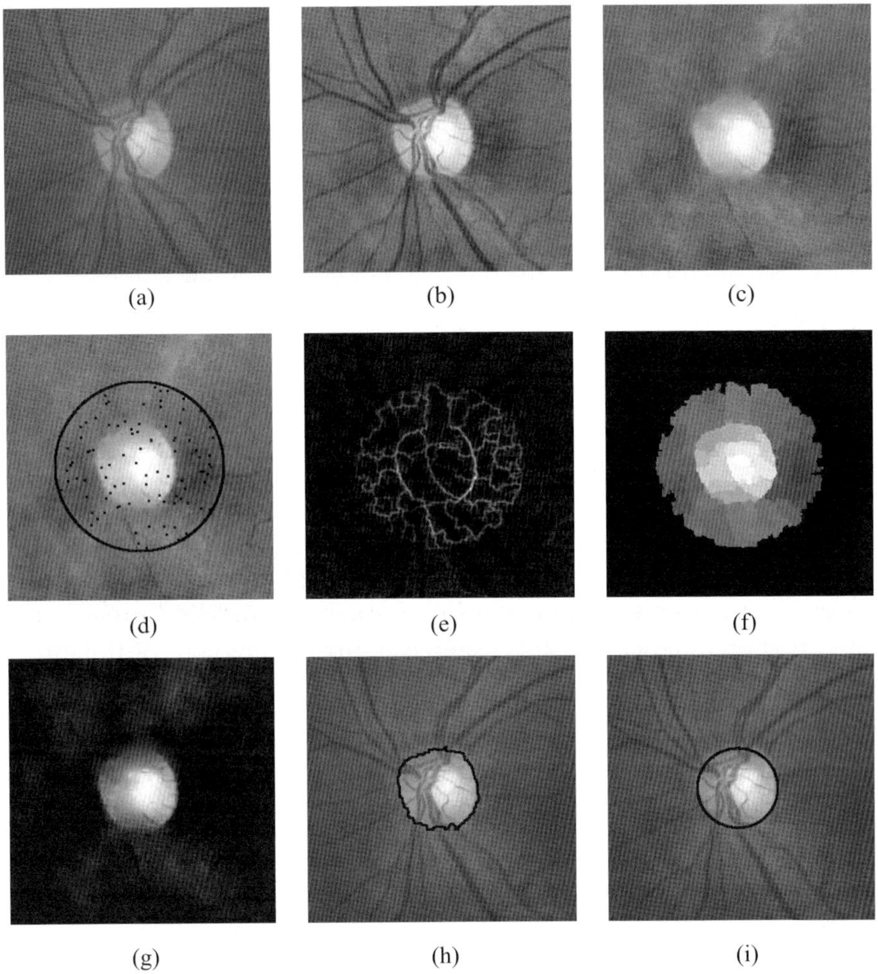

Fig. 3. OD segmentation process: (a) Original image, (b) Enhancement of first principal component, (c) Inpainted image, (d) Uniform random markers, (e) Probability density function of contours using 15 simulations and 100 internal markers, (f) Average intensity of the watershed regions, (g) Residue of close-hole operator, (h) Contour of final OD segmentation and (i) Circular approximation of the OD contour.

removal helps to extract the OD-boundary more precisely and to reduce the existing borders within the OD which increase the risk of sub-segmentation. To perform the vessel removal, an inpainting technique is applied.[47]

4.2. *Processing*

As mentioned above, the segmentation method makes use of the stochastic watershed. This transformation uses random markers to build a probability density function (*pdf*) of contours, according to Eq. (8), which is then segmented by volumic watershed for defining the most significant regions. However, in the marker definition not only internal markers (that specify what is the object of interest) are needed, but also an external marker which limits the area to be segmented.

On one hand, the chosen external marker, f_{ext}, will be a circle of constant diameter centred on the centroid of the image. The centroid of a grey-level image can be calculated through the generalized distance function (GDF).[48] This way for calculating the grey-image centroid combines the centrality of the image with respect to edge distance (i.e. purely geometric) but penalizing this distance in relation to the intensities. Thus, note that it cannot be defined as the center of mass of the intensities or as the center of the brighter and larger zone, since the two effects are combined.

On the other hand, the internal markers, f_{int}, will be uniform random markers generated within the area limited by f_{ext}. Hence, the final set of markers (external and internal), f_m is the logical OR of both of them, $f_m = f_{int} \vee f_{ext}$.

In particular, the *pdf* is built from 15 marker-controlled-watershed realizations, as shown in Section 2.2, using as input the gradient of the inpainted image [Fig. 3(c)]. f_{int} is generated for each simulation while f_{ext} is the same in all of them. The number of internal markers used is $N = 100$. An example of f_m can be observed in Fig. 3(d).

Obtaining a *pdf* of the contours of the watershed regions [Fig. 3(e)] facilitates the final segmentation, providing robustness and reliability since the arbitrariness in choosing the markers is avoided. Afterwards, the *pdf* can be combined with the initial gradient in order to reinforce the gradient contours which have a high probability resulting a probabilistic gradient.[43]

Finally, a last marker-controlled watershed is applied on the *pdf* using a new set of markers $f_{m'}$. In this case, stratified markers are employed instead of random markers. Specifically, stratified markers are uniform markers generated within an area. The reason for using this type of markers is to make sure that every pixel within the area in question belongs to a watershed region. Due to the fact that there are markers located outside the OD, not all regions obtained by the watershed transformation are wanted. The next stage is to discriminate which resulting regions are significant and which ones are not and should be filtered out. The discrimination between the significant and non-significant regions is based on the average intensity of the region. In Fig. 3(f), the average intensity of the watershed region is depicted. The regions belonging to the optic disc are light regions around darker regions therefore the residue of a close-hole operator is calculated to obtain the regions that accomplish this condition [Fig. 3(g)]. Afterwards, a threshold is applied on the resulting image to select the valid regions. This operation leads to the final OD segmentation. The value of the threshold is $u = m - 2s$, being m and s the mean and the standard deviation of the residue of the close-hole operator.

4.3. *Post-processing*

Once OD region has been obtained, the result must be fitted to eliminate false contours, which are detected due generally to the blood vessels that pass through the OD. The inpainting technique was performed to remove most of them, as previously mentioned, however some irregularities can still be appreciated in the final region contour [Fig. 3(i)].

In this case, the OD-contour has been estimated as a circle [Fig. 3(h)] in the same way that in Refs. [11, 28, 29] although a elliptical shape could also have been chosen. The fit is performed by means of Kasa's method[49] which lets us calculate the center and the radius of the circle that better is adapted to a binary region through least squares.

5. Results

5.1. *Retinal Vessel Centerline*

The validation of the vessel centerline extraction method has been carried out on two public databases widely used: DRIVE[50] and STARE.[14] Although, in both databases, manual segmentations are included, the complete vasculature has been detected, not only the vessel centerline which is the goal of our work. For that reason, the homotopic skeleton[51] associated to the manual segmentations was obtained for future comparisons. In Fig. 4, the results of

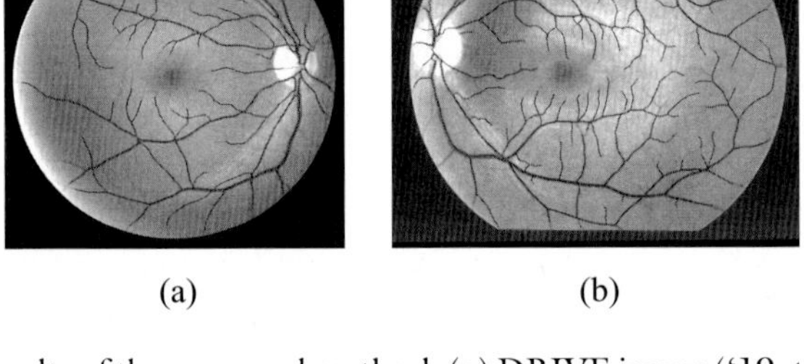

(a) (b)

Fig. 4. Skeleton results of the proposed method: (a) DRIVE image ('19_test') and (b) STARE image ('im0255').

the proposed method on two images of DRIVE and STARE databases can be observed.

The validation has been performed in two ways. One of them is based on comparing the results of this work with methods that first segment the vessels and after performing a skeletization process and the other compares it with algorithms that obtain the skeleton directly.

On one hand, regarding methods that require a previous segmentation, the presented algorithm has been compared with two methods published previously. The local maxima over scales of the magnitude of the gradient and the maximum principal curvature of the Hessian tensor are used in a multiple pass region growing procedure in the first work.[12] The other method,[52] as the presented work, is based on mathematical morphology and curvature evaluation although the morphological operations used are different as well as the obtained result. In the same way as explained above, the homotopic skeleton was performed after the segmentation process in both cases. On the other hand, as for the methods that obtain directly the retinal vessel centreline, the analysis has been focused on other two approaches based also on watershed transformation.[25,26] In Figs. 5 and 6, the strengths and weaknesses of the proposed method can be observed in two examples of both databases.

Avoiding complete vessel segmentation supposes an improvement in the automatic fundus processing since the skeleton is not dependent of a previous stage and the computational cost is reduced by decreasing the number of required steps. Apart from this fact, it must be stressed that an important advantage of the proposed method is its performance in pathological images or with large changes in illumination, as was observed in Figs. 4, 5 and 6. In those cases, the algorithm presented in this paper works properly and reduces over-segmentation problems which can be found in methods based on a previous segmentation.[12,52] With regard to other methods that obtain the skeleton in a direct way and use the watershed transformation[25,26] instead of the stochastic watershed, the proposed work achieves a more robust detection and decreases the number of spurs. Despite good results, it must be mentioned that the main disadvantage of the method is that some vessels can lose their continuity if some part of them are not detected and it should be corrected in a post-processing stage.

5.2. *Optic Disc*

The validation of the method has been carried out on five public databases: DRIONS,[53] DIARETDB1,[54] DRIVE,[50] MESSIDOR,[55] and ONHSD.[33,56]

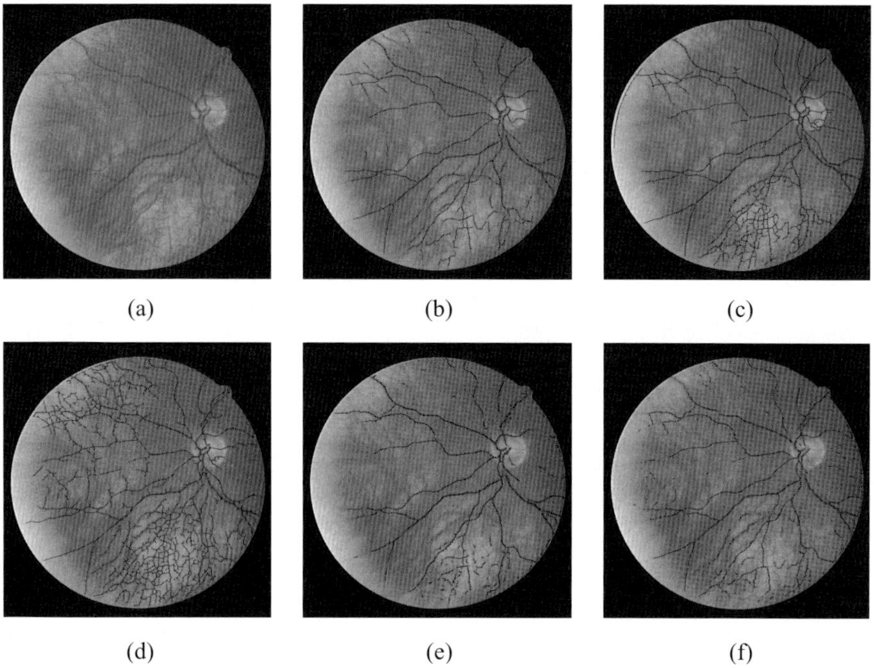

Fig. 5. Comparison between different methods on DRIVE image ('23_training'): (a) Original image, (b) Proposed method, (c) Martinez *et al.* method,[12] (d) Morales *et al.* method,[52] (e) Bessaid *et al.* method[26] and (f) Walter and Klein method.[25]

The performance of the method has been evaluated based on different concepts. Jaccard's (JC) and Dice's (S) coefficients describe similarity degree between two compared elements being equal to 1 when segmentation is perfect. Accuracy (Ac) is determined by the sum of correctly classified pixels as OD and non-OD divided by the total number of pixels in the image. True positive fraction (TPF) is established by dividing the correctly classified pixels as OD by the total number of OD pixels in the gold standard. False positive fraction (FPF) is calculated by dividing the misclassified pixels as OD by the total number of non-OD pixels in the gold standard. Finally, in order to be able to compare more with other authors' works, another measure was calculated: the mean absolute distance (MAD),[57] whose aim is to measure the accuracy of the OD-boundary.

In Table 1, the results achieved on the 5 databases can be observed. On one hand, in order to analyse the results on DRIONS database, the first observer images of this database have been taken as reference (gold standard) to calculate similarity degree between them and our segmentation. Regarding MESSIDOR database, the OD rim of these 1200 images has been hand segmented and it is currently available online to facilitate performance comparison between

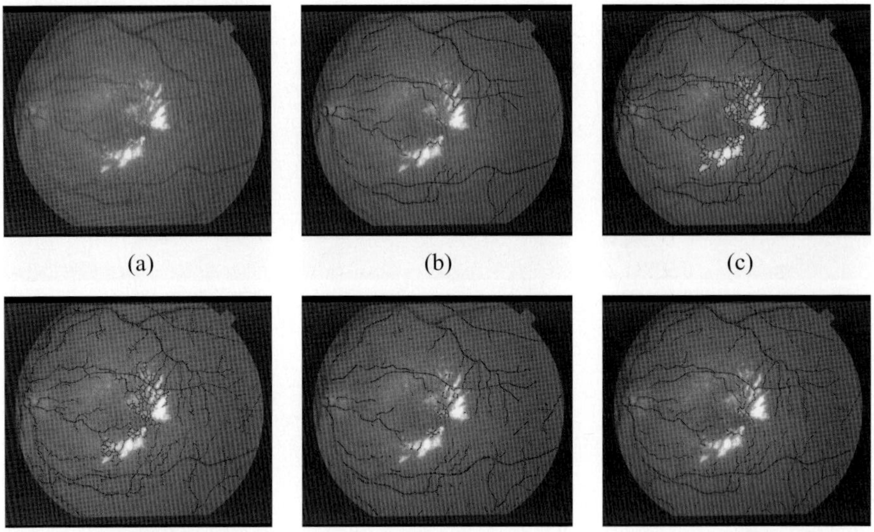

(a) (b) (c) (d) (e) (f)

Fig. 6. Comparison between different methods on STARE image ('im0001'): (a) Original image, (b) Proposed method, (c) Martinez *et al.* method,[12] (d) Morales *et al.* method,[52] (e) Bessaid *et al.* method[26] and (f) Walter and Klein method.[25]

Table 1. Results (average values and standard deviations) obtained by the proposed method using the DRIONS, DIARETDB1, DRIVE, MESSIDOR, and ONHSD databases. Jaccard's (JC) and Dice's (S) coefficients, accuracy (Ac), true positive (TPF) and true negative fractions (FPF), and mean absolute distance (MAD).

	DRIONS	DIARETDB1	DRIVE	MESSIDOR	ONHSD
JC	0.8424 (0.1174)	0.8173 (0.1308)	0.7163 (0.1880)	0.8228 (0.1384)	0.8045 (0.1175)
S	0.9084 (0.0982)	0.8930 (0.0913)	0.8169 (0.1712)	0.8950 (0.1056)	0.8867 (0.0776)
Ac	0.9934 (0.0051)	0.9957 (0.0039)	0.9903 (0.0134)	0.9949 (0.0050)	0.9941 (0.0042)
TPF	0.9281 (0.1177)	0.9224 (0.1058)	0.8544 (0.1938)	0.9300 (0.1239)	0.9310 (0.1046)
FPF	0.0040 (0.0041)	0.0028 (0.0029)	0.0061 (0.0085)	0.0035 (0.0041)	0.0043 (0.0042)
MAD	4.1098 (3.4684)	9.6759 (8.4836)	7.9981 (9.9957)	5.8387 (6.5215)	4.4826 (3.0962)

different methods.[58] Concerning ONHSD dataset, the average of the edges marked by the four experts has been used to generate the reference images. On the other hand, neither DIARETDB1 nor DRIVE database have the OD segmented publicly available. In those cases, we have compared our results with the same ground truth used in Ref. [37], where the contour of each image was labelled by four ophthalmologists, and then, only the mean of those contours is considered as ground truth.

The OD-segmentation method presented in this chapter has been compared with other morphological algorithms of the state of the art. On one

Table 2. Comparison of the parameters of Table 1 achieved by the proposed method, by the 2nd observer and by other marker-controlled-watershed algorithm on DRIONS database.

	Proposed method	2nd observer	Walter *et al.*[35]
JC	0.8424 (0.1174)	0.9202 (0.0455)	0.6227 (0.3695)
S	0.9084 (0.0982)	0.9578 (0.0265)	0.6813 (0.3854)
Ac	0.9934 (0.0051)	0.9970 (0.0017)	0.9689 (0.0492)
TPF	0.9281 (0.1177)	0.9498 (0.0537)	0.6715 (0.3980)
FPF	0.0040 (0.0041)	0.0012 (0.0009)	0.0210 (0.0417)
MAD	4.1098 (3.4684)	1.8887 (1.1455)	29.0645 (48.0576)

Table 3. Comparison of the method presented for OD-segmentation with the other state-of-the-art works in based on Jaccard's coefficient (JC) and mean absolute distance (MAD) on DIARETDB1 and DRIVE databases.

	DIARETDB1		DRIVE	
	JC	MAD	JC	MAD
Sopharak *et al.*[59]	0.2979 (0.0981)	16.31 (5.35)	0.1798 (0.0623)	20.94 (15.57)
Walter *et al.*[35]	0.3725 (0.1186)	15.52 (5.32)	0.3003 (0.1322)	12.39 (8.27)
Seo *et al.*[60]	0.3533 (0.0765)	9.74 (4.65)	0.3160 (0.0971)	11.19 (4.06)
Kande *et al.*[61]	0.3318 (0.0529)	8.35 (3.20)	0.2868 (0.0788)	17.42 (8.06)
Stąpor *et al.*[62]	0.3410 (0.0998)	6.02 (5.64)	0.3247 (0.1517)	9.85 (6.00)
Lupaşcu *et al.*[63]	0.3095 (0.1348)	13.81 (9.11)	0.4035 (0.0843)	8.05 (7.61)
Welfer *et al.*[37]	0.4365 (0.1091)	8.31 (4.05)	0.4147 (0.0833)	5.74
Morales *et al.*[45]	0.8173 (0.1308)	9.6759 (8.4836)	0.7163 (0.1880)	7.9981 (9.9957)

hand, Table 2 is focused on analysing further DRIONS database at the same time that the performance of our work is contrasted. Therefore, first, the segmented images by the second observer have also been compared with the gold standard to obtain inter-expert differences, and secondly, other existing technique based on marker-controlled-watershed transformation[35] has been implemented and compared with ours. On the other hand, the concepts of Jaccard's coefficient (also known as area overlap) and the MAD included in Table 1 allow us to compare with the method proposed in Ref. [37] as well as with other state-of-the-art algorithms that were analysed in it (see Table 3). According to these data, our method obtains a mean overlap greater than 70% for the five databases which signifcantly improves the results of the compared methods inasmuch as the best results were around 40%. As for MAD values, it can be observed that the method proposed in Ref. [45] gets the second best results on DRIVE database although its results on DIARETDB1 are not so good. However, it must be taken into account that in Ref. [37], the DIARETDB1 images along with their ground truth were resized from 1500 × 1152 pixels to 640 × 480. As MAD is a measure in pixels, it is logical that the results of Morales *et al.* were higher since they were calculated on the original size of DIARETDB1 images. Moreover, due to the fact that the DIATRETDB1 images are the largest images of the five analysed databases, it makes sense that the MAD of this database was higher than in the rest of databases. A deeper validation of the method can be found in Ref. [45], where it was also compared with template-based methods and deformable models.

6. Conclusions

Although watershed transformation is a known segmentation technique, the use of the stochastic watershed is not widely extended in spite of avoiding sub-segmentation problems related to classical watershed. In this chapter, two different applications of the stochastic watershed have been presented with clinical purposes. In particular, the main retinal structures have been segmented: the retinal vascular network and the optic disc. The detection of these structures is nowadays a key process in a lot of retinal and systemic disease screening systems.

Regarding the detection of vascular network centerline, experimental results show qualitative improvements if the proposed method is compared with other state-of-the-art algorithms, particularly with pathological images or with large changes in illumination. As for the optic disc segmentation, the obtained results (a Jaccards and Dices coefficients of 0.8200 and 0.8932, respectively, an accuracy of 0.9947, and a true positive and false positive fractions of 0.9275 and 0.0036) demonstrate that the presented algorithm is a robust tool that works properly in images with different casuistry. Therefore, it can be concluded that the stochastic watershed is an efficient and effective segmentation technique that can be applied with clinical purposes and could be useful for other further applications.

References

1. N. Patton, T. M. Aslam, T. MacGillivray, I. J. Deary, B. Dhillon, R. H. Eikelboom, K. Yogesan, and I. J. Constable, "Retinal image analysis: Concepts, applications and potential," *Progress in Retinal and Eye Research* **25**, 99–127 (2006).
2. M. J. Cree and H. F. Jelinek, "Image analysis of retinal images," ed. G. Dougherty, *Medical Image Processing: Techniques and Applications*, Biological and Medical Physics, Biomedical Engineering, chapter 11, 249–268. Springer (2011).

3. M. Abramoff, M. Garvin, and M. Sonka, "Retinal imaging and image analysis," *Biomedical Engineering, IEEE Reviews in* **3**, 169–208 (2010).
4. H. M. Herbert, K. Jordan, and D. W. Flanagan, "Is screening with digital imaging using one retinal view adequate?" *Eye*, 497–500 (2003).
5. L. Verma, G. Prakash, and H. K. Tewari, "Diabetic retinopathy: time for action. No complacency please!" *Bulletin of the World Health Organization* **80**, 419–419 (2002).
6. J. Anitha, C. Kezi Selva Vijila, and D. Jude Hemanth, "An overview of computational intelligence techniques for retinal disease identification applications," *Int J Rev Computing* **5**, 29–46 (2011).
7. American Diabetes Association, "Economic costs of diabetes in the U.S. in 2007," *Diabet Care* **31**, 596–615 (2008).
8. M. Fraz, P. Remagnino, A. Hoppe, B. Uyyanonvara, A. Rudnicka, C. Owen, and S. Barman, "Blood vessel segmentation methodologies in retinal images: A survey," *Computer Methods Programs Biomed* **108**, 407–433, (2012).
9. J. Kanski and B. Bowling, *Clinical Ophthalmology: A Systematic Approach, 7th Edition.* Elsevier Health Sciences (2011).
10. Y. Hatanaka, A. Noudo, C. Muramatsu, A. Sawada, T. Hara, T. Yamamoto, and H. Fujita, "Automatic measurement of vertical cup-to-disc ratio on retinal fundus images," In *Medical Biometrics*, vol. 6165," *Lecture Notes in Computer Science*, 64–72. Springer Berlin/Heidelberg (2010).
11. M. Niemeijer, M. D. A. Moff, and B. van Ginneken, "Fast detection of the optic disc and fovea in color fundus photographs," *Medical Image Analysis* **13**, 859–870, (2009).
12. M. E. Martinez-Perez, A. D. Hughes, S. A. Thom, A. A. Bharath, and K. H. Parker, "Segmentation of blood vessels from red-free and fluorescein retinal images," *Medical Image Analysis* **11**, 47–61, (2007).
13. X. Jiang and D. Mojon, "Adaptive local thresholding by verification-based multithreshold probing with application to vessel detection in retinal images," *IEEE Trans Pattern Anal Mach Intell* **25**, 131–137 (January, 2003).
14. A. Hoover, V. Kouznetsova, and M. Goldbaum, "Locating blood vessels in retinal images by piecewise threshold probing of a matched filter response," *IEEE Transactions on Medical Imaging* **19**, 203–210 (2000).
15. M. Al-Rawi, M. Qutaishat, and M. Arrar, "An improved matched filter for blood vessel detection of digital retinal images," *Computers Biol Med* **37**, 262–267 (2007).
16. C. Sinthanayothin, J. F. Boyce, H. L. Cook, and T. H. Williamson, "Automated localisation of the optic disc, fovea, and retinal blood vessels from digital colour fundus images," *Brit J Ophthalmology* **83**, 902–910 (1999).
17. E. Ricci and R. Perfetti, "Retinal blood vessel segmentation using line operators and support vector classification," *Medical Imaging, IEEE Transactions on* **26**, 1357–1365 (2007).
18. D. Marín, A. Aquino, M. E. Gegúndez-Arias, and J. M. Bravo, "A new supervised method for blood vessel segmentation in retinal images by using gray-level and moment invariants-based features," *Medical Imaging, IEEE Transactions on* **30**, 146–158 (2011).
19. G. B. Kande, P. V. Subbaiah, and T. S. Savithri, "Unsupervised fuzzy based vessel segmentation in pathological digital fundus images," *J Med Syst* **34**, 849–858 (2010).

20. F. Zana and J. C. Klein, "Segmentation of vessel-like patterns using mathematical morphology and curvature evaluation," *IEEE Transactions on Image Processing* **10**, 1010–1019 (2001).
21. K. Sun, Z. Chen, S. Jiang, and Y. Wang, "Morphological multiscale enhancement, fuzzy filter and watershed for vascular tree extraction in angiogram," *J Med Syst* **35**, 811–824 (2011).
22. L. Chen, Y. Ju, S. Ding, and X. Liu, "Topological vascular tree segmentation for retinal images using shortest path connection," *Image Processing (ICIP), 2011 18th IEEE International Conference on*, 2137–2140 (2011).
23. M. Sofka and C. Stewart, "Retinal vessel centerline extraction using multiscale matched filters, confidence and edge measures," *IEEE TMI* **25**, 1531–1546 (2006).
24. C. Wu, J. Kang Derwent, and P. Stanchev, "Retinal vessel radius estimation and a vessel center line segmentation method based on ridge descriptors," *J Signal Process Syst* **55**, 91–102 (2009).
25. T. Walter and J. C. Klein, "A computational approach to diagnosis of diabetic retinopathy," *Proceedings of the 6th Conference on Systemics Cybernetics and Informatics (SCI)*, 521–526 (2002).
26. A. Bessaid, A. Feroui, and M. Messadi, "Detection of blood vessels from retinal images using watershed transformation," *J Mechanics Med Biol* **09**, 633–642 (2009).
27. M. Park, J. S. Jin, and S. Luo. "Locating the optic disc in retinal images," *Proceedings of the International Conference on Computer Graphics, Imaging and Visualisation*, 141–145. IEEE Computer Society (2006).
28. A. Aquino, M. E. Gegúndez-Arias, and D. Marín, "Detecting the optic disc boundary in digital fundus images using morphological, edge detection, and feature extraction techniques," *Medical Imaging, IEEE Transactions on* **29**, 1860–1869 (2010).
29. M. Lalonde, M. Beaulieu, and L. Gagnon, "Fast and robust optic disc detection using pyramidal decomposition and hausdorff-based template matching," *Medical Imaging, IEEE Transactions on* **20**, 1193–1200 (2001).
30. T. Kauppi and H. Kälviäinen, "Simple and robust optic disc localisation using colour decorrelated templates," *Proceedings of the 10th International Conference on Advanced Concepts for Intelligent Vision Systems*, ACIVS '08, 719–729, Berlin, Heidelberg (2008). Springer-Verlag.
31. A. Osareh, M. Mirmehdi, B. Thomas, and R. Markham, "Comparison of colour spaces for optic disc localisation in retinal images," *Pattern Recognition, 2002. Proceedings. 16th International Conference on* **1**, 743–746 **1** (2002).
32. H. Li and O. Chutatape, "Automated feature extraction in color retinal images by a model based approach," *Biomedical Engineering, IEEE Transactions on* **51**, 246–254 (2004).
33. J. Lowell, A. Hunter, D. Steel, A. Basu, R. Ryder, E. Fletcher, and L. Kennedy, "Optic nerve head segmentation," *IEEE Trans Med Imaging* **23**, 256–264 (2004).
34. J. Xu, O. Chutatape, E. Sung, C. Zheng, and P. Chew Tec Kuan, "Optic disk feature extraction via modified deformable model technique for glaucoma analysis," *Pattern Recognition* **40**, 2063–2076 (2007).
35. T. Walter, J. C. Klein, P. Massin, and A. Erginay, "A contribution of image processing to the diagnosis of diabetic retinopathy-detection of exudates in color fundus images of the human retina," *Medical Imaging, IEEE Transactions on* **21**, 1236–1243 (2002).

36. C. Eswaran, A. Reza, and S. Hati, "Extraction of the contours of optic disc and exudates based on marker-controlled watershed segmentation," *Computer Science and Information Technology, 2008. ICCSIT '08. International Conference on*, 719–723 (2008).
37. D. Welfer, J. Scharcanski, C. M. Kitamura, M. M. D. Pizzol, L. W. Ludwig, and D. R. Marinho, "Segmentation of the optic disk in color eye fundus images using an adaptive morphological approach," *Computers in Biology and Medicine* **40**, 124–137 (2010).
38. R. C. Gonzalez, R. E. Woods, and S. L. Eddins, *Digital Image Processing using MATLAB*. Pearson Prentice Hall (2004).
39. J. Hajer, H. Kamel, and E. Noureddine, "Localization of the optic disk in retinal image using the 'watersnake'," *Computer and Communication Engineering, 2008. ICCCE 2008. International Conference on*, 947–951 (2008).
40. R. J. Qureshi, L. Kovacs, B. Harangi, B. Nagy, T. Peto, and A. Hajdu, "Combining algorithms for automatic detection of optic disc and macula in fundus images," *Computer Vision Image Understanding* **116**, 138–145 (2012).
41. J. Serra, *Image Analysis and Mathematical Morphology* vol. I, Ac. Press, London (1982).
42. S. Beucher and F. Meyer, *Mathematical Morphology in Image Processing*. E. Dougherty Ed. (1992).
43. J. Angulo and D. Jeulin, "Stochastic watershed segmentation," *Proc. of the 8th International Symposium on MathematicalMorphology (ISMM'2007)*, 265–279 (2007).
44. R. O. Duda and P. E. Hart, *Pattern Classification and Scene Analysis*. John Wiley & Sons Inc (1973).
45. S. Morales, V. Naranjo, J. Angulo, and M. Alcañiz, "Automatic detection of optic disc based on pca and mathematical morphology," *Medical Imaging, IEEE Transactions on* **32**, 786–796 (2013).
46. I. T. Jolliffe, *Principal Component Analysis*. Second edition, Springer (2002).
47. T. F. Chan and J. Shen, "Mathematical models for local nontexture inpaintings," *SIAM J Appl Math* **62**, 1019–1043 (2002).
48. L. Vincent, "Minimal path algorithms for the robust detection of linear features in gray images," *Proceedings of the Fourth International Symposium on Mathematical Morphology and its Applications to Image and Signal Processing*, ISMM '98, 331–338 (1998).
49. C. A. Corral and C. S. Lindquist, "On implementing kasa's circle fit procedure," *IEEE Transactions on Instrumentation and Measurement* **47**, 789–795 (1998).
50. J. Staal, M. Abramoff, M. Niemeijer, M. Viergever, and B. van Ginneken, "Ridge-based vessel segmentation in color images of the retina," *Medical Imaging, IEEE Transactions on* **23**, 501–509 (2004).
51. P. Soille, *Morphological Image Analysis: Principles and Applications*. Second edition, Springer-Verlag New York, Inc. (2003).
52. S. Morales, V. Naranjo, J. Angulo, J. Fuertes, and M. A. Niz, "Segmentation and analysis of retinal vascular tree from fundus images processing," *International Conference on Bio-inspired Systems and Signal Processing (BIOSIGNALS 2012)*, 321–324 (2012).
53. E. J. Carmona, M. Rincón, J. García-Feijoó, and J. M. Martínez-de-la-Casa, "Identification of the optic nerve head with genetic algorithms," *Artif Intell Med* **43**, 243–259 (2008).
54. T. Kauppi, V. Kalesnykiene, J.-K. Kamarainen, L. Lensu, I. Sorri, A. A. Raninen, R. Voutilainen, H. Uusitalo, H. Kälviäinen, and J. Pietilä, "The DIARETDB1 diabetic retinopathy database and evaluation protocol," *British Machine Vision Conference (BMVC2007)*, 252–261 (2007).

55. Messidor Techno-Vision Project. MESSIDOR: Digital retinal images. France (2008). http://messidor.crihan.fr/download-en.php. Last access on 24th September, 2012.
56. Retinal Image Computing & Understanding. ONHSD — Optic Nerve Head Segmentation Dataset. University of Lincoln, United Kingdom (2004). http://reviewdb.lincoln.ac.uk/Image Datasets/ONHSD.aspx. Last access on 24th September, 2012.
57. V. Chalana, D. T. Linker, D. R. Haynor, and Y. Kim, "A multiple active contour model for cardiac boundary detection on echocardiographic sequences," *IEEE Transactions on Medical Imaging* **15**, 290–298 (1996).
58. Expert system for early automated detection of dr by analysis of digital retinal images project website. Univ. Huelva, Spain. http://www.uhu.es/retinopathy/muestras.php. Last access on 24th September, 2012.
59. A. Sopharak, B. Uyyanonvara, S. Barman, and T. H. Williamson, "Automatic detection of diabetic retinopathy exudates from non-dilated retinal images using mathematical morphology methods," *Computerized Med Imag Graphics* **32**, 720–727 (2008).
60. J. Seo, K. Kim, J. Kim, K. Park, and H. Chung, "Measurement of ocular torsion using digital fundus image," *Engineering in Medicine and Biology Society, 2004. IEMBS '04. 26th Annual International Conference of the IEEE* **1**, 1711–1713 (2004).
61. G. Kande, P. Subbaiah, and T. Savithri, "Segmentation of exudates and optic disk in retinal images," *Computer Vision, Graphics Image Processing, 2008. ICVGIP '08. Sixth Indian Conference on*, 535–542 (2008).
62. K. Stąpor, A. Świtonski, R. Chrastek, and G. Michelson, "Segmentation of fundus eye images using methods of mathematical morphology for glaucoma diagnosis," *Computational Science — ICCS 2004* **3039**, *Lecture Notes in Computer Science*, 41–48. Springer Berlin Heidelberg (2004).
63. C. Lupaşcu, D. Tegolo, and L. Di Rosa, "Automated detection of optic disc location in retinal images," *Computer-Based Medical Systems, 2008. CBMS '08. 21st IEEE International Symposium on*, 17–22 (2008).

Chapter 12

Automatic Segmentation of Retinal Images for Glaucoma Screening

Jun Cheng, Fengshou Yin, Damon Wing Kee Wong and Jiang Liu

*Institute for Infocomm Research, A*STAR*
1 Fusionopolis Way, #21-01 Connexis, Singapore 138632
E-mail: jcheng, fyin, wkwong, jliu@i2r.a-star.edu.sg

Glaucoma is a chronic eye disease in which the optic nerve is progressively damaged. As the disease often progresses silently without symptoms, early detection of glaucoma via screening is important. Cup to disc ratio (CDR) computed from monocular retinal fundus images may provide an option for low cost large-scale glaucoma screening programme. In the chapter, we introduce the Automatic RetinA cup to disc Ratio AssessmenT (ARARAT) system for glaucoma screening. ARARAT uses superpixel classification to segment the optic disc and optic cup from monocular retinal fundus images and computes the CDR values for the screening. The method is validated using two data sets from different races. The areas under curve of the receiver operating characteristic curves are 0.827 and 0.822 from the two data sets. From the discussion with clinicians, the results are promising for large-scale glaucoma screening.

1. Introduction

Glaucoma is a chronic eye disease. It is the second leading cause of blindness, and is predicted to affect around 80 million people by 2020.[1] However, many patients with glaucoma are unaware of the disease until it has reached its advanced stage. Therefore, screening of people at high risk for the disease is vital. Clinically, the intraocular pressure (IOP), visual field and optic nerve head are often used in glaucoma assessment. However, the IOP measurement provides low accuracy and a visual field examination requires special equipment only present in specialized hospitals. The optic nerve head or the optic disc (in short, disc) is the location where ganglion cell axons exit the eye to form the optic nerve. A low cost way for glaucoma screening is to compute the cup to disc ratio (CDR) from a monocular 2D fundus images because: (1) CDR is well-accepted and commonly used as a good indicator for glaucoma assessment;

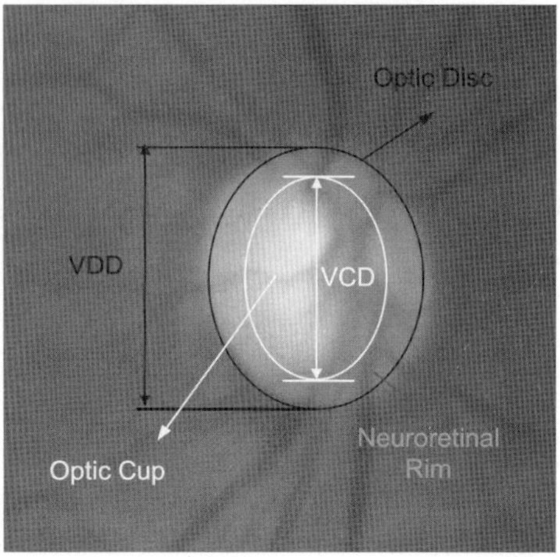

Fig. 1. Structure of an optic disc: optic disc boundary (dark); optic cup (white); neuroretinal rim (gray). CDR is computed as VCD/VDD.

(2) Fundus camera is widely available in hospitals, polyclinics, optical shops, etc. In 2D images, the disc can be divided into a central bright zone called the optic cup (in short, cup) and a peripheral region called the neuroretinal rim. Figure 1 shows the major structures of the disc. The CDR is clinically described as the ratio of the vertical cup diameter (VCD) to vertical disc diameter (VDD) clinically.

The chapter introduces Automatic RetinA cup to disc Ratio AssessmenT (ARARAT) for confidence based glaucoma screening. It includes a disc segmentation followed by a cup segmentation using superpixel classification. Centre surround statistics are computed from superpixels and combined with histograms for disc and cup segmentation. Prior knowledge of the cup is incorporated by including location information for cup segmentation. CDR is computed from the segmented disc and cup for glaucoma screening. A confidence score is computed for self-assessment of the computed CDR. Self-assessment is an important issue that has seldom been discussed previously. In practice, an automated segmentation method might work well for most images while working poorly for the rest. Therefore, it is important to have self-assessment where users are warned of cases with potentially large errors.

2. Optic Disc Segmentation

2.1. *Background*

Disc segmentation estimates the disc boundary, which is a challenging task due to many reasons such as blood vessel occlusions, pathological changes around the disc and variable imaging conditions. Many methods have been proposed for disc segmentation and they are generally classified into three types. The first type is based on template matching.[2–4] In these methods, template matching is applied to find the disc. Clinical studies show that a disc has a slightly oval shape with the vertical diameter being about 7%–10% larger than the horizontal one.[5] As a result, ellipse fitting is shown to be better than circular fitting.[4] The second type is based on deformable models.[6–10] Various deformable models are proposed and applied to find the disc boundary such as active contour model,[6] modified active snake model,[7] level set,[8] modified Chan-Vese model,[9] active shape model.[10] These methods find the disc boundary by contour deformation. The third type is based on pixel classification.[11,12] Classification-based methods use various features such as intensity and texture from each pixel and its surroundings to classify each pixel as disc or non-disc. Muramatsu *et al.*[13] showed that the pixel classification-based methods and the deformable model-based methods perform similarly. Recent studies[4] show that one challenge in disc segmentation is the differentiation of edges of the disc from edges of other surrounding structures, such as peripapillary atrophy (PPA). An example of PPA is shown as the area between the dark and light lines in Fig. 2(a). The PPA region is often confused as part of disc due to the similar color and shape that make it form another ellipse (often stronger) together with the disc. Deformable models are sensitive to poor initialization. Very often, the deformation cannot exclude PPA from the segmented disc if it has been included in the initialization. For example, the dark contour in Fig. 2(b) is the boundary detected by the active shape model-based method[10] due to poor initialization. To overcome this problem, we previously proposed a template-based approach with PPA elimination.[4] By using a PPA detection module based on texture, the chance of mistaking PPA as part of the disc is reduced. However, it does not work

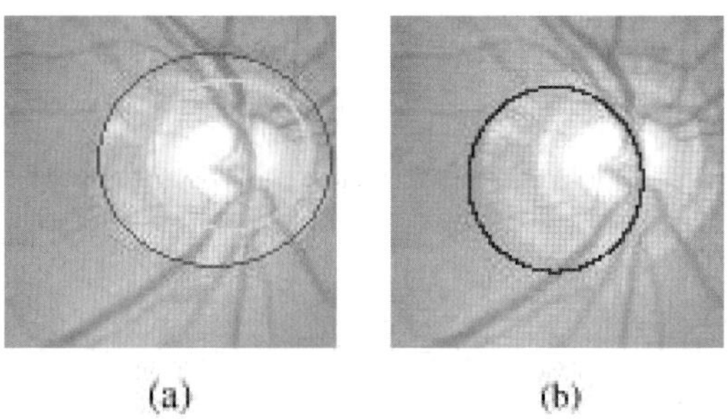

Fig. 2. An example of PPA. (a) gray: PPA boundary, light: Manual Disc (b) dark: Disc by a deformable model based method.

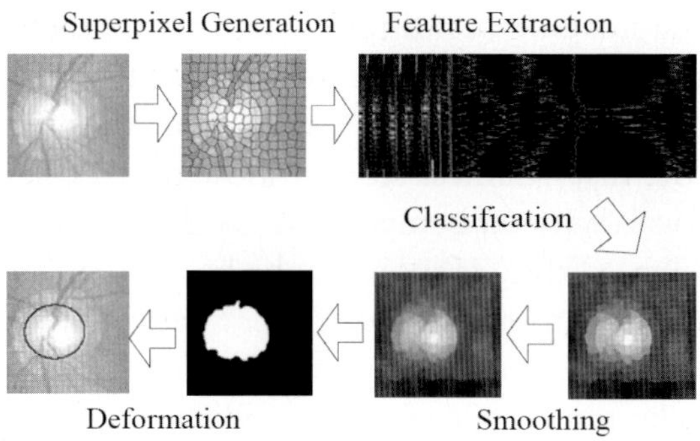

Fig. 3. Superpixel based optic disc segmentation in ARARAT.

well when the PPA area is small, or when the texture is not significantly predominant.

ARARAT uses a superpixel classification-based method for disc segmentation. Superpixels are local, coherent and provide a convenient primitive to compute local image features. They capture redundancy in the image and reduce the complexity of subsequent processing. In the method, superpixel classification is used for an initialization of disc boundary and then a deformable model using active shape model[10] is used to fine tune the disc boundary, i.e., a superpixel classification-based disc initialization for deformable models. The flow chart of the proposed disc segmentation method is summarized in Fig. 3.

2.2. *Superpixel Generation*

Many superpixel algorithms[14–18] have been proposed for the segmentation of scenes, animals, and human. The simple linear iterative clustering[18] algorithm (SLIC) is used here to aggregate nearby pixels into superpixels in retinal fundus images. SLIC is used because it is fast, memory efficient and excellent in boundary adherence. It is simple to use with only one parameter, i.e., the number of desired superpixels k. In SLIC, k initial cluster centres C_k are sampled on a regular grid spaced by $S = \sqrt{N/k}$ pixels apart from the image with N pixels. The centres are first moved towards the lowest gradient position in a 3×3 neighborhood. Then clustering is applied from these centres. For each C_k, SLIC iteratively searches for its best matching pixel from the $2S \times 2S$ neighborhood around C_k based on color and spatial proximity and then computes the new cluster centre based on the pixel found. The iteration continues until the distance between the new centres and previous ones is small enough. Finally, a post-processing is applied to enforce connectivity. More details of the SLIC algorithm can be found in the SLIC paper.[18]

2.3. *Feature Extraction*

2.3.1. *Contrast enhanced histogram*

Many features can be used for superpixel classification including color, appearance, gist, location and texture.[19] Color histogram of superpixels is an intuitive choice as the disc is often the brightest in the retina. Histogram equalization is first applied to red r, green g, and blue b channels from RGB color space respectively to enhance the contrast. The hue h and saturation s from HSV color space are also included to keep the image's color balance. The histogram of each superpixel is computed from all five channels: the histogram equalized r, g, b as well as the original h, s. The histogram computation uses 256 bins and $256 \times 5 = 1280$ dimensional feature $HIST_j = [\hbar_j(HE(r))\ \hbar_j(HE(g))\ \hbar_j(HE(b))\ \hbar_j(h)\ \hbar_j(s)]$ is computed for the jth superpixel SP_j, where $HE(\cdot)$ denotes the function of histogram equalization and $\hbar_j(\cdot)$ the function to compute histogram from SP_j.

2.3.2. *Centre surround statistics*

As the PPA region looks similar to the disc, it is necessary to include features that reflect the difference between the PPA region and the disc region. One main difference between the two regions is texture: the PPA region contains blob-like structures while the disc region is relatively more homogeneous. Centre surround statistics (CSS)[20,21] are proposed as important features to distinguish PPA from disc.

To compute CSS, nine spatial scale dyadic Gaussian pyramids[22] are generated with a ratio from 1:1 (level 0) to 1:256 (level 8). Then centre surround operation between centre (finer) levels $c = 2, 3, 4$ and surround (coarser) levels $s = c + d$, with $d = 3, 4$ is applied to obtain six maps empirically computed at levels of 2–5, 2–6, 3–6, 3–7, 4–7, and 4–8 from an image channel.[23–25] Denoting the feature map in centre level c as $I(c)$ and the feature map in surround level s as $I(s)$, the centre surround difference is computed as $|I(c) - f_{s-c}(I(s))|$, where $f_{s-c}(\cdot)$ denotes the interpolation from level s to level c. All the difference maps are resized to be the same size as the original. The above operation is applied on r, g and b channels to get $6 \times 3 = 18$ maps. The CSS features are then computed as the first and second moments of these maps within superpixels. Denoting M_i, $i = 1, 2, \ldots, 18$, as the ith map, the feature CSS_j consists of the mean μ_j and variance v_j of maps within the superpixels, i.e., $CSS_j = [\mu_j\ v_j]$, where μ_j and v_j from superpixel SP_j with n_j pixels are computed by:

$$\mu_j(i) = \frac{1}{n_j} \sum_{(x,y)\in SP_j} M_i(x,y) \tag{1}$$

$$v_j(i) = \frac{1}{n_j} \sum_{(x,y)\in SP_j} (M_i(x,y) - \mu_j(i))^2 \tag{2}$$

2.3.3. *Context feature*

Since the texture feature from the PPA region is often included in a large region, the features from neighboring superpixels are also considered in the classification of the current superpixel. Four neighboring superpixels SP_{j1}, SP_{j2}, SP_{j3} and SP_{j4} are empirically determined for SP_j, where SP_{j1} is determined as the first superpixel by moving out of the current superpixel horizontally to the left from its centre. Similarly, SP_{j2}, SP_{j3} and SP_{j4} are determined by moving right, up and down. The CSS feature for SP_j would then be expanded to: $\widehat{CSS}_j = [CSS_j \;\; CSS_{j1} \;\; CSS_{j2} \;\; CSS_{j3} \;\; CSS_{j4}]$, which has a dimension of $18 \times 2 \times 5 = 180$. We combine $HIST_j$ and $\widehat{CSS}_j$ to form the proposed feature $[HIST_j \;\; \widehat{CSS}_j]$.

2.4. *Initialization and Deformation*

A support vector machine is used as the classifier. The LIBSVM[26] toolbox with linear kernel is used in our experiments. The linear kernel is used instead of non-linear radial basis function (RBF) kernel as the feature dimensionality is already high. It is found that nonlinear mapping using the RBF kernel does not improve the performance. In the training step, the same number of superpixels from the disc and non-disc region are randomly obtained from a set of training images with manual disc boundary. One challenge to find a good classifier is that samples from the non-disc region are often from different clusters with unbalanced numbers. A typical example is PPA. There are often fewer superpixels from the PPA region compared with the other non-disc regions, and the trained classifier is often dominated by superpixels from the latter. Therefore, a bootstrapping strategy[27] is adopted: an active training data set is first restricted to be a sub-set of the available training data set (pool) and extended iteratively. In every iteration, the training is performed on the active set and returns a preliminary classifier. The classifier is then used to evaluate the pool. In every round of training, the active training set is extended by examples misclassified in the previous round, thus emphasizing samples close to the decision boundary. The iteration is repeated until there is no improvement in the classification accuracy or the maximum number of iterations has been reached. After that, the trained classifier is used for subsequent testing.

Instead of directly using the binary classification results from LIBSVM, the output values from the SVM decision function are used. The output value for each superpixel is used as the decision values for all pixels in the superpixel as shown in Fig. 3. Smoothing using a mean filter is then applied on the decision values to achieve smoothed decision values, which are then binarized using a threshold to get a matrix with 1 as object and 0 as background. The largest connected object, i.e., the connected component with largest number of pixels, is obtained through morphological operation and its boundary is used as the raw estimation of the disc boundary. The best fitted ellipse using elliptical Hough transform[4] is computed as the fitted estimation. Finally, the active shape model[10] is used to fine tune the disc boundary.

3. Optic Cup Segmentation

Detecting the cup boundary from 2D fundus images without depth information is a challenging task as depth is the primary indicator for the cup boundary. In 2D fundus images, one landmark to determine the cup region is the pallor, defined as the area of maximum colour contrast inside the disc.[7] Another landmark is the vessel bends at the boundary of the cup.[5] Compared with disc segmentation, fewer methods have been proposed for cup segmentation from 2D fundus images. Thresholding is used to determine the cup by Joshi *et al.*,[29] relying on intensity difference between cup and neuroretinal rim. A level set-based approach[8] is also proposed. It relies on the edges between cup and neuroretinal rim. This method and thresholding-based methods are essentially based on pallor information. However, in many subjects from screening data, there is no obvious pallor or edge within the disc to mark the cup boundary. Figure 4 shows an example of such a disc. The contrast between the cup and the neuroretinal rim in the example is much weaker than that in Fig. 1. Wong *et al.*[28]

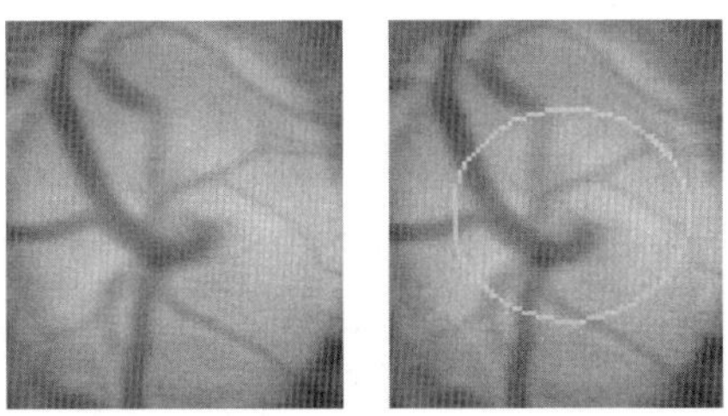

Fig. 4. An example disc without obvious pallor: the line is the manual cup boundary.

detect small vessel bends ("kinks") from the vicinity of the initial estimated cup to aid the cup segmentation. The challenge is to exclude vessel bends from a non-cup boundary, especially when the initial estimation is inaccurate. A similar concept is used to locate relevant-vessel bends ("*r*-bend") at the vicinity of a pallor region determined by bright pixels.[9] This method, again, requires pallor information to find a good initial estimation of the cup boundary. Moreover, it requires at least a few bends in nasal, inferior and superior angular of the disc for the cup boundary fitting, which is not necessarily true for many images from our experience. Xu *et al.* proposed a sliding window and regression-based method.[30] Although it performs better than earlier methods, the sliding window strategy requires heavy computational cost. Recently, Yin *et al.*[31] developed a deformable model-based method for cup segmentation, where the initialization of the cup boundary is based on pallor combined with prior knowledge of the cup.

The main challenge in cup segmentation is to determine the cup boundary when the pallor is non-obvious or weak. In such scenarios, even marking the cup boundary manually is challenging. Although vessel bends are potential landmarks, they can occur at many places within the disc region and only one sub-set of these points defines the cup boundary. In addition, combining the vessel bends with pallor information is a challenging task that often requires a set of heuristic parameters, which raises the concern of the robustness of the method. The chapter introduces the superpixel classification-based method for cup segmentation. It incorporates prior knowledge into the training of superpixel classification instead of relying on vessel bends. The procedure is similar to the superpixel classification-based disc segmentation.

3.1. *Feature Extraction*

After obtaining the disc, the minimum bounding box of the disc is used for cup segmentation. The feature extraction is similar to that for disc segmentation, except that the red channel is no longer used. This is because there is little information about the cup in the red channel. Because of the additional challenge in cup segmentation where the pallor is non-obvious, a new feature, the distance D_j between the centre of superpixel SP_j and the centre of the disc as location information is also included. To adapt the variation of disc size, D_j is the normalized distance using the height and width of the disc. Mathematically, D_j is computed as:

$$D_j = \sqrt{\left(\frac{x_c - x_j}{h}\right)^2 + \left(\frac{y_c - y_j}{w}\right)^2} \tag{3}$$

where (x_c, y_c) denotes the coordinate of the disc centre, (x_j, y_j) denotes the coordinate of the centre of SP_j, and h and w denote the height and width of the disc, respectively. The use of D_j is inspired by the prior knowledge that the cup usually lies at the centre section of the disc. Thus, the feature vector for cup segmentation is computed as $[HIST_j^c \widehat{CSS_j^c} D_j]$.

3.2. *Superpixel Classification for Optic Cup Estimation*

The classification is similar to that for the disc. The difference is highlighted below. First, the boostrapping strategy is not necessary here. Contour deformation or fine tuning using a deformable model is also avoided. This is because many cases do not have an obvious/strong contrast between the cup and the rim for deformable models. A deformation in these cases often leads to an over-estimated cup. However, an ellipse fitting using direct least squares fitting[32] is applied to get the cup boundary. Ellipse fitting is beneficial for overcoming noise introduced by vessels, especially from the inferior and superior sector of the cup which are important for CDR computation.

3.3. *Cup to Disc Ratio*

After obtaining the disc and cup, various clinical/diagnostic features can be computed. We follow the clinical convention to compute the CDR. As mentioned in the introduction, CDR is an important indicator for glaucoma computed as

$$CDR = \frac{\text{VCD}}{\text{VDD}}. \tag{4}$$

The computed CDR is used for glaucoma screening, in which CDR greater than a threshold indicates a higher risk of glaucoma.

3.4. *Confidence Score*

An automated algorithm fails or works poorly in some images inevitably. However, most algorithms fail without warning. ARARAT presents a confidence score calculation method for this particular application, which represents the reliability of the automated output. Since disc segmentation is a critical step affecting the disc and cup diameters, the accuracy of disc segmentation affects the performance of the system. Therefore, the confidence score is computed from the evaluation of disc segmentation. As the disc shape is often close to an ellipse, the raw disc boundary before ellipse fitting should be approximately an ellipse if the superpixel classification works well. Inspired by this, the confidence score is computed as follows. Defining the set of points from the raw estimation as X and the set of points from the fitted estimation as $\Upsilon = f(X)$, for each point x in X, we find its nearest point in Υ and their distance is computed as

$$d_f(x) = \inf\{d(x, y)|y \in \Upsilon\} \tag{5}$$

where inf represents the infimum and $d(x, y)$ the Euclidean distance between x and y. Then, the self-assessment confidence score is computed as the ratio of the number of x with $d_f(x) < T$ to the total number of x, i.e,

$$r(X) = \frac{Card(\{x|d_f(x) < T, x \in X\})}{Card(X)}, \tag{6}$$

where $Card(Z)$ is the cardinality of the set Z, and T is a threshold empirically determined.

4. Experimental Results

4.1. *Data Sets*

The experiments used images from two population-based studies: the Singapore Malay Eye Study (SiMES) with 3280 subjects and the Singapore Chinese Eye Study (SCES) with 1677 subjects, aged 40 to 80 years. A sub-set of 650 images with a resolution of 3072 × 2048 pixels from SiMES had been selected for manual marking of the disc and cup boundaries previously.[33] In the chapter, these images were randomly divided into 325 training images and 325 validation images based on subjects. The training images were used to train the classifiers for superpixel classification in disc and cup segmentation. The validation images were used to compute the agreement between automated and manual disc, cup, and CDR. After excluding subjects used in the training and subjects without a visible optic disc in their fundus images, the remaining 2801 SiMES subjects and 1676 SCES subjects were used in the glaucoma screening test. Following clinical practice, only the right eyes of these subjects were used. The SiMES images were acquired using a digital retinal camera with 45 degree field of view (Canon CR-DGi with a 10D SLR digital camera backing; Canon, Tokyo, Japan). The SCES images were acquired using the Canon CR-1 Mark-II Nonmydriatic Digital Retinal Camera, Canon, Japan. The images were stored in TIFF format originally and were converted to JPEG format for less storage. The SiMES images have a resolution of 3072×2048 pixels and the SCES images have resolutions of either 3504 × 2336 or 3888 × 2592 pixels. Glaucoma was diagnosed according to International Society of Geographical and Epidemiological Ophthalmology criteria.

To train the disc and cup segmentation, we use the 325 training images with manual disc and cup boundaries. The validation of ARARAT is done in two major approaches. The first approach is through the agreement between the automated and manual disc, cup, and CDR in the validation images. The agreements between the automated and manual disc and cup are evaluated separately using the overlapping error:

$$E = 1 - \frac{Area(S \cap M)}{Area(S \cup M)}, \tag{7}$$

where S and M denote the segmented and manual disc and cup respectively. The agreement between the automated and manual CDR is evaluated by the Pearson's correlation coefficient, Spearman's correlation coefficient and the CDR error

$$\delta = |CDR_A - CDR_M|, \tag{8}$$

where CDR_A and CDR_M denotes the automated and manual CDR from trained professionals.

The second approach is through the performance of the proposed method in population-based glaucoma screening. Sensitivity and specificity are often used as measures of accuracy in diagnosis tests. There is a tradeoff between the specificity and sensitivity of a test. This is usually expressed on a receiver operating characteristic (ROC) curve, which plots sensitivity against 1-specificity for all possible values. Often, the area under the curve (AUC) is calculated as the overall measure of diagnostic strength of a test. In our analysis, we evaluate the methods through their AUCs.

4.2. *Agreement Between Automated and Manual Disc, Cup and CDR*

The agreement between the automated and manual disc, cup and CDR in ARARAT is computed using the 325 vaidation images from the SiMES data set. Table 1 shows ARARAT's average overlapping error between the automated and manual discs in the 325 validation SiMES images. The agreement for images with PPA and images without PPA is calculated separately as the disc

Table 1. Automated Disc vs. Manual Disc.

	w/o PPA	With PPA	All
HIST	9.2%	11.5%	10.0%
HIST + CSS	9.1%	10.3%	9.5%

segmentation in these two types of images are different. To illustrate the effectiveness of different features, we show the performance when different features are used. It is observed that the combination of CSS with the histograms (HIST) improves the disc segmentation especially for the cases with PPA with a relative reduction of overlapping error by $(11.5 - 10.3)/11.5 = 10.4\%$. There is little improvement for images without PPA as the disc segmentation in these images is much easier and HIST is sufficient. Figure 5 shows results of the segmented disc from four samples with PPA absent in the first sample and present in the rest of three samples to visualize the effects of different features used in the superpixel classification. In general, ARARAT achieves excellent agreement compared with manual ones. However, since ARARAT is obtained by training, it may not be able to work well for cases with irregular shapes compared with those used in the training data set. For example, the last row in Fig. 5 shows a failed disc segmentation result due to the irregular disc shape and the presence of PPA. Table 2 shows the accuracy of cup segmentation using the overlapping error between the automated and manual cup, the mean CDR error, the Pearson's correlation coefficient and the Spearman's correlation coefficient between the automated CDR and manual CDR in the 325 validation SiMES images. It is observed that both CSS and location information D are beneficial for cup segmentation and CDR computation. Figure 6 shows five samples with first three samples from normal subjects and last two samples from glaucomatous subjects. From top to bottom, the manual CDRs for the five examples are 0.54, 0.55, 0.35, 0.68 and 0.83 respectively. The automated CDR by ARARAT are 0.53, 0.58, 0.52, 0.61 and 0.66 respectively. ARARAT performs well for examples with medium CDRs. However, it over-estimated the very small cup in the third example and under-estimated the very large cup in the last example. There are two reasons for this bias. The first reason is the contrast between cup and rim is very weak especially for the last example with poor image quality. The second reason is a limitation inherited from the high proportion medium cups in the training. Since most cups are medium sized, the ARARAT system learns from the training samples and gives a result biased toward the medium sizes.

4.3. *Population-Based Glaucoma Screening Using ARARAT*

The population-based glaucoma screening is conducted using the 2801 SiMES images and 1676 SCES images. The ROC curves are obtained and the AUCs are computed. Figure 7 shows the ROC curves of ARARAT, as well as those when only a sub-set of features are used in the SiMES and SCES data sets.

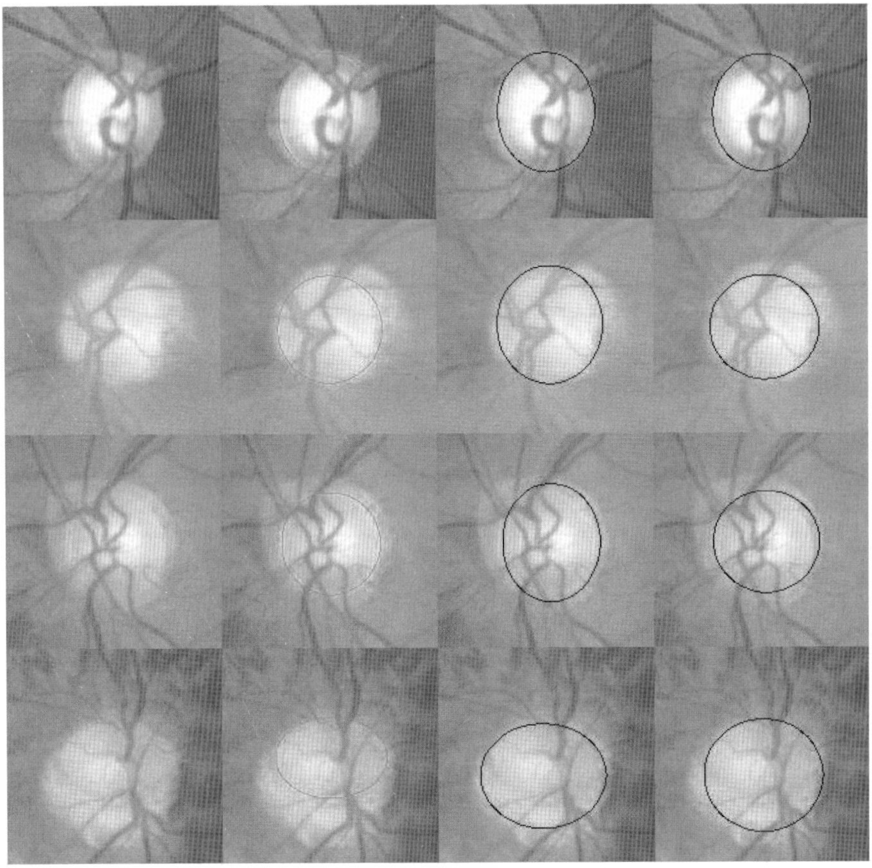

Fig. 5. Sample results of optic disc segmentation in ARARAT. From left to right, the original image, the manual disc, the automated disc using HIST only, and the disc using both HIST and CSS in the superpixel classification. From top to bottom, PPA is absent in the first sample and present in the rest of samples.

Table 2. Automated Cup/CDR vs. Manual Cup/CDR.

	Overlapping Error	CDR Error Error	Pearson's Correlation	Spearman's Correlation
HIST	53.6%	0.122	$0.12(p < 0.005)$	$0.12(p < 0.005)$
HIST + CSS	27.0%	0.091	$0.36(p < 0.001)$	$0.40(p < 0.001)$
HIST + CSS + D	24.1%	0.080	$0.59(p < 0.001)$	$0.59(p < 0.001)$

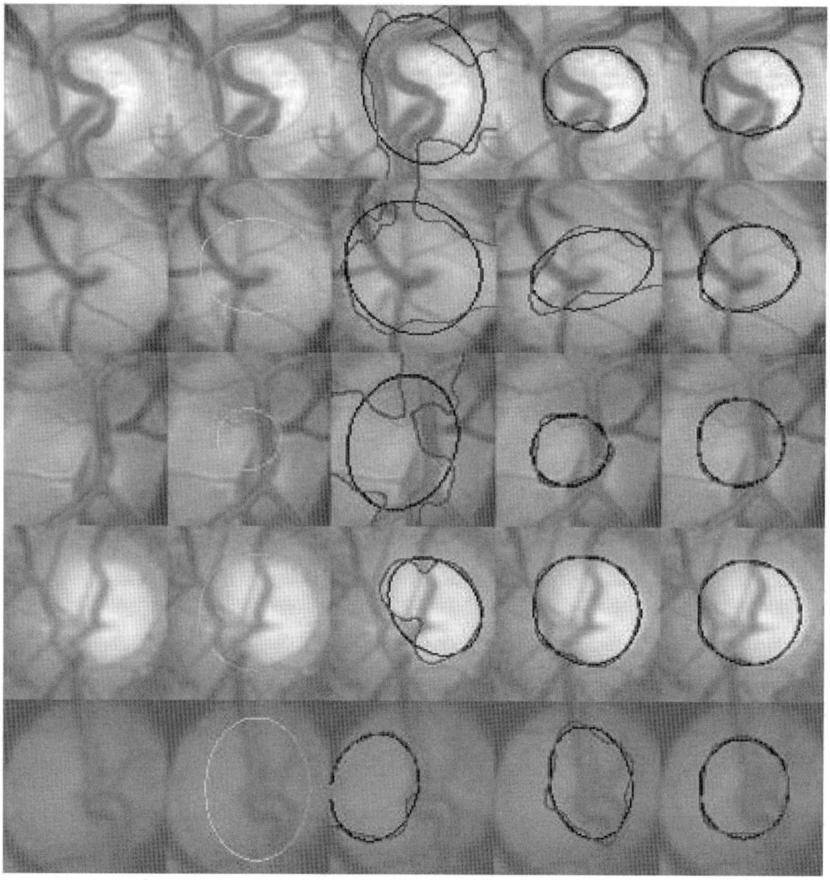

Fig. 6. Sample results of optic cup segmentation in ARARAT. From left to right, the original image, the manual cup boundary, the results by superpixel classification using HIST only, both HIST and CSS, and all features in the classification. Gray: raw contour; Dark: best fitted ellipse.

Table 3 shows the AUCs of the ROC curves for glaucoma screening in the two population-based studies. The results clearly show the degree of positive influence of the CSS and location feature D. Speed of ARARAT is also evaluated. It takes about 14s per image in a dual core 3.0 GHz PC with 3.25 GB RAM.

4.4. *Comparison With Other Methods*

Next, we also compare the ARARAT CDR-based screening method with previous methods including the threshold method, the active shape model (ASM) method and the IOP measurement. Figure 8 shows the respective

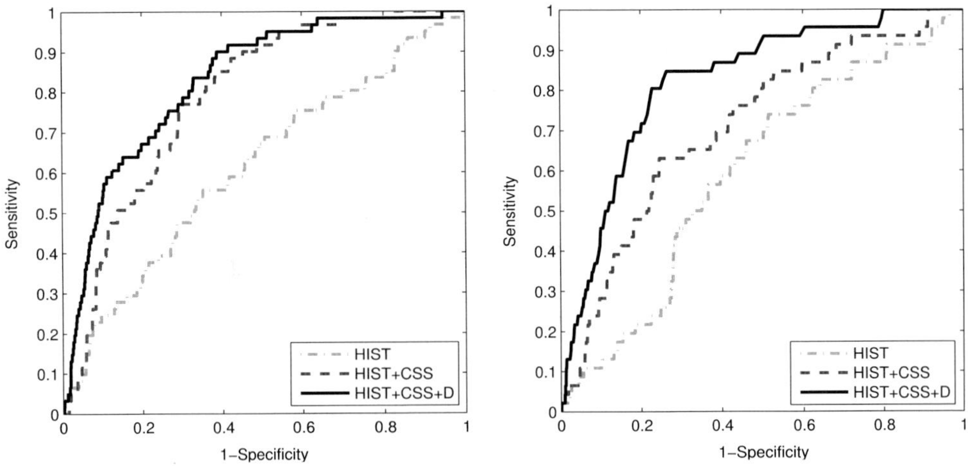

Fig. 7. ROC plots in SiMES and SCES data set by using various features in superpixel classification.

Table 3. AUC of the ROC curves in glaucoma screening by ARARAT using various features.

Data Set	HIST	HIST + CSS	HIST + CSS + D
SiMES	0.611	0.768	0.827
SCES	0.597	0.710	0.822

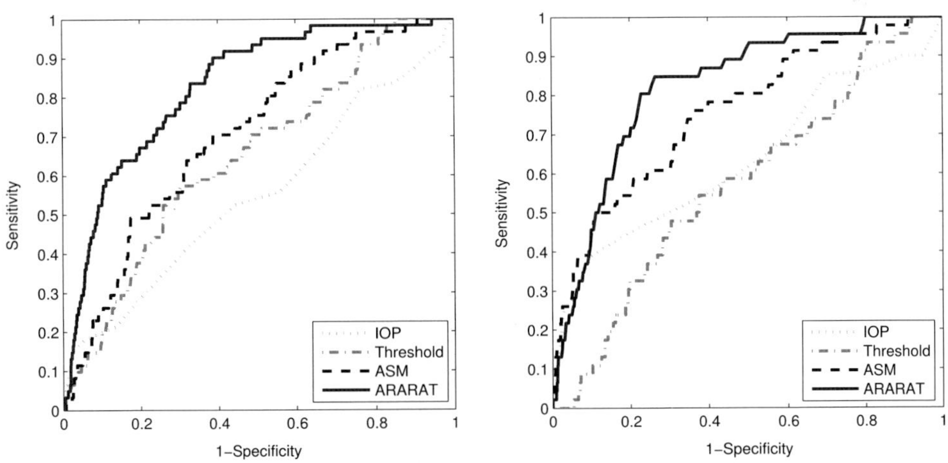

Fig. 8. The ROC plots in SiMES and SCES data set by various methods.

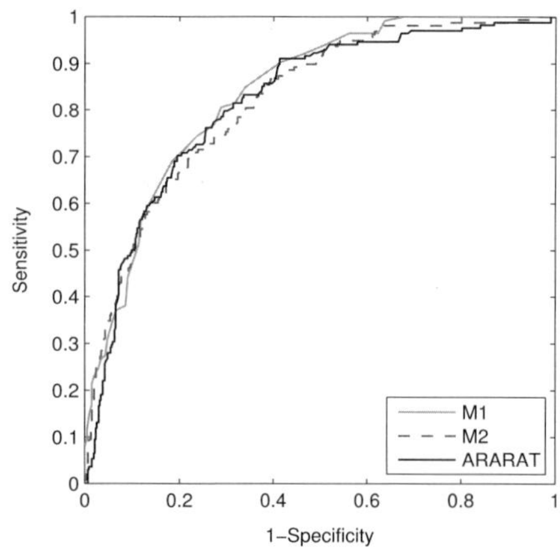

Fig. 9. ROC curves by GT1, GT2 and ARARAT in validation images.

Table 4. AUCs of the ROC curves in glaucoma screening by various methods.

Data Set	IOP	Threshold	ASM	ARARAT
SiMES	0.547	0.646	0.702	0.827
SCES	0.660	0.574	0.756	0.822

ROC curves. Table 4 shows AUCs of the corresponding ROC curves. Clearly, ARARAT outperformed the other methods.

It is particularly important to point out that the proposed method achieves AUC of 0.827 and 0.822 on SiMES and SCES image sets respectively, which are better than the current clinical practice of using IOP. From the discussions with clinicians, the obtained results show that ARARAT has potential for large-scale glaucoma screening.

4.5. *Confidence-based Screening*

Finally, we evaluate how the confidence score affects the screening accuracy in ARARAT. Table 5 shows the percentages of the images at different confidence levels from 0.8 to 0.95. It is observed that there are more results with high confidence in SiMES than SCES. This is likely due to the fact that the 325 images used in the training are from SiMES data set. Therefore, the trained classifiers are slightly biased towards the rest of SiMES images captured using the same camera with the same setting. Table 6 shows the corresponding AUCs of the ROC curves in glaucoma screening. Generally, ARARAT performs better

Table 5. The percentages of the images above different confidence levels.

	$r \geq 0.95$	$r \geq 0.90$	$r \geq 0.85$	$r \geq 0.80$
SiMES	47%	68%	81%	89%
SCES	29%	49%	66%	79%

Table 6. AUC of the ROC in glaucoma screening at different confidence levels.

	$r \geq 0.95$	$r \geq 0.90$	$r \geq 0.85$	$r \geq 0.80$	All
SiMES	0.877	0.843	0.836	0.832	0.827
SCES	0.950	0.903	0.874	0.853	0.822

in images with higher confidence. For example, it achieves an AUC of 0.877 for 47% of SiMES images and 0.950 for 29% of SCES images. The consideration of this confidence score may be an important factor when designing an automated glaucoma screening program based on ARARAT. It can be very useful in practice. For example, one may set a confidence level to achieve a higher accuracy for the subjects with high confidence scores and request confirmation for results with low confidence scores.

4.6. *Inter-observer Errors*

To evaluate how the ARARAT system compares with the manual demarcations by a different person, an independent ophthalmologist marked the disc and cup boundary for the 325 validation images. Therefore, the overlapping error between the two manual disc and cup boundaries, the CDR errors, the diagnosis ROC curves and their AUCs are also obtained. Table 7 shows the results where M1 and M2 denote the first and second sets of manual boundaries. Results show that the disc overlapping error between ARARAT and M1 is slightly larger than that between M1 and M2, i.e., the inter-observer error. The cup overlapping error between ARARAT and M1 is smaller than the inter-observer error. ARARAT is more biased to M1 as it is trained according to M1. In terms of CDR, the CDR errors among M1, M2 and ARARAT are close. The Pearson's correlation coefficient between M1 and M2 is higher than that between ARARAT and M1 or M2 while the Spearman's correlation coefficients among the three are close.

Figure 8 shows the ROC curves using the CDRs from M1, M2 and ARARAT using the 325 validation images. The AUCs by M1, M2 and

Table 7. Inter-Observer Error.

	Disc Error	Cup Error	CDR Error	Pearson's Correlation	Spearman's Correlation
M1 vs. M2	8.7%	25.6%	0.078	$0.62(p < 0.001)$	$0.61(p < 0.001)$
ARARAT vs M1	9.5%	24.1%	0.080	$0.59(p < 0.001)$	$0.59(p < 0.001)$
ARARAT vs M2	11.9%	28.1%	0.077	$0.59(p < 0.001)$	$0.58(p < 0.001)$

ARARAT are 0.839, 0.819 and 0.820 respectively. The ROC curves show that the manual marking works slightly better than ARARAT when specificity is close to 0 or 1. However, their performances are quite close in the middle range of the specificities. This is intuitively correct as ARARAT has a bias of underestimating the very high CDRs while overestimating the very small CDRs.

5. Discussions and Conclusions

We have presented ARARAT, which uses fast superpixel classification-based methods for disc and cup segmentation to automatically compute CDR for glaucoma screening. Results show that ARARAT achieves good agreement between automated and manual disc and cup. In addition, the Spearman's correlation coefficients between the automated and two manual CDRs and the ROC curves by the three CDRs are comparable. This suggests that the CDR from ARARAT is comparable with that by manual grading in glaucoma detection. The results also show that CSS is effective for both disc and cup segmentation. In disc segmentation, CSS provides better differentiation between PPA and disc compared with histograms only. In cup segmentation, the benefit of CSS is even greater than that in disc segmentation. This is because the color change from the cup to the neuroretinal rim is small and as such the uneven illumination across disc has a large effect. The CSS is less sensitive to it and thereby improves the result. Confidence score is an important indicator of the automated results. From our experience, results with $r > 0.85$ is likely to be very reliable. Further, the relatively higher accuracy of ARARAT against airpuff IOP and other previous CDR-based methods show good potential for the system to be used for screening in polyclinics and eye centres.

There is still room for improvement for ARARAT. Although we have utilized CSS features to improve the disc segmentation in cases with PPA, ARARAT may fail if the shape of disc and PPA is irregular. The second limitation is that the trained cup classifier is slightly dominated by cups with medium sizes. Therefore, ARARAT under-estimates the very large cups (CDR > 0.8)

and over-estimates the very small cups (CDR < 0.4) for discs with non-obvious contrast between the cup and the neuroretinal rim (see third and fifth example in Fig. 6). This is partly due to the use of the location feature D. However, the advantage of using D is to help avoid very poor results. Both the cup segmentation and glaucoma screening accuracies show improvement by including D as a feature. One possible solution to overcome this trade-off is to collect more samples with very small and very large cups to train a better classifier. Another possibility is to use a different classifier such as k-nearest neighbors (kNN). However, the limitation is that kNN is less robust to noise. The third solution is to use vessel bends to correct the bias. For example, we can obtain the vessel bends from the vicinity of the cup boundary from ARARAT to fine-tune the cup boundary. As it requires some heuristics in vessel tracking and bending detection, a robust algorithm is important for future development.

In summary, ARARAT achieves constant and fast performance on two large databases and better accuracy than airpuff. It is able to achieve good classification accuracy between glaucoma cases and healthy subjects. Its limitations are that it under-estimates the very large cups, while over-estimating the very small cups when pallor is not obvious. Despite that, the obtained CDRs for very large cups are still relatively high and the CDRs for very small cups are relatively small. In addition, the confidence score provides a possibility to build a confidence-based glaucoma screening programme. As mentioned, one may set a confidence level to achieve a higher accuracy for the subjects with high confidence scores and request confirmation for results with low confidence scores. There are still many features that can be improved in the proposed method. ARARAT is trained using one set of disc and cup boundaries and therefore is potentially biased to this set of manual demarcations. It can be helpful if multiple sets of disc and cup boundaries are obtained to further improve the accuracy. Screening based on CDR only also has some limitations. Therefore, combining CDR with other factors is expected to further improve the performance. There is potential for ARARAT to be deployed in widely available 2D retinal cameras for fast and automatic glaucoma screening. Future work will explore the integration of other factors to improve diagnostic outcomes towards a more reliable and efficient glaucoma screening system.

Acknowledgments

This work was supported in part by the Agency for Science, Technology and Research, Singapore, under SERC grant 121-148-0007. We would like to thank those who provided materials used in this article.

References

1. H. A. Quigley and A. T. Broman, "The number of people with glaucoma worldwide in 2010 and 2020," *Br J Ophthalmol* **90**, 262–267 (2006).
2. X. Zhu and R. M. Rangayyan, "Detection of the optic disc in images of the retina using the hough transform," *Int Conf of IEEE Eng in Med and Bio Soc*, 3546–3549 (2008).
3. A. Aquino, M. Gegundez-Arias, and D. Marin, "Detecting the optic disc boundary in digital fundus images using morphological, edge detection, and feature extraction techniques," *IEEE Trans Med Imag* **29**, 1860–1869 (2010).
4. J. Cheng, J. Liu, D. W. K. Wong, F. Yin, C. Cheung, M. Baskaran, T. Aung, and T. Y. Wong, "Automatic optic disc segmentation with peripapillary atrophy elimination," *Int Conf of IEEE Eng in Med and Bio Soc*, 6624–6627 (2011).
5. J. B. Jonas, W. M. Budde, and S. Panda-Jonas, "Ophthalmoscopic evaulation of the optic nerve head," *Surv Ophthalmol*, 293–320 (1999).
6. J. Lowell, A. Hunter, D. Steel, A. Basu, R. Ryder, E. Fletcher, and L.Kennedy, "Optic nerve head segmentation.," *IEEE Trans Med Imag* **23**, 256–264 (2004).
7. J. Xu, O. Chutatape, E. Sung, C. Zheng, and P. C. T. Kuan, "Optic disk feature extraction via modified deformable model technique for glaucoma analysis," *Pattern Recognition* **40**, 2063–2076 (2007).
8. D. W. K. Wong, J. Liu, J. H. Lim, X. Jia, H. Li F. Yin and, and T. Y. Wong, "Level-set based automatic cup-to-disc ratio determination using retinal fundus images in argali," *Conf Proc IEEE Eng Biol Soc*, 2266–2269 (2008).
9. G. D. Joshi, J. Sivaswamy, and S. R. Krishnadas, "Optic disk and cup segmentation from monocular color retinal images for glaucoma assessment," *IEEE Trans Med Imag* **30**, 1192–1205 (2011).
10. F. Yin, J. Liu, S. H. Ong, Y. Sun, D. W. K. Wong, N. M. Tan, C. Cheung, M. Baskaran, T. Aung, and T. Y. Wong, "Model-based optic nerve head segmentation on retinal fundus images," *Int Conf of IEEE Eng in Med and Bio Soc*, 2626–2629 (2011).
11. M. D. Abràmoff, W. L. M. Alward, E. C. Greenlee, L. Shuba, C. Y. Kim, J. H. Fingert, and Y. H. Kwon, "Automated segmentation of the optic disc from stereo color photographs using physiologically plausible features," *Invest Ophthalmol Vis Sci* **48**, 1665–1673 (2007).
12. D. W. K. Wong, J. Liu, N. M. Tan, F. Yin, B. H. Lee, and T. Y. Wong, "Learning-based approach for the automatic detection of the optic disc in digital retinal fundus photographs," *Int Conf of IEEE Eng in Med and Bio Soc*, 5355–5358 (2010).
13. C. Muramatsu, T. Nakagawa, A. Sawada, Y. Hatanaka, T. Hara, T. Yamamoto, and H. Fujita, "Automated segmentation of optic disc region on retinal fundus photographs: Comparison of contour modeling and pixel classification methods," *Comp Methods Prog Biomed* **101**, 23–32 (2011).
14. L. Vincent and P. Soille, "Watersheds in digital spaces: An efficient algorithm based on immersiion simulations," *IEEE Trans Pattern Anal Mach Intell* **13**, 583–598 (1991).
15. D. Comaniciu and P. Meer, "Mean shift: A robust approach toward feature space analysis," *IEEE Trans Pattern Anal Mach Intell* **24**, 603–619 (2002).
16. A. Moore, S. Prince, J. Warrell, U. Mohammed, and G. Jones, "Superpixel lattices," *Proc IEEE Conf Computer Vision and Pattern Recognition*, 1–8 (2008).

17. A. Levinshtein, A. Stere, K. Kutulakos, D. Fleet, S. Dickinson, and K. Siddiqi, "Turbopixels: Fast superpixels using geometric flows," *IEEE Trans Pattern Anal and Mach Intell* **31**, 2290–2297 (2009).
18. R. Achanta, A. Shaji, K. Smith, A. Lucchi, P. Fua, and S. Susstrunk, "Slic superpixels compared to state-of-the-art superpixel methods," *IEEE Trans Pattern Anal and Mach Intell* **34**, 2274–2281 (2012).
19. J. Tighe and S. Lazebnik, "Superparsing: Scalable nonparametric image parsing with superpixels," *European Conf on Computer Vision* **5**, 352–365 (2010).
20. J. Cheng, J. Liu, Y. Xu, F. Yin, D. W. K. Wong, N. M. Tan, C. Y. Cheng, Y. C. Tham, T. Y. Wong, "Superpixel classification based optic disc segmentation," *Asian Conf on Computer Vision ACCV Part II LNCS 7725*, 293–304 (2013).
21. J. Cheng, J. Liu, Y. Xu, F. Yin, D. W. K. Wong, N. M. Tan, D. Tao, C. Y. Cheng, T. Aung and T. Y. Wong, "Superpixel classification based optic disc and optic cup segmentation for glaucoma screening," *Trans on Med Imaging* **32**, 1019–1032 (2013).
22. E. H. Adelson, C. H. Anderson, J. R. Bergen, P. J. Burt, and J. M. Ogden, "Pyramid methods in image processing," *RCA Engineer* **29**, 33–41 (1984).
23. L. Itti, C. Koch, and E. Niebur, "A model of saliency-based visual attention for rapid scene analysis," *IEEE Trans Pattern Anal and Mach Intell* **20**, 1254–1259 (1998).
24. D. Song and D. Tao, "Biologically inspired feature manifold for scene classification," *IEEE Trans Image Processing* **19**, 174–184 (2010).
25. J. Cheng, D. Tao, J. Liu, D. W. K. Wong, N. M. Tan, T. Y. Wong TY, and S. M. Saw, "Peripapillary atrophy detection by sparse biologically inspired feature manifold," *IEEE Trans Med Imaging* **31**, 2355–2365 (2012).
26. C. C. Chang and C. J. Lin, "LIBSVM: A library for support vector machines," Software available at http://www.csie.ntu.edu.tw/~cjlin/libsvm (2001).
27. Z. Kalal, J. Matas, and K. Mikolajczyk, "Weighted sampling for large- scale boosting," *British Machine Vision Conference* (2008).
28. D. W. K. Wong, J. Liu, J. H. Lim, H. Li, and T. Y. Wong, "Automated detection of kinks from blood vessels for optic cup segmentation in retinal images," *Proc SPIE 7260*, 72601J (2009).
29. G. D. Joshi, J. Sivaswamy, K. Karan, and R. Krishnadas, "Optic disk and cup boundary detection using regional information," *Proc IEEE Int Symp. Biomed Imag*, 948–951 (2010).
30. Y. Xu, D. Xu, S. Lin, J. Liu, J. Cheng, C. Y. Cheung, T. Aung, and T. Y. Wong, "Sliding window and regression based cup detection in digital fundus images for glaucoma diagnosis," *MICCAI 2011 Part III LNCS*, 1–8 (2011).
31. F. Yin, J. Liu, D. W. K. Wong, N. M. Tan, C. Cheung, M. Baskaran, T. Aung, and T. Y. Wong, "Automated segmentation of optic disc and optic cup in fundus images for glaucoma diagnosis," *IEEE Int Symp on Computer-Based Medical Systems*, 1–6 (2012).
32. A. Fitzgibbon, M. Pilu, and R. B. Fisher, "Direct least squares fitting of ellipses," *IEEE Trans Pattern Anal and Mach Intell* **21**, 476–480 (1999).
33. Z. Zhang, F. Yin, J. Liu, W. K. Wong, N. M. Tan, B. H. Lee, J. Cheng, and T. Y. Wong, "Origa-light: An online retinal fundus image database for glaucoma analysis and research," *Int Conf IEEE Eng Med Biol Soc*, 3065–3068 (2010).

Chapter 13

Blind Source Separation in Assessing Tumor Pharmacokinetics

Hatef Mehrabian[*,†]

[*] *Department of Medical Biophysics, University of Toronto, Toronto, ON, Canada*

[†] *Department of Physical Sciences, Sunnybrook Research Institute, Toronto, ON, Canada*

E-mail: hatef.mehrabian@sri.utononto.ca

Dynamic contrast enhanced (DCE)-MRI combined with pharmacokinetic (PK) modeling of a tumor tissue provides information about its perfusion and vascular permeability. Most PK models require the intravascular contrast agent concentration as an input, which is inseparable from DCE-MRI data. Thus, it is approximated with an arterial input function (AIF), measured outside of the tissue of interest. Variations and error in calculation of AIF is a major source of discrepancy between PK parameters reported in different studies. An algorithm is developed, using blind source separation, to identify and separate the intravascular signal from the DCE-MRI data at the tissue of interest. The performance of the algorithm is assessed using numerical and physical tissue-mimicking phantom as well as clinical DCE-MRI of prostate cancer. The results show the algorithm is capable of accurately separating the intravascular signal, and its PK parameters provide better separation of normal and tumor tissues. Thus, the proposed algorithm could replace AIF-based methods, and more importantly could be used in cases an AIF cannot be measured.

1. Introduction

Personalized therapy is becoming more viable as our understanding of cancer biology is increasing. Given the complexity and high cost of these therapies, it is of upmost importance to identify responding and non-responding patients as early as possible in the course of the treatment.[1] However, there is large heterogeneity in tumors and although they present apparently similar clinical characteristics, tumor response to therapy is a fundamental but not well-understood concept in clinical oncology. The two main approaches that are used in clinical practice to assess tumor response to therapy are measuring markers secreted by cancer cells, and measuring tumor size using medical imaging.

Some malignant tumors produce serum molecules at a level sufficient for monitoring,[2,3] however; the secretion of these biomarkers is not controlled by the tumor alone and several other factors affect their level, which limits their application for therapy monitoring. Thus, tumor size measurement, using the response evaluation criteria in solid tumors (RECIST),[4] has become the main response assessment approach in clinical practice.[5] RECIST assumes reduction in tumor size after therapy shows better prognosis than no change or increase in tumor size. Despite its broad adoption, this assumption is not necessarily correct[6] and has some limitations, as some molecular targeting agents may result in improved clinical response while making no significant change in tumor size.[7]

Thus, there has been significant interest in functional and molecular imaging techniques. Molecular imaging with PET, when combined with compartmental modeling enables studying biological changes in the tumor.[8] Contrast enhanced ultrasound provides quantitative information about tumor vasculature.[9] Dynamic contrast enhanced (DCE)-computed tomography (CT) is used to quantify vascular permeability and blood flow.[10] Non-contrast T_1-weighted or T_2-weighted MRI provides information about morphological changes in the tumor or changes in its fluid content. Diffusion- and perfusion-weighted MRI provide promising tools for response assessment.[11] DCE-MRI, similar to DCE-CT, provides information about the vascular permeability and tumor perfusion,[12] and is used in the chapter to obtain quantitative information about the tumor.

Pharmacokinetic (PK) modeling DCE-MRI of a tissue models the passage of a bolus of contrast agent (CA) through its vasculature and provides quantitative information about its physiology, such as the exchange rate of substances through the vasculature into the extravascular extracellular space. This quantitative information can be used in detecting and diagnosing tumors as well as assessing their response to therapy.

DCE-MRI involves intravenous injection of a low molecular weight CA followed by repeated imaging of the tissue of interest over time. The CA can diffuse through the vessel walls into the extravascular space. However, its molecules are too large to cross the cell membrane and can only diffuse into the extravascular extracellular space (EES). The rate by which the CA diffuses from blood plasma to the EES is determined by blood flow, vascular permeability, and surface area of the vessel. PK modeling of DCE-MRI data provides quantitative information about these characteristics of the tumor vasculature, which have been shown to correlate with prognostic factors.

PK analysis of a tumor tissue requires information about the CA concentration in the intravascular space, while in DCE-MRI studies this signal is mixed with the EES signal and cannot be measured directly. Thus, it is approximated using an arterial input function (AIF)[13–16] which is calculated outside of the tissue of interest. AIF is measured using a major feeding artery adjacent to the tissue,[13] a theoretical AIF which usually takes the form of a bi-exponential curve,[14] a population-average AIF measured experimentally through blood sampling or high temporal resolution imaging at a major artery,[15] a reference-tissue AIF using the known PK parameters in a normal tissue,[16] or a dual bolus AIF which first injects a low dose bolus for AIF measurement.[17] These methods introduce error to the system as they do not measure the intravascular signal at the tissue of interest and also in many cases there are difficulties in measuring an appropriate AIF due to the several limitations of these methods. Thus, more sophisticated techniques are required to identify the intravascular signal at the tissue of interest and separate it from the EES signal.

There exist several blind source separation (BSS) techniques, such as principal component analysis (PCA),[18] non-negative matrix factorization (NMF),[19] factor analysis of dynamic structures (FADS),[20] and independent component analysis (ICA),[21] that could be used to perform the separation and have been previously applied to dynamic contrast enhanced series to separate their underlying structures. These methods, which make no prior assumption about the physiology of the underlying structure and treat the time-series data as random variables, have been shown to segment them efficiently.[21] The CA concentration in each MR voxel is the sum of the amount of CA that is intravascular and the amount that is in EES (linear mixture of the signal in the two spaces). In addition, these two spaces (intravascular space and EES) are anatomically separate and independent (spatially independent). These characteristics of DCE-MRI data satisfy the assumptions for spatial independent component analysis (ICA). Thus, ICA is used in the chapter to separate the intravascular and EES signals in DCE-MRI to be used in PK analysis.

2. Pharmacokinetic Modeling

The extended Tofts-Kety (ETK) model is the most commonly used PK model in tumor characterization.[22] The governing equations ETK are:

$$\mathbf{c}_t(t) = v_p\mathbf{c}_p(t) + v_e\mathbf{c}_e(t) \quad \& \quad v_e\frac{d\mathbf{c}_e}{dt}(t) = K^{trans}(\mathbf{c}_a(t) - \mathbf{c}_e(t)) \qquad (1)$$

where $\mathbf{c}_t$ is the concentration of the CA in the tissue, $\mathbf{c}_e$ is the concentration in the EES, $\mathbf{c}_p$ is the CA concentration in the plasma space, $\mathbf{c}_a$ is the CA concentration in the plasma space at the arterial input of the tissue which in ETK model is equal to $\mathbf{c}_p$ ($\mathbf{c}_p = \mathbf{c}_a$), K^{trans} is the volume transfer constant describing the rate by which the CA diffuses from plasma into the EES, v_e is the EES per unit volume of tissue, and v_p is the blood plasma space per unit volume of tissue. Solving the ETK model equations requires tissue CA concentration (derived from MRI data), and intravascular CA concentration in the tumor (vascular input function or VIF) which cannot be measured and is approximated using an AIF.

An ICA-based algorithm is developed to measure this VIF and separate it from the EES signal of the tumor.[23,24] Such separation does not require an artery, accounts for variability between subjects and simplifies the analysis as some of the parameters are eliminated. An introduction to ICA and the ICA-based algorithm, called adaptive complex ICA (AC-ICA),[24] is presented here. The chapter uses capital bold letters for 2D matrices, lowercase bold letters for column vectors, non-bold letters for scalars, and bold italic letters for functions.

3. Spatial Independent Component Analysis (ICA)

ICA is a statistical signal processing algorithm that attempts to split a dataset into its underlying features, assuming these features are statistically spatially independent, and without having any knowledge of their mixing processes.[25] Having a linear mixture of the features, the spatial ICA model is expressed as:

$$\mathbf{Z} = \mathbf{AS} \tag{2}$$

where $\mathbf{A} \in \mathbb{R}^{N\times M}$ is the mixing matrix, $\mathbf{Z} = [\mathbf{z}_0, \mathbf{z}_1, \ldots, \mathbf{z}_{N-1}]^T$ represents the complex-valued time-series dataset (DCE-MRI data in our case) such that $\mathbf{x}_i$ represents the MRI image acquired at time point i, N is the number of time points in the DCE-MRI sequence, $\mathbf{S} = [\mathbf{s}_0, \mathbf{s}_1, \ldots, \mathbf{s}_{M-1}]^T$ is a matrix containing the M structures known as independent components or ICs (usually $M \leq N$), which in this study are the images representing intravascular space and EES of the tissue. Having the observed mixed signal $\mathbf{Z}$, the ICA algorithm attempts to estimate the ICs, $\mathbf{S}$, and the mixing matrix $\mathbf{A}$. This is achieved by estimating the unmixing matrix $\mathbf{W}$, and the IC matrix $\mathbf{Y}$ such that:

$$\mathbf{Y} = \mathbf{WZ} \tag{3}$$

where $\mathbf{W} \in \mathbb{R}^{M\times N}$, the rows of $\mathbf{Y} = [\mathbf{y}_0, \mathbf{y}_1, \ldots, \mathbf{y}_{M-1}]^T$ are statistically independent with zero mean and unit variance (i.e. $\boldsymbol{E}\{\mathbf{YY}^{\boldsymbol{H}}\} = \boldsymbol{I}$ where $\boldsymbol{H}$ is the Hermitian transform) and, $\boldsymbol{E}\{.\}$ is the expectation operator. The IC's can be recovered up to a scaling and permutation.[25] Although we assume there are only 2 spaces in our model (intravascular and EES), since ICA makes no assumption about the spatial distribution of these spaces, it might split each space into several components. In practice, more than 2 ICs are required to achieve accurate separation, i.e. each space (intravascular space or EES) might be represented with more than one IC.

3.1. *Adaptive Complex Independent Component Analysis (AC-ICA)*

According to the central limit theorem, the distribution of a sum of independent random variables with finite support probability density functions (pdf) tends towards a Gaussian distribution.[26] Thus, by maximizing the non-Gaussianity of the estimated components, the independent components can be identified. One way of measuring non-Gaussianity of a random variable ($\mathbf{y}$) is to measure its Negentropy,[25] which is approximated using the following equation:

$$J_{negentropy}(\mathbf{w}) = [E\{G(\mathbf{y})\} - E\{G(\mathbf{y}_{\mathbf{gauss}})\}]^2 \quad (4)$$

where $\mathbf{y} = \mathbf{w}^H\mathbf{Z}$ is a complex-valued random variable ($\mathbf{w}$ is a column of unmixing matrix $\mathbf{W}$), $G(\mathbf{y}) = -log(p(\mathbf{y}^R, \mathbf{y}^I))$ is the contrast function and $p(\mathbf{y}^R, \mathbf{y}^I)$ is the joint pdf of real ($\mathbf{y}^R$) and imaginary ($\mathbf{y}^I$) parts of $\mathbf{y}$,[27] and $\mathbf{y}_{\mathrm{gauss}}$ is a Gaussian random variable with the same variance as $\mathbf{y}$. Assuming that $G(\mathbf{y}) = |C(\mathbf{y})|^2$ in which $C(.)$ is the non-linearity function, the ICA cost function[27] is expressed as $J_{negentropy}(\mathbf{w}) = E\{|C(\mathbf{w}^T\mathbf{Z})|^2\}$. Maximizing $\mathbf{J}_{negentropy}$ with respect to $\mathbf{w}$ (subject to constraint $\|\mathbf{w}\| = 1$), using a quasi-Newton algorithm, results in the following update rule:

$$\begin{aligned}\mathbf{w}_{\mathrm{k}+1} = &-E\{C^*(\mathbf{w}_{\mathrm{k}}^H\mathbf{Z})C'(\mathbf{w}_{\mathrm{k}}^H\mathbf{Z})\mathbf{Z}\} + E\{C'(\mathbf{w}_{\mathrm{k}}^H\mathbf{Z})C'^*(\mathbf{w}_{\mathrm{k}}^H\mathbf{Z})\}\mathbf{w}_{\mathrm{k}} \\ &+ E\{\mathbf{Z}\mathbf{Z}^T\}E\{C^*(\mathbf{w}_{\mathrm{k}}^H\mathbf{Z})C''(\mathbf{w}_{\mathrm{k}}^H\mathbf{Z})\}\mathbf{w}_{\mathrm{k}}^* \end{aligned} \quad (5)$$

where C^*, C' and C'' are complex conjugate, first and second derivatives of C respectively. Each column of $\mathbf{W}$ is estimated iteratively using this update rule.

3.2. *Selecting Non-linearity Function for AC-ICA*

In order to solve the AC-ICA problem the non-linearity function is required, which is not known in ICA and has to be estimated. We have observed that the distributions of real and imaginary parts of MR images of each component fit well into the generalized Gaussian distribution (GGD) formulation given as:

$$g(\mathbf{y}; \alpha, \beta) = \frac{\beta}{2\alpha\Gamma(1/\beta)} exp\left(-\frac{|\mathbf{y}|^\beta}{\alpha^\beta}\right) \quad (6)$$

where $\Gamma(.)$ is the gamma function defined as $\Gamma(\mathbf{x}) = \int_0^\infty e^{-t}t^{\mathbf{x}-1}dt$, and β and α are the model parameters. We modeled the intravascular signal with a sum of a number of GGDs, and the parameters (α, β) were calculated at each ICA iteration using an expectation maximization (EM) framework.

3.3. *Expectation Maximization (EM)*

The AC-ICA algorithm first models the pdf of independent component **y**, estimated in the last iteration, as a sum of a number (usually 3 to 5) of GGDs:

$$f(\mathbf{y},\boldsymbol{\Theta}) = \sum_{i=1}^{K} p_i \mathcal{g}(\mathbf{y};\alpha_i,\beta_i) \tag{7}$$

Where $\boldsymbol{\Theta} = [\boldsymbol{\theta}_1,\boldsymbol{\theta}_2,\ldots,\boldsymbol{\theta}_i] = [(p_1,\alpha_1,\beta_1),\ldots,(p_i,\alpha_i,\beta_i)]$ is the parameter space of the GGDs, and p_i is the membership probability of the ith GGD. The algorithm calculates $\boldsymbol{\Theta}$ through maximum log-likelihood estimation, given as:

$$\hat{\boldsymbol{\Theta}} = \underset{\boldsymbol{\Theta}}{\boldsymbol{argmax}}\{\boldsymbol{\Lambda}(\mathbf{y},\boldsymbol{\Theta})\} \tag{8}$$

where $\boldsymbol{\Lambda}(\mathbf{y},\boldsymbol{\Theta}) = \boldsymbol{log}\prod_{n=1}^{N_y} f(\mathbf{y},\boldsymbol{\Theta})$ and N_y represents the number of samples in **y**. Solving this system using EM leads to calculating the (p_i,α_i,β_i) using Eqs. (9), (10) and (11) at each iteration. The membership probabilities, $p_i^{(k)}$, are calculated at iteration k using (9):

$$p^{(k)}(i|n) = \frac{p_i^{(k)}\mathcal{g}(y_n;\alpha_i^{(k)},\beta_i^{(k)})}{\sum_{m=1}^{K} p_m^{(k)}\mathcal{g}(y_n;\alpha_m^{(k)},\beta_m^{(k)})} \quad \& \quad \sum_{i=1}^{K} p^{(k)}(i|n) = 1 \tag{9}$$

The parameters $\alpha_i^{(k)}$ of the GGDs are calculated at iteration k using (10):

$$\alpha_i^{(k)} = \left[\frac{\beta_i^{(k)}\sum_{n=1}^{N_y}(p^{(k)}(i|n)|y_n|^{\beta_i^{(k)}})}{N_y}\right]^{1/\beta_i^{(k)}} \tag{10}$$

and the parameters $\beta_i^{(k)}$ of the GGDs are calculated by solving (11) using an optimization algorithm. We used the fzero function of MATLAB software (The MathWorks Inc., Natick, USA) to find the value of β_i at iteration k:

$$\frac{1}{\beta_i^{(k)}}\left[1+\frac{1}{\beta_i^{(k)}}\boldsymbol{\psi}\left(\frac{1}{\beta_i^{(k)}}\right)\right]\sum_{n=1}^{N_y} p^{(k)}(i|n) - \sum_{n=1}^{N_y} p^{(k)}(i|n)\left(\frac{|y_n|}{\alpha_i^{(k)}}\right)^{\beta_i^{(k)}} \boldsymbol{log}\left(\frac{|y_n|}{\alpha_i^{(k)}}\right) = 0 \tag{11}$$

where $\boldsymbol{\psi}(\mathbf{x}) = \boldsymbol{d}(\mathbf{log}(\boldsymbol{\Gamma}(\mathbf{x})))/\boldsymbol{dx}$ is the polygamma function. The GGD with the highest membership probability is selected as the probability distribution of the intravascular signal at that iteration. This GGD was then used to derive the ICA non-linearity which is given as:

$$\boldsymbol{C}(\mathbf{y}) = (\mathbf{y}/\alpha)^{\beta/2} \tag{12}$$

3.4. *AC-ICA Implementation and VIF Identification*

Dimensionality reduction and Whitening were performed as pre-processing steps in order to reduce noise and make the DCE-MRI signal zero mean and unit variance. Singular value decomposition was performed on the dataset and the significant eigenvalues (the eigenvalues that were bigger than 0.1% of the largest eigenvalue) were kept. AC-ICA was then applied and all of the ICs, which were equal to the number of eigenvalues kept at the dimensionality reduction step, were estimated. The intravascular components were selected heuristically such that the curves with a uniform pre-contrast uptake phase, an uptake phase in which the intensity increased rapidly, and a washout phase in which the intensity dropped to less than 60% of the peak value were considered intravascular.

The intravascular image and its corresponding time-intensity curve that were calculated using AC-ICA algorithm have to be converted into CA concentration before being used in PK analysis. In order to convert the signal intensity of a voxel at time $t = t_0$ into its CA concentration, both the pre-contrast signal intensity and the MR signal intensity at $t = t_0$ are required. As ICA is a data-driven algorithm which does not make any assumption about the physiology of the data it is processing, some structures, e.g. intravascular space, might split into several ICs. These ICs have to be first combined to represent the entire intravascular signal. We can rewrite (2) in expanded form as:

$$\begin{bmatrix} \mathbf{z}_0 \\ \vdots \\ \mathbf{z}_{N-1} \end{bmatrix} = [\mathbf{a}_0, \ldots, \mathbf{a}_{IV}^{(1)} \ldots, \mathbf{a}_{IV}^{(K)}, \ldots, \mathbf{a}_{M-1}][\mathbf{s}_0, \ldots, \mathbf{s}_{IV}^{(1)}, \ldots, \mathbf{s}_{IV}^{(K)}, \ldots, \mathbf{s}_{M-1}]^T \tag{13}$$

where $\mathbf{a}_i$ is a column of mixing matrix $\mathbf{A}$, and K is the number of ICs that are identified as intravascular. The time series data corresponding to the intravascular signal, $\mathbf{Z}_{IV}$, can be written as:

$$\mathbf{Z}_{IV} = [\mathbf{z}_{IV,0}, \mathbf{z}_{IV,2}, \ldots, \mathbf{z}_{IV,N-1}]^T = \mathbf{a}_{IV}^{(1)}\mathbf{s}_{IV}^{(1)} + \cdots + \mathbf{a}_{IV}^{(K)}\mathbf{s}_{IV}^{(K)} \tag{14}$$

where $\mathbf{z}_{IV,t_0}$ is intravascular portion of the DCE-MRI data at $t = t_0$. The change in the intravascular signal due to the passage of CA between $t = 0$ and $t = t_0$ is:

$$\Delta\mathbf{z}_{IV,t_0} = \mathbf{z}_{IV,t_0} - \mathbf{z}_{IV,0} \tag{15}$$

adding $\Delta\mathbf{z}_{IV,t_0}$ to the DCE-MRI frame corresponding to $t = 0$ (which is $\mathbf{z}_0$), a DCE-MRI time-series data in which the only enhancement is due to the CA arrival and passage through the intravascular space can be generated. The signal intensity is the magnitude of the complex-valued MRI signal and thus we have:

$$\mathbf{SI}_{IV}(0) = |\mathbf{z}_0|, \quad \& \quad \mathbf{SI}_{IV}(t_0) = |\mathbf{z}_0 + \Delta\mathbf{z}_{IV,t_0}| \tag{16}$$

having $\mathbf{SI}_{IV}(0)$ and $\mathbf{SI}_{IV}(t_0)$, intravascular CA concentration is calculated using standard conversion method for spoiled gradient recalled (SPGR) pulse sequence.

4. Numerical Phantom

A numerical study was conducted to simulate DCE-MRI of a leaky phantom using finite element analysis (FEA) and the classical description of MRI physics (Bloch equations), and was used to evaluate performance of AC-ICA algorithm.

4.1. *Contrast Agent (CA) Concentration Modeling*

Comsol Multiphysics (Comsol Inc., Burlington, USA) FEA software was used to construct the numerical phantom (Fig. 1). This phantom was comprised of a grid of 10×10 leaky tubes (through which water was flowing) that ran in parallel through a chamber of agar gel (0.5% agar gel). The tubes had an internal diameter of 200 μm, wall thickness of 30 μm, and center-to-center spacing of 300 μm. To model our physical phantom (explained in Section 5), some of the tubes were removed to simulate the blocked or damaged tubes. The study simulated passage of a bolus of CA (injected into the tubes) through the tubes and its leakage from the tubes into the agar gel over time.

The 2D CA distribution of the phantom was simulated for an imaging plane at the middle of the phantom in x-direction [Fig. 1(a)] for 6.48 min with a temporal resolution of 3.3 s. As the CA arrived in the imaging plane, it diffused into the surrounding gel. The imaging plane was split into 2555 subdomains [Fig. 1(b)], and proper diffusion coefficients were assigned to the subdomains of the tubes (1×10^{-3} mm^2.s^{-1}) which model water flow, the tube walls ($2 \times 10^{-5} \pm 10^{-6}$ mm^2.s^{-1} with uniform distribution), and the gel ($2.08 \times 10^{-4} \pm 10^{-5}$ mm^2.s^{-1} with uniform distribution), to account for variability of diffusion in the gel and generate a heterogeneous leakage space.

4.2. *Generating DCE-MRI Data (Bloch Equations)*

The geometry and CA concentrations, calculated in the FEA, were fed to the MRI simulation software that solved Bloch equations for each voxel at every time point (120 frames) to generate the DCE-MRI data. The simulator assumed each voxel was comprised of 2 isochromates[28] corresponding to the

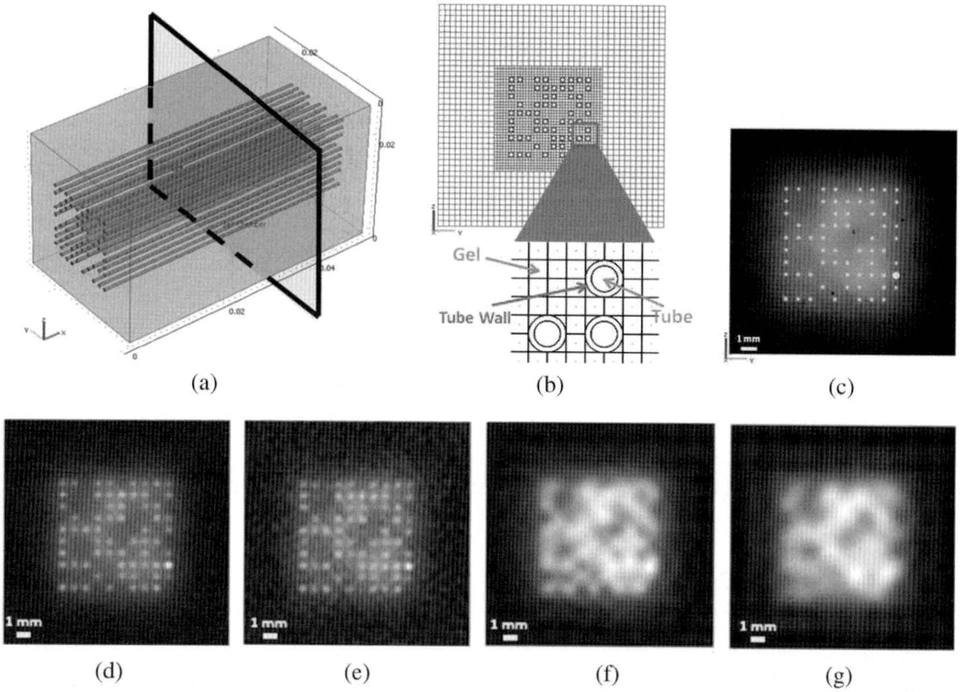

Fig. 1. (a) 3D view of the numerical phantom showing the imaging plane located in yz-plane halfway through the phantom in x-direction. (b) The MR imaging plane showing the arrangement of the tubes as well as the blocked tubes, and 2555 subdomains of the phantom used in FEA. As shown in the enlarged region, the tubes, their walls, and their surrounding gel areas are separated and proper diffusion coefficients are assigned to them. (c) The CA distribution in the imaging plane (resulted from FEA), at t = 2.5 min after CA injection, and the corresponding simulated MR image for in-plane resolutions of (d) 150 μm, (e) 300 μm (f) 600 μm, and (g) 800 μm.

tubes and gel compartments and assigned proton density ρ (derived from FEA step), pre-contrast longitudinal relaxation T_1 (3000 ms for water and 2100 ms for gel) and transverse relaxation T_2 (250 ms for water and 65 ms for gel), to each isochromate of every voxel.[29,30] The post-contrast T_1 and T_2 values were calculated using their pre-contrast values, the CA concentration of the voxel at each time point, and the relaxivities of the CA (Omniscan).[31] The imaging parameters used in the simulator for 2D SPGR sequence were: B_0 = 1.5 T (1 ppm inhomogeneity), single coil RF pulse, Field-of-View (FOV) = 19.2 mm, TR/TE = 12.5/2.9 ms, FA = 20°, Nx/Ny = 128/128, Slice Thickness = 5 mm.

Gaussian noise was added to the k-space data such that an SNR of 20 was achieved in the image space. The data was reconstructed at four different in-plane resolutions (150 μm, 300 μm, 600 μm and 800 μm), as shown in Fig. 1(d)–(g), which were used to assess robustness of the algorithm. Data of each resolution was generated 10 times, which differed in the distribution of noise and B_0 inhomogeneity, to assess the reproducibility of the separation results.

4.3. AC-ICA Separation Results (Numerical Phantom)

The AC-ICA algorithm for intravascular time-intensity curve calculation was applied to all simulated datasets (four different resolutions) and the signal from inside the tubes (intravascular signal) was extracted. Dimensionality reduction was performed on each dataset where 8 to 15 eigenvalues were kept. The data was then Whitened to make it zero mean and unit variance. In all cases, all IC's were estimated and the IC (or ICs) that corresponded to the tubes' signal was selected using the heuristic criterion.

Figure 2(a)–(d) show the IC images of the tubes for the four in-plane resolutions. The corresponding time-intensity curves of the tubes are shown

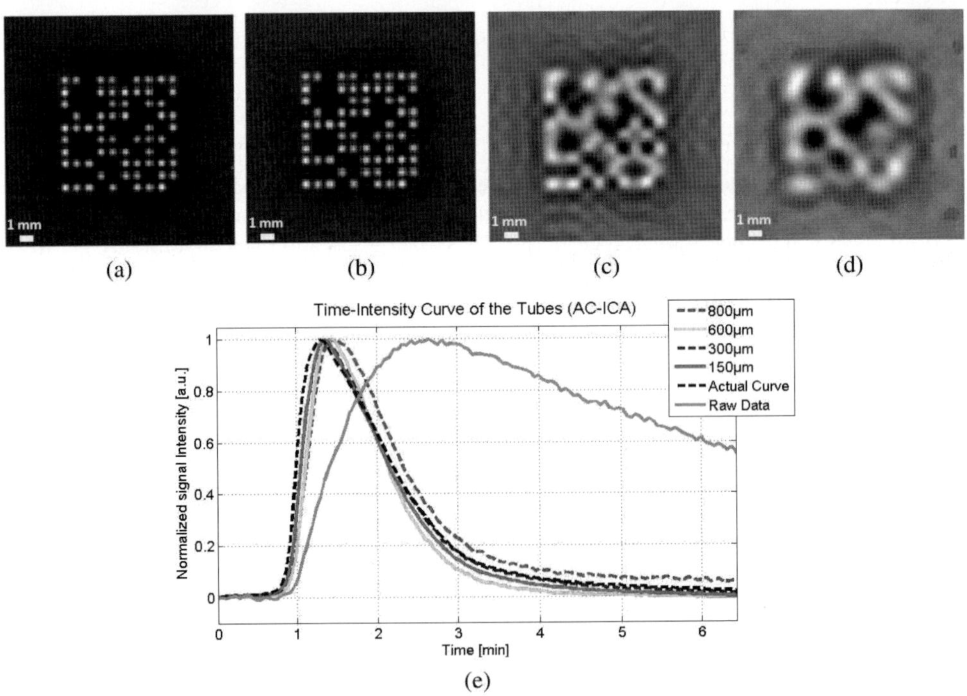

Fig. 2. The separated tubes' image and the time-intensity curves of the tubes calculated using AC-ICA for the four simulated DCE-MRI datasets. Tubes images for datasets with in-plane resolutions of (a) 150 μm, (b) 300 μm, (c) 600 μm, (d) 800 μm. (e) Calculated time-intensity curves of the tubes corresponding to the four simulated datasets, the actual time-intensity curve of the tubes (Actual Curve), and the curve corresponding to the mean across the entire raw (not analyzed) DCE-MR images over time (Raw Data).

Table 1. RMSE and correlation coefficients between estimated (AC-ICA) tubes' and actual time intensity curve, for all four resolutions of the numerical phantom, using 10 different implementations of the phantom (calculated after setting baseline value of the curves to zero and normalizing them).

In-plane Resolution	150 μm	300 μm	600 μm	800 μm
	Root Mean Square Error (RMSE)			
AC-ICA	0.04 ± 0.01	0.04 ± 0.01	0.07 ± 0.01	0.08 ± 0.01
	Correlation Coefficient			
AC-ICA	0.99 ± 0.001	0.99 ± 0.001	0.97 ± 0.01	0.96 ± 0.01

in Fig. 2(e). These curves represent the average signal intensity over time of all the voxels that were separated by ICA as the intravascular space (tubes). Figure 2(e) also shows the actual intravascular time-intensity curve as well as the raw data curve calculated by averaging the signal across the raw DCE-MR images. All time-intensity curves are normalized with respect to their maximum and their pre-contrast signal intensities are set to zero to enable comparison.

For each in-plane resolution, 10 DCE-MRI data sets of the phantom were simulated with SNR = 20 and the AC-ICA algorithm was applied to all datasets. Table 1 reports the root mean square error (RMSE) between the estimated time-intensity curves of the tubes obtained using AC-ICA and the actual curve for all four in-plane resolutions. Table 1 also reports the correlation coefficient between the estimated and actual time-intensity curves of the tubes.

The results presented in Fig. 2 and Table 1 demonstrate that AC-ICA algorithm is capable of separating time-intensity curve of the tubes with high accuracy, for DCE-MRI data with different resolutions, in both spatial and temporal domains. Note that in lower resolutions although the tubes could not be visualized in the spatial domain, their time-intensity curves were calculated with high accuracy. There were small differences between the time-intensity curves of the tubes calculated using AC-ICA for different resolutions and even in the lowest resolution the error in the enhancement curve was small.

5. Physical Phantom

A physical phantom was built to mimic CA dynamics in tumor microvasculature[32] (Fig. 3), which was similar to our numerical phantom. It was comprised of a grid of 10 $\times$ 10 dialysis tubing (Diapes PES-150, Baxter) embedded in a chamber of agar gel (0.5 wt%, Sigma-Aldrich Canada Ltd., Canada).[32] The dialysis tubing had inner diameter of 200 μm, wall thickness of 30 μm, and were

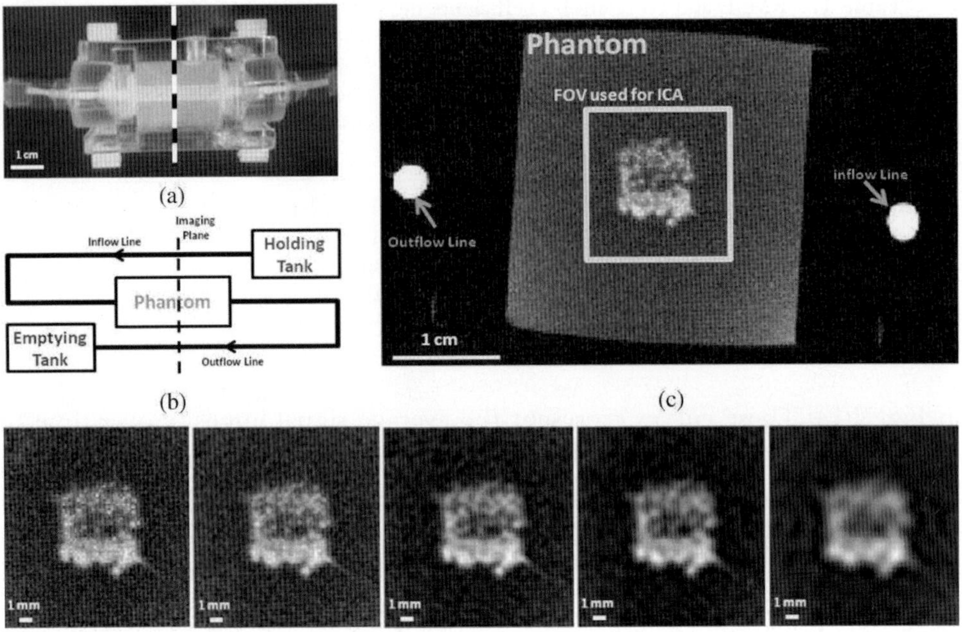

(a) (b) (c) (d) (e) (f) (g) (h)

Fig. 3. (a) Photograph of the physical phantom in which the DCE-MR imaging was performed across the dashed line, in a plane perpendicular to view shown in the photo. (b) Schematic of the tissue-mimicking phantom set up. Water was flowing from the holding tank to the emptying tank and the contrast agent bolus was injected into the inflow line. The phantom was imaged at the imaging plane which included the phantom, as well as the inflow and outflow lines as shown in this figure. (c) An MR image of the full imaging FOV at time = 1.8 min after CA injection showing the inflow and outflow lines, the phantom, and the FOV that was used in ICA analysis. The corresponding MR image of the ICA FOV (time = 1.8 min), reconstructed with in-plane resolutions of (d) 170 μm, (e) 225 μm, (f) 340 μm, (g) 450 μm, and (h) 680 μm.

aligned parallel to each other in a square grid with center-to-center spacing of 300 μm over a 5 cm distance.[32]

The pore sizes of the dialysis tubing were such that low-molecular weight CA could diffuse from the tubes into the surrounding gel. Water was flowing through the tubes at a constant rate of 0.047 ml/s (achieving a flow velocity within physiological range of arterioles[33]). A bolus of Gd-DTPA contrast agent was injected into the flow line, which was capable of leaking from the tubes as it reached the gel chamber. DCE-MR images were obtained at an imaging plane transverse to the tubes (Fig. 3), and the inflow and outflow lines of the flow through the chamber were oriented such that they passed through the imaging plane [Fig. 3(b)–(c)]. The enhancement curves of these two flow lines were used to evaluate the separation algorithm.

DCE-MR imaging was performed using a 2D fast SPGR sequence with the following imaging parameters: TR/TE = 12.5/2.9 ms, BW = 15.63 kHz, FA = 20°, Nx/Ny/NEX = 256/256/1, FOV = 45 mm, Slice Thickness = 5 mm. A total of 120 images were acquired over about 6.48 min with a temporal resolution of 3.3 s. The DCE-MR images was reconstructed at five different in-plane resolutions (170 μm, 225 μm, 340 μm, 450 μm and 680 μm), to assess the performance and robustness of the AC-ICA algorithm in dealing with different imaging resolutions, particularly in low resolution data that are commonly in clinical studies. Moreover, two identical phantoms were built, imaged, and analyzed to assess the reproducibility of the AC-ICA algorithm. A sample frame of each dataset (for five in-plane resolutions) is shown in [Fig. 3(d)–(h)].

5.1. *AC-ICA Separation Results for Physical Phantom*

The AC-ICA algorithm was applied to DCE-MRI of the physical tissue-mimicking phantom and the signal of the tubes was separated. The phantom data was reconstructed at five different in-plane resolutions and the AC-ICA algorithm was applied to all five datasets. Similar to the numerical study, dimensionality reduction and Whitening were first performed, and then AC-ICA was applied to the DCE-MRI data. The IC images corresponding to the tubes' signal of the five datasets are shown in Fig. 4(a)–(e).

The separated time-intensity curves of the tubes for the five datasets, as well as the actual time-intensity curve of the tubes that was measured at the inflow line of the phantom, the time-intensity curve at the outflow line of the phantom, and the raw data curve calculated by averaging the signal across the raw MRI images (not analyzed) over time are shown in Fig. 4(f). The baseline values of these enhancement curves are set to zero and they are normalized with respect to their maximum values.

Two physical phantoms were built and DCE-MRI imaging was performed on both phantoms to assess the reproducibility of the results for the intravascular time-intensity curve calculation algorithms. Table 2 reports the root mean square error (RMSE) between the estimated and the actual time-intensity curves of the tubes (inflow line) for all five datasets of both phantoms. This table also reports the correlation coefficient between the estimated and actual time-intensity curves of the tubes for AC-ICA algorithm in all five in-plane.

Similar to the numerical study, the separation results obtained for the DCE-MRI data of the physical phantoms, as shown in Fig. 4 and also reported in Table 2, show that the tubes were separated accurately in both spatial and

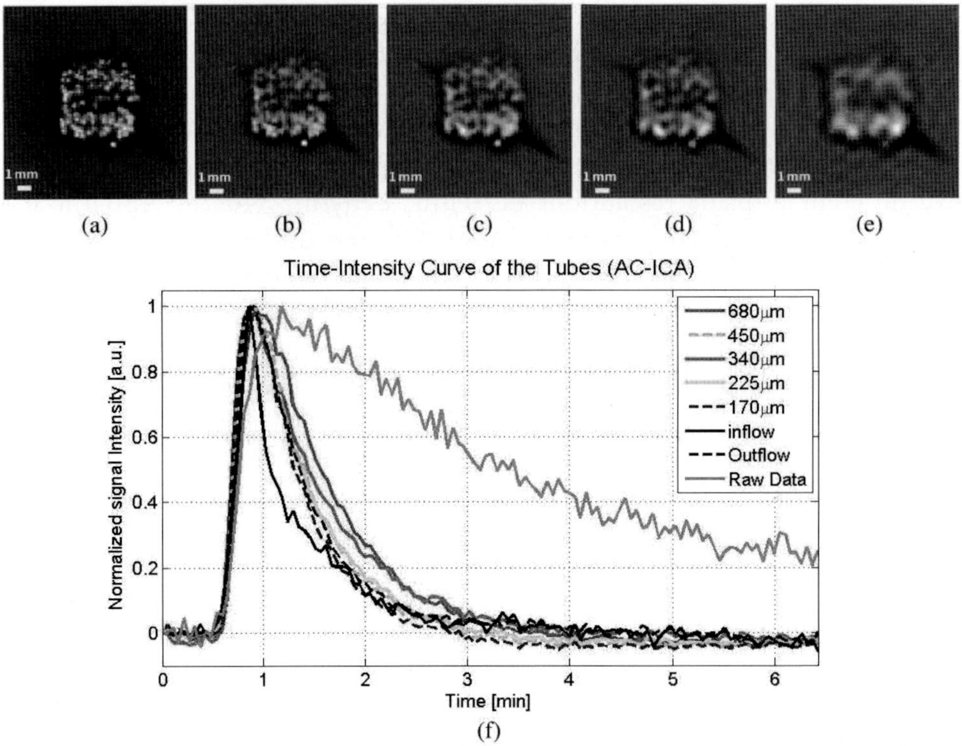

Fig. 4. The separated tubes' image and their time-intensity curves calculated using AC-ICA for the five DCE-MRI datasets of the physical tissue-mimicking phantom. Tubes' images for datasets with in-plane resolutions of (a) 170 μm, (b) 225 μm, (c) 340 μm, (d) 450 μm, and (e) 680 μm. (f) Calculated time-intensity curves of the tubes corresponding to the five datasets, the actual time-intensity curve of the tubes (inflow line), the curve of the tubes at the outflow line, and the curve corresponding to mean across the raw (not analyzed) DCE-MR images over time (Raw Data).

Table 2. RMSE and correlation coefficients between the estimated (AC-ICA) and the actual (inflow) time-intensity curves of the tubes for all 5 resolutions (using both physical phantoms). The values are calculated after setting the baseline values of the curves to zero and normalizing them).

In-plane Resolution	170 μm	225 μm	340 μm	450 μm	680 μm
	Root Mean Square Error (RMSE)				
AC-ICA	0.07 ± 0.01	0.09 ± 0.02	0.08 ± 0.03	0.08 ± 0.01	0.11 ± 0.03
	Correlation Coefficient				
AC-ICA	0.97 ± 0.004	0.96 ± 0.02	0.97 ± 0.01	0.97 ± 0.02	0.95 ± 0.03

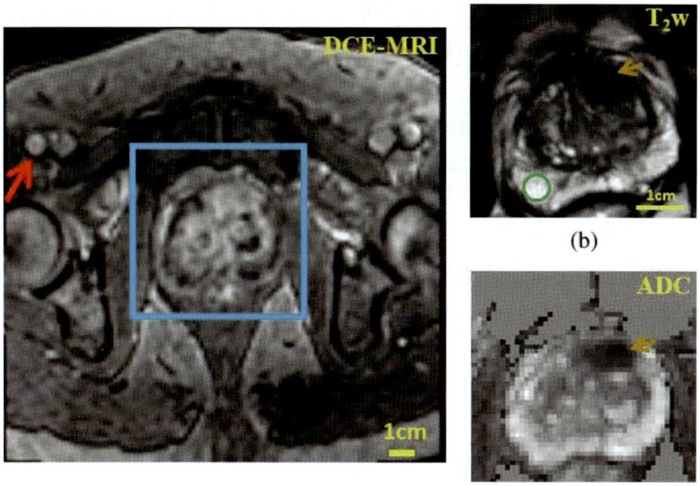

(a) (b) (c)

Fig. 5. (a) Full FOV of the prostate DCE-MR images showing femoral artery (red arrow) and the prostate region used in ICA analysis (blue box). (b) T_2-weighted MRI of the prostate showing the tumor (arrow) and a region of normal peripheral zone tissue (green circle). (c) The ADC map of the prostate showing the tumor (arrow).

temporal domains. As the pixel size increased, it became more difficult to visualize the tubes in the IC images such that in the two lowest resolutions it was impossible to see them separately from the leakage. However, the time-intensity curves of the tubes were estimated with high accuracy, and similar to the numerical study the AC-ICA algorithm demonstrated high accuracy in dealing with lower resolution data and there were small differences between time-intensity curves of the tubes at varying resolutions.

Having developed and evaluated the AC-ICA algorithm that is capable of separating the intravascular signal, the next step is to assess its performance in clinical data and also compare the PK parameters calculated using its VIF to the commonly used AIF-based methods.

6. Prostate Cancer Assessment

DCE-MRI of a cohort of 27 prostate cancer patients (28 MRI dataset where one patient was imaged twice) were acquired and used to assess the performance of the VIF calculated using the AC-ICA algorithm in PK analysis of prostate DCE-MRI. The calculated PK parameters were compared to PK parameters calculated using an AIF, measured at the femoral artery. In addition to DCE-MRI, T_2-weighted and diffusion weighted MRI of the prostate were acquired which are used for tumor detection (Fig. 5).

MR imaging was performed on a 3T Achieva Philips scanner (Philips Medical Systems). DCE-MR imaging was performed using a 3D SPGR sequence with TE/TR = 3.91/1.81 ms, FA = 8, FOV = 20 cm, slice thickness = 3.5 mm, spacing between slices = 3.5 mm, and temporal resolution = 4.8 s, where contrast agent, Magnevist (Gd-DTPA), was injected intravenously with a dose of 0.1 mM/Kg. T_2-weighted MRI was performed using a spin echo sequence, followed by axial diffusion weighted MRI with b-values = 0, 1000 s.mm^{-2}, which were used to generate apparent diffusion coefficient (ADC) maps. Multiple flip angle (FA = 5, 15) T_1-weighted MRI were also acquired to generate pre-contrast T_1-map that is required to convert MRI signal into CA concentration.

6.1. *Vascular Input Function (VIF) Calculation in Prostate*

Each prostate DCE-MRI dataset contained 20 slices. The slices in which the prostate was visible were first identified and a rectangular region of interest [blue box in Fig. 5(a)] was selected around the prostate gland. The AC-ICA algorithm was applied to each individual slice and the intravascular component was separated. The separated intravascular component, for the prostate slice which was shown in Fig. 5, in spatial and temporal domains is shown in Fig. 6(a)–(b).

The signal intensity in each voxel of the separated intravascular signal was converted into contrast agent concentration, using the method explained in Section 3.4, and then averaged over the entire image for each time point to generate the VIF curve. The conversion results in temporal domain (representing the VIF curve), and in spatial domain (representing prostate vasculature) are shown in Fig. 6(c)–(d).

The scaling of the VIF curve depends on the size of the ROI that was initially selected for ICA analysis, which in turn depends on the size of the prostate cross section in that slice, and thus is operator-dependent. These issues make the calculated PK parameters highly dependent on the manually selected ROI. However, it can be proved that if two VIFs satisfy the governing equations of the two-compartment ETK model, their AUC have to be equal. Thus, in order to remove the operator dependence and also enable comparison of VIF-based and AIF-based analyses, we normalized the VIF and the AIF with respect to their area under the curve (AUC) as shown in Fig. 7(a).

6.2. *Pharmacokinetic (PK) Analysis Results*

PK modeling was performed using the ETK model for each voxel of the prostate gland in all patients, using the VIF (AC-ICA), and the AIF (artery).VIF-based

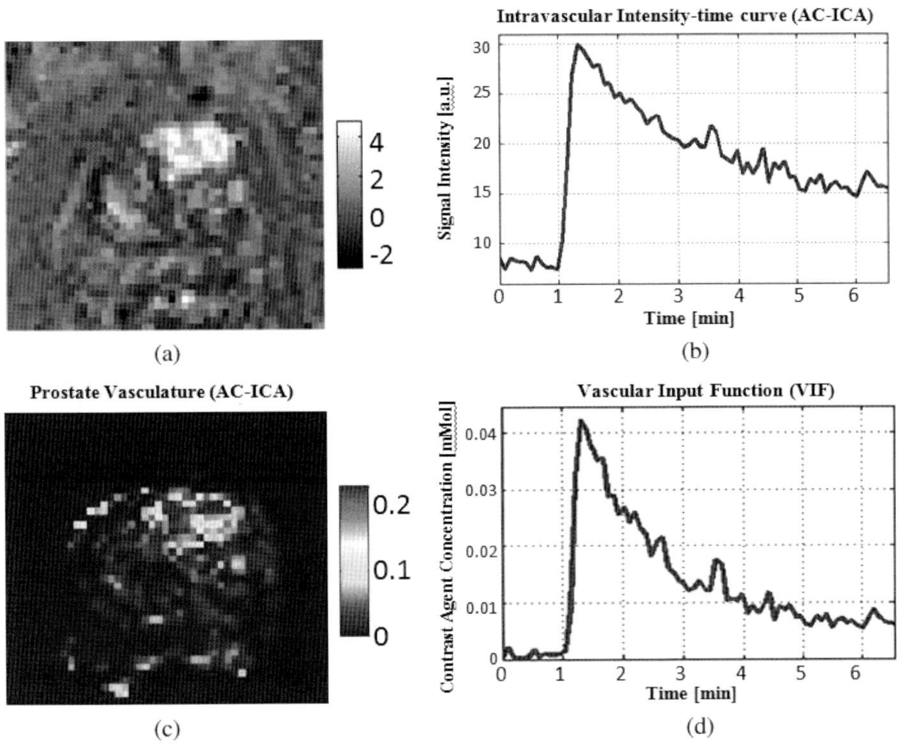

Fig. 6. The IC corresponding to prostate vasculature separated by AC-ICA in (a) spatial and, (b) temporal domains. Conversion of AC-ICA results into CA concentration in (c) spatial domain (showing the intravascular CA concentration at each voxel) and, (d) temporal domain (representing the VIF curve generated by averaging CA concentration in the intravascular space of each frame).

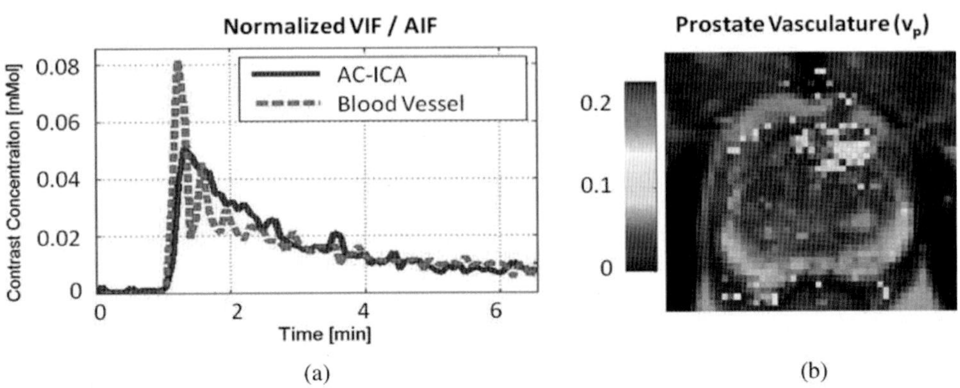

Fig. 7. (a) The VIF and the AIF after normalization, and (b) the vascular map corresponding to the VIF (calculated using AC-ICA).

analysis was performed using the prostate vasculature map which was estimated by AC-ICA, as the v_p parameter and subtracting the $v_p\mathbf{c}_p(t)$ term from the DCE-MRI data, and then calculating the remaining two model parameter (K^{trans} and v_e) through curve fitting. For the AIF-based PK analysis, curve fitting was performed to calculate all three model parameters.

The K^{trans} value is a characteristic of the tissue as it represents the vascular permeability and perfusion of the tissue, and thus, for a specific tissue type K^{trans} should be the same regardless of the VIF (or AIF) calculation method. Thus, both AIF-based and VIF-based methods should result in similar K^{trans} values for the normal peripheral zone (PZ) tissue in prostate [Fig. 5(b)], and the method that results in smaller variation in its K^{trans} has better performance.

The calculated PK parameters for the patient (which was shown in Fig. 5), are shown in Fig. 8 as parametric maps. As can be seen in this figure, the VIF-based and AIF-based K^{trans} maps have small values in the normal PZ tissue, and large values in the tumor. Thus, the performances of the methods in detecting the tumor are similar. Moreover, the similarity between the v_p map calculated directly from ICA and the v_p map that resulted from AIF-based PK analysis proves that the component that was separated by ICA as the intravascular component is actually the intravascular component, and more importantly the v_p map, which could be used in assessing anti-vascular therapies, can be directly obtained using AC-ICA algorithm without any PK modeling.

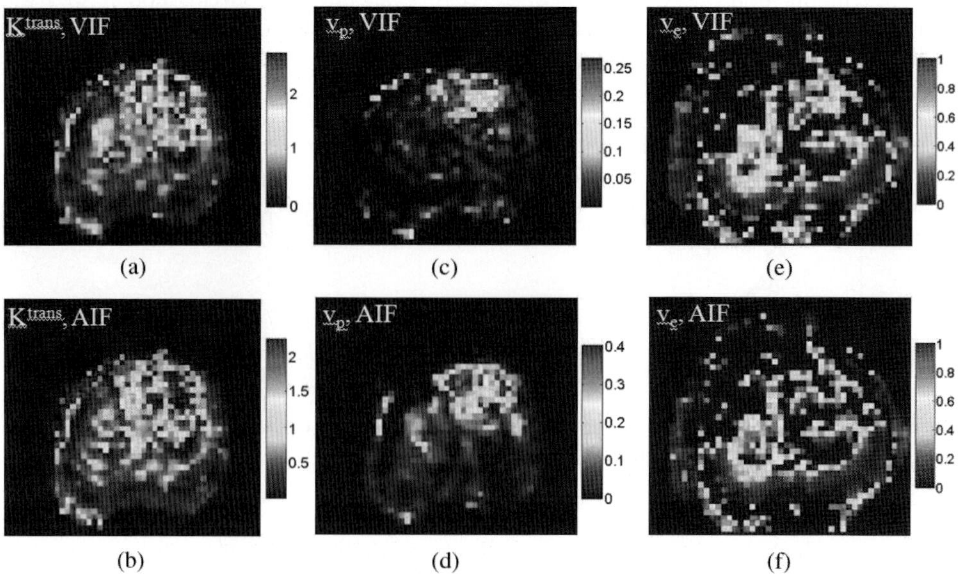

Fig. 8. The K^{trans} maps (a, b), v_p maps (c, d), and v_e maps (e, f) calculated using the normalized VIF and normalized AIF for ETK model.

Table 3. The mean and standard deviation of the K^{trans} in normal PZ tissue, calculated from the distribution of the mean values for each patients (the mean value for each patient was calculated by averaging K^{trans} values of all normal PZ tissue voxels in that patient). These values were calculated using all the patients in which normal PZ tissue was identified (20 patients).

Method	TissueType	VIF [min^{-1}]	AIF [min^{-1}]
With Normalization	Normal PZ	**0.21** ± 0.05	**0.26** ± 0.11
Without Normalization	Normal PZ	**1.09** ± 0.53	**0.29** ± 0.34

Table 4. The median and inter-quartile ranges of the K^{trans} value calculated using pooled distribution (for all patients) of all voxels in normal PZ and tumor regions (both distributions were positively skewed). The K^{trans} values were calculated using VIF and AIF (normalized and not normalized) for the normal PZ tissue (for 20 patients) and for tumor tissue (for 27 patients). The table also reports several prostate K^{trans} values from literature.

Method	Tissue Type	VIF [min^{-1}]	AIF [min^{-1}]
With Normalization	Normal PZ	**0.13** [0.07 0.22]	**0.15** [0.07 0.28]
	Tumor	**0.59** [0.40 0.88]	**0.97** [0.61 1.47]
Without Normalization	Normal PZ	**0.51** [0.22 1.29]	**0.07** [0.02 0.20]
	Tumor	**2.29** [1.01 4.28]	**0.31** [0.15 0.78]
Moradi[34]	Normal PZ	—	**0.07** ± 0.047
	Tumor	—	**0.148** ± 0.071
Langer[35]	Normal PZ	—	**0.29** [0.09 0.87]
	Tumor	—	**0.36** [0.16 1.28]
Ocak[36]	Normal PZ	—	**0.23** ± 0.25
	Tumor	—	**0.47** ± 0.57
Korporral[37]	Normal PZ	—	**0.10** [0.04 0.21]
	Tumor	—	**0.44** [0.25 0.75]
Li[38]	Normal PZ	—	**0.09** ± 0.07
	Tumor	—	**0.32** ± 0.23

The mean and standard deviation of the K^{trans} values for normal PZ tissue (distribution of the mean values), using the ETK model, are reported in Table 3 for AIF-based and VIF-based PK analyses. These values were calculated for the entire patient population in which normal PZ tissue was identifiable (20 datasets). This table also reports the K^{trans} value for normal PZ tissue using the VIF and AIF without normalization which shows normalization results in smaller variation in the K^{trans} value. This table shows after normalization the mean K^{trans} value of the AIF-based and VIF-based methods are close to each other, indicating that both methods are calculating the same value for the normal PZ tissue (these mean values correspond to two samples of the same population as assessed by ANOVA). However, the VIF-based method provides smaller variation compared to the AIF-based method and thus, is working better.

Table 4 reports the median and inter-quartile ranges of the K^{trans} obtained for the tumor and normal PZ tissues (these distributions were positively skewed and thus inter-quartile ranges are used) for the VIF-based and AIF-based PK analyses as well as the K^{trans} values of five studies reported in the literature. Comparing the results obtained using AIF and VIF with normalization, to those obtained using AIF and VIF without normalization and the values that were reported in the literature, shows that using the VIF with normalization provides clear separation of the normal PZ and tumor tissues.

7. Conclusions

Pharmacokinetic modeling of tumor tissues using their DCE-MRI requires information about the CA concentration in the intravascular space. This signal is inseparable from the DCE-MRI data, and thus it is approximated using an AIF. An ICA-based algorithm (AC-ICA) was developed to separate this intravascular signal locally at the tissue of interest and calculate the vascular input function (VIF), and also to assess the effects of using this VIF in PK analysis.

The performance of the AC-ICA algorithm in separating the intravascular signal was first evaluated using numerical and physical tissue-mimicking phantoms, which showed the algorithm was capable of separating this signal with high accuracy and could efficiently handle low resolution DCE-MR images that are commonly encountered in clinics. The VIF calculated using the AC-ICA algorithm was then used in PK analysis of prostate cancer and its results were compared to the commonly used AIF-based method. The results showed that the PK parameters calculated using the VIF were comparable to those calculated using the AIF, and also there was smaller variation in the calculated PK parameters in VIF-based analysis which shows its better performance. Thus, the proposed VIF could replace the currently used AIFs in PK analyses, and more importantly it could be used in cases where it is impossible or very difficult to measure an AIF, e.g. in small animal studies or in studying tissues like breast tumors.

Acknowledgments

The author would like to thank Anne L. Martel, PhD, Rajiv Chopra, PhD, Masoom A. Haider, MD, Michael Da Rosa, MD, Chaitanya Chandrana, PhD, and Ian Pang, MSc, for their contributions in the presented research.

References

1. E. A. Handorf EA, S. McElligott, A. Vachani, C. J. Langer, M. B. Demeter, K. Armstrong, and D. A. Asch, "Cost effectiveness of personalized therapy for first-line treatment of stage IV and recurrent incurable adenocarcinoma of the lung," *J Oncol Pract* **8**, 267–274 (2012).
2. H. Lilja, D. Ulmert, and A. J. Vickers, "Prostate-specific antigen and prostate cancer: Prediction, detection and monitoring," *Nat Rev Cancer* **8**, 268–278 (2008).
3. I. Jacobs, D. Oram, J. Fairbanks, J. Turner, C. Frost, and J. G. Grudzinskas, "A risk of malignancy index incorporating CA 125, ultrasound and menopausal status for the accurate preoperative diagnosis of ovarian cancer," *Br J Obstet Gynaecol* **97**, 922–929 (1990).
4. L. C. Michaelis and M. J. Ratain, "Measuring response in a post-RECIST world: from black and white to shades of grey," *Nat Rev Cancer* **6**, 409–414 (2006).
5. W. A. Weber, "Assessing tumor response to therapy," *J Nucl Med* **50**, 1S–10S (2009).
6. A. B. Miller, B. Hoogstraten, M. Staquet, and A. Winkler, "Reporting results of cancer treatment," *Cancer* **47**, 207–214 (1981).
7. A. Forner, C. Ayuso, M. Varela, J. Rimola, A. J. Hessheimer, L. Bianchi, J. M. Llovet, and J. Bruix, "Evaluation of tumor response after locoregional therapies in hepatocellular carcinoma: Are response evaluation criteria in solid tumors reliable?" *Cancer* **115**, 616–623 (2009).
8. M. Muzi, F. O'Sullivan, D. Mankoff, R. K. Doot, L. Pierce, B. F. Kurland, H. M. Linden, and P. E. Kinahan, "Quantitative assessment of dynamic PET imaging data in cancer imaging," *Magn Reson Imaging* **30**, 1203–1215 (2012).
9. J. M. Hudson, R. Williams, R. Karshafian, L. Milot, M. Atri, P. N. Burns, and G. A. Bjarnason, "Quantifying vascular heterogeneity using microbubble disruption-replenishment kinetics in patients with renal cell cancer," *Invest Radiol* **49**, 116–123 (2013).
10. J. H. Naish, D. M. McGrath, L. J. Bains *et al.*, "Comparison of dynamic contrast enhanced (DCE)-MRI & DCE-CT biomarkers in bladder cancer," *Magn Reson Med* **66**, 219–226 (2011).
11. J. J. Smith, A. G. Sorensen, and J. H. Thrall, "Biomarkers in imaging: Realizing radiology's future," *Radiology* **227**, 633–638 (2003).
12. N. Hylton, "Dynamic contrast-enhanced magnetic resonance imaging as an imaging biomarker," *J Clin Oncol* **24**, 3293–3298 (2006).
13. D. M. McGrath, D. P. Bradley, J. L. Tessier, T. Lacey, C. J. Taylor, and G. J. M. Parker, "Comparison of model-based arterial input functions for dynamic contrast-enhanced MRI in tumor bearing rats," *Magn Reson Med* **61**, 1173–1184 (2009).
14. R. Lawaczeck, G. Jost, and H. Pietsch, "Pharmacokinetics of contrast media in humans model with circulation, distribution, and renal excretion," *Invest Radiol* **46**, 576–585 (2011).
15. A. Shukla-Dave, N. Lee, H. Stambuk, Y. Wang, W. Huang, H. T. Thaler, S. G. Patel, J. P. Shah, and J. Koutcher, "Average arterial input function for quantitative dynamic contrast enhanced magnetic resonance imaging of neck nodal metastases," *BMC Med Phys* **9**, 4 (2009).
16. Y. Yu, Q. Jiang, Y. Miao *et al.*, "Quantitative analysis of clinical dynamic contrast enhanced MRI for evaluating treatment response in human breast cancer," *Radiology* **257**, 47–55 (2010).

17. L. E. Kershaw and M. H.-L. Cheng, "A general dual-bolus approach for quantitative DCE-MRI," *Magn Reson Imaging* **29**, 160–166 (2011).
18. B. C. Moore, "Principal component analysis in linear-systems — controllability, observability, and model-reduction," *IEEE Trans Automat Contr* **26**, 17–32 (1981).
19. D. D. Lee and H. S. Seung, "Learning the parts of objects by non-negative matrix factorization," *Nature* **401**, 788–791 (1999).
20. A. L. Martel, S. J. Allder, G. S. Delay, P. S. Morgan, and A. R. Moody, "Perfusion MRI of infarcted and noninfarcted brain tissue in stroke: A comparison of conventional hemodynamic imaging and factor analysis of dynamic studies," *Invest Radiol* **36**, 378–385 (2001).
21. H. Mehrabian, L. Lindvere, B. Stefanovic, and A. L. Martel, "A constrained independent component analysis technique for artery-vein separation of two-photon laser scanning microscopy images of the cerebral microvasculature," *Med Image Anal* **16**, 239–251 (2012).
22. M. O. Leach, K. M. Brindle, J. L. Evelhoch *et al.*, "The assessment of antiangiogenic and antivascular therapies in early-stage clinical trials using magnetic resonance imaging: Issues and recommendations," *Br J Cancer* **92**, 1599–1610 (2005).
23. H. Mehrabian, C. Chandrana, I. Pang, R. Chopra, and A. L. Martel, "Arterial input function calculation in dynamic contrast-enhanced MRI: An in vivo validation study using co-registered contrast-enhanced ultrasound imaging," *Eur Radiol* **22**, 1735–1747 (2012).
24. H. Mehrabian, R. Chopra, and A. L. Martel, "Calculation of intravascular signal in dynamic contrast enhanced-MRI using adaptive complex independent component analysis," *IEEE Trans Med Imaging* **32**, 699–710 (2013).
25. P. Comon, "Independent component analysis, A new concept?" *Signal Processing* **36**, 287–314 (1994).
26. A. Araujo, and E. Ginei, *The Central Limit Theorem for Real and Banach Valued Random Variables.* Wiley, (1980).
27. M. Novey and T. Adali, "Complex ICA by negentropy maximization," *IEEE Trans. Neural Networks* **19**, 596–609 (2008).
28. P. Latta, M. L. H. Gruwel, V. Jellúš, and B. Tomanek, "Bloch simulations with intra-voxel spin dephasing," *J Magn Reson* **203**, 44–51 (2010).
29. H. Benoit-Cattin, G. Collewet, B. Belaroussi, H. Saint-Jalmes, and C. Odet, "The SIMRI project: a versatile and interactive MRI simulator," *J Magn Reson* **173**, 97–115 (2005).
30. L. Cochlin, A. Blamire, and P. Styles, "Dependence of T1 and T2 on high field strengths in doped agarose gels; facilitating selection of com- position for specific T1/T2 at relevant field," *Int Soc Magn Reson Med* 885 (2003).
31. R. E. Hendrick and E. M. Haacke, "Basic physics of MR contrast agents and maximization of image contrast," *J Magn Reson Imaging* **3**, 137–148 (1993).
32. I. Pang, "Design and characterization of a multi-modality phantom for contrast enhanced ultrasound & magnetic resonance imaging," MSc thesis,University of Toronto, Canada (2011).
33. W. A. Ritschel. and G. L. Kearns, *Handbook of Basic Pharmacokinetics — Including Clinical Applications.* American Pharmaceutical Association (1999).
34. M. Moradi, S. E. Salcudean, S. D. Chang, E. C. Jones, N. Buchan, R. G. Casey, S. L. Goldenberg, and P. Kozlowski, "Multiparametric MRI maps for detection and grading of dominant prostate tumors," *J Magn Reson Imaging* **35**, 1403–1413 (2012).

35. D. L. Langer, A. J. Evans, A. Plotkin, J. Trachtenberg, B. C. Wilson, and M. A. Haider, "Prostate tissue composition and MR measurements: Investigating the relationships between ADC, T2, Ktrans, Ve and corresponding histologic features," *Radiology* **255**, 485–494 (2010).
36. I. Ocak, M. Bernardo, G. Metzger, T. Barrett, and P. L. Choyke, "Dynamic contrast enhanced MRI of prostate cancer at 3T: Study of pharmacokinetic parameters," *AJR* **189**, 849 (2007).
37. J. G. Korporaal, C. A. T. van den Berg, G. Groenendaal, and U. van der Heide, "Phase-based arterial input function measurements in femoral arteries for quantification of dynamic contrast enhanced (DCE)-MRI and comparison with DCE-CT," *Magn Reson Med* **66**, 1267–1274 (2011).
38. C. Li, M. Chen, S. Li, X. Zhao, C. Zhang, and C. Zhou, "Diagnosis of prostate cancer: Comparison of MR diffusion tensor imaging, quantitative dynamic contrast enhanced MRI & the two techniques combined at 3T," *Int Soc Magn Reson Med* **19**, 3069 (2011).

Chapter 14

Computer-Aided Tumor Detection in Automated Breast Ultrasound Images

Chung-Ming Lo and Ruey-Feng Chang*,†*

**Department of Computer Science and Information Engineering*
National Taiwan University, Taipei, Taiwan

†Graduate Institute of Biomedical Electronics and Bioinformatics
National Taiwan University, Taipei, Taiwan
E-mail: rfchang@csie.ntu.edu.tw

Automated breast ultrasound (ABUS) is developed to automatically scan the whole breast for breast imaging on clinical examination. Hundreds of slices compose an image volume in a scanning to establish the volumetric structure of breasts. Reviewing the image volumes is a time-consuming task for radiologists. In this chapter, a computer-aided detection (CADe) system is proposed to automatically detect suspicious abnormalities in ABUS images. The database used included 122 abnormal and 37 normal cases. In abnormal cases, 58 are benign and 78 are malignant lesions. A Hessian-based multi-scale blob detection was used to segment blob-like structures into tumor candidates. The blobness, echogenicity, and morphology features were then extracted and combined in a logistic regression model to classify tumors and nontumors. The CADe system achieved the sensitivity of 100%, 90%, and 70% with false positives per case of 17.4, 8.8, and 2.7, respectively. The performance provides a promising use in tumor detection of ABUS images.

1. Introduction

Ultrasound (US) has been used in evaluating suspicious abnormalities in breast tissues. For women with dense breasts, US can improve cancer detection compared with using mammography alone.[1] The advantages of US examination compared to mammography are that it is radiation-free and makes the patients experience less pain. Automated breast US (ABUS) systems have been developed to be more suitable in screening than conventional hand-held US.[2,3] With less operator dependence, breast volumes can be completely scanned in a shorter time and can be reproduced easily. The automatic scanning procedure reduces possible oversight errors caused by operators. The standardized construction of whole breast provides more detailed three-dimensional (3D) information for reviewing. Substantial interobserver agreement is obtained on lesion detection and characterization in the review of ABUS images by radiologists.[4] Other studies such as breast tumor diagnosis[5,6] and breast density analysis[7,8] are accomplished based on ABUS systems. Although the use of ABUS for clinical breast examination is demonstrated to be practical and reliable, reviewing thousands of patients in a screening database is a time-consuming task. An ABUS scanning generates an image volume composed of two to three hundred slices. For each patient with two breasts, thousands of slices are generated. To deal with the enormous image data, efficient computer-aided analysis is expected to be helpful.

Computer-aided detection (CADe) is one of the emerging tools to automatically discover suspicious abnormalities in breast tissues.[9–11] Advanced CADe systems construct a sequence of quantitative procedures including image analysis, pattern recognition, and artificial intelligence. After image processing, various quantitative features are extracted from tissues and combined together to estimate the likelihood of being tumors. With the assistance of CADe, additional potential carcinomas may be detected to reduce oversight errors. The following section introduces a novel CADe system[12] based on multi-scale blob detection for breast tumor detection in ABUS images.

The detection algorithm in the system used Hessian analysis which has been widely used in detecting objects with certain geometric structures such as vessels and plates.[13–17] Frangi used Hessian analysis to calculate the second order derivatives in an image for vessel measurement.[14] The prostate tumors in magnetic resonance imaging can be detected by Hessian analysis with high sensitivity.[16] In the observation of ABUS images, breast tumors presenting blob-like shape and hypo-echogenicity can be characterized using Hessian. Moreover, the detection of tumors with low contrast boundaries or nearby shadows may be improved.

2. Computer-Aided Tumor Detection Algorithm

The algorithm in the CADe system includes a series of steps as shown in Fig. 1. The first step was speckle noise reduction to remove the inherent speckle noises in ABUS images. The enhanced quality would lead to a better segmentation result. Multi-scale blob detection was then used to extract blob-like objects in an ABUS image. More than one scale was used to detect various sizes of tumors. To save computation time, a preliminary tumor candidate extraction was used to remove too small or big regions. Quantitative features including blobness, echogenicity, and morphology features were extracted from the

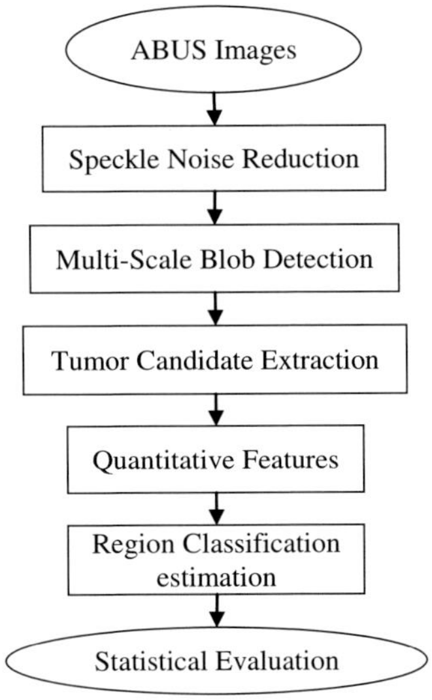

Fig. 1. The flowchart of the CADe system.

tumor candidates for region classification. The performance of the classification result was evaluated using statistical analysis in the end.

2.1. *Patients and ABUS Acquisition*

The tumor detection algorithm introduced in this chapter used the ABUS images acquired by a SomoVu ScanStation (U-system, San Jose, CA). A total of 136 biopsy-proven lesions from 122 patients included 58 benign and 78 malignant lesions. Size ranged from 0.5 to 6.5 cm with mean = 2.00 cm and standard deviation (SD) = 1.28 cm. Benign lesions included 27 fibroadenomas and 31 fibrocystic lesions while malignant lesions included 71 infiltrating carcinomas and 7 ductal carcinoma in situ. Patients underwent ABUS examination in the supine position with 10-MHz, 15.4 cm transducer. Two or three passes were performed to completely scan each breast. A total of 159 passes including 122 abnormal passes with lesions and 37 normal passes were included to evaluate the tumor detection algorithm. The approval of this study was obtained from our institutional review board and informed consent was waived.

2.2. *Speckle Noise Reduction*

Diagnostic US uses high frequency sound waves propagating through human tissues for imaging. The return echo composed of the reflection, absorption, and scattering from various acoustic interfaces is measured to construct US images. Speckle patterns as the constructive and destructive interference in the return echo from microstructure scatterers are inherent noises in US images. For image preprocessing, edge-preserving noise reduction filters were commonly used in reducing speckle noise and enhancing the image quality simultaneously.[18,19] Here, sigma filter[19] was used as the image preprocessing before tumor detection. In the sigma filter, image distribution in a symmetric mask can be presented as a Gaussian distribution with mean μ and SD σ. In the range $[\mu - 2\sigma, \mu + 2\sigma]$, the two-sigma average value is defined as the sum of pixel values divided by the pixel number M adjacent to the mask center. While M is larger than a predefined threshold K, the center pixel value is replaced by the two-sigma average value. Otherwise, it is replaced by the neighbor's average value. A mask of $3 \times 3 \times 3$ and $K = 3$ was used in the experiment to remove speckle noises.

2.3. *Multi-Scale Blob Detection*

Breast tumors are ellipse-like masses in ABUS images. To detect this kind of object, Hessian analysis which can evaluate geometric shapes such as blob, tube, and plate was used.[14–16] Convoluting the images with derivatives of a Gaussian kernel generates the second derivatives in the 3D dimensions. The Hessian matrix can be shown as follows:

$$H_\sigma(x, y, z) = \begin{pmatrix} I_{xx} & I_{xy} & I_{xz} \\ I_{yx} & I_{yy} & I_{yz} \\ I_{zx} & I_{zy} & I_{zz} \end{pmatrix} \tag{1}$$

In the matrix, each element I_{ij} means the second deviation in the dimension i and j. The standard deviation of Gaussian distribution is σ, which is used as a parameter of blob radius. By solving the Hessian matrix on each pixel the eigenvectors and eigenvalues are obtained. Eigenvectors are three orthogonal directions of a detected blob and eigenvalues are the corresponding curvature degrees along the directions. The likelihood of being a blob, R_B, using eigenvalues $(|\lambda_1| \leq |\lambda_2| \leq |\lambda_3|)$ and the eigenvalue magnitude, M, are formulated as follows:

$$R_B = \frac{|\lambda_1|}{\sqrt{|\lambda_2||\lambda_3|}}, \tag{2}$$

$$M = \sqrt{\sum_{n=1}^{3} \lambda_n^2} \tag{3}$$

While the detected object is more like a blob, the curvatures are expected to be higher and close to each other. R_B should be the maximum in this situation. Similarly, M as the eigenvalue magnitude should be larger in blob-like objects than background. Consequently, a blob-like object can be determined using the formula as follows:

$$B_\sigma(\boldsymbol{\lambda}_\mathbf{p}) = \begin{cases} \left(1 - e^{-\frac{R_B}{2\alpha^2}}\right)\left(1 - e^{-\frac{M}{2\beta^2}}\right) & \text{if } \lambda_1 > 0, \lambda_2 > 0, \text{ and } \lambda_3 > 0 \\ 0 & \text{otherwise} \end{cases} \tag{4}$$

For a pixel $\mathrm{p} = (x, y, z)$, λ_p is the eigenvalues, α and β are sensitivity parameters of R_B and M to adjust the weights of terms. In the experiment, $\alpha = 0.5$ and $\beta = 0.5$. The criteria of $\lambda_1 > 0, \lambda_2 > 0$, and $\lambda_3 > 0$ were used to detect hypo-echogenic objects. Lesions are different sizes. To detect various sizes of lesions, multi-scale blob detection was used. The defined range is as follows:

$$Blobness(\boldsymbol{\lambda}_\mathbf{p}) = \max_{\sigma_{min} \leq \sigma \leq \sigma_{max}} B_\sigma(\boldsymbol{\lambda}_\mathbf{p}) \tag{5}$$

where σ_{max} and σ_{min} are the maximum and minimum scales to be detected.

The scale parameters used in the experiment were from 1.2 to 3.2 mm with an increasing scale of 0.1 mm. Another advantage of multi-scale over single-scale blob detection is for lesions with substantial sizes. Large-scale blob detection encompassed most area of a lesion with coarse contour. Small-scale blob detection benefited from the detailed information on the boundary and resulted in finer region contour while a lesion may be separated into several parts. Consequently, multi-scale blob detection can combine the detection areas from large-scale and small-scale blob detection to provide better lesion interpretation. 3D connected component[20] was used to integrate the detected areas into a more complete object.

2.4. *Tumor Candidate Extraction*

Suspicious abnormalities close to the blob-like structures were detected after the multi-scale blob detection. Among these detected regions, some of them can be eliminated before further processing to reduce computation time and potential FPs. In tumor candidate extraction, blobness value was used to filter out nontumor regions. Higher blobness value representing darker blob-like structure is expected to appear more frequently in tumors than nontumors. The maximum and mean blobness values were calculated from a region as the criteria for tumor candidate extraction. The formulas were defined as below:

$$Blobness_{mean}(R) = \frac{\sum_{\mathbf{p}\in R} Blobness(\boldsymbol{\lambda}_{\mathbf{p}})}{N_R} \tag{6}$$

$$Blobness_{\max}(R) = \max_{\mathbf{p}\in R} Blobness(\boldsymbol{\lambda}_{\mathbf{p}}) \tag{7}$$

For each region, R, p is a voxel within R and the number of all voxels is N_R. Size was another criterion for tumor candidate extraction. Many regions detected by Hessian-based blob detection were little intensity variations and were much smaller than true lesions. Combining the three criteria in a linear regression model[21] is the classification method in tumor candidate extraction. The likelihood being a tumor of a region can be estimated using the following expression:

$$Z(R) = \beta_0 + \sum_{i=1}^{N_f} \beta_i x_i \tag{8}$$

$$L_S(R) = \frac{1}{1 + e^{-Z(R)}} \tag{9}$$

where the number of features is N_f. For each feature value, x_i, there is a coefficient β_i. The constant coefficient is β_0. $L_S(R)$ is the linear regression model for likelihood estimation. A probability threshold is then defined as:

$$L_S(R) \geq TH \tag{10}$$

With the threshold, TH, the regions detected by the multi-scale blob detection were classified into two groups according to their features. Only regions with equal to or higher probabilities than the threshold were extracted to be tumor candidates. Probabilities less than the threshold were regarded as nontumors and removed. The threshold used in the experiment was 0.5.

2.5. *Quantitative Features*

Tumor candidate extraction is a preliminary step to filter out regions with low likelihoods of being tumors. The remaining candidates are basically the regions needed to be recognized. As an efficient way, various quantitative features were extracted and integrated together for region characterization. Logistic regression model was used again in distinguishing tumors from nontumors. The proposed features included three groups: blobness, echogenicity, and morphology features.

2.5.1. *Blobness features*

As mentioned before, breast tumors are blob-like structures with more hypo-echogenicity than surrounding normal tissues. Different echogenicities belong to different tissues makes the basic discrimination in breast tumor detection. By Hessian matrix analysis, the statistical blobness features including the maximum, the mean, and the standard deviation of the blobness values were calculated to describe the echogenicity level. Higher blobness value indicates more hypo-echogenicity. In a real tumor, a voxel closer to the tumor center may have higher blobness value. If a tumor candidate is a real tumor, the distance between the center and the blobness centroid should be smaller than normal tissues. Following equation defines the distance measurement:

$$Dis = \sqrt{(x_c - x_{bc})^2 + (y_c - y_{bc})^2 + (z_c - z_{bc})^2}. \tag{11}$$

where (x_c, y_c, z_c) indicates the center of a tumor candidate as follows:

$$x_c = \frac{1}{N_T}\sum_{i=1}^{N_T} x_i, \quad y_c = \frac{1}{N_T}\sum_{i=1}^{N_T} y_i, \quad \text{and} \quad z_c = \frac{1}{N_T}\sum_{i=1}^{N_T} z_i \tag{12}$$

(x_i, y_i, z_i) is a voxel position and N_T is the total number of voxels in a tumor candidate.

(x_{bc}, y_{bc}, z_{bc}) is the blobness centroid as defined below:

$$\begin{aligned} x_{bc} &= \frac{1}{Sum_{Blob}}\sum_{i=1}^{N_T} x_i \times Blobness(\boldsymbol{\lambda}_\mathbf{p}) \\ y_{bc} &= \frac{1}{Sum_{Blob}}\sum_{i=1}^{N_T} y_i \times Blobness(\boldsymbol{\lambda}_\mathbf{p}) \\ z_{bc} &= \frac{1}{Sum_{Blob}}\sum_{i=1}^{N_T} z_i \times Blobness(\boldsymbol{\lambda}_\mathbf{p}) \end{aligned} \tag{13}$$

In a tumor candidate, each voxel p has λ_p as the eigenvalues and the summation of all blobness values is Sum_{Blob}.

2.5.2. *Echogenicity features*

Transmission of ultrasound waves through the tissue results in return echoes composed of the reflection, absorption, and scattering from various acoustic interfaces. The magnitude of return echo was measured to be echogenicity for tissue interpretation. In ABUS images, the echogenic intensity of each voxel was expressed using gray-scale values. The statistical echogenicity features extracted from the gray-scale intensity distribution including mean, SD, skewness, and kurtosis[22] were used as the echogenicity features in distinguishing tumors from nontumors as defined below:

$$I_{mean} = \frac{1}{N_T} \sum_{\mathbf{p} \in T} I_{\mathbf{p}} \quad (14)$$

$$I_{std} = \sqrt{\frac{1}{N_T} \sum_{\mathbf{p} \in T} (I_{\mathbf{p}} - I_{mean})^2} \quad (15)$$

$$I_{skewness} = \frac{1}{N_T} \sum_{\mathbf{p} \in T} \left(\frac{I_{\mathbf{p}} - I_{mean}}{I_{std}} \right)^3 \quad (16)$$

$$I_{kurtosis} = \frac{1}{N_T} \sum_{\mathbf{p} \in T} \left(\frac{I_p - I_{mean}}{I_{std}} \right)^4 \quad (17)$$

where $I_{\mathbf{p}}$ is the voxel intensity in the position **p** in a tumor candidate with a total of N_T voxels. Additionally, more echogenicity features such as the mean and SD of intensity gradient, and intensity gradient around lesion boundary were also quantified to be echogenicity features.

2.5.3. *Morphology features*

Similar tissues were gathered together to become a mass structure. Rather than echogenicity patterns used in showing the internal distribution of a mass, morphology features were used to describe the external boundary. The analysis of region contour is useful in tissue characterization. As defined in the standard BI-RADS lexicon,[23] various shape-correlated descriptors such as microlobulation and spiculation have been suggested to be sonographic findings. Further quantification of morphology features has been used in computer-aided diagnosis systems.[24,25]

After Hessian-based blob detection, various mass-like structures were segmented to be tumor candidates. The morphology features extracted from the regions to distinguish tumors from nontumors included two groups: shape and ellipse-fitting features.[25] Shape features were volume, compactness,[26] radius, and speculation.[27] Region volume can be used to filter out extremely small noises or large shadows. Compactness was used to calculate the ratio of region volume and surface for roundness estimation. Radius and spiculation were detailed margin properties on the boundary to show if a region is aggressive. The two used compactness formulas included conventional C_c and novel C_n are expressed as follows:

$$C_c = \frac{Surface^{1.5}}{Volume^2} \tag{18}$$

$$C_n = \frac{Volume - \frac{Surface}{6}}{Volume - Volume^{1.5}} \tag{19}$$

where *Volume* and *Surface* are the volume and surface extracted from a tumor candidate.

Instead of using original tumor properties, the ellipse-fitting features were extracted from a best-fit ellipse. Because tumors have ellipse-like shapes, a best-fit ellipse can be used to estimate tumor characters using the length ratio between the axes of the best-fit ellipse and surface comparison between the best-fit ellipse and the tumor. The degree of regularity on the boundary can also be obtained from the difference. More details were described in the previous study.[25]

2.6. *Region Classification*

Quantitative features were extracted from the tumor candidates and combined in a logistic regression model[21] to generate the likelihood being a tumor for each region. Backward elimination was used in relevant feature selection in the classifier. The step-wise backward elimination[28] evenly separated all regions into the training set and testing set in each step. Regions from one case only belonged to one set to make sure the independence between the training and testing sets. That is, one case was not in both training set and testing set simultaneously in the same evaluation. An equalized sampling method was then used to achieve the size balance between the tumors and nontumors. Because the number of tumors was much less than that of nontumors, total tumors were used in the training set. Equal size of nontumors was then sampled in the training set. After constructing the training model of logistic regression, regions in the testing set were used to test the model. In each step of the backward elimination, one feature with the least contribution was determined and removed from the features until the removal does not achieve significant residual sum of squares of the performance by a partial-F test. After feature selection, the likelihood of being a tumor was estimated using the trained model. Regions in the tumor candidates with probabilities equal to or higher than a probability threshold were regarded as tumors.

2.7. *Statistical Evaluation*

The performance of the quantitative features used in the logistic regression classifier was evaluated using a 10-fold cross-validation (10-fold CV) and a leave-one-out cross validation (LOOCV).[29] Under cross validation, the cases used in the experiment were divided into K disjoint partitions that were approximately equal in size. K iterations of case training were used in the validation. For 10-fold CV, the value of K is 10. LOOCV uses the number of cases to be K to provide a more generalized result with more iterations. In each iteration, one partition was picked from the K partitions to test the model trained by the remaining K-1 partitions. The performance of K iterations was averaged to be the final evaluated result. Although LOOCV provides more generalization validation, it is time-consuming to train and test thousands of tumor candidates. The performances of 10-fold CV and LOOCV were compared later to show the difference. Additionally, a blind test was used to evaluate the performance using independent data sets. The cases were divided into two disjoint sets i.e. training and testing sets. After the training of the classification model by only the training set, the testing was accomplished by only the testing set. The evaluation simulated the procedure in future clinical use for unknown tumors. As mentioned before, blobness and size features were combined in the classifier for tumor candidate extraction. According to the features, each region was given a probability of being a tumor. A probability threshold was then determined to filter out nontumor regions and keep all true tumors for further classification. More quantitative features including blobness, echogenicity, and morphology features were extracted from the tumor candidates obtained after the preliminary classification. The most relevant features selected from the two classifications were based on the training set. In the testing, the trained model and determined probability threshold were applied to the testing set for performance evaluation. After exchanging the training and testing sets, the procedure was executed again for cross validation. Such validation was performed three times to accomplish the blind test. Each time, the training and test sets were randomly composed from the total cases.

The classification result was obtained using various feature sets. To investigate the contribution of each feature set, free-response operating characteristics (FROC) curve and jackknife alterative of FROC-1 (JAFROC-1) figure of merit (FOM) were used.[30] FOM is a probability to show if the estimated likelihood of a true tumor higher than that of all nontumors. High FOM indicates the estimation for a region being a tumor is reliable. The definition is as follows:

$$FOM = \frac{\sum_{i=1}^{N_C} \sum_{j=1}^{N_C} \sum_{l=1}^{N_L(i)} \psi(\max_{k \in N_K(j)}(P(k)), P(l))}{N_C \times N_{T\_total}} \tag{20}$$

$$\psi(X, \Upsilon) = \begin{cases} 1, & \Upsilon > X \\ 0.5, & \Upsilon = X \\ 0, & \Upsilon < X \end{cases} \tag{21}$$

N_C is the number of used cases, $N_L(i)$ is the number of true lesions in i-th case, $N_K(j)$ is the number of non-tumors in j-th case, N_{T_total} is the number of true lesions in all cases. The function P means the estimated probability being a tumor for a non-tumor k or a tumor l. In the function ψ, X and Υ are the tumor likelihood of a non-tumor and a tumor, respectively.

The FOM comparisons between feature sets were evaluated using JAFROC-1 FOM. The area under FROC curve was calculated for a comprehensive evaluation with the trade-offs between sensitivities and FPs. The area value is between 0 and 1. The value closer to 1 means better classification in higher sensitivity with less FPs simultaneously. p-value less than 0.05 indicates a statistically significant comparison result. For multiple comparisons, Bonferroni-Holm correction[31] was used to adjust p-values under increased type I error.

3. Results

The proposed CADe algorithm was applied to 159 cases including 122 abnormal cases and 37 normal cases without lesions. Using an Intel Core 2 Q6600 2.4 GHz processor and 3 GB RAM in Windows 7 operating system (Microsoft, Seattle, WA, USA), the average execution time for each case was 13.02 minutes. The detection sensitivity achieved 100%, that is, 58 benign and 78 malignant tumors in the 122 abnormal cases were all detected. The average FPs/case corresponding to different features are listed in Table 1.

Table 1. The average FPs/case corresponds to different features.

Validation	Features	FPs/case
10 fold-CV	None	1044.89
	Size	777.71
	$\text{Blobness}_{\text{max}}$	214.21
	$\text{Blobness}_{\text{mean}}$	133.71
	$\text{Blobness}_{\text{mean}}$ & Size	116.92
LOOCV	$\text{Blobness}_{\text{mean}}$ & Size	117.11

Table 2. Different sensitivities and the corresponding FPs/case using 10-fold CV and LOOCV.

10-fold CV				LOOCV			
Sensitivity (%)	FPs/case			Sensitivity (%)	FPs/case		
	Abnormal	Normal	All		Abnormal	Normal	All
0.00	0.00	0.00	0.00	0.00	0.00	0.00	0.00
56.62	1.43	1.35	1.42	60.29	1.43	1.35	1.41
69.85	2.82	2.16	2.67	72.06	2.80	2.24	2.67
77.21	4.10	3.14	3.87	77.94	4.02	3.00	3.79
85.29	5.30	4.24	5.05	82.35	5.30	4.35	5.08
85.29	6.64	5.27	6.32	87.50	6.60	5.35	6.32
87.50	7.89	6.35	7.53	88.24	7.77	6.51	7.48
91.18	9.11	7.76	8.80	88.24	9.30	7.57	8.91
92.65	10.46	9.24	10.18	89.71	10.52	9.08	10.23
93.38	12.11	10.68	11.77	93.38	12.19	10.70	11.87
96.32	13.80	12.54	13.50	95.59	13.89	12.51	13.57
99.26	15.76	14.22	15.40	99.26	15.73	14.27	15.42
100.00	17.66	16.24	17.33	100.00	17.82	16.22	17.45

Originally, the detected regions in the ABUS images had mean = 1044.89, maximum = 1699, and minimum = 494, respectively. Figure 2 shows an example of ABUS image before and after speckle noise reduction and Fig. 3 illustrates the corresponding initial result of multi-scale blob detection. Tumor candidate extraction reduced the FPs/case to 116.92 with 10-fold CV, and 117.11 with LOOCV. In this step, about 90% nontumors were filter out with all true tumors kept. The further region classification using blobness, echogenicity, and morphology features reduced the rest FPs. The FPs/case for different sensitivities under 10-fold CV or LOOCV are listed in Table 2. The sensitivity of 100%, 90%, and 70% achieved 17.33, 8.80, and 2.67 FPs/case in 10-fold CV which is slightly better than 17.45, 10.23, and 2.67 FPs/case in LOOCV. Normal cases had slightly less FPs/case than abnormal cases in the result.

Table 3 lists the JAFROC-1 FOM comparisons of different combinations of feature sets. All single feature set performed worse than multiple feature set. The lowest FOM is 0.16 achieved by the morphology feature set. Combining all feature sets including blobness, echogenicity, and morphology features achieved the best FOM = 0.47. For both 10-fold CV and LOOCV, the performance was evaluated to be consistent. The p-values showed the same result. Combining more feature sets together obtained significantly better FOMs i.e. p-value < 0.05. Also, the difference between 10-fold CV and LOOCV was not significant, p-value $= 0.73$. Figure 4 shows the FROC curves and FOMs of all features with different cross validations.

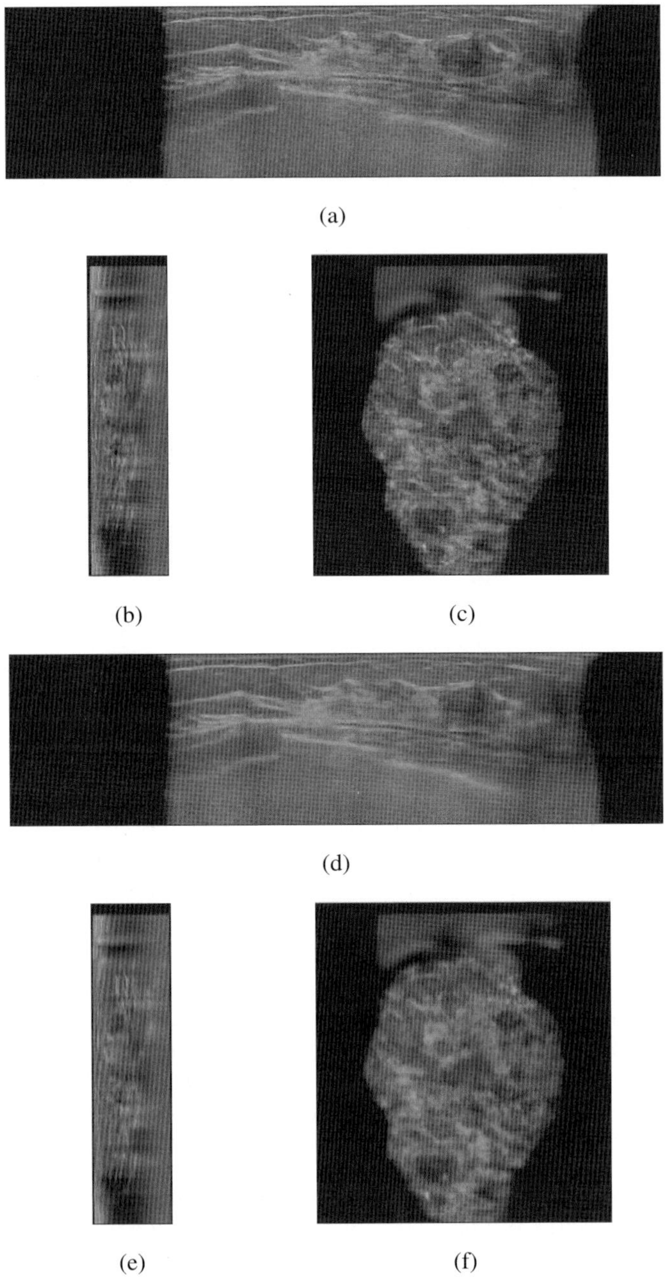

Fig. 2. An example of speckle noise reduction with a tumor circled (a) Axial view (b) Sagittal view (c) Coronal view (d), (e), and (f). The views after speckle noise reduction.

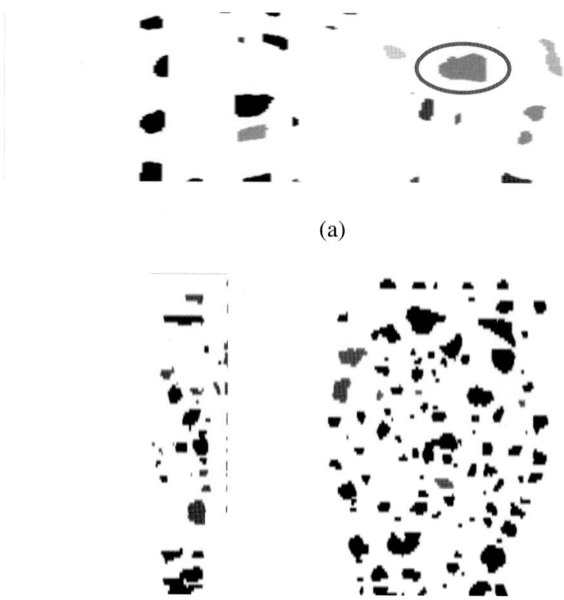

(a) (b) (c)

Fig. 3. The multi-scale blob detection of Fig. 2 with a true positive circled (a) Axial view (b) Sagittal view (c) Coronal view.

Table 3. The JAFROC-1 FOM comparisons of different combinations of feature sets with cross validations.

Feature sets (FOM)			Adjusted p-value
Blobness (0.28)	vs.	Echogenicity (0.23)	0.39
Blobness (0.28)	vs.	Morphology (0.16)	<0.05
Echogenicity (0.23)	vs.	Morphology (0.16)	0.08
Echogenicity (0.23)	vs.	Blobness & Echogenicity (0.33)	<0.05
Morphology (0.16)	vs.	Blobness & Morphology (0.36)	<0.05
All features with 10-fold CV (0.47)	vs.	Blobness & Echogenicity (0.33)	<0.05
All features with 10-fold CV (0.47)	vs.	Blobness & Morphology (0.36)	<0.05
All features with 10-fold CV (0.47)	vs.	Echogenicity & Morphology (0.43)	0.39
All features with 10-fold CV (0.47)	vs.	All features with LOOCV (0.47)	0.73

With respect to the size issue, the number and likelihoods of benign and malignant tumors for five size categories are listed in Table 4. Most malignant tumor (38/78) sizes were 1 to 2 cm with the average likelihoods of 0.94. Most benign tumor (32/58) sizes were less than 1 cm with the average likelihoods

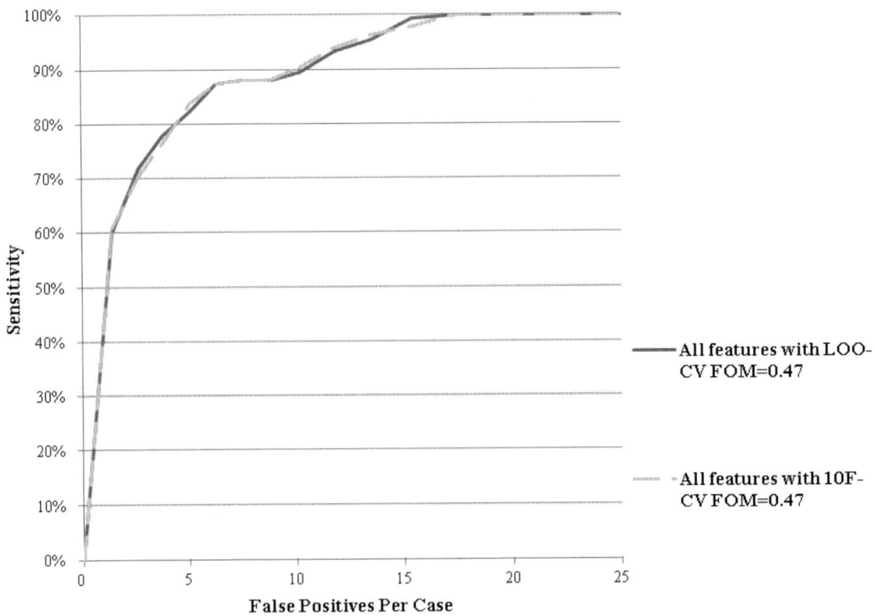

Fig. 4. FROC curves and FOMs of all features with different cross validations.

Table 4. The number and likelihoods of benign and malignant tumors for five size categories.

Category	Size	<1 cm	1–2 cm	2–3 cm	3–4 cm	≧4 cm
Likelihood (Number)	Benign	0.88 ± 0.15 (32)	0.86 ± 0.20 (17)	0.86 ± 0.16 (6)	0.92 ± 0.13 (1)	0.99 ± 0.01 (2)
	Malignant	N/A	0.94 ± 0.10 (38)	0.90 ± 0.17 (16)	0.94 ± 0.09 (8)	0.83 ± 0.17 (8)

Table 5. The results of FOMs and adjusted *p*-values of the corresponding three tests in the blind test.

Test Number (FOM)	Adjusted *p*-value
Test 1 (0.37) vs. Test 2 (0.37)	0.97
Test 1 (0.37) vs. Test 3 (0.38)	1.21
Test 2 (0.37) vs. Test 3 (0.38)	1.21

of 0.88. Table 5 shows the result of the blind test. The three tests obtained FOMs of 0.37, 0.37, and 0.38, respectively. The difference of any two tests was not significant (p-value > 0.05). Among the tests, the best sensitivity without missing malignant tumors was 97.80% with 12.28 FPs/case and the worst one was 97.80% with 16.92 FPs/case.

4. Discussions and Conclusion

ABUS systems are becoming more and more popular for screening breast cancers. Various CADe systems were developed to provide quantitative and efficient assistance to reduce oversight errors.[9–11] This chapter introduces a novel tumor detection algorithm for breast tumors using multi-scale blob detection. The algorithm combined different parameters of Hessian analysis to include blob-like structures. Small-scale blob detection detected the details on the tumor boundary which resulted in better morphology description. On the other side, large-scale blob detection enclosed the major area of tumor to become a region for internal echogenicity analysis. However, using only small-scale detection would obtain too many fragments while large-scale detection cannot delineate the accurate tumor contour. The proposed multi-scale blob detection detected potential abnormalities using both small-scale and large-scale. 3D connected component was then used to integrate the detected regions into a complete object with the advantages of both small-scale and large-scale. The scale range used in the experiment was from 1.2 mm to 3.2 mm. After blob detection, many blob-like nontumor regions such as fats and ribs were also detected. Take the cases used in the experiment as an example, one case had at most 3 tumors in hundreds of slices but the average number of detected regions was 1044.89. Size and blobness features were used in tumor candidate extraction to remove about 90% noise. Then, multiple feature sets were extracted from the tumor candidates to distinguish tumors from nontumors.

The Hessian-based blob detection separated the blob-like regions with low contrast boundaries or nearby shadows from ABUS images. In Hessian analysis, intensity variation around tumor boundaries was detected as second-order local derivatives. According to the analysis, breast tumors known as ellipse-like shape and hypo-echogenic in ABUS images were successfully discovered with 100% sensitivity in the experiment. The CADe system spent the average time of 13 minutes for each case to do region segmentation and feature calculation. The time-consuming task can be done via parallel processing methods to reduce the execution time in future studies. Another limitation in the CADe system is that the likelihood estimation for malignant tumors over 4 cm is not as good as those of other sizes. One possible reason is that the scale range used in the multi-scale blob detection did not include the 4 cm scale. In the result observation, enlarging the scale range may cause over-segmentation. A better way for various tumor sizes is executing the multi-scale blob detection several times with different scale ranges. Besides, no tumor in the collected database is smaller than 1 cm. Breast tumors in the early-stage are usually small in size. Whether the proposed CADe system can detect tumors smaller than 1 cm should be tested in further studies.

More and more women are diagnosed with breast cancer. To reduce the mortality, early detection and treatment are helpful. Especially for women with dense breasts, US is a necessary imaging tool to observe abnormalities. Using ABUS systems on screening would be more reliable than conventional hand-held US for breast cancer detection. The CADe system proposed in this chapter quantifies the examination procedure in ABUS to become automatic. The high sensitivity would assist radiologists in tumor detection. Whether radiologists can improve their sensitivities with the CADe system will need to be explored. Moreover, a computer-aided diagnosis system can be combined with the CADe system to estimate the malignancy of the detected tumors. The computer-aided technologies would be promising in clinical use to reduce oversight errors and time-consuming tasks in ABUS reviewing.

References

1. W. A. Berg, J. D. Blume, J. B. Cormack, E. B. Mendelson, D. Lehrer, M. Bohm-Velez, E. D. Pisano, R. A. Jong, W. P. Evans, M. J. Morton, M. C. Mahoney, L. H. Larsen, R. G. Barr, D. M. Farria, H. S. Marques, K. Boparai and A. Investigators, "Combined screening with ultrasound and mammography vs mammography alone in women at elevated risk of breast cancer," *Jama-J Am Med Assoc* **299**, 2151–2163 (2008).
2. K. M. Kelly, J. Dean, W. S. Comulada and S. J. Lee, "Breast cancer detection using automated whole breast ultrasound and mammography in radiographically dense breasts," *Eur Radiol* **20**, 734–742 (2010).
3. J. M. Chang, W. K. Moon, N. Cho, J. S. Park and S. J. Kim, "Radiologists' performance in the detection of benign and malignant masses with 3D automated breast ultrasound (ABUS)," *Eur J Radiol* **78**, 99–103 (2011).
4. H. J. Shin, H. H. Kim, J. H. Cha, J. H. Park, K. E. Lee and J. H. Kim, "Automated ultrasound of the breast for diagnosis: Interobserver agreement on lesion detection and characterization," *Am J Roentgenol* **197**, 747–754 (2011).
5. W. K. Moon, C. M. Lo, J. M. Chang, C. S. Huang, J. H. Chen and R. F. Chang, "Computer-aided classification of breast masses using speckle features of automated breast ultrasound images," *Med Phys* **39**, 6465 (2012).
6. W. K. Moon, Y. W. Shen, C. S. Huang, L. R. Chiang and R. F. Chang, "Computer-aided diagnosis for the classification of breast masses in automated whole breast ultrasound images," *Ultrasound Med Biol* **37**, 539–548 (2011).
7. W. K. Moon, C. M. Lo, J. M. Chang, M. S. Bae, W. H. Kim, C. S. Huang, J. H. Chen, M. H. Kuo and R. F. Chang, "Rapid breast density analysis of partial volumes of automated breast ultrasound images," *Ultrason Imaging* **35**, 333–343 (2013).

8. W. K. Moon, Y. W. Shen, C. S. Huang, S. C. Luo, A. Kuzucan, J. H. Chen and R. F. Chang, "Comparative study of density analysis using automated whole breast ultrasound and MRI," *Med Phys* **38**, 382 (2011).
9. R. F. Chang, K. C. Chang-Chien, H. J. Chen, D. R. Chen, E. Takada and W. K. Moon, "Whole breast computer-aided screening using free-hand ultrasound," *Int Congr Ser* **1281**, 1075–1080 (2005).
10. Y. Ikedo, D. Fukuoka, T. Hara, H. Fujita, E. Takada, T. Endo and T. Morita, "Development of a fully automatic scheme for detection of masses in whole breast ultrasound images," *Med Phys* **34**, 4378–4388 (2007).
11. R. F. Chang, K. C. Chang-Chien, E. Takada, C. S. Huang, Y. H. Chou, C. M. Kuo and J. H. Chen, "Rapid image stitching and computer-aided detection for multipass automated breast ultrasound," *Med Phys* **37**, 2063–2073 (2010).
12. W. K. Moon, Y. W. Shen, M. S. Bae, C. S. Huang, J. H. Chen and R. F. Chang, "Computer-aided tumor detection based on multi-scale blob detection algorithm in automated breast ultrasound images," *IEEE Trans Med Imaging* **32**, 1191–1200 (2013).
13. P. Perona and J. Malik, "Scale-space and edge-detection using anisotropic diffusion," *IEEE Trans Pattern Anal Mach Intell* **12**, 629–639 (1990).
14. A. F. Frangi, W. J. Niessen, K. L. Vincken and M. A. Viergever, "Multiscale vessel enhancement filtering," *Lect Notes Comput Sci* **1496**, 130–137 (1998).
15. Y. Sato, S. Nakajima, N. Shiraga, H. Atsumi, S. Yoshida, T. Koller, G. Gerig and R. Kikinis, "Three-dimensional multi-scale line filter for segmentation and visualization of curvilinear structures in medical images," *Med Image Anal* **2**, 143–168 (1998).
16. P. C. Vos, J. O. Barentsz, N. Karssemeijer and H. J. Huisman, "Automatic computer-aided detection of prostate cancer based on multiparametric magnetic resonance image analysis," *Phys Med Biol* **57**, 1527–1542 (2012).
17. X. Ye, X. Lin, J. Dehmeshki, G. Slabaugh and G. Beddoe, "Shape-based computer-aided detection of lung nodules in thoracic CT images," *Biomed Eng IEEE Trans* **56**, 1810–1820 (2009).
18. P. Perona and J. Malik, "Scale-space and edge detection using anisotropic diffusion," *IEEE Trans Pattern Anal Mach Intell* **12**, 629–639 (1990).
19. J.-S. Lee, "Digital image smoothing and the sigma filter," *Comput Vision Graph* **24**, 255–269 (1983).
20. M. B. Dillencourt, H. Samet and M. Tamminen, "A general approach to connected-component labeling for arbitrary image representations," *JACM* **39**, 253–280 (1992).
21. D. W. Hosmer, *Applied Logistic Regression. 2nd edition.* Wiley, New York, (2000).
22. R. A. Groeneveld and G. Meeden, "Measuring skewness and kurtosis," *The Statistician*, 391–399 (1984).
23. American College of Radiology, *Breast Imaging Reporting and Data System, 4th ed.* American College of Radiology (2003).
24. W. K. Moon, C. M. Lo, J. M. Chang, C. S. Huang, J. H. Chen and R. F. Chang, "Computer-aided classification of breast masses using speckle features of automated breast ultrasound images," *Med Phys* **39**, 6465–6473 (2012).
25. W. K. Moon, Y. W. Shen, C. S. Huang, L. R. Chiang and R. F. Chang, "Computer-aided diagnosis for the classification of breast masses in automated whole breast ultrasound images," *Ultrasound Med Biol* **37**, 539–548 (2011).

26. E. Bribiesca, "An easy measure of compactness for 2D and 3D shapes," *Pattern Recognit* **41**, 543–554 (2008).
27. L. A. Meinel, A. H. Stolpen, K. S. Berbaum, L. L. Fajardo and J. M. Reinhardt, "Breast MRI lesion classification: Improved performance of human readers with a backpropagation neural network computer-aided diagnosis (CAD) system," *J Magn Reson Imaging* **25**, 89–95 (2007).
28. R. Kohavi and G. H. John, "Wrappers for feature subset selection," *Artif Intell* **97**, 273–324 (1997).
29. R. R. Picard and R. D. Cook, "Cross-validation of regression models," *J Am Statist Assoc* **79**, 575–583 (1984).
30. D. P. Chakraborty, E. S. Breatnach, M. V. Yester, B. Soto, G. Barnes and R. Fraser, "Digital and conventional chest imaging: A modified ROC study of observer performance using simulated nodules," *Radiology* **158**, 35–39 (1986).
31. A. F. Frangi, W. J. Niessen, K. L. Vincken and M. A. Viergever, "Multiscale vessel enhancement filtering," in *Medical Image Computing and Computer-Assisted Interventation — MICCAI'98,* Springer (1998), pp. 130–137.

Part 3

Emerging Methods and Medical Imaging Systems

Chapter 15

Histomorphometry of Digital Pathology: Case Study in Prostate Cancer

Robert W. Veltri,[*,‡] *Ph.D., Guangjing Zhu,*[*] *M.D., Ph.D., George Lee,*[†] *Ph.D., Sahirzeeshan Ali,*[†] *M.S. and Anant Madabhushi,*[†,§] *Ph.D.*

[*]*James Buchanan Brady Urological Institute, The Johns Hopkins University School of Medicine, Baltimore MD 21287*

[†]*Center for Computational Imaging and Personalized Diagnostics, Case Western Reserve University, Cleveland, OH 44106*

[‡]*rveltri1@jhmi.edu*

[§]*anantm@case.edu*

This review utilizes prostate cancer (CaP) as a case study to assess the application of quantitative histomorphometry to characterize the aggressive phenotype and also to make predictions of outcome like recurrence, metastasis and survival. Dr. Robert Veltri describes the use of a microspectrophotometry microscope and novel software to capture nuclear morphometry of Feulgen (DNA) stained features and successfully identify indolent and aggressive CaP as well as predict outcomes such as biochemical recurrence, metastasis and survival. His research also indicates that quantitative nuclear morphometry by this method indicates a field effect nearby the can that also has predictive value. However, the original technology was bottle-necked by the fact that it could not be extended to whole slide images. Subsequently, the initiation of a collaboration with Dr. Anant Madabhushi who has developed high throughput quantitative image and histomorphometric tools that are amenable to work on whole slide digitized images, has allowed for confirmation of Dr. Veltri's prior and published observations that nuclear size, shape and texture as well as the glandular structure or architecture of prostate cancer are critical in predicting disease aggressiveness. Dr. Madabhushi's algorithms take advantage of advanced machine vision imaging images for diagnosis and prognosis. Additionally Dr. Madabhushi's group has also been developing machine learning tools to combine image based and molecular measurements for creating unified predictors of disease aggressiveness and patient outcome. It is hoped that the additional development and validation of these tools will set the stage for creation of decision tools to aid the pathologist to predict severe outcomes early so that appropriate interventions can be made by the urologist and patient.

1. Introduction

Prostate Cancer (CaP) is the second most common cause of cancer-specific mortality among men in the United States, with an anticipated 238,590 newly diagnosed cases and 29,720 CaP deaths in 2012.[1] The use of Prostate Specific Antigen (PSA) as a screening tool has been in place in the United States for more than 25 years. PSA testing (screening) remains quite controversial even though it has been shown to have changed the natural history for the pathology and pathogenesis of CaP.[2] The current American Urological Association (AUA) guidelines are quite specific and recommend an age-specific, patient-physician shared decision making process.[3,4] Prior to the widespread use of PSA for screening, more than half of the men presenting with CaP had aggressive, incurable (locally advanced or distant metastatic) disease. PSA testing has resulted in lower grade and stage at diagnosis of CaP.[3,5–7] Today, a substantial proportion of newly diagnosed cases represent CaP that would never have been detected during a lifetime had a PSA test not been used and has resulted in over-diagnosis and over-treatment of CaP.[3,8] Consequently, there remains a need for "early identification" of men with high risk (more aggressive) CaP who will benefit from early definitive personalized treatment. There is evidence that high risk CaP clinicopathological features can predict aggressive disease that is in danger of early progression and may require early aggressive treatment.[9] However, further improvement in accuracy of this prediction should include the discovery and development of additional automated and quantitative morphological and molecular biomarkers for early detection of high risk CaP will therefore have a major impact on the personalized management of CaP.

2. Hallmarks of Prostate Cancer

Several early initiation events seem to be required for CaP that includes chronic infections, inflammation and genomic instability.[10–12] Published results indicate that several such hallmark biological events occur in the multiple step process; they include sustaining proliferative signaling, evading growth suppressors, resisting cell death, enabling replicative immortality, inducing angiogenesis, and activating invasion and metastasis.[10] In conjunction with these oncogenic molecular hallmarks, there are additional pathways that drive the etiopathogenesis of cancer progression. These additional events include the bioenergetics of metabolism,[13–15] evasion of the immune surveillance system[16–18] and establishment of a unique ecological niche or "tumor microenvironment" required to sustain the invasive and metastatic phenotype[19–22] and these latter physiological factors (metabolism, immunity and tumor microenvironment) may also serve as new targets for treatment. Furthermore, the National Comprehensive Cancer Network (NCCN) has provided a description for low to high risk CaP based upon clinicopathologic features.[23] Early prediction of high risk CaP may involve several unique prognostic tissue morphologic,[24–26] molecular[27–35] as well as clinicopathologic features,[36–41] that may be implicated in high risk CaP and hence useful to stratify such patients for treatment. In order to understand the basic pathology of CaP, we must comprehend the fundamental biology and histology of the disease.

3. The Staging of Prostate Cancer

3.1. *The Gleason System*

The Gleason system for CaP histopathologic grading is based on how much the cancer looks like healthy (benign) tissue when viewed under a low power microscope (10–20 ×) by an expert pathologist. Less dangerous prostate tumors have an appearance of normal glandular tissue, and more aggressive tumors that are more likely to invade and spread to other parts of the body look much less like normal tissue with respect to their loss of normal glandular architecture (size, shape, and organization) as well as other histologic features including changes in the cell's nuclear structure.[42,43] To assign a Gleason score (GS), the pathologist first looks for a dominant (primary) pattern of cell growth or grade (area where the cancer is most prominent) and then looks for a less widespread pattern or grade (secondary) of growth, and gives each one a grade number. GS is the sum of the dominant or primary tissue pattern grade (representing the majority of tumor) and the less dominant or secondary tissue pattern grade (assigned to the minority of the tumor). Today, pathologists tend to describe a GS of 5, 6 as a low-grade cancer, 7 (3 + 4 or 4 + 3) as a medium-grade, and 8, 9, or 10 as a high-grade cancer. Occasionally, a pathologist may note a small area of a higher grade pattern in a biopsy or radical prostatectomy (RP) specimens known as a "tertiary pattern" and may record this result.[44] A lower-grade cancer tends to grow more slowly and is less likely to spread than a cancer with a higher grade. Some limitations for the GS system involve interpretation when comparing biopsy to RP specimens, pathologist to pathologist reproducibility, and difficulty in diagnosing small acinar atypical lesions.

3.2. *The Clinical Stage*

The clinical stage is based on the urologist's clinical examination of the patient's prostate (via palpation or digital rectal exam, DRE) and this is combined with other results of clinical tests (i.e. PSA) done prior to definitive treatment (i.e. surgery or irradiation). The DRE involves digital palpation of the gland for size and any abnormalities. Based on these results, the urologist may suggest performance of a systematic biopsy of the gland to determine a diagnosis. Additionally, the urologist may suggest possibly X-rays, CT scans, and bone scans, but these tests may not always be needed. They are usually recommended based on high levels of serum PSA as well as the biopsy Gleason score and/or volume (size) of the cancer. The clinical stage of the CaP is generally described below:

(1) **T1**: The tumor cannot be felt during the DRE and is not seen during imaging (any test that produces pictures of the inside of the body, such as a CT scan). It may be found when surgery is done for another reason, usually for benign prostate hypertrophy (BPH), or abnormal growth of benign prostate cells.

    (a) **T1c**: The tumor is found during a needle biopsy, usually because the patient has an elevated PSA level.

(2) **T2**: The tumor is found only within the prostate, not other areas of the body. It is large enough to be felt during the DRE.

    (a) **T2a**: The tumor has invaded one-half of one lobe (part or side) of the prostate and may be palpated during the DRE.
    (b) **T2b**: The tumor has spread to more than one-half of one lobe of the prostate, but not to both lobes and may be palpated during the DRE.
    (c) **T2c**: The tumor has invaded both lobes of the prostate and may be palpated during the DRE.

3.3. *Pathological Stage*

Following surgery to remove the prostate gland, an expert uropathologist will assign the Gleason score and stage (extent of the size and spread of the cancer). They utilize the standardized T, N, and M classification to define TNM combinations to describe each stage of prostate cancer. The TNM is an abbreviation for tumor (T), lymph node (N), and metastasis (M) to lymph nodes and/or bone or other organs. Urologists look at these three parameters to determine the stage (extent) of cancer (Table 1):

Table 1. Prostate cancer pathologic stage grouping chart (current system).

Stage	Tumor	Nodes	Metastasis
I	T1a, T1b, or T1c	N0	M0
	T2a	N0	M0
	Any T1 or T2a	N0	M0
IIA	T1a, T1b, or T1c	N0	M0
	T1a, T1b, or T1c	N0	M0
	T2a	N0	M0
	T2b	N0	M0
	T2b	N0	M0
IIB	T2c	N0	M0
	Any T1 or T2	N0	M0
	Any T1 or T2	N0	M0
III	T3a or T3b	N0	M0
IV	T4	N0	M0
	Any T (lymph nodes +)	N1	M0
	Any T	Any N	M1

4. Quantitative Image Analysis of Nuclear Morphometry

4.1. *Manual Digital Image (Planimetry) Analysis Technology*

In 1982, David Diamond *et al.*[45] was the first to utilize Graphpad and a Zeiss Planapochromatic 100× oil immersion objective with a 12.5× ocular (total magnification 1, 250×) to trace 300 malignant and benign nuclei from each CaP case. Based upon this approach he easily separated the benign (normal) nuclei from the malignant nuclei. Next, he compared nuclear size and shape in all Stage B CaP cases that had long-term follow-up and determined that he could with high accuracy separate those with a good prognosis from those with a poor prognosis (metastasis) ($p < 0.005$). Using a circle = 1.0, he calculated nuclear roundness factor (NRF) using the formula described in Eq. (1) and (2).

$$NRF = \frac{\left(\frac{C}{2\pi}\right)}{\sqrt{\frac{A}{\pi}}} \tag{1}$$

Whereas the circularity form factor

$$C = \frac{4\pi A}{e^2} \tag{2}$$

Subsequently, the authors at the Brady Urological Institute of Johns Hopkins University School of Medicine (JHUSOM) used Nuclear Roundness Variance

(NRV) seen in Eq. (3) to predict CaP heterogeneity and tumor aggressiveness.[46,47]

$$Nuclear\ roundness = \frac{Radius\,(circumference)}{radius\,(area)} = \frac{R}{r} = \frac{\left(\frac{P}{2\pi}\right)}{\sqrt{\frac{A}{\pi}}} \quad (3)$$

Eventually a commercially available hardware and software program became available and the clinical value of NRV measurements were validated using a Zeiss inverted IM microscope (Carl Zeiss, Inc., Thornwood, NY) equipped with a Zeiss planapachromatic 100× oil immersion objective at a total magnification of 2440×. The images were analyzed with the DynaCELL Motility Morphometry Measurement workstation (JAW Associates, Inc., Annapolis, MD). By this method, measurements differed by less than 5% among examiners and the authors could confirm that this variable readily predicts progressive disease and mortality of CaP.[48–50] As further improvement, Alan Partin *et al.*[51] was able to combine NRV with Gleason score, clinical stage and age to create the "Prognostic Factor Score (PFS)" to predict three risk groups based on Kaplan-Meier plots. Also, using a multivariate model, the PFS predicted disease-free survival with statistical accuracy ($p < 0.0001$) for 100 CaP patients treated surgically without adjuvant therapy, regardless of pathologic stage. Finally, Veltri *et al.*[52] confirmed that accuracy of NRV is significantly higher than Gleason score to predict metastasis and CaP-specific death in men with long term follow-up (median follow-up: 19 years). Hence, NRV alone and in combinations with other clinical and pathologic features acts as a quantitative measure of not only pleomorphisms which reflects CaP heterogeneity — but when combined with other parameters predict CaP progression. Hence, NRV is better able to identify aggressive phenotypes of CaP than Gleason score and is associated with an increase in irregularity of the nuclear border; however, currently there is no commercially viable tool to automatically measure this NRV feature available.

4.2. *Tissue Digital Imaging using Feulgen Stained Nuclei*

The Feulgen staining reagent specifically and quantitatively binds to DNA in cellular material. The reagent binds to DNA by uncovering the free aldehyde groups in the DNA during the acid hydrolysis process, which then reacts with the Feulgen reagent via a Shiff-Base interaction to form a stable, colored compound (blue) that absorbs light at 560 nm.[53,54] Figure 1 illustrates examples of matched H&E and Feulgen histochemical stains of histology and cytology tissue preparations.

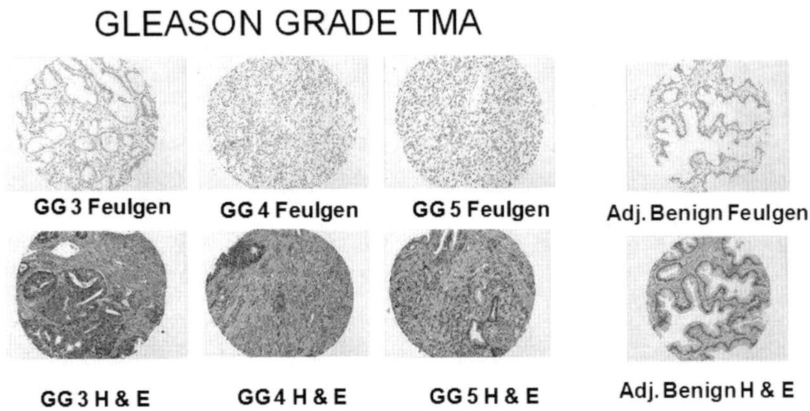

Fig. 1. Feulgen (upper row) and H&E (lower row) staining of prostate cancer with different Gleason grades (GG) or adjacent benign prostate tissue in a tissue microarray.

4.3. *The AutoCyte™ Pathology Workstation (AWP)*

The AutoCyte™ Pathology Workstation (AWP) (TriPath Inc, Burlington, NC) process starts with a calibrator slide made with normal rat liver tetraploid nuclei that has been stained at the same time as the study tissue sections; the APW imaging system (Fig. 2) is calibrated for the integrated optical density (IOD). This is done by analyzing an external rat hepatocyte standard from which a minimum of 500 tetraploid nuclei are captured, resulting in a peak with a CV <2.0% and an IOD somewhere between 6500–8500, depending on the intensity of the Feulgen stain lot. Next using the QUIC-DNA v1.201software, we capture nuclear images of malignant Feulgen stained Active Surveillance (AS) biopsy nuclei from a pathologist-marked biopsy slide (~150–200 per area). The QUIC-DNA v1.201software employs nuclear morphometric descriptors (NMDs) and ~40 selected nuclear features including size, shape, and/or DNA content (pg DNA, IOD, intensity, and mean Gray level) will be used for data analysis. Additional software employs QUIC-Immuno to quantify immunohistochemical (qIHC) chromagen-based staining for molecular biomarkers in cancer tissues.

4.4. *Quantitative Nuclear Grade using AutoCyte™*

A digital imaging approach described by Veltri *et al.* uses the AutoCyte™ Pathology Workstation (TriPath Inc., Burlington, NC, USA) and Feulgen stained prostate nuclei to study the CaP in biopsy and RP specimens. By capturing 150–200 nuclei (benign or cancer) and calculating variance of the NMDs above using the AutoCyte™ DNA QUIC DNA v1.201 software. We

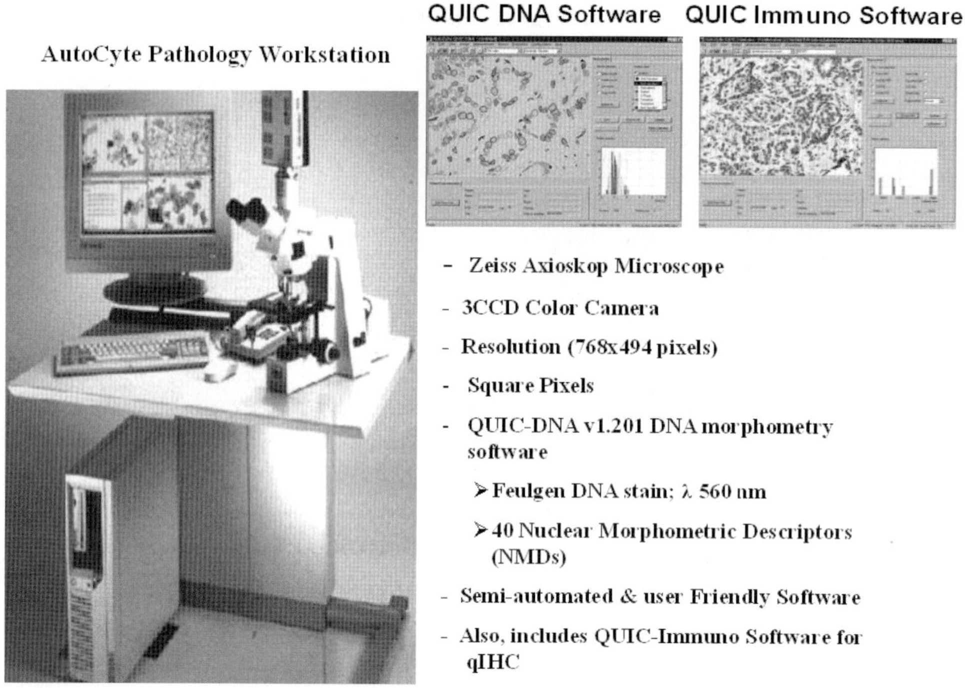

Fig. 2. AutoCyte™ Pathology Workstation equipment (left), software and important features (right).

devised methods to calculate a "Quantitative Nuclear Grade" (QNG) to make predictions of grade, stage, metastasis and survival (Fig. 3). The method of calculation we have applied is Multivariate Logistic Regression (MLR).[26] Alternative statistical analysis identifying critical NMDs from among the 40 NMDs that reliably distinguish higher risk from persistently very low risk patients involves two stages: (1) high dimension reduction to reduce the number of NMDs to a smaller subset, and (2) comparison of correlated receiver operating characteristic (ROC) curves.[55] Dimension reduction borrows from filtering techniques developed for the analysis of very high-dimensional microarray data, and will apply the correlation analysis of microarrays approach developed by Dr. Kowalski to obtain a subset of markers selected as commonly,[56] between high and low groups, reproducible within each group.[55,56] When QNG is calculated, the best NMD features are selected that are most predictive and least redundant NMDs that assist in differentiating the two classes of patients (i.e. progressors and non-progressors). Figure 3 shows an example of how QNG solutions are derived from the NMDs. Included are a Feulgen stain and 3D artificially color pixel maps of three individual nuclei.

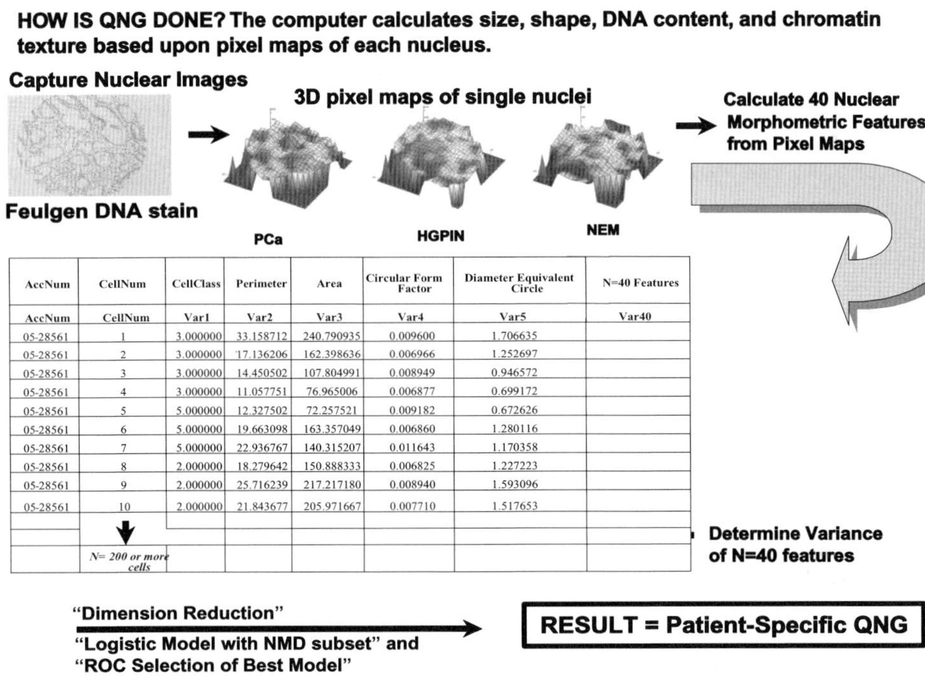

AccNum	CellNum	CellClass	Perimeter	Area	Circular Form Factor	Diameter Equivalent Circle	N=40 Features
AccNum	CellNum	Var1	Var2	Var3	Var4	Var5	Var40
05-28561	1	3.000000	33.158712	240.790935	0.009600	1.706635	
05-28561	2	3.000000	17.136206	162.398636	0.006966	1.252697	
05-28561	3	3.000000	14.450502	107.804991	0.008949	0.946572	
05-28561	4	3.000000	11.057751	76.965006	0.006877	0.699172	
05-28561	5	5.000000	12.327502	72.257521	0.009182	0.672626	
05-28561	6	5.000000	19.663098	163.357049	0.006860	1.280116	
05-28561	7	5.000000	22.936767	140.315207	0.011643	1.170358	
05-28561	8	2.000000	18.279642	150.888333	0.006825	1.227223	
05-28561	9	2.000000	25.716239	217.217180	0.008940	1.593096	
05-28561	10	2.000000	21.843677	205.971667	0.007710	1.517653	
	↓						
	N= 200 or more cells						

Fig. 3. Example of QNG solutions based on AutoCyte™ Pathology Workstation.

4.4.1. *QNG to study Gleason grade differences*

Veltri *et al.*[57] used the AutoCyte™ Pathology Workstation (TriPath, Inc., Burlington, NC) digital imaging system and Feulgen stained prostatic nuclei to study Gleason grade (GG) in RP specimens. A Gleason grade TMA-471 prepared by an expert uropathologist at JHUSOM, contained sets of four cores (0.6 mm) per case of GG3, GG4 and GG5 CaP patterns. The concept was to use the AutoCyte™ nuclear features on pools of 1100 nuclei from these three GGs to determine the optimal variables to discriminate the three GGs (3, 4, and 5) and is based on the MLR analysis in order to make comparisons. Nine NMD features (perimeter, area, Feret X, Feret Y, Maximum Feret, Intensity, Median OD, StdDev OD, and DNA ploidy) were selected for all GG comparisons. The results yielded areas of ROC curve (ROC-AUC) that distinguished differences among benign cancer-adjacent nuclei and GG3 (ROC-AUC = 0.78); GG4 (ROC-AUC = 0.86) and GG5 (ROC-AUC = 0.88) cancer areas with accuracies of 73%, 78% and 80% respectively.[57] By calculating the predictive probability (PP) values, we noted significant variations (i.e. marked heterogeneity) among the three GG patterns. Also, using the CAS-200 system, Venkataraman *et al.*[58] separated GG3 and GG4 by evaluating prostate biopsies and the method yielded a 85% classification accuracy using a three nuclear feature set (minimum diameter, angularity and sum optical density) determined by decision tree analysis. The latter provides one approach to determine GG based on quantitative nuclear morphometry. Furthermore, our approach provides data to improve our understanding of morphological variability in nuclear structure and its role in CaP during the establishment of heterogeneity among Gleason grades. Hence, the importance of automated computer-assisted quantitative nuclear morphometry to estimate CaP Gleason grade is clearly illustrated by these methods.

4.4.2. *QNG to predict CaP outcomes: biochemical recurrence*

In 1996, Veltri *et al.*[59] used the CAS-200 imaging system and only 38 NMDs to predict CaP biochemical recurrence (BCR). The patient cohort included 115 patients with clinically localized CaP and the mean follow-up period in 70/115 patients without disease progression was 10.4 ± 1.7 years. Using backward stepwise multivariate logistic regression (MLR) at a variable feature selection stringency of $p < 0.05$, the variances of 11/38 of the NMDs were found to be multivariately significant for predicting BCR ($p < 0.00001$; ROC-AUC 86%; sensitivity of 78%; specificity of 83%). Further, QNG and the postoperative Gleason score when combined, yielded a MLR model for the prediction of BCR yielding an ROC-AUC = 92% and having a sensitivity of 89% and specificity of 84%. These two parameters (QNG and Gleason score) separated the 115 patients into three statistically significant "risk groups" (low to high) based upon Kaplan-Meier analysis. Subsequently, employing an NCI Cooperative Prostate Cancer Tissue Resource (CPCTR) tissue microarray (TMA) of 92 cases with long term follow-up (56 non-recurrences and 36 recurrences), we showed that by combining nuclear features i.e. circular form factor (rho -0.26; $p = 0.012$) and minimum Feret (rho -0.21; $p = 0.048$) with the p300 (acetyltransferase) protein biomarker expression, we were able to predict BCR both as a continuous or dichotomous variable and can be combined with Gleason score for BCR risk stratification.[60] Hence, by combining QNG produced with Feulgen stained tissue preparations and a computer-assisted image analysis system, we can enhance predictive accuracy for CaP outcomes.

4.4.3. *QNG to predict CaP metastasis and CaP-specific survival*

The prediction of high risk CaP requires having long-term patient follow-up data to predict serious CaP outcomes like BCR, metastasis and survival. Khan *et al.*[61] working in our laboratory developed QNG signatures that predicted progression to metastasis and/or CaP-mortality in 227 men that have undergone RP. He also employed the AutoCyte™ Pathology Workstation and

QUIC-DNA v1.201 morphology software to calculate QNG solutions. Khan showed that a multivariate MLR model including routine pathology variables and prostatectomy Gleason score yielded a ROC-AUC of 75% with an accuracy of 59% at 90% sensitivity. The best QNG solution yielded an ROC-AUC of 84% and an accuracy of 70% at 90% sensitivity. The combined pathology-QNG model retained LN status, prostatectomy Gleason score, and QNG and yielded an ROC-AUC of 86% with an accuracy of 76% at 90% sensitivity. Also, his data was also assessed via a Cox proportional hazards model and produced the following univariately and multivariately significant hazard ratios (HR): QNG = 3.5 and 2.9, respectively; LN = 2.7 and 1.8, respectively; and prostatectomy Gleason score, 2.8 and 2.1, respectively. The QNG variable proved to be a strong predictor of CaP progression to metastasis and/or mortality in this study of advanced high risk CaP. Later, Veltri *et al.*[62] confirmed these results using a TMA consisting of 186 CaP cases with matched cancer and adjacent benign normal-appearing areas ("field effects") and employed the same AutoCyte™ imaging technology to re-evaluate the use of QNG alone and with pathological and clinical variables to predict metastasis and CaP death. The routine pathology model yielded an ROC-AUC of 72.5%. Alternatively, the QNG-benign and QNG-cancer area solutions yielded an ROC-AUC of 81.6% and 79.9%, respectively. Kaplan-Meier plots for the routine clinicopathologic variables; the QNG-benign and QNG-cancer area solutions were combined with pathology to define three statistically significantly distinct risk groups (low to high) to predict distant metastasis and/or death ($p < 0.0001$). Hence, in both the cancer epithelial and the benign cancer-adjacent ("field effects") nuclear area, QNG solutions could predict metastasis and/or CaP death and the Kaplan-Meier plots partitioned the patients into three groups and with very significant log ranks to separate the risk groups. Therefore, QNG can be combined with molecular biomarkers and clinicopathological features to create a "combination signature" to predict recurrence, metastasis and survival of high risk CaP patients.[60–62] The future is to automate a commercially viable operating system and apply these imaging tools by combining the best QNG and protein biomarker solution to generate to predict those high risk cancers that will progress so that appropriate early intervention can be instituted.

5. Engineering Approaches to Quantitative Histomorphometry

Today, the emergence of the rapid and high resolution scanning microscopy and the development of novel machine vision imaging techniques (virtual pathology) are aiding pathologists to improve the analysis of histologic tissue images for diagnosis and prognosis.[63,64] Automated computer-assisted image applications have been the recent focus for CaP and other cancers. The development of machine vision techniques have been applied to routine H&E stained tissue sections, aiding pathologists to analyze CaP tissue images and accurately and reproducibly evaluate tissue histomorphometry of CaP pathology. Rapid and steady progress during the past decade has seen novel applications of automated quantitative image analysis including improved cancer cell nuclear segmentation and tissue texture analysis to assess different Gleason grading patterns based on H&E and Feulgen histochemical stained tissue images have been reported.[24–26,57,63–66] Numerous approaches to quantify nuclear size, shape and texture analysis of these CaP images have been successfully employed as shown in Table 2. The biomedical and electrical engineers have used Wavelet and multiwavelet transforms, fractal analysis, Voronoi and Delaunay graph tessellations, and other novel image computational tools for tissue feature extraction and classification in studies of the automated quantitative histologic tumor grading. Below we have summarized collaborative efforts to demonstrate the potential value of this newer approach to automated computer-assisted pathology.

5.1. *Wavelet Transforms*

Previous work by Jafari-Khouzani *et al.*[77] has used wavelet transforms for the grading of histopathology images of prostate cancer. These transforms are overlaid onto the image to identify textures. Wavelet transforms have been popular for characterizing image texture and have been used to extract energy and entropy features for identifying prostate cancer malignancy.[68,77] Furthermore, multi-wavelet transforms have been used to extend upon single wavelet transforms via simultaneous representation of orthogonally, symmetry, and moments.[77] For multi-wavelet features, energy can describe the amount of signal in a given resolution, while entropy describes differences in the submatrices.

Fractal analysis of wavelets has been also been investigated by Almuntashri *et al.*[68] for classifying Gleason grade from prostate histology images. Wavelet coefficients are obtained from each decomposition level measure spatial architecture. The corresponding submatrices from the decomposition each contain a fractal dimension which can be aggregated to obtain an averaged wavelet-based fractal dimension for the image. This type of fractal dimension analysis has been shown to correctly classify grade 3 cancers at a 90% classification rate.[68]

Table 2. Image derived histologic features to model disease patterns on histology.

Feature Class	Derived attributes	Relevance to histology
Voronoi Tessellation	Number of nodes, number of edges, cyclomatic number, number of triangles, number of k-walks, spectral radius, eigenexponent, Randic index, area, roundness factor, area disorder, roundness factor homogeneity.[67]	Tissue architecture and arrangement of nuclei.
Delaunay Triangulation	Number of nodes, edge length, degree, number of edges, cyclomatic number, number of triangles, number of k-walks, spectral radius, Eigen exponent, Wiener index, eccentricity, Randic index, fractal dimension.[67]	
Minimum Spanning Tree	Number of nodes, edge length, degree, number of neighbors, Wiener index, eccentricity, Randic index, Balaban index, fractal dimension.[68]	
Cell-Graph (local)	Giant Connected Component, eccentricity, number of edges, Connected Component C,D, E.[24,69–72]	
Nuclear, Glandular Morphology	Margin spicularity, fractal dimension, height to width ratio, roundness factor, area overlap ratio, area disorder, perimeter, diameter, explicit shape descriptors (medial axis based shape modeling of individual glands).[73,74]	Nuclear and glandular size boundary, appearance
Cell Orientation Entropy/ Co-occurring Gland Tensors	Contrast energy, Contrast inverse moment, Contrast average, Contrast variance, Contrast entropy, Intensity average, Intensity variance, Intensity entropy, Entropy, Energy, Correlation, 2 measures of information.[75,76,81]	Second-order descriptors of nuclear orientation in local neighborhoods

5.2. *Intensity Co-occurrence Texture*

Another method of describing texture in images is via intensity co-occurrence matrices. Second order co-occurrence features[78] are calculated from a symmetric co-occurrence matrix which aggregates the frequency in which two pixel intensities co-occur within a pre-determined window distance around each pixel. The size of the co-occurrence matrix is determined by the maximum possible intensity value in the image, which for 8-bit images is $2^8 = 256$. Subsequent features such as Haralick texture features[79] can be computed from each window.

Co-occurrence matrix based features have been used to describe textures for prostate histopathology. Diamond *et al.*[74] showed that Haralick features could be used to discriminate stroma from prostate cancer in 100×100 pixel regions. However, they also noted that improvement to discrimination could be achieved via the use of nuclear morphology. Results using a combination of both morphological and co-occurrence texture features showed 89% classification accuracy on a three class case (stroma, normal, and cancerous regions).

5.3. *Nuclear Shape, Orientation, and Architectural Features for Grading and Assessing Aggressive Prostate Cancers*

5.3.1. *Adaptive active contour model (AdACM) for nuclei segmentation*

Useful nuclear features to be extracted for the purpose of identifying CaP progression include that of nuclear morphology, texture, orientation, and arrangement. Extraction of these features rely heavily on the ability to accurately detect and segment nuclei on digitized prostate histology samples. However, in prostate histology, overlapping nuclei is a common occurrence. These overlapping objects (nuclei, lymphocytes, etc.) often appear clumped together as one single object. There is a need to resolve multiple overlapping nuclei and accurately segment them for the subsequent feature extraction. Ali *et al.* used an Adaptive Active Contour Model (AdACM),[25] which uses a shape prior to aid in the identification of individual nuclei. The ability of the model to selectively invoke energy terms in the variational functional allows for resolving (a) overlaps between nuclei and (b) significant computational savings.[25] Segmentation schemes such as AdACM (see Fig. 4) allow for

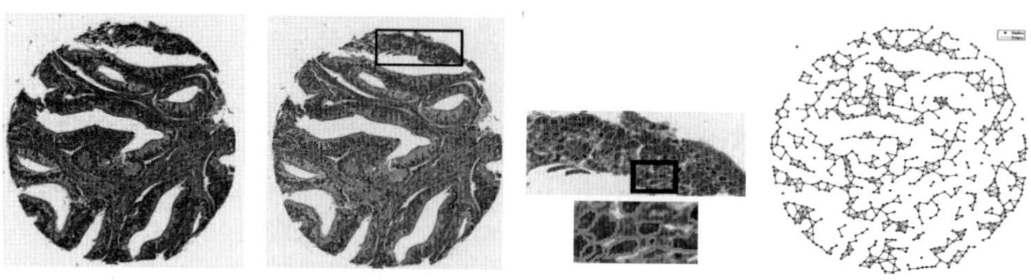

(a) (b) (c) (d)

Fig. 4. (a) Original Gleason grade 4 CaP TMA, (b) automated nuclear segmentation by the AdACM scheme, (c) Magnification of a ROI on the TMA reveals that the scheme is able to accurately resolve overlaps between nuclei, and (d) Delaunay triangulation graph obtained by connecting nuclear centers [segmented in (b)].

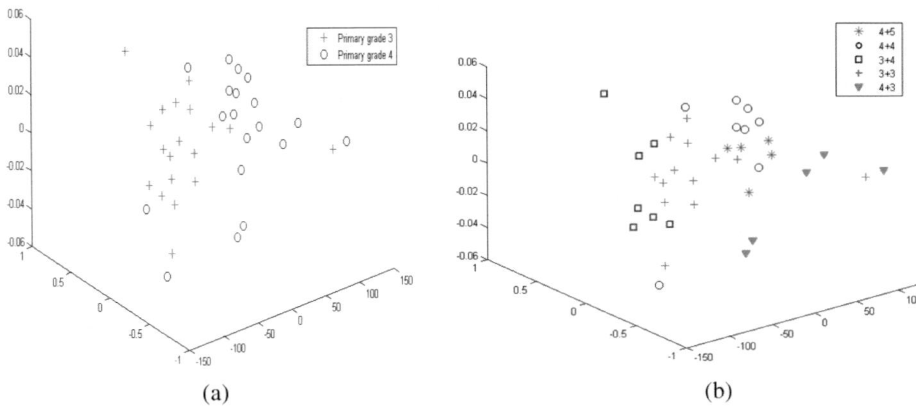

Fig. 5. Low dimensional representation of histomorphometric features shows separation of (a) grades 3, 4 and (b) Gleason scores 6, 7, 8, 9.

extraction of sophisticated histomorphometric features (e.g. characterizing the precise spatial distribution of nuclei [see Fig. 4(d)]) to distinguish different Gleason patterns of CaP (Fig. 4).

In previous work[25] a predictor based on nuclear features derived from prostate TMAs was able to discriminate intermediate Gleason grades [See Fig. 5(a)] as well as Gleason scores [See Fig. 5(b)]. Figures 5(a), (b) reveal low dimensional projections of morphologic features derived from TMAs from 40 different patient studies. The clustering clearly shows very good discrimination between Gleason grades 3, 4 [Fig. 5(a)] with a classification accuracy >85% and Gleason scores. Figure 5(b) shows the low dimensional representation of 40 patients with different Gleason scores (3+3, 3+4, 4+3, 4+4, 4+5). Note in Fig. 5(b), the separation between 3 + 4 and 4 + 3 Gleason scores; clinically the most challenging problem.

5.3.2. *Nuclear orientation*

Recent work by Lee *et al.*[75] has suggested that the information in nuclear orientations can be used to predict prostate cancer progression. Cell orientation entropy (COrE) aggregates co-occurrences of similarly orientated nuclei within local neighborhoods defined by local cell graphs and calculates second order statistics to determine characteristics of the tissue (Fig. 6). Statistics such as entropy are used to quantify the disorder of nuclear orientation within the tissue. Mean and standard deviations of these statistics across neighborhoods provide features for identifying CaP progressors. These methods were shown to accurately predict biochemical recurrence in 74% of CaP patients following radical prostatectomy, and found to be complementary to architectural and

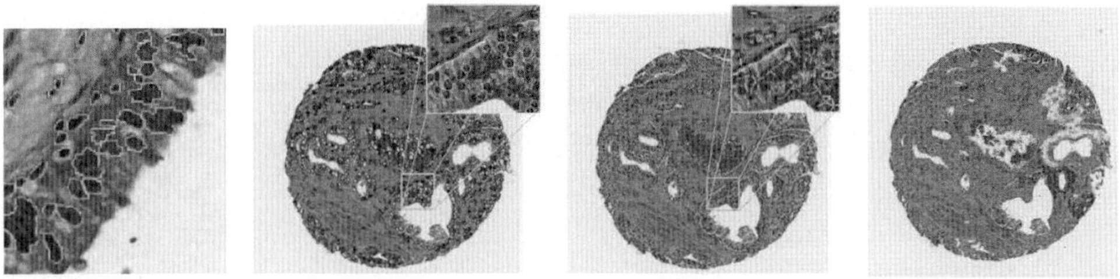

(a) (b) (c) (d)

Fig. 6. (a) Automated cell segmentation by AdACM on CaP TMA core, (b) capturing cell orientation, (c) subgraph localization of nuclear neighborhoods, (d) second order co-occurrence features by COrE methodology.

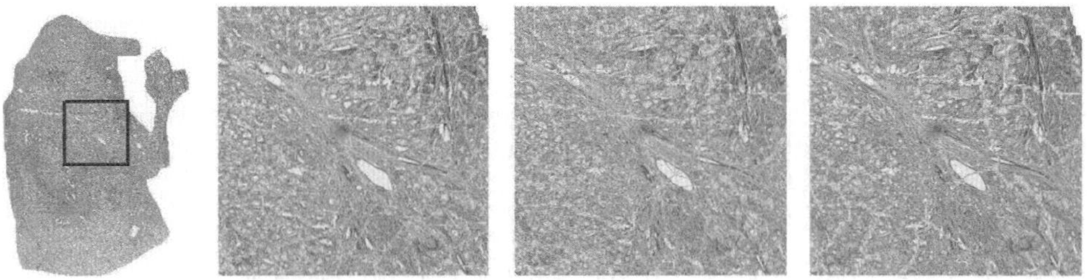

(a) (b) (c) (d)

Fig. 7. Different graph tessellations can be used to extract architectural information across objects such as glands or nuclei. Common tesselations used are based on (a) Voronoi, (b) Delaunay, and (c) Minimum spanning trees.

morphological features for predicting CaP progression, correctly identifying biochemical recurrence (82% accuracy) in the CaP patients following radical prostatectomy.

5.3.3. *Nuclear architecture*

Formally, a simple graph is an undirected and un-weighted graph without self-loops, with V and E being the node and edge set of graph G, respectively. Graphs are effective techniques to represent structural information by defining a large set of topological features. These features are quantified by definition of computable metrics. Features will be calculated that describe the spatial location of nuclei within the histological image. Nuclear centers will be used to calculate a set of features such as the number and density of the nuclei in the image. Graph-based algorithms (e.g. Delaunay Triangulation, Voronoi, Minimum spanning tree)[67,68] can then be directly computed from the original image, using the nuclear, glandular centroids as vertices of the graphs. Figure 7(d) shows a minimum spanning tree graph-based representation of intermediate Gleason grade prostate histology image.

While these methods focus on global architecture, researchers have developed methods for extracting features which describe local architecture which can differentiate between stroma and epithelial regions of the prostate. Gunduz *et al.*[70] noted a natural clustering of cells and utilized cell graphs to model gliomas and differentiate cancerous, healthy, and non-neoplastic inflamed tissue. These graphs are created via edges between nearest neighbors between nuclei as nodes. Demir *et al.*[71] and others[24,69–72] have developed a set of graph features using features such as connected component size and eccentricity to quantify the local cell-graphs. Features were extracted from simple, probabilistic, and hierarchical cell-graphs, as well as a hybrid combination of simple and hierarchical approaches. Similarly, Ali *et al.*[24,72] utilized attributes of probabilistic cell-cluster graphs for extracting features from prostate cancer tissue microarrays. Modeling prostate cancer via subgraphs offers the advantage of being able to explicitly and independently model spatial architecture of nuclei within the epithelial and stromal regions and 83% classification accuracy was found by combining features extracted from these regions independently.[72]

5.4. *Gland Based Features Grading and Assessing Aggressiveness in Prostate Cancers*

5.4.1. *Markov random fields for automated gland segmentation*

Monaco *et al.* previously developed a novel Markov Random field (MRF) segmentation algorithm[80] for identifying CaP regions from whole mount histologic section. Glands are first automatically segmented and then classified as benign or cancerous based on features extracted from the gland (area, morphology). The MRF then identifies cancerous glands based on the assumption that CaP glands tend to be closer to other CaP glands. We showed that this automated segmentation scheme was able to more precisely segment CaP regions compared to the rough annotation provided by the pathologist. Furthermore, this methodology was shown to identify cancerous regions on whole mount prostate histology with 93% accuracy.[80]

5.4.2. *Gland morphology*

Additionally, others have used gland lumen segmentation to characterize prostate cancer for the purpose of differentiating different tissue types and identifying aggressive CaP.[74,76] From the segmented boundaries of each

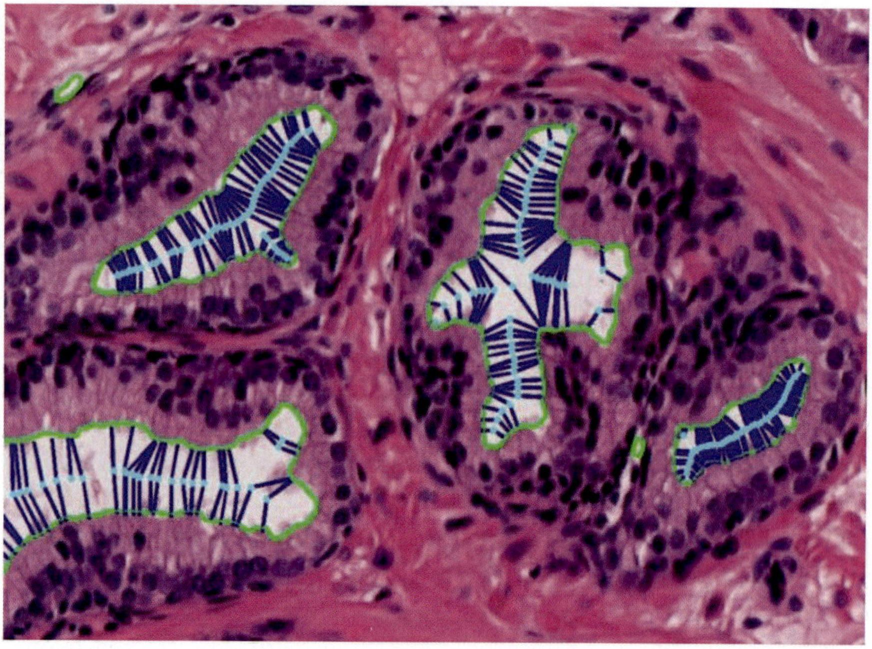

Fig. 8. Medial axis shape (MAS) model (cyan) and surface vectors (dark blue) for a set of glands (green). MAS allows for extraction of glandular morphological features, then used to train the image based classifier then used to discriminate good/bad outcome CaP.

gland, morphological features such as Area Ratio, Distance Ratio, Standard Deviation of Distance, Variance of Distance, Distance Ratio, Perimeter Ratio, Smoothness, Invariant Moment 1–7, Fractal Dimension, Fourier Descriptor 1–10 (Mean, Std. Dev, Median, Min/Max of each) can be extracted to identify cancer progressors.[64] These methods have been shown to be able to differentiate between different Gleason grades[64] as well as CaP progressors.[76]

Sparks *et al.* has developed Explicit Shape Descriptors (ESDs)[73] to determine subtle differences between object morphology. ESDs describe gland morphology via fitting a medial axis shape model (MASM) to each gland (see Fig. 8). ESDs were shown to distinguishing glands from grades 3 and 4 with an accuracy of over 80%.

5.4.3. *Gland orientation*

Normal benign glands align themselves with respect to the fibromusclar stroma, and thus display a coherent directionality.[81] Malignant prostate glands, however, lose their capability to orient themselves and display no preferred directionality. Additionally with increasing degree of malignancy and disease

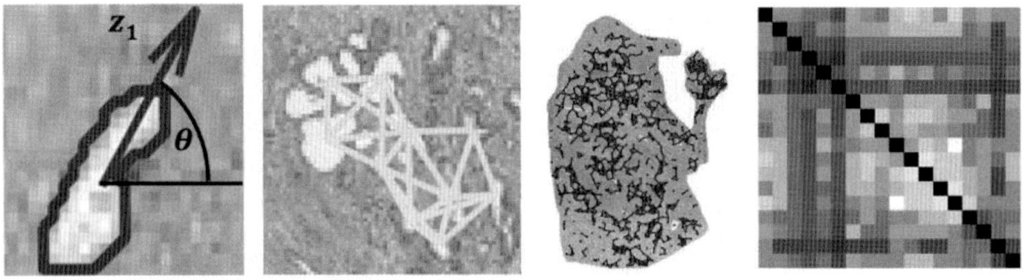

(a) (b) (c) (d)

Fig. 9. (a) Gland orientations are quantified via a 1st order tensor. Local gland neighborhoods are identified via subgraph construction. (c) Subgraphs create local clusters of neighboring glands from which to extract neighborhood tensor co-occurrence information. (d) Tensor co-occurrence matrix is descriptive of the gland tensor entropy as brighter co-occurrence values in the off-diagonal cells, suggest higher co-occurrence of differing orientations.

aggressiveness, the coherence of gland orientations within localized regions is completely disrupted. In such cases, the entropy (which captures disorder) in gland orientations is shown to increase as a function of malignancy. Co-occurring gland tensors (CGTs) provide a means to quantify this disorder.[76] Figure 9 illustrates the use of gland orientation in local subgraphs to construct tensor co-occurrence matrices. These co-occurrence matrices capture the disorder in the gland orientations, and second order statistics of these matrices allow for the differentiation of aggressive and non-aggressive CaP.

For a cohort of 40 intermediate-risk (mostly Gleason sum 7) surgically cured CaP patients where half suffered biochemical recurrence, the CGT features were able to predict biochemical recurrence with 73% accuracy. Additionally, for 80 regions of interest chosen from the 40 studies, corresponding to both normal and cancerous cases, CGT features yielded a 99% accuracy. CGTs were shown to be statistically significantly ($p < 0.05$) better at predicting biochemical recurrence compared to state-of-the-art quantitative histomorphometric methods such as gland morphology, and intensity texture and postoperative Kattan prostate cancer nomogram.

6. Summary

In summary, this chapter demonstrates how prostate cancer quantitative histomorphometry can be used to extract and employ computer-assisted image features and hence serve as a potential new and innovative predictive tool to improve determination of aggressive phenotypes of cancer. The prior semi-automated approach of Dr. Veltri using a spectrophotometer microscope, though accurate and capable of predicting stage, recurrence and progression of prostate cancer, it has deficiencies that limit its extension to whole slide image. The AutoCyte Pathology Workstation is no longer commercially available and new approaches had to be sought to prove the value of computer-assisted histomorphometry. Dr. Veltri is currently employing commercially available image analysis software to evaluate Feulgen (DNA) and H&E histochemical stains. However, the collaboration started a few years ago with Dr. Madabhushi and his team at Case Western Reserve University has afforded the opportunity to develop and validate new methods that can be applied for high throughput quantification and feature analysis from whole slide images. These novel tools could form the basis of future software tools to conduct, in cooperation with the pathologist, automated, rapid and reproducible identification and quantification of tissue histology morphologic and molecular events, enabling machine based predictions of tumor aggressiveness and outcomes such as recurrence, metastasis and survival.

References

1. R. Siegel, D. Naishadham, & A. Jemal, "Cancer statistics," 2013. *CA* **63**, 11–30 (2013).
2. B. E. Sirovich, L. M. Schwartz, & S. Woloshin, "Screening men for prostate and colorectal cancer in the United States: Does practice reflect the evidence?" *JAMA* **289**, 1414–1420 (2003).
3. H. B. Carter *et al.*, "Early detection of prostate cancer: AUA Guideline," *J Urology* **190**, 419–426 (2013).
4. A. W. Partin, "Early detection of prostate cancer continues to support rational, limited screening," *J Urology* **190**, 427–428 (2013).
5. R. Etzioni *et al.*, "Overdiagnosis due to prostate-specific antigen screening: lessons from U.S. prostate cancer incidence trends," *J Nat Cancer Institute* **94**, 981–990 (2002).
6. R. Etzioni *et al.*, "Quantifying the role of PSA screening in the US prostate cancer mortality decline," *Cancer Causes Control* **19**, 175–181 (2008).
7. S. A. Strope & G. L. Andriole, "Prostate cancer screening: Current status and future perspectives," *Nat Rev Urology* 7, 487–493 (2010).
8. G. Draisma *et al.*, "Lead times and overdetection due to prostate-specific antigen screening: estimates from the European Randomized Study of Screening for Prostate Cancer," *J Nat Cancer Institute* **95**, 868–878 (2003).
9. D. Sundi *et al.*, "Very-high-risk localized prostate cancer: Definition and outcomes," *Prostate Cancer Prostatic Dis* **17**, 57–63 (2014).
10. T. Atsumi *et al.*, "Inflammation amplifier, a new paradigm in cancer biology," *Cancer Research* **74**, 8–14 (2014).
11. E. A. Platz & A. M. De Marzo, "Epidemiology of inflammation and prostate cancer," *J Urology* **171**, S36–40 (2004).

12. A. J. Schetter, N. H. Heegaard & C. C. Harris, "Inflammation and cancer: Interweaving microRNA, free radical, cytokine and p53 pathways," *Carcinogenesis* **31**, 37–49 (2010).
13. C. V. Dang, "Rethinking the Warburg effect with Myc micromanaging glutamine metabolism," *Cancer Res* **70**, 859–862 (2010).
14. C. V. Dang, A. Le & P. Gao, "MYC-induced cancer cell energy metabolism and therapeutic opportunities," *Clinical Cancer Res* **15**, 6479–6483 (2009).
15. J. L. Spratlin, N. J. Serkova & S. G. Eckhardt, "Clinical applications of metabolomics in oncology: a review," *Clinical Cancer Res* **15**, 431–440 (2009).
16. S. I. Grivennikov, F. R. Greten & M. Karin, "Immunity, inflammation, and cancer," *Cell* **140**, 883–899 (2010).
17. N. Rajarubendra, N. Lawrentschuk, D. M. Bolton, L. Klotz & I. D. Davis, "Prostate cancer immunology — an update for Urologists," *BJU Int* **107**, 1046–1051 (2011).
18. M. J. Rutkowski, M. E. Sughrue, A. J. Kane, S. A. Mills & A. T. Parsa, "Cancer and the complement cascade," *Mol Cancer Res* **8**, 1453–1465 (2010).
19. C. C. Sprenger, S. R. Plymate & M. J. Reed, "Aging-related alterations in the extracellular matrix modulate the microenvironment and influence tumor progression," *In J Cancer. J Int du Cancer* **127**, 2739–2748 (2010).
20. O. E. Franco & S. W. Hayward, "Targeting the tumor stroma as a novel therapeutic approach for prostate cancer," *Adv Pharmacology* **65**, 267–313 (2012).
21. D. Gao, L. T. Vahdat, S. Wong, J. C. Chang & V. Mittal, "Microenvironmental regulation of epithelial-mesenchymal transitions in cancer," *Cancer Res* **72**, 4883–4889 (2012).
22. M. A. Swartz *et al.*, "Tumor microenvironment complexity: Emerging roles in cancer therapy," *Cancer Res* **72**, 2473–2480 (2012).
23. J. Mohler *et al.*, "NCCN clinical practice guidelines in oncology: prostate cancer," *J Nat Comprehensive Cancer Network* **8**, 162–200 (2010).
24. S. Ali, R. Veltri, J. A. Epstein, C. Christudass & A. Madabhushi, "Cell cluster graph for prediction of biochemical recurrence in prostate cancer patients from tissue microarrays," *Proc Spie* **8676** (2013).
25. S. Ali, R. Veltri, J. I. Epstein, C. Christudass & A. Madabhushi, "Adaptive energy selective active contour with shape priors for nuclear segmentation and gleason grading of prostate cancer," *Medical Image Computing and Computer-assisted Intervention International Conference on Medical Image Computing and Computer-Assisted Intervention* **14**, 661–669 (2011).
26. R. W. Veltri, C. S. Christudass & S. Isharwal, "Nuclear morphometry, nucleomics and prostate cancer progression," *Asian J Andrology* **14**, 375–384 (2012).
27. M. J. Carmichael *et al.*, "Deoxyribonucleic acid ploidy analysis as a predictor of recurrence following radical prostatectomy for stage T2 disease," *J Urology* **153**, 1015–1019 (1995).
28. S. M. Falzarano & C. Magi-Galluzzi, "Prostate cancer staging and grading at radical prostatectomy over time," *Adv Anatomic Pathology* **18**, 159–164 (2011).
29. M. Fiorentino, E. Capizzi & M. Loda, "Blood and tissue biomarkers in prostate cancer: State of the art," *Urologic Clinics North Am* **37**, 131–141, Table of Contents (2010).
30. Y. Fradet, "Biomarkers in prostate cancer diagnosis and prognosis: beyond prostate-specific antigen," *Curr Opin Urology* **19**, 243–246 (2009).

31. S. Isharwal *et al.*, "Prognostic value of Her-2/neu and DNA index for progression, metastasis and prostate cancer-specific death in men with long-term follow-up after radical prostatectomy," *Int J Cancer J Int du Cancer* **123**, 2636–2643 (2008).
32. S. Isharwal *et al.*, "DNA Ploidy as surrogate for biopsy gleason score for preoperative organ versus nonorgan-confined prostate cancer prediction," *Urology* **73**, 1092–1097 (2009).
33. D. V. Makarov, S. Loeb, R. H. Getzenberg & A. W. Partin, "Biomarkers for prostate cancer," *Annual Rev Med* **60**, 139–151 (2009).
34. G. Ploussard & A. de la Taille, "Urine biomarkers in prostate cancer," *Nat Rev Urology* **7**, 101–109 (2010).
35. G. Sardana, B. Dowell & E. P. Diamandis, "Emerging biomarkers for the diagnosis and prognosis of prostate cancer," *Clin Chem* **54**, 1951–1960 (2008).
36. D. Sundi *et al.*, "Identification of men with the highest risk of early disease recurrence after radical prostatectomy," *Prostate* **74**, 628–636 (2014).
37. H. B. Carter *et al.*, "Prostate-specific antigen and all-cause mortality: Results from the Baltimore longitudinal study On aging," *J Nat Cancer Institute* **96**, 557–558 (2004).
38. S. E. Eggener *et al.*, "Predicting 15-year prostate cancer specific mortality after radical prostatectomy," *J Urology* **185**, 869–875 (2011).
39. J. Fang *et al.*, "Low levels of prostate-specific antigen predict long-term risk of prostate cancer: Results from the Baltimore Longitudinal Study of Aging," *Urology* **58**, 411–416 (2001).
40. C. G. Rogers, M. A. Khan, M. Craig Miller, R. W. Veltri & A. W. Partin, "Natural history of disease progression in patients who fail to achieve an undetectable prostate-specific antigen level after undergoing radical prostatectomy," *Cancer* **101** (2004).
41. E. J. Wright *et al.*, "Prostate specific antigen predicts the long-term risk of prostate enlargement: Results from the Baltimore Longitudinal Study of Aging," *J Urology* **167**, 2484–2487; discussion 2487–2488 (2002).
42. D. F. Gleason, "Classification of prostatic carcinomas," *Cancer Chemotherapy Reports* **50**, 125–128 (1966).
43. D. F. Gleason, "Histologic grading of prostate cancer: A perspective," *Hum Pathology* **23**, 273–279 (1992).
44. J. I. Epstein, "An update of the Gleason grading system," *J Urology* **183**, 433–440 (2010).
45. D. A. Diamond, S. J. Berry, C. Umbricht, H. J. Jewett & D. S. Coffey, "Computerized image analysis of nuclear shape as a prognostic factor for prostatic cancer," *Prostate* **3**, 321–332 (1982).
46. M. C. Benson, D. C. McDougal & D. S. Coffey, "The application of perpendicular and forward light scatter to assess nuclear and cellular morphology," *Cytometry* **5**, 515–522 (1984).
47. M. C. Benson, D. C. McDougal & D. S. Coffey, "The use of multiparameter flow cytometry to assess tumor cell heterogeneity and grade prostate cancer," *Prostate* **5**, 27–45 (1984).
48. J. I. Epstein, S. J. Berry & J. C. Eggleston, "Nuclear roundness factor. A predictor of progression in untreated Stage A2 prostate cancer," *Cancer* **54**, 1666–1671 (1984).

49. J. L. Mohler, A. W. Partin, J. I. Epstein, W. D. Lohr & D. S. Coffey, "Nuclear roundness factor measurement for assessment of prognosis of patients with prostatic carcinoma. II. Standardization of methodology for histologic sections," *J Urology* **139**, 1085–1090 (1988).
50. J. L. Mohler, A. W. Partin, W. D. Lohr & D. S. Coffey, "Nuclear roundness factor measurement for assessment of prognosis of patients with prostatic carcinoma. I. Testing of a digitization system," *J Urology* **139**, 1080–1084 (1988).
51. A. W. Partin *et al.*, "Use of nuclear morphometry, gleason histologic scoring, clinical stage, and age to predict disease-free survival among patients with prostate cancer," *Cancer* **70**, 161–168 (1992).
52. R. W. Veltri, S. Isharwal, M. C. Miller, J. I. Epstein & A. W. Partin, "Nuclear roundness variance predicts prostate cancer progression, metastasis, and death: A prospective evaluation with up to 25 years of follow-up after radical prostatectomy," *Prostate* **70**, 1333–1339 (2010).
53. J. E. Gill & M. M. Jotz, "Further observations on the chemistry of pararosaniline-Feulgen staining," *Histochemistry* **46**, 147–160 (1976).
54. E. Schulte & D. Wittekind, "Standardization of the Feulgen-Schiff technique. Staining characteristics of pure fuchsin dyes; a cytophotometric investigation," *Histochemistry* **91**, 321–331 (1989).
55. E. R. Delong, D. M. Delong & D. I. Clarkepearson, "Comparing the areas under 2 or more correlated receiver operating characteristic curves — a nonparametric approach," *Biometrics* **44**, 837–845 (1988).
56. J. Kowalski, A. Blackford, C. Feng, A. J. Mamelak & D. N. Sauder, "Nested, nonparametric, correlative analysis of microarrays for heterogenous phenotype characterization," *Stat Med* **26**, 1090–1101 (2007).
57. R. W. Veltri *et al.*, "Significant variations in nuclear structure occur between and within Gleason grading patterns 3, 4, and 5 determined by digital image analysis," *Prostate* **67**, 1202–1210 (2007).
58. G. Venkataraman *et al.*, "Morphometric signature differences in nuclei of Gleason pattern 4 areas in Gleason 7 prostate cancer with differing primary grades on needle biopsy," *J Urology* **181**, 88–93; discussion 93–84 (2009).
59. R. W. Veltri, M. C. Miller, A. W. Partin, D. S. Coffey & J. I. Epstein, "Ability to predict biochemical progression using Gleason score and a computer-generated quantitative nuclear grade derived from cancer cell nuclei," *Urology* **48**, 685–691 (1996).
60. S. Isharwal *et al.*, "p300 (histone acetyltransferase) biomarker predicts prostate cancer biochemical recurrence and correlates with changes in epithelia nuclear size and shape," *Prostate* **68**, 1097–1104 (2008).
61. M. A. Khan *et al.*, "Quantitative alterations in nuclear structure predict prostate carcinoma distant metastasis and death in men with biochemical recurrence after radical prostatectomy," *Cancer* **98**, 2583–2591 (2003).
62. R. W. Veltri *et al.*, "Ability to predict metastasis based on pathology findings and alterations in nuclear structure of normal-appearing and cancer peripheral zone epithelium in the prostate," *Clin Cancer Res* **10**, 3465–3473 (2004).

63. S. Doyle, M. Feldman, J. Tomaszewski & A. Madabhushi, "A boosted Bayesian multiresolution classifier for prostate cancer detection from digitized needle biopsies," *IEEE Trans Bio-medical Eng* **59**, 1205–1218 (2012).
64. A. Madabhushi, S. Agner, A. Basavanhally, S. Doyle & G. Lee, "Computer-aided prognosis: Predicting patient and disease outcome via quantitative fusion of multi-scale, multi-modal data," *Computerized Medical Imaging Graphics* **35**, 506–514 (2011).
65. M. Gao, P. Bridgman & S. Kumar, "Computer aided prostate cancer diagnosis using image enhancement and JPEG2000," *P Soc Photo-Opt Ins* **5203**, 323–334 (2003).
66. P. Tiwari, S. Viswanath, G. Lee & A. Madabhushi, "Multi-modal data fusion schemes for integrated classification of imaging and non-imaging biomedical data," *I S Biomed Imaging* 165–168 (2011).
67. W. A. ChristensBarry & A. W. Partin, "Quantitative grading of tissue and nuclei in prostate cancer for prognosis prediction," *J Hopkins Apl Tech D* **18**, 226–233 (1997).
68. A. Almuntashri *et al.*, "Gleason grade-based automatic classification of prostate cancer pathological images," *IEEE Sys Man Cybern* 2696–2701 (2011).
69. C. Demir, S. H. Gultekin & B. Yener, "Augmented cell-graphs for automated cancer diagnosis," *Bioinformatics* **21**, 7–12 (2005).
70. C. Gunduz, B. Yener & S. H. Gultekin, "The cell graphs of cancer," *Bioinformatics* **20**, 145–151 (2004).
71. C. Gunduz-Demir, "Mathematical modeling of the malignancy of cancer using graph evolution," *Math Biosci* **209**, 514–527 (2007).
72. S. Ali, J. Lewis & A. Madabhushi, "Spatially aware cell cluster(SpACCl) graphs: predicting outcome in oropharyngeal p16+ tumors," *Medical Image Computing Computer-Assisted Intervention 2013 Lecture Notes in Computer Science* **8149**, 412–419 (2013).
73. R. Sparks & A. Madabhushi, "Explicit shape descriptors: Novel morphologic features for histopathology classification," *Med Image Anal* **17**, 997–1009 (2013).
74. J. Diamond, N. H. Anderson, P. H. Bartels, R. Montironi & P. W. Hamilton, "The use of morphological characteristics and texture analysis in the identification of tissue composition in prostatic neoplasia," *Hum Pathology* **35**, 1121–1131 (2004).
75. G. Lee *et al.*, "Cell orientation entropy (COrE): Predicting biochemical recurrence from prostate cancer tissue microarrays," *Medical Image Computing Computer-assisted Intervention Int Conf Medical Image Computing Computer-Assisted Intervention* **16**, 396–403 (2013).
76. G. Lee *et al.*, "Co-occurring gland tensors in localized cluster graphs: Quantitative histomorphometry for predicting biochemical recurrence for intermediate grade prostate cancer," *2013 IEEE 10th International Symp Biomedical Imaging (Isbi)*, 113–116 (2013).
77. K. Jafari-Khouzani & H. Soltanian-Zadeh, "Multiwavelet grading of pathological images of prostate," *IEEE Trans Bio-medical Eng* **50**, 697–704 (2003).
78. S. Doyle, M. D. Feldman, N. Shih, J. Tomaszewski & A. Madabhushi, "Cascaded discrimination of normal, abnormal, and confounder classes in histopathology: Gleason grading of prostate cancer," *BMC Bioinformat* **13**, 282 (2012).
79. R. M. Haralick, K. Shanmuga & I. Dinstein, "Textural features for image classification," *IEEE T Syst Man Cyb* **Smc3**, 610–621 (1973).

80. J. P. Monaco *et al.*, "High-throughput detection of prostate cancer in histological sections using probabilistic pairwise Markov models," *Med Image Anal* **14**, 617–629 (2010).
81. G. Lee, R. Sparks, S. Ali, N. N. Shih, M. D. Feldman, E. Spangler, T. Rebbeck, J. E. Tomaszewski, A. Madabhushi, "Co-occuring gland angularity in localized subgraphs: predicting biochemical recurrence in intermediate-risk prostate cancer patients," *PLOS ONE* **9**, e97954 (2014).

Chapter 16

Automated Diagnosis of Diabetic Retinopathy: Fundamentals, Current State of Art and Perspectives

Arturo Aquino

Control and Robotics Research Group,
High Technical School of Engineering,
University of Huelva, La Rábida (Palos de la Frontera),
Huelva, Andalusia, Spain
E-mail: arturo.aquino@diesia.uhu.es

Diabetic retinopathy (DR) is the first cause of blindness in people of working age in the developed countries. In spite of DR not being a curable illness, it can be treated if it is detected in its early stages. However, this early detection is not always possible since DR patients do not perceive symptoms until the illness is in advance stages, when treatment is less effective. This is why diabetic patients are periodically examined in the frame of preventive screening programs. Nevertheless, effectiveness of these preventive protocols is compromised due to the human and material resources needed to manage a huge number of patients needing revisions. This is why, especially over the last two decades, a great effort has been carried out by the scientific community to develop reliable and accurate systems for the automated detection of DR.

On the one hand, this chapter describes the medical and technical fundamentals of the automated detection of DR. On the other hand, outstanding comprehensive systems tested within the frame of screening programs as clinical trials are reviewed in order to assess the current state of art of the topic and its perspectives.

1. Introduction

Diabetic retinopathy (DR) is a chronic retinal disease which nowadays constitutes one of the most common causes of vision loss and blindness.[1,2] Actually, statistics of incidence indicates that DR is the first cause of blindness in people of working age in the industrialized world.[3] DR is a consequence of diabetes-mellitus, illness which produces glucose concentration elevation in blood. This abnormal high glucose concentration damages the eye vessel endothelium provoking the set of damages associated to the illness. Although diabetes affection does not necessarily involve vision impairment, about 2% of the patients affected by this disorder are blind and 10% undergo vision degradation after 15 years of diabetes[4,5] as a consequence of DR complications. The estimated prevalence of diabetes for all age groups worldwide was 2.8% in 2000 and 4.4% in 2030.[6]

Despite DR being not a curable disease, visual impairment can be avoidable in 98% of cases if the illness is detected and treated in its early stages.[7] In this respect, laser photocoagulation has demonstrated to be an effective treatment for preventing major vision loss produced by DR.[8,9] In spite of it, the early illness detection is a difficult task since affected people do not perceive symptoms until visual loss develops, and this usually happens in the later disease stages, when treatment is less effective. This is why population potentially at risk of being affected by DR, i.e. diabetic population, has to be periodically examined by their public health systems in search of early DR signs. However, this preventive action involves a huge challenge for health systems due to the high number of ophthalmologists and material resources needed to attend so many patients needing ophthalmologic revision. Furthermore, this fact ends up being a limiting factor.[10]

DR is diagnosed by means of digital retinal image inspection, and the use of digital images provides the chance of increasing effectiveness of preventive protocols by means of the use of a computerized approach. Concretely, the successful development of a system to automatically filtrate cases of patients not affected by the disease or, even, to automatically grade the illness stage, would reduce the specialists' workload and increase the effectiveness of preventive protocols and early therapeutic treatments. That is why an intensive research has been carried out over the last two decades towards the development of such a system sufficiently accurate and reliable to be included in the mentioned preventive protocols.

This chapter has the aim of being a comprehensive overview of the automated detection of DR. Firstly, the topic is widely described and motivated from a medical point of view. Secondly, the goal of the automated detection of DR is formulated in terms of engineering as it has been faced by the scientific community over the years. Then, once the topic is introduced and formulated, comprehensive systems for the automated detection of DR tested within the frame of screening programs recently presented in the literature are reviewed. Finally, the chapter ends by discussing about short term perspectives of the topic under study.

2. The Retina

The retina is the main eye's membrane involved in the process of vision. It is approximately 0.5 mm thick, lines the internal back of the eye and is composed of a set of layers. The retina is smooth and semi-transparent; it modifies its opacity when is exposed to direct sunlight.

Studying the retinal surface, its frontal view shows three main anatomical features: the optic disc [number (4) in Fig. 1], macula [the macula center, called the fovea, is number (3) in Fig. 1] and vascular tree [numbers (1), (2), (5) and (6) in Fig. 1]. The description of these retinal components is the following:

- Optic disc: the optic disc [see diagram in Fig. 2(a) to follow the description], also called the optic nerve head or papilla, is located on the nasal side of the macula and represents the location where the nerve fibers come together, form the optic nerve, and exit the eye. It is slightly elliptical in shape, with a diameter varying between 1.5 and 2 mm. The optic disc is also the entrance and exit site of the blood vessels that feed the retina. There are no photoreceptors in the optic disc, so it represents the blind spot in the retina. The optic nerve fibers do not occupy the whole area of the optic nerve head as they are located at the optic nerve head border, which leads to an excavation in the center; this excavation resembles a small "cup." When it is visible, the cup appears in white color as a result from exposure of the hyper reflective tissue, the lamina cribrosa. The lamina cribrosa is a continuation of the sclera and provides support to nerve fibers and blood vessels.
- Macula: a round area in the central region of the retina that measures between 3 to 4 mm in diameter. The macula contains mainly cones, so this area is the one providing the most distinct vision and is responsible of central vision.

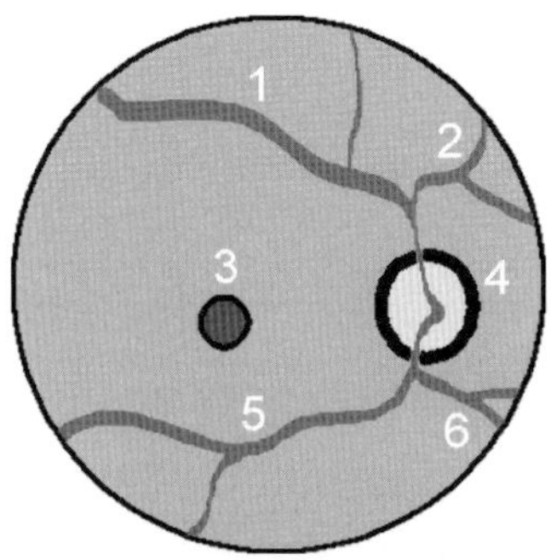

Fig. 1. Diagram of the retinal surface: (4) optic disc, (3) macula center (fovea) and (1), (2), (5), (6) retinal vascular tree: (1) upper temporal blood vessels, (2) upper nasal blood vessels, (5) lower temporal blood vessels and (6) lower nasal blood vessels.

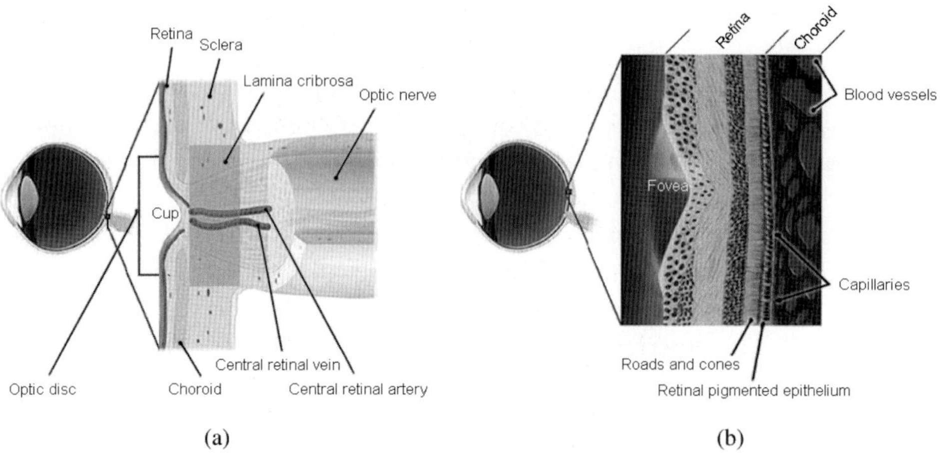

Fig. 2. (a) Cross-sectional optic nerve diagram, (b) cross-sectional macula diagram.

There is a small depression in the center of the macula measuring about 1 mm in diameter and visible as a round dark area called the fovea [see diagram in Fig. 2(b)]. The fovea contains the largest concentration of cone cells and do not contain rods, so it is in charge of our sharp central vision and it is also the main portion of the retina used for color discrimination.

- Vascular tree: is a vascular tree-like connected structure, which nourishes the inner parts of the retina. This vascular structure originates in the optic disc with the central retinal artery and vein [see Fig. 2(a)], which progressively split into many other smaller vessels for covering the retina. Structurally, the retinal vascular tree can be divided into four types of vessels: upper temporal blood vessels [number (1) in Fig. 1], upper nasal blood vessels [number (2) in Fig. 1], lower temporal blood vessels [number (5) in Fig. 1] and lower nasal blood vessels [number (6) in Fig. 1].

A digital image of the retinal surface showing the optic disc, macula and vascular tree is presented in Fig. 3.

3. Diabetic Retinopathy

Metabolism is the process of converting the food we eat into energy. It begins when food is broken down during digestion to create glucose, which is the main source of fuel for the body. Glucose metabolism in the body is controlled by insulin, a hormone produced by the pancreas. When glucose passes into the bloodstream, insulin allows it to get into the cells.

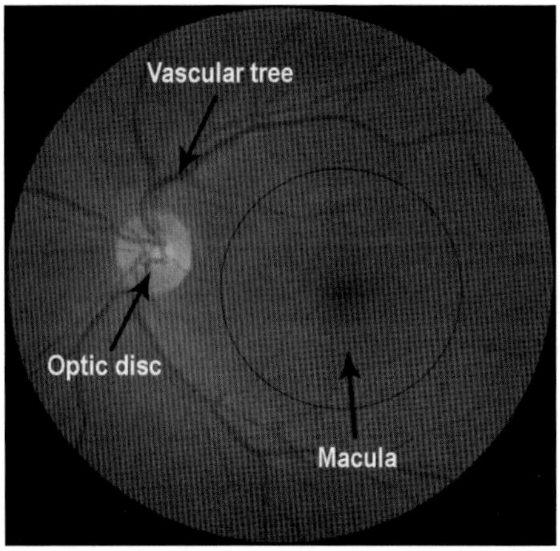

Fig. 3. Digital retinal image showing the optic disc, macula and vascular tree.

Diabetes mellitus, commonly known as diabetes, is a metabolic disorder that interferes with the body's ability to use and store glucose. The determining factor in diabetes is insulin, and people with diabetes present glucose concentration elevation in blood as a consequence of low insulin production, abnormal cell response to insulin or both reasons.

The excess of glucose in blood produced by diabetes damages the macro- and microvascular system, and usually the eye is one of the first places where this becomes apparent. DR is the retinal disease derived from complications caused by the abnormally high level of glucose in blood produced by diabetes and is the most frequent microvascular complication of this disease. When the microvascular system in the eye is progressively damaged, vision loss and, ultimately, blindness can occur. In fact, DR is nowadays the leading ophthalmic pathological cause of blindness among people of working age in the developed countries.[3]

All people affected by diabetes are at risk for the development of DR and most of them will eventually develop the illness. Indeed, although the presence of diabetes does not necessarily involve vision impairment, about 2% of patients affected by this disorder are blind and 10% undergo vision degradation after 15 years of diabetes[4,5] as a consequence of DR complications. The estimated prevalence of diabetes for all age groups worldwide was 2.8% in 2000 and 4.4% in 2030, meaning that the total number of diabetic patients is forecasted to rise from 171 million in 2000 to 366 million in 2030.[6] These figures of incidence make DR, besides a great public health problem, a great economic problem for Administrations since, for instance, costs of ophthalmic chronic complications caused by diabetes exceeded 1 billion dollars in 2007 only in the U.S.[11]

As previously mentioned, DR damages the eye's vascular system due to the abnormally high level of glucose in blood. This vascular damage consists in the deterioration of the vessel endothelium, which results in vessel permeability and fragility increasing. As a consequence, with the progression of the illness and this damage, a set of characteristic and univocal clinical signs of the illness may appear on the retinal surface. Accurate assessment of DR requires the ability to detect and identify the clinical features described as follows (see Fig. 4 for recognizing each feature described below):

- Microaneurysms: these lesions are the first manifestation of DR. Microaneurysms are capillary dilations produced by local weakening of capillary walls that make them to emerge in a balloon-like fashion. They are visible on the retinal surface as tiny round dark red dots and their size varies from 10 to 100 microns in diameter.
- Hemorrhages: the disease and damage progression can produce the burst of microaneurysms, which leaks blood and therefore causes hemorrhages. Retinal hemorrhages can be discernible either as small red dots or blots indistinguishable from microaneurysms, or as larger red flame-shaped patches.
- Exudates: besides the leaking of blood, vessels also leak lipids and proteins causing the appearance of bright spots called exudates. These are typically manifested as yellowish/whitish patches of varying sizes, shapes and locations. The leaking of fluid from vessels can progress producing large exudative areas in the macula, which can provoke its swelling. This complication is called diabetic macular edema (ME) and can seriously affect central vision.

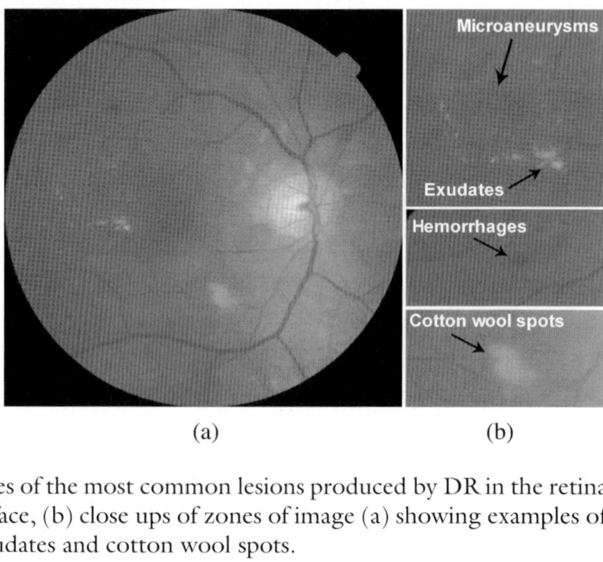

(a) (b)

Fig. 4. Examples of the most common lesions produced by DR in the retina: (a) photography of the retinal surface, (b) close ups of zones of image (a) showing examples of microaneurysms, hemorrhages, exudates and cotton wool spots.

- Cotton wool spots: with the progression of DR and its associated lesions, parts of the retina can be deprived of blood and consequently can suffer ischemia. These ischemic areas are called cotton wool spots and are visible on the retina as fluffy whitish blobs.
- Neovascularization: the appearance of ischemic areas in the retina provokes as response the growing of new vessels to supply the retina with more oxygen. These new vessels are called neovascularizations and have a greater risk of rupturing and causing larger hemorrhages than normal vessels.

In the later stages of DR, as a consequence of the great produced damage, the retina can detach from its supporting tissues, phenomenon known as retinal detachment. This is a serious situation what can lead to permanent vision loss if it is not shortly repaired.

DR is not a curable disease, but it can be treated and controlled if it is detected in its early stages.[3,9] Currently, treatment of DR is still predominantly based on laser photocoagulation. It consists in the application of a strong light beam to certain areas of the retina. For instance, the laser can be directly applied to leaking microaneurysms to prevent further hemorrhaging. Another example is that it can also be applied in a grid pattern over a larger part of the retina with the purpose of reducing the overall need for oxygen and diminishing the load on the damaged microvasculature.

Laser photocoagulation can prevent major vision loss although it cannot restore visual acuity already lost. Therefore, the detection of the illness in its early stages is of vital importance to apply the treatment in the most effective possible way. The main problem of this early illness detection is that DR patients do not perceive symptoms until visual loss develops, and this usually occurs in the later disease stages. This fact has motivated a widely accepted preventive protocol based on the periodical retinal examination of diabetic patients (typically yearly examination),[12–15] which is the population potentially at risk. Concretely, this plan consists in screening sessions where the retinas of both eyes are examined by physicians looking for early signs of DR. If any sign of the illness is found, the patient is referred to an ophthalmologist who decides the necessary treatment. Otherwise, the patient continues attending to the periodical examinations.

The retina is the only part of the human body where the blood vessels can be directly inspected in a non-invasive manner.[16] In the context of DR detection, it is carried out by means of mainly two types of screening methods: ophthalmoscopy and retinal photography. Ophthalmoscopy consists in the direct examination of the retina through the pupil by means of a portable instrument called ophthalmoscope, composed of a light source and a set of

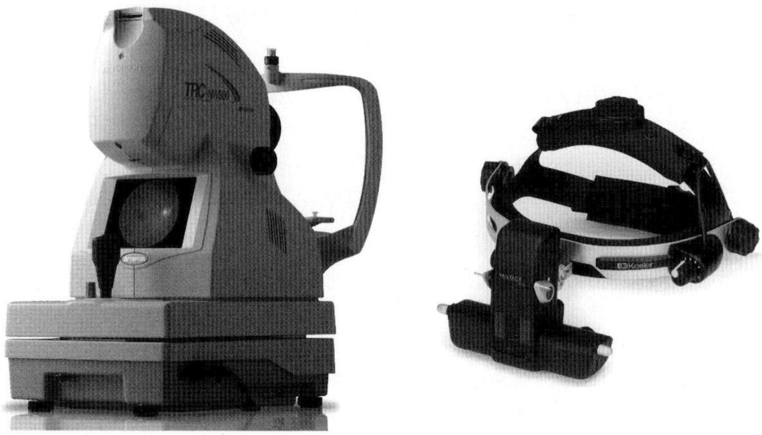

(a) (b)

Fig. 5. Main instruments used for retinal inspection: (a) non-mydriatic retinograph manufactured by Topcon Corporation, (b) indirect ophthalmoscope manufactured by Keeler Instruments Inc.

lenses [Fig. 5(b)]. On the other hand, retinal photography is the procedure of taking digital photos of the retinal surface (retinographies) by using special CCD based digital cameras, called retinographs, with special optics that allow to make color photographs of the eye fundus through the pupil [Fig. 5(a)]. Since the pupil is narrow and does not allow much light to enter the eye, a good strategy to facilitate the retinal visualization is to lower the ambient light intensity. Besides this, ophthalmoscopy and retinal photography can also be performed with mydriasis (dilation of the pupil with eye drops). However, it is important to point out that mydriasis is not needed with modern retinographs in the majority of cases.

Retinal photography offers outstanding advantages for large scale retinal screening. This modality allows instantaneous examination of the retina and quick storage and access of the images. Furthermore, since digital retinographs offer interfaces for connecting them to PCs, acquisition and interpretation stages of the screening can be decoupled. The images can be acquired anywhere and sent instantaneously to a specialized institution for their interpretation. An example of such a screening program is the Andalusian Comprehensive Plan for the Prevention of Diabetes.[17] This plan includes periodical retinal examinations of the diabetic population. Thus, this large population is screened in primary health care centers of the Andalusian Health Service by physicians. Images are acquired on site and sent over the internet to a central server. Then, a trained reader specialized in DR logs into this server for grading the images.

Patients needing to be attended by an ophthalmologist for further investigation or needing to attend the screening sessions more frequently are notified.

Regarding classification of DR, two different approaches have emerged during the last years. They may be called: full disease classifications and population screening classifications. The main differences between both types of classifications are their aim and complexity. A brief description of both types of classifications is the following:

- Full disease classifications: classifications in this category are aimed to be used by ophthalmologists. They are complex classifications considering a great number of levels of DR condition to cover the full range of the illness exhaustively. The main classification in this group is the extended Airlie House classification developed by the "Early Treatment Diabetic Retinopathy Study Research Group."[18] Other full disease classifications are mainly modifications of this one. The cited classification distinguishes a great number of DR stages grouped into two global stages of severity. The first stage, called Non-proliferative Diabetic Retinopathy (NPDR), refers to the earliest retinal changes caused by DR. In this stage, a person affected by DR can present microaneurysms, retinal hemorrhages, exudates and cotton wool spots. Vision loss can develop in this stage as a consequence of ME or macular isquemia. On the other hand, the appearance of neovascularization marks the beginning of the second and severe stage of DR called Proliferative Diabetic Retinopathy (PDR). In this stage, hemorrhages in the vitreous and, ultimately, retinal detachment can occur.
- Population screening classifications: these classifications are designed to be used in large screening programs. They are simplified gradings based on the previous ones that allow to be more efficient in the context of such programs. The main goal of these classifications is not to grade DR accurately, but to assess when a patient presents the illness in a stage sufficiently severe to merit referral for expert ophthalmological opinion and possible treatment. Typically, these classifications are designed by countries depending on their needs to make their screening programs viable.

An example of this type of classification is the one designed within the framework of the MESSIDOR-Techno-Vision Project. This classification grades DR into four stages and, additionally, proposes a classification to evaluate the risk of ME. The two simplified gradings were elaborated by experts from the recommendations provided by: Alfediam (French association for the study of diabetes and metabolic diseases),[19,20] ETDRS (Early Treatment Diabetic Retinopathy Study)[18] and Diabetic Retinopathy Screening Services in

Scotland.[21] The descriptions of the proposed gradings are:

- DR grade:
  - $*$ 0 (Normal): $(\mu A = 0)$ and $(H = 0)$.
  - $*$ 1: $(0 < \mu A <= 5)$ and $(H = 0)$.
  - $*$ 2: $((5 < \mu A < 15)$ or $(0 < H < 5))$ and $(NV = 0)$.
  - $*$ 3: $(\mu A >= 15)$ or $(H >= 5)$ OR $(NV = 1)$.

where μA is the number of microaneurysms, H is the number of hemorrhages, and $NV = \{0; 1\}$ denotes the absence or presence of neovascularization, respectively.

- Risk of ME:
  - $*$ 0 (No risk): no visible hard exudates.
  - $*$ 1: shortest distance between macula and hard exudates $>$ one optic disc diameter.
  - $*$ 2: shortest distance between macula and hard exudates $<=$ one optic disc diameter.

4. Automated Detection of Diabetic Retinopathy

The benefits and cost-effectiveness of screening programs for early detection of DR are well-recognized.[22] However, their effective development is a great challenge for health systems as a consequence of the great amount of human and material resources needed to put them into place.[10] These difficulties, and the generalized use of retinal photography in screening programs, has motivated during the last 20 or 25 years an outstanding effort in the investigation of algorithms for the diagnosis of DR sufficiently accurate to be able to implement them into these programs. If an automated system could be able to exclude a large number of those patients not affected by DR, it would reduce the workload of the specialists and thus would enhance preventive protocols. Actually, this reduction could reach about 70%, since normal fundi predominates in DR-screened populations approximately in this magnitude. Furthermore, it would also result in economic benefits for public health systems, since cost-effective treatments associated to early illness detection lead to remarkable cost savings.[23,24]

The construction of a generic comprehensive system for the diagnosis of DR may be structurally and logically divided into four general phases. Each of these phases produces as a result a logical module of the system which gives support to its underlying modules. Figure 6 shows a flow diagram of

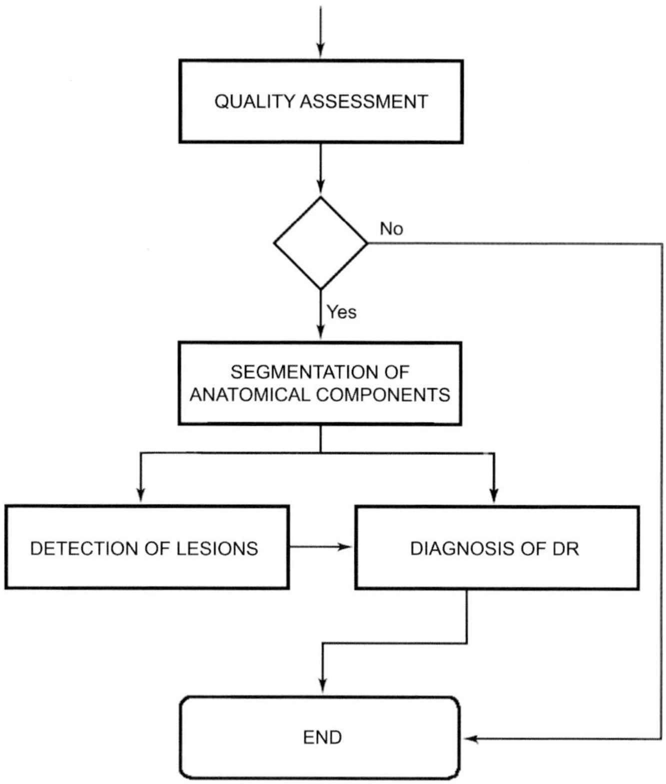

Fig. 6. Flow diagram of a generic system for the automated diagnosis of DR.

a generic comprehensive system for the automated diagnosis of DR based on the four phases, which are detailed below. This structure results in a strong unidirectional coupling between modules, what argues for a bottom-up development of the system. In this diagram, the modules resulting from the phases can be identified and it can be checked how these modules interact in an unidirectional way from the bottom to the top.

The four phases for the construction of a system for DR diagnosis are described as follows:

4.1. *Image Quality Assessment*

Since retinal images are taken using retinographs, the image acquisition is completely decoupled from the system. Many factors can affect negatively the acquisition process and can give as result images without enough quality to be processed (see Fig. 7). For example, eye movement at the moment of retinography capture may lead to blurred images, or insufficient pupil dilation

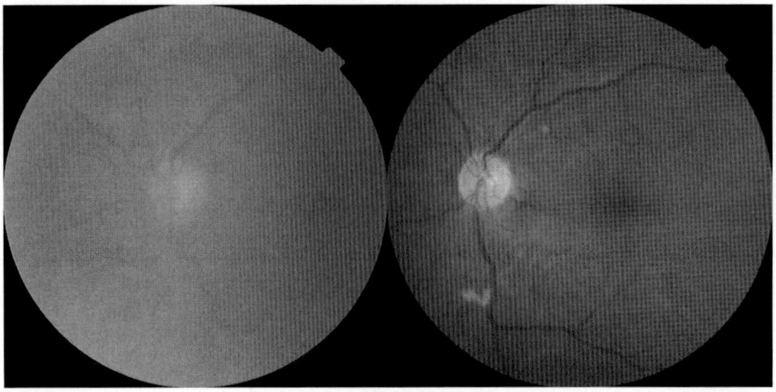

(a) (b)

Fig. 7. Examples of different image quality as consequence of the acquisition process: (a) blurred image, (b) image suitable to be processed.

as a consequence of inappropriate illumination or inefficient mydriasis (if it is needed) may produce too dark and low contrasted images. With all these considerations, this phase defines the preconditions of the system and its entry point. The way the system receives an image, and the decision rules to assess if this one has enough quality to be successfully processed, are designed and implemented in this phase.

In spite of the availability of general purpose algorithms for image quality assessment which can be used for the goal of this phase, specific algorithms for assessing quality of retinal images have been developed and can be found in the literature.[25–33]

4.2. *Segmentation of the Main Anatomical Components of the Retina*

The success key for the construction of an automated system for DR diagnosis is the accurate detection and identification of lesions produced by the illness (this is faced in the following phase). These lesions must be detected on a highly variable retinal image that includes: the optic disc, vascular tree, macula, and distractors such as choroidal vessels, laser scars or light artifacts, among other. Furthermore, other features inherent to the retina, such as differences of pigmentation in different ethnic races, increase this variability.[34] This fact has motivated a widely used structured approach in which the main anatomical components in the retina are segmented and used as landmarks. Thus, their *a priori*-known anatomical features and relationships between them are exploited to increase confidence in the classification of each object.

4.2.1. *Optic disc segmentation*

Segmentation of the optic disc plays an important role in many algorithms designed to identify other retinal features. For example, its segmentation and identification is valuable to locate the macula by making use of the known relatively constant distance between them.[35–37] Since the vascular tree emerges from the optic disc, knowledge about its location can also help identify the vasculature origin.[37,38] Another example of the use of the optic disc in the mentioned structured approach is that, since color features of the optic disc can be similar to those of retinal exudates, optic disc segmentation can be exploited to decrease false positives in the detection of these lesions.[39]

For the reasons explained above, many optic disc segmentation algorithms have been developed and published, increasing progressively the robustness and accuracy of the task (Fig. 8 shows an example of OD segmentation).[35,38,40–49]

4.2.2. *Vascular tree segmentation*

Regarding retinal vessels segmentation, it is also a key preprocessing in the development of automated DR diagnosis systems. For instance, the vasculature origin can be used to locate the optic disc.[50–52] Another outstanding application of the vascular tree segmentation is that it provides valuable information about the approximated location of the fovea. It is a known anatomical feature that the fovea is approximately located at a known distance from the optic disc following an imaginary line separating the upper and lower regions of the retina, being this line determined by the upper and lower vessels of the vascular tree. Therefore, the segmentation of the vascular tree provides that line and can be

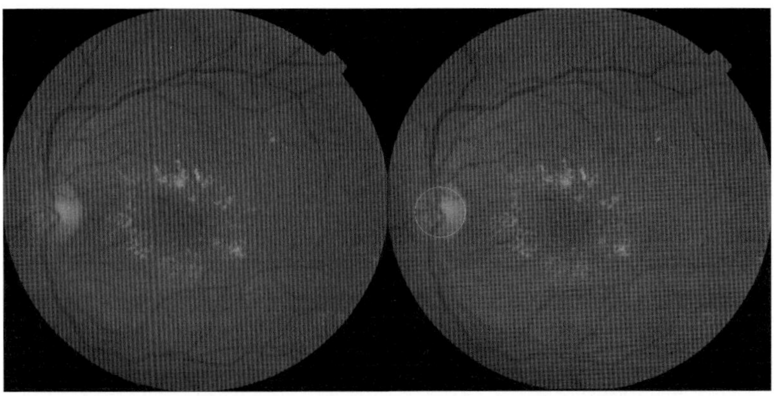

(a) (b)

Fig. 8. Optic disc segmentation: (a) original retinal image, (b) image (a) with the optic disc segmented.

used to locate the fovea.[36,53] On the other hand, vascular tree segmentation also provides knowledge about blood vessels location. This information can be used to reduce the number of false positives in microaneurysm and hemorrhage detection due to color similarity.[54–57] Besides these applications, vascular tree segmentation can also be valuable to detect advanced signs of the illness such as the presence of neovascularization or vessels tortuosity increasing.[58]

Retinal vessels segmentation may be the topic within the frame of automated DR detection that has generated more publications in the literature (a recent and detailed review of the state of art can be found in Ref. [59]). Some of the most relevant works are those in Refs. [35], [60]–[73]. A vascular tree segmentation example can be checked in Fig. 9.

4.2.3. *Macula segmentation*

As was previously commented, the macula is responsible for central vision and, concretely, the fovea is in charge of sharp central vision. Because of this important function of the macula in vision, the distance at which lesions produced by DR are located from this area influences their clinical relevance. This is why the macula segmentation is not a preprocessing, but an unavoidable requirement in the development of DR diagnosis systems. Some outstanding works related to macula segmentation are those presented in Refs. [35]–[37], [53], [74]–[77].

It should be highlighted that, at this point, a tool for assisting ophthalmologists to grade DR more comfortably and can quickly be obtained. These specialists place a grading grid in the image centered on the fovea (this grid

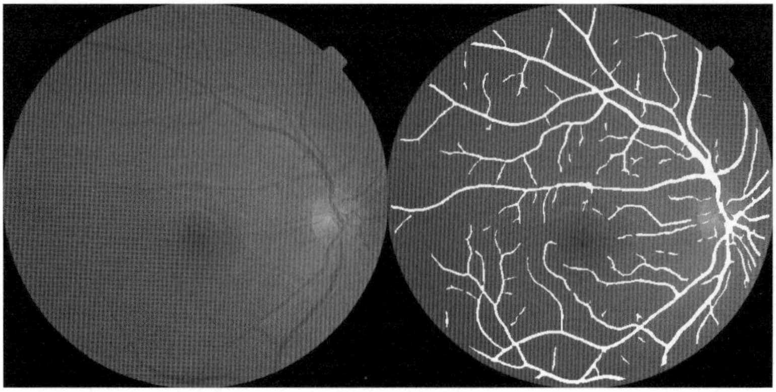

(a) (b)

Fig. 9. Vascular tree segmentation: (a) original retinal image, (b) image resulting from the segmentation of the vascular tree.

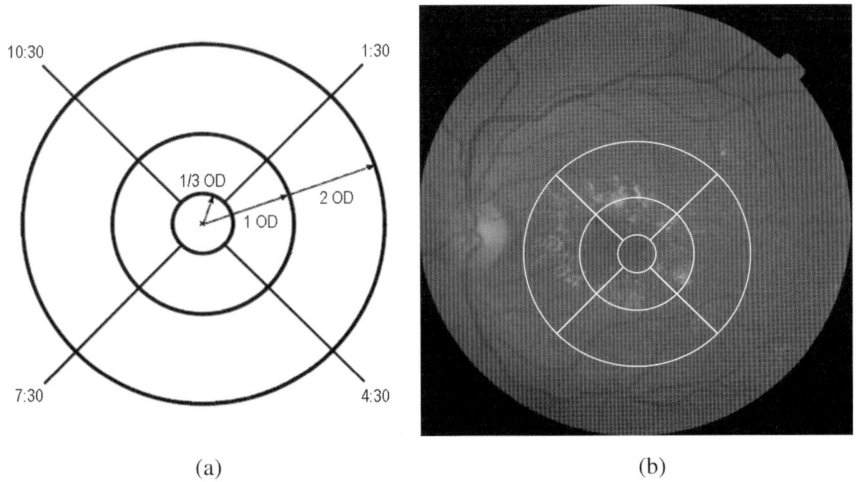

Fig. 10. Automated macular grading grid placing: (a) macular grading grid, (b) macular grading grid automatically placed thanks to the information obtained from the segmentation of the main retinal anatomical components.

was defined by the ETDRS research group[18]). This grading grid divides the retinal image into ten subfields as presented in Fig. 10(a). The radii of the three fovea-centered circles from the innermost to the outermost correspond to (1/3) optic disc diameter, 1 optic disc diameter, and 2 optic disc diameter, respectively. Once the grading grid is placed, illness condition is assessed by counting lesions, taking into account that their relevance varies according to where they are located. This relevance decreases from the central subfield to the far temporal subfield. Since at the end of the phase is being described, the optic disc, vascular tree and macula are segmented, a tool for automatically placing the macular grading grid can be easily obtained. By this way, ophthalmologists could automatically get the image in Fig. 10(b) for its manual diagnosis.

4.3. *Detection of Lesions Produced by DR*

Taking advantage of the information previously obtained, the aim of this phase is the identification of DR signs by means of the analysis of the image. As was discussed, automated detection of DR is especially interesting in its early stages, when lesions are not still too severe and evident to non-expert eyes. Thus, the system could help physicians in the preventive protocols to decrease the number of patients unnecessarily referred to ophthalmologists, producing, by this way, the benefits already discussed here. Taking this into account, the main goal in this phase is the detection of microaneurysms, hemorrhages and exudates.

There are two main challenges to overcome in the present task. The first one is the development of algorithms capable of identifying the mentioned lesions. The second challenge derives from the fact that the image to be analyzed may come from a healthy patient or from a patient affected by the illness. Therefore, the system can produce false positives, if it detects non-existing lesions, and false negatives in the contrary case. Therefore, the second challenge is the minimization of both types of errors.

4.3.1. *Detection of microaneurysms*

Microaneurysms are the earliest signs of DR, hence, their accurate detection and segmentation are of vital importance for automated early DR detection. They look like very small red dots on the retinal surface. On one hand, their invariable shape and color are very clear — usable features to discover them and have been widely used in the literature. Nonetheless, their tiny size makes their accurate detection a very challenging task (see Fig. 11). Some outstanding published works on microaneurysms detection are in Refs. [54], [55], [78]–[82].

4.3.2. *Detection of hemorrhages*

Hemorrhages occur due to microaneurysms explosion or vessels breaking. This is why they are very unspecific in shape and size, being their only *a priori*-known feature their red color. Moreover, tiny hemorrhages may be very difficult to

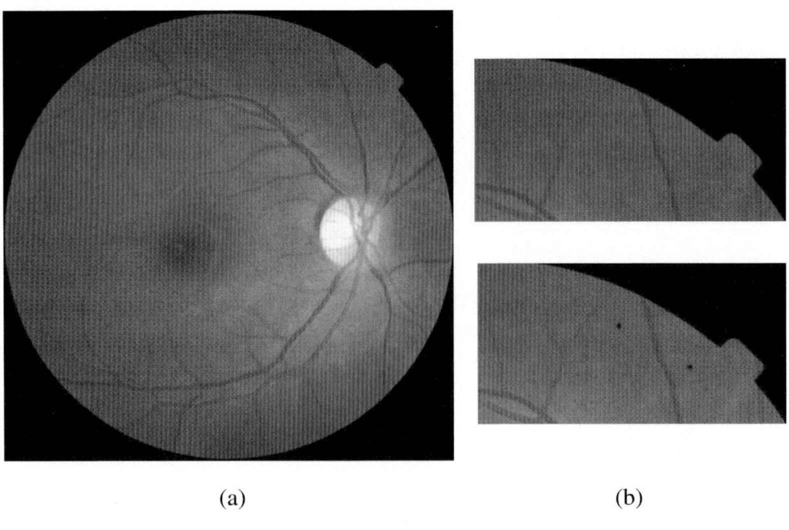

(a) (b)

Fig. 11. Detection of microaneurysms: (a) retinography of a patient affected by DR in early stages, (b) the upper image on the right is a fragment of (a), and the bottom image on the right is the same subimage with two microaneurysms segmented.

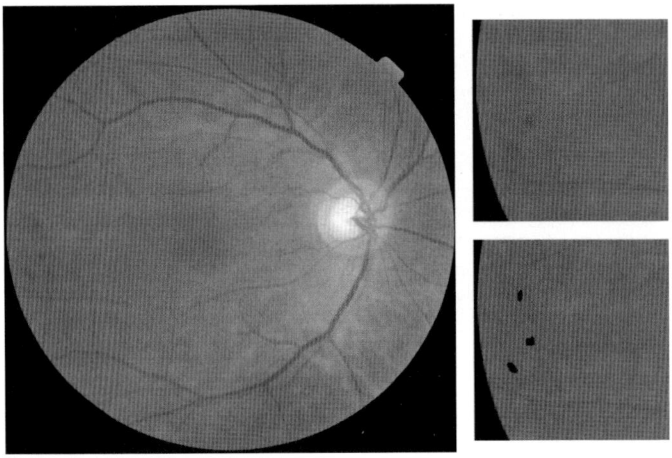

(a) (b)

Fig. 12. Detection of hemorrhages: (a) original image of a patient affected by DR, (b) the upper image on the right shows a hemorrhage-containing subimage, and the bottom image on the right shows segmentation of the lesions.

distinguish from microaneurysms. Probably for these reasons, the literature is sparse in specific works for detecting and segmenting only hemorrhages, and existing works use to face the problem along with the segmentation of microaneurysms; it is usually known as detection of red lesions.[56,57,83] An example of hemorrhage detection is shown in Fig. 12.

4.3.3. *Detection of exudates*

These lesions appear on the retinal surface as yellowish or whitish patches well contrasted from the retinal tissue with variable size. As was commented, their color may be similar to that of the optic disc, but in this phase, this anatomical component is segmented and therefore can be discarded. Therefore, attending to exudate features, this is probably the lesion produced by DR less challenging to be segmented. However, this aspect does not underestimate the importance of exudates detection since, besides being important for DR detection, it also plays a key role in assessing risk of ME. Some works focused on exudates detection can be found in Refs. [39], [44], [53], [83]–[90], and an example is presented in Fig. 13.

4.4. *Implementation of an Expert System*

This is the last development phase of the system. At this point, the image was accepted to be processed, the retinal anatomical components were segmented

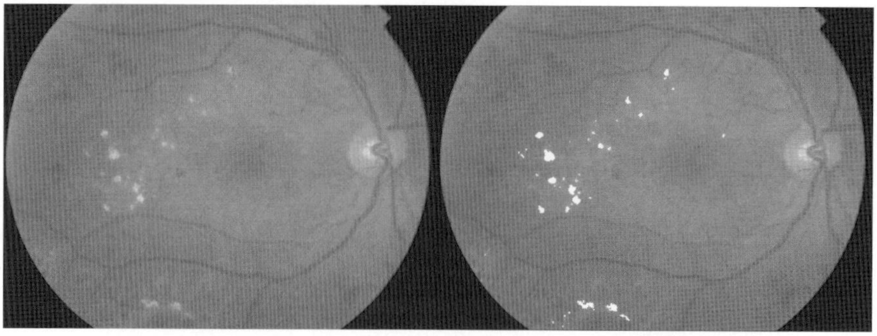

(a) (b)

Fig. 13. Detection of exudates: (a) original image, (b) image with the exudates segmented.

and results of the image analysis for the identification of lesions are available. Therefore, in this phase, an expert system for the identification of DR is designed and implemented. Taking all the information resulting from the previous phases, this expert system has to provide a diagnosis of the illness. The complexity of this system is the main design decision. It can be implemented simply as a "disease/no disease" decision system, as a system based on any population screening classification or, even, as a system based on any complex full disease classification.

5. Current State of Art of Comprehensive Automated Systems for DR Detection

The aim of this section is to assess the current maturity level achieved by the scientific community in automated segmentation of DR. To this effect, complete systems (those implementing the generic system described in Fig. 6) that have been checked on large populations within the frame of screening programs as clinical trials are reviewed here. It is important to point out that, the no inclusion here of all other commendable works that have contributed along the years to obtain advances in the field, should only be understood only as a consequence of the goal of this study.

A "disease/no disease" decision system was presented by Philip *et al.*[91] in 2007. The system implemented a neural network for patient classification attending to the presence or absence of red lesions (microaneurysms and hemorrhages) to produce a "disease/no disease" response. This system was tested on images acquired in the Grampian Diabetes Retinal Screening Program in North-East Scotland. Two sets of images were collected from screening sessions between the years 2003 and 2004. A first set of 1067 retinographies was used to train the neural network, and another set of 14406 separate images from 6722 patients was employed to test the system; 29.3% of those patients were DR-affected. The system obtained 0.97 sensitivity and 0.875 specificity detecting image technical failures. With respect to disease detection excluding technical failures, results were 0.802 sensitivity, this is, 19.8% of images from DR-affected eyes wrongly classified, and 0.879 specificity, implies that 12.1% of images from healthy eyes were erroneously classified. The area under ROC curve of the system was not reported. Authors calculated that these results would allow a grading workload reduction of 60%. Fleming *et al.*[92] presented in 2010 a larger evaluation of this system with the goal of evaluating its performance when used in other Scottish screening centers. 78601 images from 33535 patients attended in screening centers in Glasgow and Fife between 1st January 2007 and 31st January 2008 were used for this purpose. The system detected 99.8% of ungradable images and obtained 0.978 sensitivity and 0.411 specificity (figures calculated from results in the paper but not reported directly therein), statistics given in terms of patients; the area under ROC curve was not reported. Authors calculated from this study that 36.3% of patients could be removed from manual grading workload.

In 2008, Abràmoff *et al.*[93] presented a system for the automated detection of DR built from algorithms previously developed and published by them. The proposal was also a "disease/no disease" system based on the detection of microaneurysms, hemorrhages, exudates and cotton wool spots. This system extracted several features from the image under evaluation and, using them, created two probabilities: the probability that an exam had sufficient quality for evaluation, and the probability that an exam showed referable DR. These probabilities were ultimately thresholded at an optimum threshold value, calculated to obtain the maximum sensitivity and specificity in the system, deciding an illness presence/absence response. The system performance was evaluated within the frame of the EyeCheck project for online DR detection in the Netherlands. It was tested on 10000 images from a group of 5692 patients. 2311 of those 10000 images were detected by the system as not having sufficient quality to be processed. The resting 7689 were analyzed by the system obtaining 0.84 sensitivity, 0.64 specificity and an area under ROC curve of 0.84. These figures indicate that 16% of images affected by DR were erroneously classified as normal, and that 36% of healthy images were erroneously recommended for ophthalmic revision as affected by DR. Authors concluded from these results that automated grading software could not yet be recommended for clinical practice, as 27% of their false negatives involved severe forms of DR or neovascularisation.

Table 1. Summarized details of complete systems for DR detection checked on large populations within the frame of screening programs as clinical trials.

Authors	Screening program/ project	Country	Images (patients)	System description	Se	Sp
Philip *et al.*[91]	Grampian Diabetes Retinal Screening Program	United Kingdom	14406 (6722)	"disease/no disease"	0.802	0.879
Fleming *et al.*[93]	Grampian Diabetes Retinal Screening Program	United Kingdom	78601 (33535)	"disease/no disease"	0.978*	0.411*
Abràmoff *et al.*[92]	EyeCheck project for online DR detection	Netherlands	7689 (5692)	"disease/no disease"	0.84	0.64
Dupas *et al.*[94]	MESSIDOR project	France	749 (-) for DR grading/581 (-) for assessing risk of ME	System based on a screening population classification. Four levels for DR and three for risk of ME	DR: 0.839/ Risk of ME: 0.728	DR: 0.727/ Risk of ME: 0.708

*Figures calculated from results in the paper but not reported directly therein.

Dupas *et al.* (2010)[94] developed a system for DR and risk of ME detection based on the population screening classification described in Section III. The system detected red lesions and exudates mainly using mathematical morphology and, according to the illness classification, graded images. This work was a result of the French MESSIDOR project, which collected a database of 1200 retinographies with the aim of developing and evaluating a computer-assisted diagnostic system for the detection and grading of DR as well as estimation of the risk of ME. The images were taken in three hospitals in Brest, Paris and Saint-Étienne. Once the system was developed, for its evaluation and improving, the 962 images acquired with pupil dilation were selected from the total 1200 in the database, since algorithms for exudates and red lesions detection were designed for this kind of images. From these 962 retinographies, 201 were selected for system improving and the resting 761 were used to evaluate the system performance for DR grading and risk of ME evaluation. With respect to DR grading evaluation, 316 images were manually classified as "normal" (DR grade >0) and the resting 445 images were classified as "abnormal" (DR grade >0). The system was able to classify 749 of the 761 images (98.4%), and obtained a sensitivity of 0.839 (16.1% of DR-affected images wrongly classified) and a specificity of 0.727 (27.3% of healthy images wrongly classified). Regarding risk of ME evaluation, 581 images were manually diagnosed as "normal" and the resting 180 images were considered to be under risk of ME. The system was able to grade all images and obtained a sensitivity and specificity of 0.728 (27.2% of images with risk of ME wrongly classified) and 0.708, respectively (29.2% of images without risk of ME wrongly classified). The area under ROC curve of the system was not reported. Authors of this work informed in their publication that the presented system was going to be integrated into the multicentre OPHDIAT telemedical network developed for DR screening in France to reduce physicians workload in manual grading.

Table 1 summarizes features and results of all systems described above.

6. Conclusion

The first work describing an automated methodology for segmenting microaneurysms in retinal images with the goal of DR detection was published in 1984 by Baudoin *et al.*[95] This early work used digitalized angiographic images. The popularization of the use of color digital retinal images and the development of digital image analysis, along with the increasing incidence of DR and the consolidation of screening programs, produced in the 90's an explosion in the automated DR detection research field. Since then, many researchers around the world have made an enormous effort for continuously increasing accuracy of algorithms for the segmentation of the retinal anatomical components and lesions associated to DR. It is clear that in the recent years, the field seems to have achieved an important maturity. Complete systems for the automated detection of the illness have been checked in “real” conditions, this is, within the frame of DR screening programs as clinical trials. Results of these experiences show that automated DR detection systems have achieved comparable performance to a single DR human expert. This fact indicates that their successful integration in screening programs will quite probably take place sooner rather than later. An evidence of this is that some groups have moved toward software commercialization.

References

1. D. Pascolini and S. P. Mariotti, “Global estimates of visual impairment: 2010,” *Brit J Ophthalmol* **96**, 614–618 (2012).
2. World Health Organization, *Action plan for the prevention of blindness and visual impairment 2009–2013.* (World Health Organization, 2010).
3. H. Taylor and J. Keeffe, “Costs of mobile screening for diabetic retinopathy: A practical framework for rural populations,” *Br J Ophthalmol* **85**, 261–266 (2001).
4. R. Klein, S. M. Meuer, S. E. Moss and B. E. Klein, “Retinal microaneurysm counts and 10-year progression of diabetic retinopathy,” *Arch Ophthalmol* **113**, 1386–1391 (1995).
5. P. Massin, A. Erginay and A. Gaudric, *Rétinopathie Diabétique.* Elsevier, Editions scientifiques of medicales, Paris (2000).
6. S. Wild, G. Roglic, A. Green, R. Sicree and H. King, “Global prevalence of diabetes: Estimates for the year 2000 and projections for 2030,” *Diabetes Care* **27**, 1047–1053 (2004).
7. H. R. Taylor, “Eye care for the community,” *Clin Exp Ophthalmol* **30**, 151–154 (2002).
8. H. R. Taylor and J. E. Keeffe, “World blindness: A 21st century perspective,” *Br J Ophthalmol* **85**, 261–266 (2001).
9. S. J. Lee, C. A. McCarty, H. R. Taylor and J. E. Keeffe, “Costs of mobile screening for diabetic retinopathy: A practical framework for rural populations,” *Aust J Rural Health* **8**, 186–192 (2001).
10. J. Mason, “National screening for diabetic retinopathy: Clear vision needed,” *Diabet Med* **20**, 959–961 (2003).
11. American Diabetes Association, “Economic costs of diabetes in the U.S. in 2007,” *Diabetes Care* **31**, 596–615 (2008).
12. G. Bresnick, D. Mukamel, J. Dickinson and D. Cole, “A screening approach to the surveillance of patients with diabetes for the presence of vision-threatening retinopathy,” *Opthalmology* **107**, 19–24 (2000).
13. Early Treatment Diabetic Retinopathy Study Research Group, “Early photocoagulation for diabetic retinopathy: Etdrs report 9,” *Ophthalmology* **98**, 766–785 (1991).

14. D. Fong, L. Aiello, T. Gardner, G. King, G. Blankenship, J. Cavallerano, F. Ferris and R. Klein, "Diabetic retinopathy," *Diabetes Care* **26**, 226–229 (2003).
15. J. Kinyoun, F. Barton, M. Fisher, L. Hubbard, L. Aiello and F. Ferris, "Ophthalmoscopy versus photography-early treatment diabetic retinopathy study report number 5," *Ophthalmology* **96**, 746–750 (1989).
16. S. Rassam, V. Patel, O. Brinchmann-Hansen, O. Engvold and E. Kohner, "Accurate vessel width measurement from fundus photographs: A new concept," *Br J Ophthalmol* **78**, 24–29 (1994).
17. M. Aguilar Diosdado, M. Amo Alfonso, C. Lama Herrera and E. Mayoral Sánchez, *II Plan Integral de Diabetes de Andalucía: 2009–2013.* Junta de Andalucía publications, Consejería de Salud, Andalucía, Spain (2009).
18. Early Treatment Diabetic Retinopathy Study Research Group, "Grading diabetic retinopathy from stereoscopic color fundus photographs — an extension of the modified airlie house classification. etdrs report number 10," *Ophthalmology* **98**, 786–806 (1991).
19. P. Massin, K. Angioi-Duprez, F. Bacin, B. Cathelineau, G. Cathelineau, G. Chaine, G. Coscas, J. Flament, J. Sahel, P. Turut, P. Guillausseau and A. Gaudric, "Recommandations de l'alfediam pour le dépistage et la surveillance de la rétinopathie diabétique," *Diabetes Metab* **22**, 203–209 (1996).
20. P. Massin, K. Angioi-Duprez, F. Bacin, B. Cathelineau, G. Cathelineau, G. Chaine, G. Coscas, J. Flament, J. Sahel, P. Turut, P. Guillausseau and A. Gaudric, "Recommandations de l'alfediam pour le dépistage et la surveillance de la rétinopathie diabétique," *J Fr Ophtalmol* **20**, 302–310 (1997).
21. Diabetic Retinopathy Screening Services in Scotland, *Diabetic retinopathy screening: Annex E. Scottish diabetic retinopathy grading scheme.* The Scottish Government Publications: http://www.scotland.gov.uk/Publications/2003/07/17638/23088, Scotland, U.K. (2003).
22. J. Javitt, L. Aiello, Y. Chiang, F. Ferris, J. Canner and S. Greenfield, "Preventative eye care in people with diabetes is cost-saving to the federal government: implications for health-care reform," *Diabetes Care* **17**, 909–917 (1994).
23. American Academy of Ophthalmology Retina Panel, *Preferred Practice Pattern Guidelines. Diabetic retinopathy.* Diabetic retinopathy, San Francisco, CA, American Academy of Ophthalmology, available at: http://www.aao.org/ppp (2008).
24. D. Lairson, J. Pugh, A. Kapadia, R. Lorimor, J. Jacobson and R. Velez, "Cost effectiveness of alternative methods for diabetic retinopathy screening," *Diabetes Care* **15**, 1369–1377 (1992).
25. S. Lee and Y. Wang, "Automatic retinal image quality assessment and enhancement," *Proc of SPIE Image Processing* (1999) 1581–1590.
26. M. Lalonde, L. Gagnon and M.-C. Boucher, "Automatic visual quality assessment in optical fundus images," *Proc of Vision Interface* (2001).
27. A. Fleming, S. Philip, K. Goatman, J. Olson, P. Sharp, "Automated assessment of diabetic retinal image quality based on clarity and field definition," *Investigat Ophthalmol Vis Sci* **47**, 1120–1125 (2006).
28. J. Lowell, A. Hunter, M. Habib and D. Steel, "Automated Quantification of Fundus Image Quality," *Proc of the 3rd European Medical and Biological Engineering Conference* 1–5 (2005).

29. M. Niemeijer, M. D. Abràmoff and B. van Ginneken, "Image structure clustering for image quality verification of color retina images in diabetic retinopathy screening," *Medical Image Analysis* **10**, 888–898 (2006).
30. J. Paulus, J. Meier, R. Bock, J. Hornegger and G. Michelson, "Automated quality assessment of retinal fundus photos," *Int J Comp Assisted Radiology Surgery* **5**, 557–564 (2010).
31. H. Davis, S. Russell, E. Barriga, M. Abramòff and P. Soliz, "Vision-based, real-time retinal image quality assessment," *Proc 22nd IEEE Int Symp Comput-Based Med Syst* 1–6 (2009).
32. H. Bartling, P. Wanger and L. Martin, "Automated quality evaluation of digital fundus photographs," *Acta Ophthalmologica* **87**, 643–647 (2009).
33. A. Hunter, J. A. Lowell, M. Habib, B. Ryder, A. Basu and D. Steel, "An automated retinal image quality grading algorithm, in: Engineering in Medicine and Biology Society," *Proc Engineering in Medicine and Biology Society* EMBC, Annual International Conference of the IEEE 5955–5958 (2011).
34. D. Usher, M. Dumskyj, M. Himaga, T. Williamson, S. Nussey and J. Boyce, "Automated detection of diabetic retinopathy in digital retinal images: A tool for diabetic retinopathy screening," *Diabet Med* **21**, 84–90 (2003).
35. C. Sinthanayothin, J. F. Boyce, H. L. Cook and T. H. Williamson, "Automated localisation of the optic disc, fovea, and retinal blood vessels from digital colour fundus images," *Br J Ophthalmol* **83**, 902–910 (1999).
36. K. Tobin, E. Chaum, V. Govindasamy and T. Karnowski, "Detection of anatomic structures in human retinal imagery," *IEEE Trans Med Imag* **26**, 1729–1739 (2007).
37. L. Gagnon, M. Lalonde., M. Beaulieu and M.-C. Boucher, "Procedure to detect anatomical structures in optical fundus images," *Proc SPIE Med Imaging: Image Processing* 1218–1225 (2011).
38. H. Li and O. Chutatape, "Automatic location of optic disc in retinal images," *Proc IEEE Int Conf Image Process* 837–840 (2001).
39. A. Osareh, M. Mirmehdi, B. Thomas and R. Markham, "Automated identification of diabetic retinal exudates in digital colour images," *Br J Ophthalmol* **87**, 1220–1223 (2003).
40. J. Lowell, A. Hunter, D. Steel, A. Basu, R. Ryder, E. Fletcher and L. Kennedy, "Optic nerve head segmentation," *IEEE Trans Med Imag* **23**, 256–264 (2004).
41. J. Xu, O. Chutatape, E. Sung, C. Zheng and P. C. T. Kuan, "Optic disk feature extraction via modified deformable model technique for glaucoma analysis," *Pattern Recognit* **40**, 2063–2076 (2007).
42. M. Lalonde, M. Beaulieu and L. Gagnon, "Fast and robust optic disk detection using pyramidal decomposition and Hausdorff-based template matching," *IEEE Trans Med Imag* **20**, 1193–1200 (2001).
43. T. Walter and J. C. Klein, "Segmentation of color fundus images of the human retina: Detection of the optic disc and the vascular tree using morphological techniques," *Proc 2nd Int Symp Med Data Anal* 282–287 (2001).
44. A. W. Reza, C. Eswaran and S. Hati, "Automatic tracing of optic disc and exudates from color fundus images using fixed and variable thresholds," *J Med Syst* **33**, 73–80 (2008).
45. M. D. Abràmoff, W. L. M. Alward, E. C. Greenlee, L. Shuba, C. Y. Kim, J. H. Fingert and Y. H. Kwon, "Automated segmentation of the optic disc from stereo color photographs using physiologically plausible features," *Invest Ophthalmol* **48**, 1665–1673 (2007).

46. A. Aquino, M. E. Gegundez-Arias and D. Marin, "Detecting the optic disc boundary in digital fundus images using morphological, edge detection, and feature extraction techniques," *IEEE Trans Med Imag* **29**, 1860–1869 (2010).
47. S. Lu, "Accurate and efficient optic disc detection and segmentation by a circular transformation," *IEEE Trans Med Imag* **30**, 2126–2133 (2011).
48. C. Muramatsu, T. Nakagawa, A. Sawada, Y. Hatanaka, T. Hara, T. Yamamoto and H. Fujita, "Automated segmentation of optic disc region on retinal fundus photographs: Comparison of contour modeling and pixel classification methods," *Comput Methods Programs Biomed* **101**, 23–32 (2011).
49. H. Yu, E. S. Barriga, C. Agurto, S. Echegaray, M. S. Pattichis, W. Bauman and P. Soliz, "Fast localization and segmentation of optic disk in retinal images using directional matched filtering and level sets," *IEEE Trans Inf Technol Biomed* **16**, 644–657 (2012).
50. A. Hoover and M. Goldbaum, "Locating the optic nerve in a retinal image using the fuzzy convergence of the blood vessels," *IEEE Trans Med Imag* **22**, 951–958 (2003).
51. M. Foracchia, E. Grisan and A. Ruggeri, "Detection of optic disc in retinal images by means of a geometrical model of vessel structure," *IEEE Trans Med Imag* **23**, 1189–1195 (2004).
52. A. A. H. A. R. Youssif, A. Z. Ghalwash, and A. R. Ghoneim, "Optic disc detection from normalized digital fundus images by means of a vessels' direction matched filter," *IEEE Trans Med Imag* **27**, 11–18 (2008).
53. H. Li and O. Chutatape, "Automated feature extraction in color retinal images by a model based approach," *IEEE Trans Biomed Eng* **51**, 246–254 (2004).
54. T. Spencer, J. A. Olson, K. C. McHardy, P. F. Sharp and J. V. Forrester, "An image-processing strategy for the segmentation and quantification of microaneurysms in fluorescein angiograms of the ocular fundus," *Comput Biomed Res* **29**, 284–302 (1996).
55. A. J. Frame, P. E. Undrill, M. J. Cree, J. A. Olson, K. C. McHardy, P. F. Sharp and J. V. Forrester, "A comparison of computer based classification methods applied to the detection of microaneurysms in ophthalmic fluorescein angiograms," *Comput Biol Med* **28**, 225–238 (1998).
56. M. Larsen, J. Godt, N. Larsen, H. Lund-Andersen, A. K. Sjølie, E. Agardh, H. Kalm, M. Grunkin and D. R. Owens, "Automated detection of fundus photographic red lesions in diabetic retinopathy," *Investigat Opht Vis Sci* **44**, 761–766 (2003).
57. M. Niemeijer, B. van Ginneken, J. J. Staal, M. S. A. Suttorp-Schulten and M. D. Abramoff, "Automatic detection of red lesions in digital color fundus photographs," *IEEE Trans Med Imag* **24**, 584–592 (2005).
58. C. Heneghan, J. Flynn, M. O'Keefe and M. Cahill, "Characterization of changes in blood vessel width and tortuosity in retinopathy of prematurity using image analysis," *Medical Image Analysis* **6**, 407–429 (2002).
59. M. M. Fraz, P. Remagnino, A. Hoppe, B. Uyyanonvara, A. R. Rudnicka, C. G. Owen and S. A. Barman, "Blood vessel segmentation methodologies in retinal images — A survey," *Comput Methods Programs Biomed* **108**, 407–433 (2012).
60. S. Chaudhuri, S. Chatterjee, N. Katz, M. Nelson and M. Goldbaum, "Detection of blood vessels in retinal images using two-dimensional matched filters," *IEEE Trans Med Imag* **8**, 263–269 (1989).
61. A. D. Hoover, V. Kouznetsova and M. Goldbaum, "Locating blood vessels in retinal images by piecewise threshold probing of a matched filter response," *IEEE Trans Med Imag* **19**, 203–210 (2000).

62. J. Staal, M. D. Abramoff, M. Niemeijer, M. A. Viergever and B. van Ginneken, "Ridge-based vessel segmentation in color images of the retina," *IEEE Trans Med Imag* **23**, 501–509 (2004).
63. J. V. B. Soares, J. J. G. Leandro, R. M. Cesar, H. F. Jelinek and M. J. Cree, "Retinal vessel segmentation using the 2-D Gabor wavelet and supervised classification," *IEEE Trans Med Imag* **25**, 1214–1222 (2006).
64. E. Ricci and R. Perfetti, "Retinal blood vessel segmentation using line operators and support vector classification," *IEEE Trans Med Imag* **26**, 1357–1365 (2007).
65. L. Xu and S. Luo, "A novel method for blood vessel detection from retinal images," *BioMedical Engineering Online* **9:14**, (2010).
66. C. A. Lupascu, D. Tegolo and E. Trucco, "FABC: retinal vessel segmentation using AdaBoost," *IEEE Trans Inf Technol Biomed* **14**, 1267–1274 (2010).
67. X. You, Q. Peng, Y. Yuan, Y.-m. Cheung and J. Lei, "Segmentation of retinal blood vessels using the radial projection and semi-supervised approach," *Pattern Recognition* **44**, 2314–2324 (2011).
68. D. Marin, A. Aquino, M. E. Gegundez-Arias and J. M. Bravo, "A new supervised method for blood vessel segmentation in retinal images by using gray-level and moment invariants-based features," *IEEE Trans Med Imag* **30**, 146–158 (2011).
69. Y. A. Tolias and S. M. Panas, "A fuzzy vessel tracking algorithm for retinal images based on fuzzy clustering," *IEEE Trans Med Imag* **17**, 263–273 (1998).
70. F. Zana and J. C. Klein, "Segmentation of vessel-like patterns using mathematical morphology and curvature evaluation," *IEEE Trans on Imag Process* **10**, 1010–1019 (2001).
71. A. M. Mendonça and A. Campilho, "Segmentation of retinal blood vessels by combining the detection of centerlines and morphological reconstruction," *IEEE Trans Med Imag* **25**, 1200–1213 (2006).
72. K. K. Delibasis, A. I. Kechriniotis, C. Tsonos and N. Assimakis, "Automatic model-based tracing algorithm for vessel segmentation and diameter estimation," *Comput Methods Programs Biomed* **100**, 108–122 (2010).
73. B. S. Y. Lam and Y. Hong, "A novel vessel segmentation algorithm for pathological retina images based on the divergence of vector fields," *IEEE Trans Med Imag* **27**, 237–246 (2008).
74. A. Fleming, K. Goatman, S. Philip, J. Olson and P. Sharp, "Automatic detection of retinal anatomy to assist diabetic retinopathy screening," *Phys Med Biol* **52**, 331–345 (2007).
75. M. Niemeijer, M. D. Abràmoff and B. van Ginneken, "Segmentation of the optic disc, macula and vascular arch in fundus photographs," *IEEE Trans Med Imag* **26**, 116–127 (2007).
76. M. Niemeijer, M. D. Abràmoff and B. van Ginneken, "Fast detection of the optic disc and fovea in color fundus photographs," *Medical Image Analysis* **13**, 859–870 (2009).
77. D. Welfer, J. Scharcanski and D. Ruschel Marinho, "Fovea center detection based on the retina anatomy and mathematical morphology," *Comput Methods Programs Biomed* **104**, 397–409 (2011).
78. T. Walter, P. Massin, A. Erginay, R. Ordonez, C. Jeulin and J. C. Klein, "Automatic detection of microaneurysms in color fundus images," *Med Image Anal* **11**, 555–566 (2007).

79. M. J. Cree, J. A. Olson, K. C. McHardy, P. F. Sharp and J. V. Forrester, "A fully automated comparative microaneurysm digital detection system," *Eye* **11**, 622–628 (1997).
80. J. H. Hipwell, F. Strachant, J. A. Olson, K. C. McHardy, P. F. Sharp and J. V. Forrester, "Automated detection of microaneurysms in digital red-free photographs: A diabetic retinopathy screening tool," *Diabetic Med* **17**, 588–594 (2000).
81. A. D. Fleming, S. Philip, K. A. Goatman, J. A. Olson and P. F. Sharp, "Automated microaneurysm detection using local contrast normalization and local vessel detection," *IEEE Trans Med Imag* **25**, 1223–1232 (2006).
82. M. Niemeijer, B. van Ginneken, M. J. Cree, A. Mizutani, G. Quellec, C. I. Sanchez, B. Zhang, R. Hornero, M. Lamard, C. Muramatsu, X. Wu, G. Cazuguel, J. You, A. Mayo, Qin Li, Y. Hatanaka, B. Cochener, C. Roux, F. Karray, M. Garcia, H. Fujita and M. D. Abramoff, "Retinopathy Online Challenge: Automatic Detection of Microaneurysms in Digital Color Fundus Photographs," *IEEE Trans Med Imag* **29**, 185–195 (2010).
83. S. Ravishankar, A. Jain and A. Mittal, "Automated feature extraction for early detection of diabetic retinopathy in fundus images," *Proc IEEE Conference on Computer Vision and Pattern Recognition* 210–217 (2009).
84. A. Sopharak, B. Uyyanonvara, S. Barman, T. H. Williamson, "Automatic detection of diabetic retinopathy exudates from non-dilated retinal images using mathematical morphology methods," *Comp Medical Imag Graphics* **32**, 720–727 (2008).
85. M. García, C. I. Sánchez, M. I. López, D. Abásolo and R. Hornero, "Neural network based detection of hard exudates in retinal images," *Comput Methods Programs Biomed* **93**, 9–19 (2009).
86. N. P. Ward, S. Tomlinson and C. J. Taylor, "Image analysis of fundus photographs. The detection and measurement of exudates associated with diabetic retinopathy," *Ophthalmology* **96**, 80–86 (1989).
87. R. Phillips, J. Forrester and P. Sharp, "Automated detection and quantification of retinal exudates," *Graefe's Arch Clin Exp Ophthalmol* **231**, 90–94 (1993).
88. T. Walter, J. C. Klein, P. Massin and A. Erginay, "A contribution of image processing to the diagnosis of diabetic retinopathy — detection of exudates in color fundus images of the human retina," *IEEE Trans Med Imag* **21**, 1236–1243 (2002).
89. C. I. Sánchez, R. Hornero, M. I. López, M. Aboy, J. Poza and D. Abásolo, "A novel automatic image processing algorithm for detection of hard exudates based on retinal image analysis," *Med Eng Phys* **30**, 350–357 (2008).
90. A. D. Fleming, S. Philip, K. A. Goatman, G. J. Williams, J. A. Olson and P. F. Sharp, "Automated detection of exudates for diabetic retinopathy screening," *Phys Med Biol* **52**, 7385–7396 (2007).
91. S. Philip, A. Fleming, K. Goatman, S. Fonseca, P. McNamee, G. Scotland, G. Prescott, P. Sharp and J. Olson, "The efficacy of automated 'disease/no disease' grading for diabetic retinopathy in a systematic screening programme," *Br J Ophthalmol* **91**, 1512–1517 (2007).
92. A. D. Fleming, K. A. Goatman, S. Philip, G. J. Prescott, P. F. Sharp, J. A. Olson, "Automated grading for diabetic retinopathy: A large-scale audit using arbitration by clinical experts," *Br J Ophthalmol* **94**, 1606–1610 (2010).
93. M. Abràmoff, M. Niemeijer, M. Suttorp-Schulten, M. Viergever, S. Russell and B. van Ginneken, "Evaluation of a system for automatic detection of diabetic retinopathy from

color fundus photographs in a large population of patients with diabetes," *Diabetes Care* **31**, 193–198 (2008).

94. B. Dupas, T. Walter, A. Erginay, R. Ordonez, N. Deb-Joardar, P. Gain, J.-C. Klein, P. Massin, "Evaluation of automated fundus photograph analysis algorithms for detecting microaneurysms, haemorrhages and exudates, and of a computer-assisted diagnostic system for grading diabetic retinopathy," *Diabetes & Metabolism* **36**, 213–220 (2010).
95. C. E. Baudoin, B. J. Lay, J. C. Klein, "Automatic detection of microaneurysms in diabetic fluorescein angiography," *Rev Epidemiol Sante Publique* **32**, 254–261 (1984).

Chapter 17

Motion Correction Techniques for MR-Guided HIFU Ablation of Abdominal Organs

Sébastien Roujol,[*,§] *Chrit Moonen*[†] *and Baudouin Denis de Senneville*[†,‡]

[*]Department of Medicine (Cardiovascular division), Beth Israel Deaconess Medical Center and Harvard Medical School, Boston, MA, USA

[†]Imaging Division, UMC Utrecht, Utrecht, Netherlands

[‡]IMB, UMR 5251 CNRS/University of Bordeaux 1/INRIA, F-33400 Talence, France

[§]E-mail: sroujol@bidmc.harvard.edu

Magnetic resonance guided high intensity focused ultrasound (MRgHIFU) ablation is a promising technique for the treatment of hepatic and renal cancers. In this approach, the HIFU system is used for ablating the tumor using local heating while the MRI scanner provides online temperature measurements which enable continuous monitoring of the delivered thermal dose. The application of MRgHIFU ablation for abdominal organs is challenging. Many technical developments have addressed the major issues associated with this procedure such as the physiological motion of abdominal organs. In this chapter, we present the different techniques which have been developed to alleviate the problem of physiological motion for MRgHIFU ablation of abdominal organs.

1. Introduction

Hepatic and renal cancers are major public health issues and account worldwide for 700 000 and 115 000 deaths/year, respectively.[1] Although surgery is generally considered as first line therapy, many patients are not eligible for this therapeutic option. Furthermore, these cancers do not respond well to chemotherapy and radiotherapy. Percutaneous ablation is one of the best alternative options, and can be achieved by inducing strong temperature increases.

To overcome the limitations associated with such minimally invasive procedures, non-invasive techniques such as high intensity focused ultrasound (HIFU) ablation[2–4] are under active investigation. The latter generally uses an extra-corporal HIFU transducer with multiple ultrasound elements and enables localized energy delivery deep into tissue. To further improve the procedure safety, magnetic resonance guided HIFU (MRgHIFU) ablation has been suggested.[5–7] MRI is a promising candidate for monitoring HIFU therapy since it provides excellent tissue contrast and enables real time *in-vivo* temperature mapping (hereafter referred to as MR-thermometry).[5,8–11] Furthermore, the delivered thermal dose can be estimated from the temporal evolution of the temperature (hereafter referred to as MR-dosimetry) and is a promising marker for the determination of the therapy endpoint.[12] The feasibility of MRgHIFU ablation has been shown in patients for the treatment of uterine fibroids[13–15] or bone metastases.[16] However, despite the progress achieved for the treatment of static tumors in patients, the application in clinics of MRgHIFU ablation to abdominal organs remains challenging.[17] A comprehensive description of these hurdles has been reviewed elsewhere.[18,19] One of the most significant limitations is the problems associated with the motion of abdominal organs.

Abdominal organs are subjected to continuous displacements and deformations induced by both the breathing and cardiac activities of the patient. Although the respiratory-induced motion is the most prominent motion component, the cardiac activity induces more complex deformation, especially in the upper part of the liver or in the vicinity of blood vessels. One possible solution is to perform the procedure with the patient undergoing a general anesthesia and passive breath-holds controlled by a ventilator.[20] Although it removes the effect of organ motion, it is less efficient and leads to risks associated with a general anesthesia. Therefore, the development of techniques compatible with free breathing conditions is desirable. In these conditions, organ motion raises significant barriers for MR-thermometry/dosimetry and accurate/precise targeted energy delivery.

MR thermometry can be performed using the proton resonance frequency (PRF) shift technique.[21,22] This method exploits the linear dependence between local temperature variations and water proton resonance frequency, and is considered as a method of choice in abdominal organs. However, the respiratory activity induces temporal variations of the local magnetic susceptibility which bias the PRF-based temperature estimates.[23] Furthermore, estimation of thermal dose maps requires voxel-wise analysis of the temperature evolution. Due to organ motion, the position of the tumor will be different

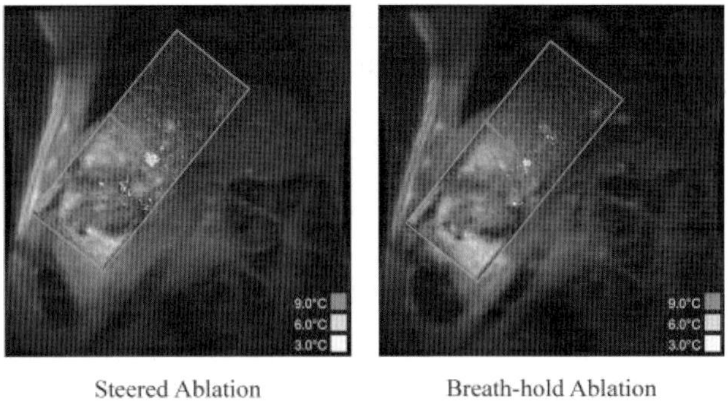

Fig. 1. *In vivo* HIFU steered and breath-hold ablations. These two images show representative images of a steered (left) and breath-hold (right) ablation *in vivo* at the time point when the maximum temperature reached 10°C above baseline. The steered ablation took 31.2 s to reach this point, whereas the breath-hold ablation took 26.7 s. The steered ablation required 16.7% more energy than the breath-hold case. Reproduced with permission of (Holbrook *et al.*, 2014).[56]

in successive MR images acquired continuously during the ablation process. Several techniques have been developed to achieve efficient and robust MR-thermometry/dosimetry in abdominal organs and are presented in the first part of this chapter.

In addition, an accurate energy deposition in the tumor is challenging in the presence of motion. Respiratory gated approaches have been proposed, and consist of intermittent sonications applied during each end-tidal phase of the respiratory cycle.[24] However, this strategy may be unfavorable to highly perfused organs such as the liver and the kidney, due to significant heat evacuation between each sonication and insufficient temperature elevation. Therefore, continuous ablation strategies are of particular interest for these organs since it would also improve the duty cycle of the sonication process, as illustrated in Fig. 1. In these conditions, more sophisticated approaches need to be employed to enable real time adjustment of the HIFU focal point based on the displacement of the targeted ablation area. Several strategies, proposed for this purpose, are presented in the second part of this chapter.

2. Motion Correction for Real Time MR-thermometry and MR-dosimetry

MR thermometry is a cornerstone for the monitoring of HIFU ablation procedures. Although many techniques have been developed for MR thermometry,[10] the PRF shift technique has been the most commonly used approach. In this technique, the phase information of gradient echo sequences is directly used to estimate pixel-wise temperature variation. Estimates of the temperature variation (ΔT) are obtained by comparing a baseline phase signal (φ_{ref}) to the phase signal obtained during the ablation procedure (φ_t) as follows:

$$\Delta T(\vec{x}, t) = k \times (\varphi_{ref}(\vec{x}) - \varphi_t(\vec{x}))$$

where k is a constant parameter (more details on the determination of k can be found in Ref. [10]) and $\vec{x}$ denotes the voxel coordinates. Due to the inhomogeneity of the signal in phase images, the reference phase signal needs to be measured on a pixel-per-pixel basis. The application of this technique to moving target is challenging since additional variations of the phase signal are induced by the patient physiological activity and the resulting organ motion,[25] as shown in Fig. 2. Therefore, if left uncorrected, these additional phase signal would lead to severe bias in temperature estimates.

MR-dosimetry is commonly based on the thermal dose model proposed by Sapareto and Dewey.[12] This model establishes an empirical relation between temperature, duration of exposure, and cell death. The accumulative effect of sustained elevated temperatures on biological tissue is computed on a

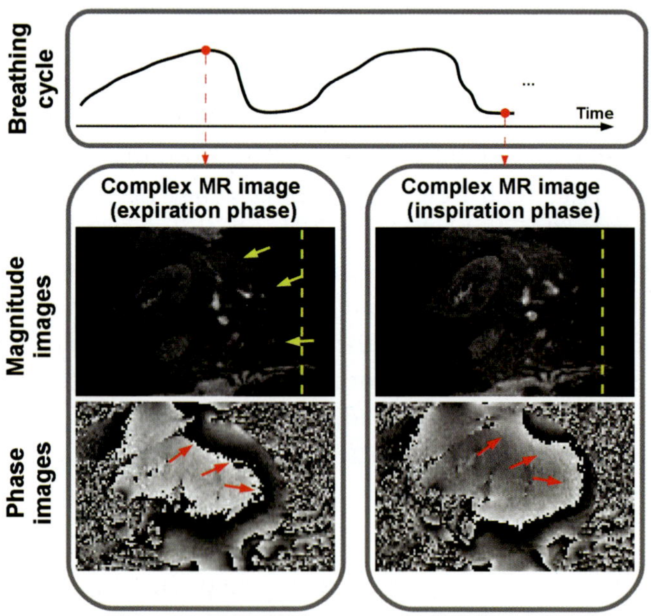

Fig. 2. Complex MR images acquired in the abdomen of a human volunteer at two different phases of the breathing cycle. MR magnitude images provide excellent tissue contrast and enable the visualization of organ motion (see yellow arrows). The overall motion is also visible in MR phase images. However, additional signal variations have been induced by the breathing activity (see red arrows).

voxel-by-voxel basis using the temporal history of past temperature measurements $T(\vec{x},t)$ in each voxel ($\vec{x}$) as follows:

$$t_{eq} = \begin{cases} \int_0^t 2^{(T(\vec{x},t)-43)}dt & if\ (T > 43°\mathrm{C}) \\ \int_0^t 4^{(T(\vec{x},t)-43)}dt & if\ (T < 43°\mathrm{C}) \end{cases} \tag{2}$$

Tissue destruction is achieved when the equivalent thermal dose t_{eq} exceeds the lethal dose (which is taken as 43°C during 240 min). The measurement of the thermal dose in abdominal organs requires additional considerations since the position of the target in temperature maps will be influenced by the breathing and cardiac activities. Therefore, the position of the targeted organ in temperature maps must be aligned to a common position to enable thermal dose estimation.

Gated and non-gated strategies have been proposed for the management of abdominal organ motion during MR thermometry and MR dosimetry under free breathing conditions. These two approaches are described in the following sections.

2.1. *Gated Acquisition Strategies*

Respiratory gated strategies consist of synchronizing the MR acquisition to a stable period of the breathing activity.[24,26–28] For this purpose, an acquisition window of ~1–2s can be exploited during the exhalation phase of the respiratory cycle. The breathing period can in principle be assessed using various types of qualitative sensors such as breathing belt,[29] or quantitative surrogates such as MR navigators[27] or ultrasound (US) echoes.[30]

These strategies substantially reduce the impact of motion-induced variations in phase images in Eq. (1), as well as the temporal misalignments between temperature maps in Eq. (2). Direct estimation of temperature maps can thus be obtained based on a static reference phase image (φ_{ref}) acquired prior heating. Excellent precision of the temperature information can be obtained when the gating strategy is employed in conjunction with state-of-the-art MR-thermometry sequences.[24,28] However, the main drawback is the limited temporal resolution of the image acquisition. While the theoretical calculation of the equivalent dose using Eq. (2) is numerically efficient for high frame-rate imaging in the range of 10 Hz, it becomes more unstable when a gating strategy is employed, since the image acquisition time is in this case generally in the range of 3–6 s. These instabilities can be further increased by remaining miss-registration errors arising from irregular breathing patterns and/or when the signal to noise ratio (SNR) of the temperature maps is reduced. In addition the obtained thermal dose information is irregular and less predictable, which prevents the use of volumetric control strategies.[31,32]

2.2. *Non-gated Acquisition Strategies*

Non-gated strategies have been recently proposed to provide continuous regular high sampling of temperature estimates during the entire respiratory cycle, which allows in turns calculating accurate and precise thermal dose maps.

2.2.1. *Non-gated MR thermometry*

Using non-gating strategies, unwanted phase shifts, generated by modified local magnetic susceptibility perturbations with motion, may induce an apparent temperature modification in Eq. (1), which can bias and even mask the true temperature estimate. Precise modeling of the inhomogeneous magnetic field *in-vivo* and under real-time conditions is however difficult to achieve. Two main approaches have been proposed obviating the need for this modeling, generally referred to as "Referenceless" and "Referenced" PRF thermometry.

In referenceless PRF thermometry, the baseline phase signal used to compute the current temperature map is directly estimated from the current MR phase image.[33] To this end, the phase signal of non-heated surrounding tissues is used to extrapolate a baseline phase signal in the targeted area.

In referenced PRF thermometry, a reference model, which establishes a relation between the variations of the baseline phase signal and the patient physiological motion, is built before heating.[27,34] To this end, both descriptors of motion patterns and MR images are continuously and simultaneously acquired during a period covering several respiratory cycles. A look-up table can then be used to store each pair of motion descriptor/MR phase image. During heating, phase artifacts due to the periodical motion of the respiration cycle are addressed by applying a phase correction based on the model of the phase variation in dependence of the current motion descriptor. Although any type of respiratory motion descriptor may be employed in principle, MR navigator echoes and MR magnitude images have been widely used for this purpose and provide reliable performance,[27,34] as shown in Fig. 3. The main limitation of referenced PRF thermometry is its inability to compensate for motion which has not been observed during the training period, as encountered with spontaneous motion.

Referenceless and referenced PRF thermometry can also be combined using hybrid techniques in order to further improve the robustness of the baseline

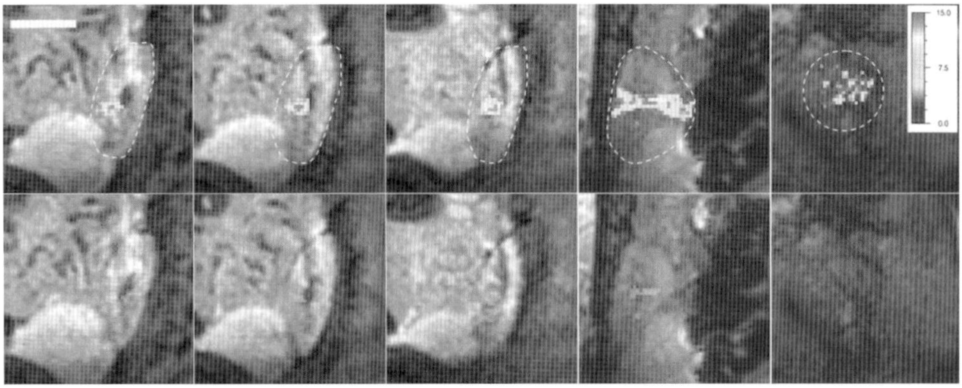

Fig. 3. Temperature (top row, with color scale on the right indicating the temperature change) and thermal dose [bottom row, with pixels colored red corresponding to a thermal dose of 240CEM43 (CEM43, equivalent minutes at 43°C) and above] images during high-intensity focused ultrasound (HIFU) ablation of the kidney. Left to right: three sagittal slices centered in the kidney, one coronal slice centered in the kidney and one sagittal slice located near the skin. The broken contours in the temperature images show the selected regions of interest (ROIs) for displaying the temperature data. The horizontal yellow bar in the top left image represents 5cm. The temperature images display the temperature distribution measured at the end of the HIFU sonication and the thermal dose images are the final images in the time series. Reproduced with permission of (Quesson *et al.*, 2011).[44]

phase image estimates.[35,36] A discussion about the inherent advantages and drawback of these methods can be found in Ref. [35].

2.2.2. *Non-gated MR dosimetry*

Spatial mismatches between the temporally acquired temperature maps, induced by organ displacement, must then be corrected to enable accurate estimation of the thermal dose with Eq. (2). The objective is now to relate the coordinates of each part of tissue in each new incoming temperature map to the corresponding one in a fixed reference position (typically the first temperature map of the temporal series).

Spatial adaption of a region of interest (ROI) position has been proposed based on the successful detection of the focal point position on the temperature maps.[37] However, since the registration accuracy depends on the choice of the ROI position, the presence of temperature artifacts during the experiment can destabilize all successive measurements. Furthermore, motion correction can only be applied after a significant temperature rise has been achieved, i.e. after the beginning of the ablation. Alternatively, the signal magnitude of gradient recalled sequences provides anatomical information such as the position and the composition of the tissue with good contrast and SNR (see Fig. 2). Therefore, these images can be used to estimate organ displacement using image-based motion estimation algorithms.[38–40] This approach enables co-registering on the fly all incoming temperature maps to a common reference position. Both rigid and non-rigid motion estimation methods have been investigated.[41–43] Recently, an optimized pipeline has been proposed to obtain registered thermal maps with a frame-rate of 10 Hz while maintaining a spatial resolution of $2.5 \times 2.5 \times 5\,\text{mm}^3$ and a thermometric precision of $\pm 2°\text{C}$.[43] In this study, MR thermometry was performed in 2D to enable a high acquisition frame-rate. To reduce the impact of through plane motion, the imaging plane was aligned along the main direction of the respiratory-induced motion of the organ (i.e. the superior-inferior orientation).[27,43] This, however, imposes severe constraints on the imaging geometry which might be unfavorable for anatomical or diagnostic reasons. Furthermore, although the motion trajectory of the kidney and the lower part of the liver can be approximated in first order by a linear shift, the true trajectory is a curve in 3D space. In particular, the upper part of the liver, which is subjected to an elastic deformation, is hard to contain in a static 2D imaging slice during the entire respiratory cycle. It is often not possible to ensure that the target area remains observable by a single static image slice during the entire motion cycle.

In principle, the acquisition of 3D images would offer a better framework for a full characterization of the true organ motion. However, this type of acquisition is difficult in practice because of technical limitations, spatial and temporal resolution trade-offs, and associated low SNR. Imaging is thus generally limited to the acquisition of 1–5 slices with modest spatial resolution in the slice direction.[44] Alternative approaches which dynamically adjust the image plane location based on real time assessment of the targeted organ position have been proposed as possible solution. The use of fast MR navigators[45] or ultrasound echoes[46] have been reported to assess the organ position. That way, it was demonstrated that it is feasible to obtain 2D thermal dose maps oriented orthogonally to the principal axis of the target motion.[45,47]

3. Motion Correction for Real-time Beam Steering

During continuous sonication in mobile organs, real time adjustment of the focal position of the HIFU-beam (hereafter referred to as beam steering) is required to "follow" the target motion. This is particularly important to avoid energy deposition in tissues surrounding the targeted area and to ensure heating within the targeted area, as illustrated in the phantom study reported in Fig. 4. To this end, imaging data acquired during sonication can be used to characterize

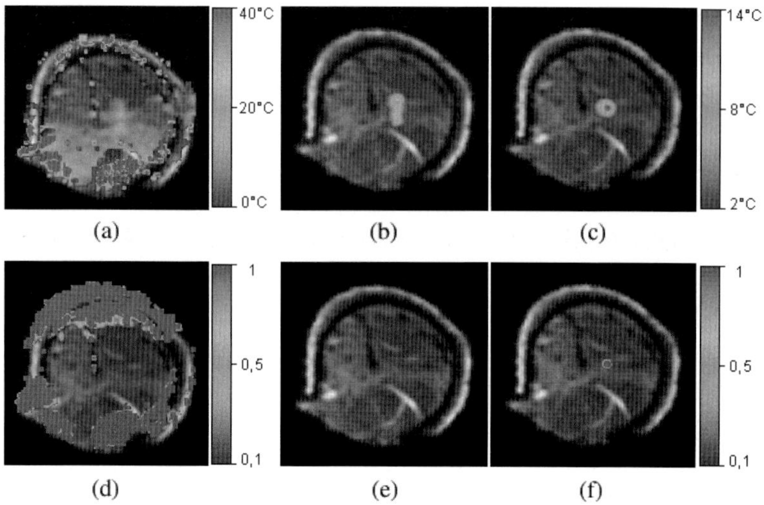

Fig. 4. Temperature variation maps (a–c) and thermal dose maps (d–f) obtained *ex vivo* during heating of a pig muscle undergoing a periodical translational motion. a and d: Uncorrected MR thermometry/dosimetry without real time beam steering. b and e: Motion corrected MR thermometry/dosimetry without real time beam steering. c and f: Motion corrected MR thermometry/dosimetry with real time beam steering. Reproduced with permission of (Denis de Senneville *et al.*, 2007).[34]

the target motion and to generate a new focal point location of the HIFU beam. The performance of a beam steering system is associated to (1) the accuracy, precision and temporal frequency of the target motion estimates, and (2) the overall latency of the system.

While the ideal accuracy and precision of the target motion estimates should be in the range of the size of the HIFU focal point (~few mm), the temporal frequency of the beam steering system needs to be sufficient to resolve the observed physiological motion. Recently, it has been shown that real time beam steering with a 10Hz frequency enables to remove the effect of physiological motion during HIFU sonication in abdominal organs.[45]

To ensure the real time feasibility of a beam steering system, the overall processing time required to compute the new location of the HIFU beam focus needs to be inferior to the time interval between two successive motion estimates. The latency of the beam steering system is defined as the time interval between the acquisition of the signal used to estimate the target motion and the actual update time of the HIFU beam. During this time interval, the target may move which would result in incorrect motion compensation of the HIFU beam focus. Therefore, the latency of the system needs also to be minimized as much as possible to reduce this consequent bias. Temporal motion prediction strategies have also been proposed to further compensate for the system latency.[34,48,49]

At this point, it is important to note that the requirements of the beam steering system and the MR thermometry/dosimetry system are different. As previously mentioned, high temporal resolution is mandatory to characterize the physiological motion of the target in the beam steering system. On the other hand, high spatial resolution and coverage are desirable for MR thermometry in order to improve the monitoring and safety of the procedure. Since both high spatial and temporal resolution together with large spatial coverage is hard to achieve using state-of-art MR scanner, several strategies have been developed to compromise between these requirements. Two paths of investigation have been proposed for target motion estimation during real time beam steering: "Direct" and "Indirect" target tracking.

3.1. *Beam Steering using Indirect Motion Estimation*

The general framework of an indirect (or model-based) motion estimation method is shown in Fig. 5. In this approach, a motion model of the target is built before heating. The model establishes a relationship between the target motion and a surrogate of the target motion. Subsequently, during heating, the surrogate of the target motion is used in conjunction to the motion model to estimate the current target position. The motion model can thus be created using imaging strategies which do not need to comply with the real time and latency constraints imposed by the beam steering system. A large variety of approaches has been proposed for model-based respiratory motion estimation and has been reviewed elsewhere.[50] In this section, we focus on the different strategies that have been proposed for motion surrogate, training data, and motion model in the scope of MRgHIFU of abdominal organs.

3.1.1. *Surrogate of the target motion*

The surrogate of the target motion is first employed before sonication to build the target motion model and then during sonication to estimate the current target motion. The surrogate signal must therefore be consistent between these two steps of the interventional process, and have sufficient temporal resolution during sonication to resolve the physiological motion.

The use of external sensors such as respiratory bellows,[24,51,52] nasal airflow prong or spirometer[51] have been suggested as potential surrogate of the respiratory motion. Optical imaging has also been proposed[53] using a shielded MR-compatible optical camera. The advantages of these techniques are their

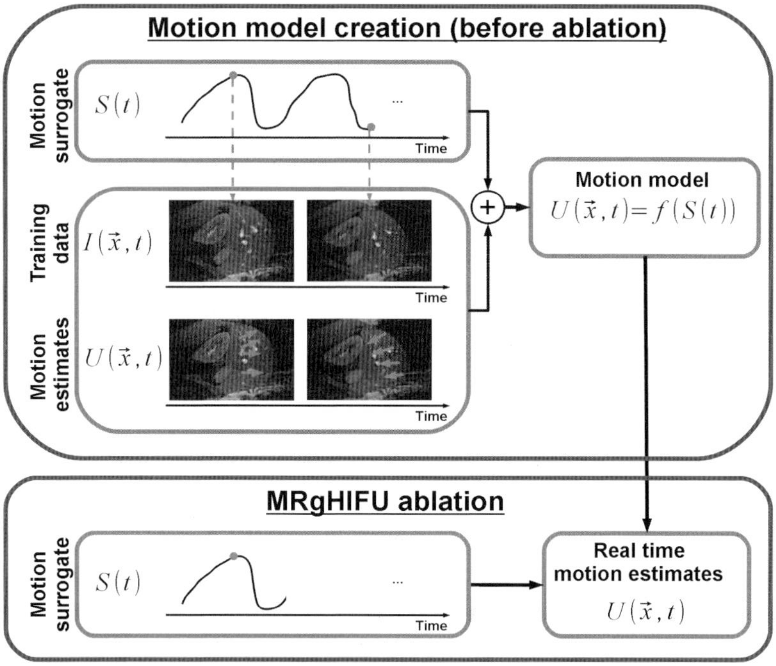

Fig. 5. Illustration of a model-based motion estimation scheme. Motion surrogate and training data are acquired simultaneously before the ablation procedure. Complex characterization of the target motion is obtained from the training data. Subsequently, the resulting motion estimates and the motion surrogate are combined to establish a model of the target motion. During the MRgHIFU ablation procedure, the incoming motion surrogate information is used together with the pre-built target motion model to generate in real time a complex description of the current target motion.

ability to provide surrogate motion information with high temporal resolution and their independency from both the MR system and the HIFU system. Therefore, the MR-thermometry sequence and the HIFU sonication protocol can be defined independently from the acquisition of the target motion surrogate. However, since these methods do not directly observe the organ of interest, the qualitative relation between the motion surrogate and the target position may become inaccurate in the presence of breathing pattern changes (abdominal breathing vs. thoracic breathing). To the best of our knowledge, none of these surrogates have yet been used in indirect beam steering MRgHIFU experiments.

The use of alternative motion surrogates which provide quantitative measurements of the target displacement (or at least tissue/organ surrounding the target) has also been investigated. Most of these quantitative motion surrogate have been extracted from MR signal[34,54–57] or US signal acquired with an external US probe.[58–63] Initial MR-based approaches used MR navigators[34,54,55] which do not require additional hardware and are easy to set up. However, the imaging pulses of MR navigators can create artifacts in subsequently acquired MR images if the fields of view of MR navigators and MR images intersect. To prevent such artifacts, MR navigators must be positioned outside the imaging field of view which limits the displacement knowledge in the targeted area. Alternatively, fat-selective navigators can be used since it does not lead to artifacts in fat-suppressed MR images[47] and allows the positioning of the navigator directly on the organ of interest. Ultrasonic echoes have also been suggested for this purpose[63] in order to obtain a 1D measure of the organ displacement.

Motion surrogate with higher dimensionality have also been proposed to increase the degrees of freedom of the motion model and to improve the characterization of more complex organ deformations. Both MR images[56,57] and US images[58–62] have been employed for this purpose. In these studies, the surrogate of the target motion was defined using either (1) a finite number of characteristic points in the images (such as a vein or the diaphragm location)[56,59,60,62] or (2) the entire or a sub-sample of the image.[57,61] MR images can be acquired with the same sequence as the one used subsequently for MR thermometry.[56,57] In this case, the MR images acquired during sonication are used for both MR thermometry/dosimetry and motion surrogate, and these two tasks are consequently performed with the same temporal resolution. Alternatively, the acquisition of US images, which requires additional hardware and careful manual positioning of the US probe, can be performed asynchronously from the MR acquisition.[58–62] In this case, the MR thermometry/dosimetry system and beam steering system can operate at different temporal resolution.

3.1.2. *Training data*

Training data must be acquired before sonication to characterize the target motion and build the motion model. This acquisition can be performed (1) immediately before sonication during the MRgHIFU procedure (hereafter referred to as intra-procedural acquisition) or (2) before the MRgHIFU procedure using a patient-specific or cross population-based approach (hereafter referred to as pre-procedural acquisition). Finally, these data should have a sufficient dimensionality (both 2D+t and 3D+t techniques have been reported) to enable accurate and precise estimates of the target motion.

Intra-procedural 2D+t training data[34,51,52,54,56–58,61,62] has been employed for the majority of studies using model-based beam steering for MRgHIFU ablation of abdominal organs.[34,56,57,61] In these studies, 2D+t training data were acquired using an imaging plane aligned along the main motion component to reduce the impact of through plane motion. This approach provides patient-specific motion patterns using data acquired immediately before sonication.

More recently, the use of 3D+t training data has been suggested to fully characterize the 3D target motion.[51,52,54,58–60,62] However, intra-procedural acquisition of 3D+t training data is challenging, time consuming and requires computationally intensive post-processing which would substantially extend the duration of the intervention. Therefore, pre-procedural acquisition of training data (i.e. before the overall MRgHIFU procedure) has been suggested to remove these constraints and to offer more flexibility for both data acquisition and post processing.[59,60] In particular, this approach should enable in principle: (1) to use different imaging modality such as MRI, US or CT, (2) to reach higher spatial/temporal resolution and higher spatial coverage, and (3) to employ most sophisticated non-real-time algorithms for the characterization of the targeted organ deformation. For this purpose, either patient specific or cross-population-based approaches can be investigated. Using patient-specific approaches, the motion model is created using data acquired from the same patient undergoing the MRgHIFU ablation. Therefore, any variations in physiological conditions such as breathing pattern and heart rate between the training period and ablation may negatively impact the value of the motion model. Using cross population-based approaches, the motion model of an organ is created as the average motion across the patient population.[59,60] The accuracy of the motion model will therefore be decreased by the significant variability of both anatomies and motion patterns across a patient population. It must be noted that the feasibility and the benefit of using 3D+t training data still remains to be shown during MRgHIFU ablation experiments.

3.1.3. *Motion model*

The motion model establishes a correspondence between surrogate data and motion estimates obtained from the training data. The correspondence can be either direct or indirect.[50]

Direct correspondence models define a function which directly relates the target motion in function of the motion surrogate. This approach has been suggested to relate motion estimates using either the phase of the respiratory cycle obtained from a respiratory sensor[52] or the 1D displacement of the diaphragm or target obtained from US images[62] or ultrasonic echoes.[63]

Indirect correspondence models parameterize during the training period the target motion with the motion surrogate. During sonication, the target motion is estimated by optimizing the model input parameters which best fit the current motion surrogate. The first reported techniques used a look-up table to store both target motion and motion surrogate obtained during the training period.[34,54,56,61] During sonication, the best match between the current motion surrogate and his counterpart in the look-up table is identified. The corresponding target motion in the look-up table is then selected and used as current estimate of the target motion. This approach has been demonstrated using 2D+t MR images for both training data and motion surrogate.[34,54,56] The technique has also been described using 2D+t MR images for the training data and 2D+t US images for motion surrogate.[61] Although these approaches have been popular in the scope of MRgHIFU ablation, it imposes several limitations including the reduced temporal sampling of the look-up table as well as the sensitivity to possible errors in motion estimates occurred during the training period. To overcome these limitations, more sophisticated indirect models have been proposed using random forest[51] or principal component analysis (PCA)-based approach.[57] In the PCA-based approach, 2D+t MR images were employed for both surrogate and training data. The PCA is employed to detect spatio-temporal coherence in the physiological organ motion, and to discard incoherent motion patterns. The organ deformation is then expressed using a small set of parameters (also called motion descriptor). During sonication, the PCA motion descriptor provides a motion field that is consistent with the learned model and robust to possible local artifacts.

3.2. *Beam Steering Using Direct Motion Estimation*

Direct motion estimation approaches estimate the target motion directly from data continuously acquired during the ablation process without the use of motion model. This approach thus allows detecting spontaneous motion events without the requirement of a calibration prior or during the intervention. Several approaches have been demonstrated during MRgHIFU ablation experiments using either real time acquisition of MRI or US.

3.2.1. *Direct motion estimation using MRI*

The use of MR navigators has been suggested to estimate and correct in real time the organ motion.[55] This type of approach is attractive due to the low acquisition time of MR-navigators and the low processing time required for motion estimation. Although the use of one or two navigators has been suggested, this technique cannot characterize complex spatial deformations, as observed in the liver. Therefore, more sophisticated approaches have been developed.

Alternatively, it has been proposed to estimate the target motion using the magnitude component of the MR images (acquired for MR thermometry) together with image-based motion estimation algorithms.[34,41,64–66] This strategy has been successfully validated for real time beam steering MRgHIFU experiment.[34] In this scenario, the acquisition, reconstruction and processing of incoming MR-images need to satisfy the real time constraint of the beam steering system and must therefore be performed with minimal overall latency. For this purpose, accelerated MR-acquisition schemes combined with efficient graphic processing unit (GPU) based reconstruction[67,68] have been shown to enable online reconstruction of 2D MR images with a high framerate and low latency.[67] Image-based motion estimation of the target can then be performed immediately after the image reconstruction using either feature-based approaches[64,69] or intensity-based approaches.[34,41,65,66] In feature-based approaches, specific vessels that were initially selected manually were automatically tracked during the procedure.[64,69] Although it does not require intensive computation, it may be limited to fully characterize complex motion. Furthermore, the additional vessel deformation induced by the cardiac activity may also bias the overall organ motion estimates. Intensity-based approaches using optical flow have also been demonstrated to offer robust motion estimates in MR-thermometry images.[34,41,65,66] Since these algorithms are generally time consuming, GPU-based acceleration has been proposed to enable their real time feasibility.[43,70] Despite the advantages of generating dense motion fields in real time which enable accurate characterization of complex motion, these techniques are still limited to 2D motion estimation since it is hard to acquire 3D MR volumes with a high frame-rate. Alignment of the imaging plane along the main direction of the motion must here again be used to minimize the effect of through plane motion.

Recently, 2D MR-images and MR-navigators have been combined to compute 3D target motion estimates in real time.[45,47] While the MR-navigator provides a measure of the target motion along one direction, MR images are used to track the target motion in the two remaining spatial dimensions using image-based motion estimation algorithms. The position of the imaging plane was also adjusted based on the MR-navigator to reduce through plane motion artifacts in the MR images. This approach has been successfully demonstrated during real time 3D beam steering MRgHIFU experiments.[45,47] Further improvements were made by using a fat-selective MR-navigator which removes potential artifacts in fat suppressed MR images caused by the imaging pulses of conventional MR navigators.[47]

Although such technique provides a robust framework for real time 3D beam steering, a high MR imaging frame-rate is mandatory (~10 Hz), which may be unfavorable for the MR thermometry/dosimetry system which would rather privilege the spatial resolution and coverage. Two alternatives strategies have been recently suggested, although not yet demonstrated for real time 3D beam steering: (1) to use lower MR imaging frame-rate required for volumetric MR thermometry/dosimetry in combination with motion prediction algorithms to improve the temporal characterization of the target motion,[71,72] or (2) to use an interleaved acquisition of one slice sweeping continuously within the desired observation area and one invariant slice.[73] While the first moving slice can be used to compute volumetric thermometry/dosimetry over the observation area, the second invariant slice may be used for high temporal estimation of the target motion.

3.2.2. *Direct motion estimation using US signal*

The simultaneous use of US imaging and HIFU is hampered by their potential mutual interference. However, although the acquisition of US signal and HIFU sonication should be interleaved, it represents a promising approach to operate the MR thermometry/dosimetry and the beam steering systems independently and with different temporal resolutions. In the settings of an MRgHIFU procedure, US signal can be acquired from two different devices: the HIFU transducer or external US probes.

US-based motion estimation of the target has been initially proposed using US echoes generated from selected elements of the HIFU transducer.[30,74,75] One dimensional displacements of the target were estimated for three different spatial directions, which enable the reconstruction of the target displacement in 3D. This technique has been validated during real time 3D beam steering HIFU experiments (without MR guidance). However, the estimation of three 1D motion can be limited to characterize the targeted organ motion when US are obstructed by ribs and air in the beam path.

The use of external US probes has also been proposed to enable the acquisition of US signal during the interventional procedure and to improve the characterization of the target motion. The feasibility of such approach has been initially demonstrated during real time beam steering MRgHIFU experiment using ultrasonic echoes obtained from a single transducer element.[63] In this study, the target motion could only be evaluated in 1D which is insufficient in practice for clinical scenario. Recent advances have demonstrated the feasibility of simultaneous acquisition of US images and MR images.[76] The potential of hybrid US-MR system to estimate the respiratory-induced motion in human heart has been shown using real time contour tracking algorithms applied to US images.[46] This strategy has also been recently evaluated during MRgHIFU experiment using optical flow algorithms to track the target motion in US images.[77]

4. Conclusions

Advanced motion correction strategies which enable continuous monitoring of the thermal dose and continuous sonication under free breathing conditions have been demonstrated in few pre-clinical studies. However, despite these progresses, additional pre-clinical studies are warranted to fully demonstrate the accuracy, safety and robustness of these techniques. In the current state, gated strategies, which are technically less challenging, may represent a reasonable compromise for initial translation to clinics.

References

1. J. Ferlay, H.R. Shin, F. Bray, D. Forman, C. Mathers, D.M. Parkin, "Estimates of worldwide burden of cancer in 2008: GLOBOCAN 2008," *Int J Cancer* **127**, 2893–2917 (2010).
2. P. Lele, "A simple method for production of trackless focal lesions with focused ultrasound: physical factors," *J Physiology* **160**, 494–512 (1962).
3. J.G. Lynn, R.L. Zwemer, A.J. Chick, A.E. Miller, "A new method for the generation and use of focused ultrasound in experimental biology," *J General Physiology* **26**, 179 (1942).
4. A. Hacker, M.S. Michel, E. Marlinghaus, K.U. Kohrmann, P. Alken, "Extracorporeally induced ablation of renal tissue by high-intensity focused ultrasound," *BJU Int* **97**, 779–785 (2006).
5. H.E. Cline, J.F. Schenck, K. Hynynen, R.D. Watkins, S.P. Souza, F.A. Jolesz, "MR-guided focused ultrasound surgery," *J Comput Assist Tomogr* **16**, 956–965. (1992).
6. K. Hynynen, N. McDannold, G. Clement *et al.*, "Pre-clinical testing of a phased array ultrasound system for MRI-guided noninvasive surgery of the brain–a primate study," *Eur J Radiol* **59**, 149–156 (2006).
7. F.A. Jolesz, K. Hynynen, "Magnetic resonance image-guided focused ultrasound surgery," *Cancer J* **8**, S100–112 (2002).
8. W. Wlodarczyk, R. Boroschewski, M. Hentschel, P. Wust, G. Monich, R. Felix, "Three-dimensional monitoring of small temperature changes for therapeutic hyperthermia using MR," *J Magn Reson Imaging* **8**, 165–174 (1998).

9. K. Kuroda, "Non-invasive MR thermography using the water proton chemical shift," *Int J Hyperthermia* **21**, 547–560 (2005).
10. V. Rieke, K. Butts Pauly, "MR thermometry," *J Magn Reson Imaging* **27**, 376–390 (2008).
11. R.J. Stafford, J.D. Hazle, "Magnetic resonance temperature imaging for focused ultrasound surgery: a review," *Top Magn Reson Imaging* **17**, 153–163 (2006).
12. S.A. Sapareto, W.C. Dewey, "Thermal dose determination in cancer therapy," *Int J Radiat Oncol Biol Phys* **10**, 787–800 (1984).
13. G.K. Hesley, K.R. Gorny, D.A. Woodrum, "MR-guided focused ultrasound for the treatment of uterine fibroids," *Cardiovasc Intervent Radiol* **36**, 5–13 (2013).
14. L. Zhang, W.Z. Chen, Y.J. Liu *et al.*, "Feasibility of magnetic resonance imaging-guided high intensity focused ultrasound therapy for ablating uterine fibroids in patients with bowel lies anterior to uterus," *Eur J Radiol* **73**, 396–403 (2010).
15. E.A. Stewart, J. Rabinovici, C.M. Tempany *et al.*, "Clinical outcomes of focused ultrasound surgery for the treatment of uterine fibroids," *Fertil Steril* **85**, 22–29 (2006).
16. D. Gianfelice, C. Gupta, W. Kucharczyk, P. Bret, D. Havill, M. Clemons, "Palliative treatment of painful bone metastases with MR imaging–guided focused ultrasound," *Radiology* **249**, 355–363 (2008).
17. A. Napoli, M. Anzidei, F. Ciolina *et al.*, "MR-guided high-intensity focused ultrasound: current status of an emerging technology," *Cardiovasc Intervent Radiol* **36**, 1190–1203 (2013).
18. J-F Aubry, K.B. Pauly, C. Moonen *et al.*, "The road to clinical use of high-intensity focused ultrasound for liver cancer: technical and clinical consensus," *J Ther Ultrasound* **1**, 13 (2013).
19. B.D. de Senneville, M. Ries, L.W. Bartels, C.T. Moonen, "MRI-guided high-intensity focused ultrasound sonication of liver and kidney," *Interv Magn Reson Imaging*: Springer, 349–366 (2012).
20. W.M. Gedroyc, "New clinical applications of magnetic resonance-guided focused ultrasound," *Top Magn Reson Imaging* **17**, 189–194 (2006).
21. Y. Ishihara, A. Calderon, H. Watanabe, K. Okamoto, Y. Suzuki, K. Kuroda, "A precise and fast temperature mapping using water proton chemical shift," *Magn Reson Med* **34**, 814–823 (1995).
22. N. McDannold, "Quantitative MRI-based temperature mapping based on the proton resonant frequency shift: review of validation studies," *Int J Hyperthermia* **21**, 533–546 (2005).
23. R.D. Peters, R.S. Hinks, R.M. Henkelman, "*Ex vivo* tissue-type independence in proton-resonance frequency shift MR thermometry," *Magn Reson Med* **40**, 454–459 (1998).
24. A. Okada, T. Murakami, K. Mikami *et al.*, "A case of hepatocellular carcinoma treated by MR-guided focused ultrasound ablation with respiratory gating," *Magn Reson Med Sci* **5**, 167–171 (2006).
25. R.D. Peters, R.M. Henkelman, "Proton-resonance frequency shift MR thermometry is affected by changes in the electrical conductivity of tissue," *Magn Reson Med* **43**, 62–71 (2000).
26. H. Rempp, S. Clasen, P.L. Pereira, "Image-based monitoring of magnetic resonance-guided thermoablative therapies for liver tumors," *Cardiovasc Intervent Radiol* **35**, 1281–1294 (2012).

27. K.K. Vigen, B.L. Daniel, J.M. Pauly, K. Butts, "Triggered, navigated, multi-baseline method for proton resonance frequency temperature mapping with respiratory motion," *Magn Reson Med* **50**, 1003–1010 (2003).
28. C. Weidensteiner, N. Kerioui, B. Quesson, B.D. de Senneville, H. Trillaud, C.T. Moonen, "Stability of real-time MR temperature mapping in healthy and diseased human liver," *J Magn Reson Imaging* **19**, 438–446 (2004).
29. S. Morikawa, T. Inubushi, Y. Kurumi *et al.*, "Feasibility of respiratory triggering for MR-guided microwave ablation of liver tumors under general anesthesia," *Cardiovas Interv Radiology* **27**, 370–373 (2004).
30. M. Pernot, M. Tanter, M. Fink, "3-D real-time motion correction in high-intensity focused ultrasound therapy," *Ultrasound Med Biol* **30**, 1239–1249 (2004).
31. C. Mougenot, B. Quesson, B.D. de Senneville *et al.*, "Three-dimensional spatial and temporal temperature control with MR thermometry-guided focused ultrasound (MRgHIFU)," *Magn Reson Med* **61**, 603–614 (2009).
32. E. Ramsay, C. Mougenot, M. Kohler *et al.*, "MR thermometry in the human prostate gland at 3.0T for transurethral ultrasound therapy," *J Magn Reson Imaging* **38**, 1564–1571 (2013).
33. V. Rieke, K.K. Vigen, G. Sommer, B.L. Daniel, J.M. Pauly, K. Butts, "Referenceless PRF shift thermometry," *Magn Reson Med* **51**, 1223–1231 (2004).
34. B.D. de Senneville, C. Mougenot, C.T. Moonen, "Real-time adaptive methods for treatment of mobile organs by MRI-controlled high-intensity focused ultrasound," *Magn Reson Med* **57**, 319–330 (2007).
35. B.D. de Senneville, S. Roujol, C. Moonen, M. Ries, "Motion correction in MR thermometry of abdominal organs: a comparison of the referenceless vs. the multibaseline approach," *Magn Reson Med* **64**, 1373–1381 (2010).
36. W.A. Grissom, V. Rieke, A.B. Holbrook *et al.*, "Hybrid referenceless and multibaseline subtraction MR thermometry for monitoring thermal therapies in moving organs," *Med Phys* **37**, 5014–5026 (2010).
37. A.B. Holbrook, J.M. Santos, E. Kaye, V. Rieke, K.B. Pauly, "Real-time MR thermometry for monitoring HIFU ablations of the liver," *Magn Reson Med* **63**, 365–373 (2010).
38. J.B. Maintz, M.A. Viergever, "A survey of medical image registration," *Med Image Anal* **2**, 1–36 (1998).
39. P. Markelj, D. Tomazevic, B. Likar, F. Pernus, "A review of 3D/2D registration methods for image-guided interventions," *Med Image Anal* **16**, 642–661 (2012).
40. A. Sotiras, C. Davatzikos, N. Paragios, "Deformable medical image registration: a survey," *IEEE Trans Med Imaging* **32**, 1153–1190 (2013).
41. S. Roujol, M. Ries, C. Moonen, B.D. de Senneville, "Robust real time motion estimation for MR-thermometry," *Biomedical Imaging: From Nano to Macro, 2011 IEEE International Symposium on: IEEE*, 508–511 (2011).
42. S. Roujol, M. Ries, C. Moonen, B.D. de Senneville, "Automatic nonrigid calibration of image registration for real time MR-guided HIFU ablations of mobile organs," *IEEE Trans Med Imaging* **30**, 1737–1745 (2011).
43. S. Roujol, M. Ries, B. Quesson, C. Moonen, B Denis de Senneville, "Real-time MR-thermometry and dosimetry for interventional guidance on abdominal organs," *Magn Reson Med* **63**, 1080–1087 (2010).

44. B. Quesson, C. Laurent, G. Maclair *et al.*, "Real-time volumetric MRI thermometry of focused ultrasound ablation *in vivo*: a feasibility study in pig liver and kidney," *NMR Biomed* **24**, 145–153 (2011).
45. M. Ries, B.D. de Senneville, S. Roujol, Y. Berber, B. Quesson, C. Moonen, "Real-time 3D target tracking in MRI guided focused ultrasound ablations in moving tissues," *Magn Reson Med* **64**, 1704–1712 (2010).
46. D.A. Feinberg, D. Giese, D.A. Bongers *et al.*, "Hybrid ultrasound MRI for improved cardiac imaging and real-time respiration control," *Magn Reson Med* **63**, 290–296 (2010).
47. M.O. Kohler, B Denis de Senneville, B. Quesson, C.T. Moonen, M. Ries, "Spectrally selective pencil-beam navigator for motion compensation of MR-guided high-intensity focused ultrasound therapy of abdominal organs," *Magn Reson Med* **66**, 102–111 (2011).
48. M. Ries, B.D. de Senneville, S. Roujol, C. Moonen, "Latency compensation for real-time 3D HIFU beam-steering on moving targets," *Proceedings 18th Scientific Meeting, International Society for Magnetic Resonance in Medicine* (2010).
49. L. Ramrath, A. Schlaefer, F. Ernst, S. Dieterich, A. Schweikard, "Prediction of respiratory motion with a multi-frequency based Extended Kalman Filter," *Proceedings of the 21st International Conference and Exhibition on Computer Assisted Radiology and Surgery (CARS'07)* (2007).
50. J.R. McClelland, D.J. Hawkes, T. Schaeffter, A.P. King, "Respiratory motion models: a review," *Med Image Anal* **17**, 19–42 (2013).
51. C. Grozea, D. Lubke, F. Dingeldey *et al.*, "ESWT-tracking organs during focused ultrasound surgery," *Machine Learning for Signal Processing (MLSP), 2012 IEEE International Workshop on: IEEE* 1–6 (2012).
52. E.-J. Rijkhorst, D. Heanes, F. Odille, D. Hawkes, D. Barratt, "Simulating dynamic ultrasound using MR-derived motion models to assess respiratory synchronisation for image-guided liver interventions," *Information Processing in Computer-Assisted Interventions*: Springer, 113–123 (2010).
53. V. Auboiroux, L. Petrusca, M. Viallon *et al.*, "Respiratory-Gated MRgHIFU in Upper Abdomen Using an MR-Compatible In-Bore Digital Camera," *BioMed Research International* (2014).
54. P. Arnold, F. Preiswerk, B. Fasel, R. Salomir, K. Scheffler, P.C. Cattin, "3D organ motion prediction for MR-guided high intensity focused ultrasound," *Med Image Comput Comput Assist Interv* **14**, 623–630 (2011).
55. J.A. de Zwart, F.C. Vimeux, J. Palussiere *et al.*, "On-line correction and visualization of motion during MRI-controlled hyperthermia," *Magn Reson Med* **45**, 128–137 (2001).
56. A.B. Holbrook, P. Ghanouni, J.M. Santos, C. Dumoulin, Y. Medan, K.B. Pauly, "Respiration based steering for high intensity focused ultrasound liver ablation," *Magn Reson Med* **71**, 797–806 (2014).
57. B.D. de Senneville, M. Ries, G. Maclair, C. Moonen, "MR-guided thermotherapy of abdominal organs using a robust PCA-based motion descriptor," *Medical Imaging, IEEE Transactions on* **30**, 1987–1995 (2011).
58. L. Petrusca, P. Cattin, V. De Luca *et al.*, "Hybrid ultrasound/magnetic resonance simultaneous acquisition and image fusion for motion monitoring in the upper abdomen," *Invest Radiol* **48**, 333–340 (2013).

59. F. Preiswerk, P. Arnold, B. Fasel, P.C. Cattin, "Robust tumour tracking from 2D imaging using a population-based statistical motion model," *Mathematical Methods in Biomedical Image Analysis (MMBIA), 2012 IEEE Workshop on: IEEE*, 209–214 (2012).
60. F. Preiswerk, V. De Lucab, P. Arnolda *et al.*, "Model-Guided Respiratory Organ Motion Prediction of the Liver from 2D Ultrasound," *Med Image Anal* (2013).
61. M. Ries, B.D. de Senneville, Y. Regard, C. Moonen, "Combined magnetic resonance imaging and ultrasound echography guidance for motion compensated HIFU interventions," *12th International Symposium on Therapeutic Ultrasound: AIP Publishing*, 202–206 (2012).
62. E.-J. Rijkhorst, I. Rivens, G.T. Haar, D. Hawkes, D. Barratt, "Effects of respiratory liver motion on heating for gated and model-based motion-compensated high-intensity focused ultrasound ablation," *Proceedings of the 14th International Conference on Medical Image Computing and Computer-Assisted Intervention-Volume Part I*: Springer-Verlag 605–612 (2011).
63. P.L. de Oliveira, B.D. de Senneville, I. Dragonu, C.T. Moonen, "Rapid motion correction in MR-guided high-intensity focused ultrasound heating using real-time ultrasound echo information," *NMR Biomed* **23**, 1103–1108 (2010).
64. J.C. Ross, R. Tranquebar, D. Shanbhag, "Real-time liver motion compensation for MRgFUS," *Med Image Comput Comput Assist Interv* **11**, 806–813 (2008).
65. S. Roujol, J. Benois-Pineau, B.D. de Senneville, B. Quesson, M. Ries, C. Moonen, "Real time constrained motion estimation for ECG-gated cardiac MRI," *Image Processing (ICIP), 2010 17th IEEE International Conference on: IEEE* 757–760 (2010).
66. S. Roujol, J. Benois-Pineau, B.D. de Senneville, M. Ries, B. Quesson, C.T. Moonen, "Robust real-time-constrained estimation of respiratory motion for interventional MRI on mobile organs," *IEEE Trans Inf Technol Biomed* **16**, 365–374 (2012).
67. S. Roujol, B.D. de Senneville, E. Vahala, T.S. Sorensen, C. Moonen, M. Ries, "Online real-time reconstruction of adaptive TSENSE with commodity CPU/GPU hardware," *Magn Reson Med* **62**, 1658–1664 (2009).
68. T.S. Sorensen, D. Atkinson, T. Schaeffter, M.S. Hansen, "Real-time reconstruction of sensitivity encoded radial magnetic resonance imaging using a graphics processing unit," *IEEE Trans Med Imaging* **28**, 1974–1985 (2009).
69. D. Kokuryo, T. Kaihara, E. Kumamoto, S. Fujii, K. Kuroda, "Method for target tracking in focused ultrasound surgery of liver using magnetic resonance filtered venography," *Engineering in Medicine and Biology Society, 2007 EMBS 2007 29th Annual International Conference of the IEEE: IEEE* 2614–2617 (2007).
70. B.D. de Senneville, K.O. Noe, M. Ries, M. Pedersen, C.T. Moonen, T. Sorensen, "An optimised multi-baseline approach for on-line MR-temperature monitoring on commodity graphics hardware," *Biomedical Imaging: From Nano to Macro, 2008 ISBI 2008 5th IEEE International Symposium on: IEEE* 1513–1516 (2008).
71. B.D. de Senneville, M. Ries, C. Moonen, "Real-time anticipation of organ displacement for MR-guidance of interventional procedures," *Biomedical Imaging (ISBI), 2013 IEEE 10th International Symposium on: IEEE* 1420–1423 (2013).
72. F. Ernst, A. Schlaefer, A. Schweikard, "Prediction of respiratory motion with wavelet-based multiscale autoregression," *Med Image Comput Comput Assist Interv* **10**, 668–675 (2007).

73. B. Denis de Senneville, S. Roujol, S. Hey, C. Moonen, M. Ries, "Extended Kalman filtering for continuous volumetric MR-temperature imaging," *IEEE Trans Med Imaging* **32**, 711–718 (2013).
74. F. Marquet, J.F. Aubry, M. Pernot, M. Fink, M. Tanter, "Optimal transcostal high-intensity focused ultrasound with combined real-time 3D movement tracking and correction," *Phys Med Biol* **56**, 7061–7080 (2011).
75. F. Marquet, M. Pernot, J.F. Aubry, M. Tanter, G. Montaldo, M. Fink, "*In-vivo* non-invasive motion tracking and correction in high intensity focused ultrasound therapy," *Conf Proc IEEE Eng Med Biol Soc* **1**, 688–691 (2006).
76. A.M. Tang, D.F. Kacher, E.Y. Lam, K.K. Wong, F.A. Jolesz, E.S. Yang, "Simultaneous ultrasound and MRI system for breast biopsy: compatibility assessment and demonstration in a dual modality phantom," *IEEE Trans Med Imaging* **27**, 247–254 (2008).
77. V. Auboiroux, L. Petrusca, M. Viallon, T. Goget, C.D. Becker, R. Salomir, "Ultrasonography-based 2D motion-compensated HIFU sonication integrated with reference-free MR temperature monitoring: a feasibility study *ex vivo*," *Phys Med Biol* **57**, N159–171 (2012).

Chapter 18

Advanced Imaging Technologies in Proton Therapy

Zhong Su, Hao Chen and Zuofeng Li*

University of Florida Proton Therapy Institute
2015 N. Jefferson St., Jacksonville, FL 32206
**suzho@ufl.edu*

Proton therapy is a key radiation therapy modality used in the treatment of cancer. With a low entrance dose and no exit dose, proton therapy has the desired physics properties to spare healthy tissues. However, uncertainties attributable to calibration of the computed tomography (CT) number-to-proton-relative stopping power, daily patient setup, and anatomical changes during a treatment course lead to proton-range uncertainties, which can be detrimental to patients. The intrinsic range uncertainty in CT-relative stopping power calibration can be minimized using proton CT; the random and systematic range variations from patient setup and anatomical changes can be monitored using positron emission tomography (PET) and prompted gamma ray imaging, which detect the byproducts from proton nuclear interactions with human tissues. This chapter reviews proton therapy physics, sources of proton-range uncertainties, and the advanced imaging technologies used to minimize or monitor these uncertainties before, during, and after proton therapy.

1. Radiation Therapy

Radiation therapy uses high-energy particles or waves, such as X-rays and gamma rays, electron beams, proton beams, and heavy ions (i.e., carbon) as part of cancer treatment to control or kill malignant cells.[1] As one of the most effective treatments for cancer, radiation therapy is intended to achieve a high probability of local tumor control (tumor control probability, TCP) with a low risk of normal tissue complications (normal tissue complication probability, NTCP).[2] The main aim of radiation therapy is to deliver a dose that is high enough to eradicate tumors while sparing surrounding normal tissues and organs at risk (OAR). Medical imaging technologies are involved in the key steps of radiation therapy to lower NTCP yet maintain high TCP.[3,4] The introduction of CT in radiation treatment planning and cone-beam CT (CBCT) for image guidance in pre-treatment target alignment are two of the major imaging technology application milestones in radiation therapy. Since 1990, when the first hospital-based proton treatment facility was built at the Loma Linda University Medical Center (LLUMC) in California,[5] proton therapy has been used to reduce normal tissue toxicity and improve tumor control due to its desirable physics properties. These properties also provide a foundation for state-of-the-art imaging technologies to be developed and applied to proton therapy treatment planning, delivery monitoring, and post-treatment evaluation.

In this chapter, we will (1) review the current state of radiation therapy using high-energy photons and protons; (2) highlight the physics of proton interactions with matter; (3) discuss factors that can affect the range of proton beams; and (4) review state-of-the-art imaging technologies that can minimize proton-range uncertainties in treatment planning and range monitoring before, during, and after proton therapy.

1.1. *High-Energy Photon Radiation Therapy*

The high-energy photons used in radiation therapy are X-rays ranging from 1 to 25 MV that deliver doses to treat deep-seated tumors located in the prostate, lung, or brain, among other organs. These high-energy photons interact with human tissues through photoelectric effect, Compton scatter, and pair production. Compton scatter, the dominant interaction within the energy range of photon radiation therapy,[6] generates a highly energetic Compton electron as well as a Compton scattered photon, which has less energy than the incident photon. The energetic electrons from Compton scatter can transfer their energy to other bonded electrons to generate more energetic free electrons. This process of ionization leads DNA chemical bonds to break; free radicals that can permanently fix the radiation breaks of DNA are also generated.[7] DNA double-strand breaks lead to cell death without regeneration. If the cell is malignant, the cancer cell is killed; if the cell is a part of healthy tissue, it is collateral damage (the normal tissue toxicity in radiation therapy).

The dose deposited in a medium by high-energy photons decreases with the increasing depth of the medium (Fig. 1). For deep tumors, a single high-energy photon beam can cause more damage to healthy tissues upstream of the tumor. Therefore, the majority of high-energy photon treatments involve targeting the tumor with multiple beams from various beam angles, thereby creating a cross-fire effect that intensifies the radiation dose to the tumor and reduces radiation toxicity to the normal tissue. This treatment technique is being used with 3-dimensional conformal therapy and intensity-modulated radiation therapy (IMRT).

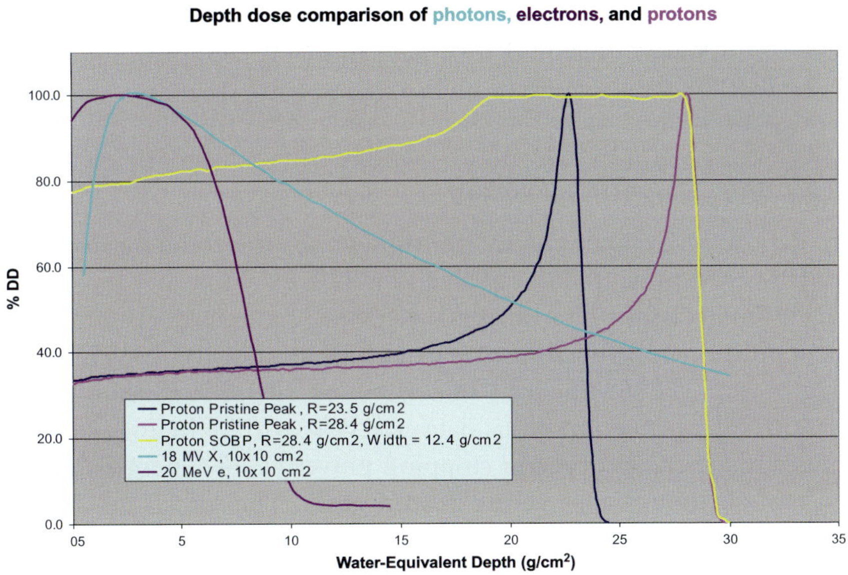

Fig. 1. Percentage depth dose curves for photon, electron, and proton beams.

In modern high-energy photon radiation therapy, X-ray radiographs/CBCT are employed before treatment to minimize uncertainties in patient setup and organ motion. After setup verification, external high energy X-rays are used to deliver the prescribed dose to the tumor.[8,9] Tumors located in the thoracic region can exhibit extensive tumor motion. The impact of this motion can be mitigated by daily pre-treatment X-ray radiographs or CBCT images. Margin expansion from the clinical target volume (CTV) to the planning target volume (PTV)[10] can account for residual setup and organ motion uncertainties. According to International Commission on Radiation Units and Measurements (ICRU) Report 62, the CTV contains malignant growth tissue and subclinical microscopic malignant disease. The PTV includes the CTV and internal variations in size, shape, and position as well as uncertainties in patient positioning and alignment. Using a population-based statistical study, Van Herk *et al.* provided a "margin recipe" that accounts for systematic and random components of target delineation, setup uncertainty, and organ motion uncertainty.[11] In the early years of radiation therapy, large PTV margins were used to account for greater setup and organ motion uncertainties without image guidance. Image-guided radiation therapy (IGRT) can reduce setup and organ motion uncertainties and improve the target alignment accuracy of the radiation field. Thus, it ensures adequate tumor coverage and minimum exposure of healthy tissue during radiation treatments.[12] Each radiation therapy institute should determine the exact margin for treatment planning while considering tumor location, image guidance, treatment modality, and planning technique. However, the PTV is not entirely applicable in proton therapy.

1.2. *Proton Radiation Therapy*

Energy deposited by high-energy photons in tissue exhibits a dose buildup followed by an exponential decay (Fig. 1). The exit dose beyond the tumor damages normal tissues. For charged particles (e.g., electrons and protons), energy deposition is a function of particle energy fluence and tissue proton stopping power. The pristine peak of a mono-energy proton beam has a sharp distal falloff. A large portion of the delivered dose within the Bragg peak is due to significantly increased proton stopping power at low energies; no dose is beyond the maximum range of the proton beam. The spread-out Bragg peak (SOBP), which is a linear combination of different mono-energy proton beams with different weights, can deliver a uniform dose into a specific area (size of tumor) located at a certain depth. The range of the proton beam is defined as 90% or 95% of distal dose falloff for the proton beam. The modulation width of the proton beam, the uniform dose region that covers tumor width in the beam direction, is defined as the plateau between 90%/95% of the distal and proximal ends.[13]

The passive-scattering mode is a proton beam delivery technique in which scattering materials spread the beam to the required field size, and range-shifting materials conform the beam to the distal portion of the treated tumor.[14] In the passive-scattering technique, 2 scatterers work together to provide a uniform lateral field profile, and the rotation of the range modulator wheel is synchronized with the current modulation of the proton beam to achieve an adjustable SOBP modulation width. An aperture is used in double-scattering proton therapy to shape the proton dose to the target laterally in the beam-eye-view, and the range compensator conforms the proton dose to the distal end of the target [Fig. 2(a)].[13] Pencil-beam scanning (PBS)[15] places pristine peaks of different proton energies throughout the target volume [Fig. 2(b)]. This 2-dimensional "layer" scanning of a proton beam in the dimension perpendicular to the beam direction can be achieved with 2 orthogonal scanning magnets. The proton dose is "painted" inside these layers located at different depths with different proton energies.

The dose delivered by a proton beam could drop from 100% down to less than 1% within 1 cm due to the sharp dose falloff at distal end of the SOBP. This property is often used by clinicians to spare OARs abutting the tumor at the distal end of the SOBP. If the proton stopping power of the tissues in the beam

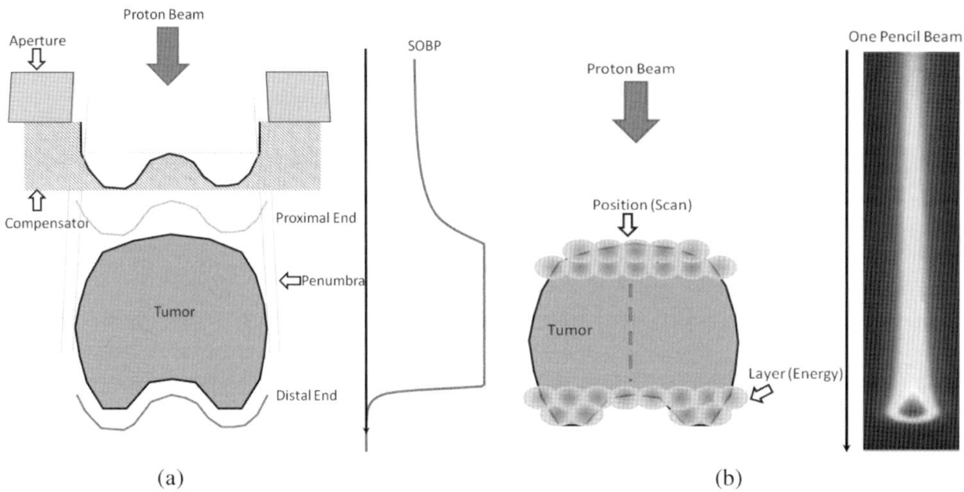

Fig. 2. Illustration of proton treatment techniques: (a) double-scattering mode; (b) pencil-beam scanning mode.

path is not accurate, the prescription dose to the tumor can be potentially deposited to the OARs. Therefore, obtaining the accurate proton stopping power for the tissues and knowing its uncertainty is essential. Moreover, the treatment beam range in patients should be actively monitored.

2. Proton Interactions with Matter

Human tissues are composed of many naturally occurring elements (Table 1); however, oxygen, carbon, hydrogen, and nitrogen account for more than 96% of human body weight. During proton therapy, high-energy protons enter the patient's body and deposit energy through either ionization or nuclear interactions with the nuclei in tissues. When protons interact with tissue electrons through electromagnetic Coulomb interactions, part of the kinetic energy of the protons is transferred to these orbital electrons of the tissue elements. The energy loss of protons through Coulomb interactions is characterized by the stopping power of protons with energy E[6]:

$$S(E) = 0.307\frac{Z}{A}\frac{1}{\beta^2}\left(\frac{1}{2}\ln\frac{2m_e c^2\beta^2 T_{\max}}{I^2(1-\beta^2)} - \beta^2\right), \tag{1}$$

where Z and A are atomic number and atomic mass of the media, respectively; $\beta = \frac{v}{c}$ is relative proton velocity; I is the mean excitation energy of the medium electron.

Table 1. Naturally occurring elements in the human body.

Symbol	Element	Atomic number	Percentage of human body weight (%)
O	Oxygen	8	65.0
C	Carbon	6	18.5
H	Hydrogen	1	9.5
N	Nitrogen	7	3.3
Ca	Calcium	20	1.5
P	Phosphorus	15	1.0
K	Potassium	19	0.4
S	Sulfur	16	0.3
Na	Sodium	11	0.2
Cl	Chlorine	17	0.2
Mg	Magnesium	12	0.1

*Trace elements (less than 0.01%): Boron (B), Chromium (Cr), Cobalt (Co), Copper (Cu), Fluorine (F), Iodine (I), Iron (Fe), Manganese (Mn), Molybdenum (Mo), Selenium (Se), Silicon (Si), Tin (Sn), Vanadium (V), and Zinc (Zn).

With an increase in incident proton energy, there is an energy threshold beyond which exists the probability of inelastic nuclear collisions of protons with tissue nuclei. During nuclear interactions, the primary protons are absorbed into tissue nuclei, creating daughter elements and emitting secondary particles (i.e., protons, neutrons, and gamma rays). We will focus on positron-emitting daughter nuclei and prompt gamma emissions in the following sections.

2.1. *Positron Emissions*

The probabilities of proton inelastic nuclear interactions are determined by the proton-induced nuclear interaction cross sections of ^{16}O, ^{12}C, and ^{14}N. Some of these interactions produce daughter elements that are radioactive; thus, they are in an unstable nuclear state. Through positron emissions, these elements are converted to stable elements. The emitted positron annihilates with an electron to create a pair of 0.511-MeV gamma rays going in opposite directions. Opposing gamma-ray detector arrays can be set up around the patient treatment section to detect these coincident photons. Positron-activity images can be reconstructed for treatment setup and range verifications. Table 2 lists some examples of positron-emitter production in proton therapy.[16]

Table 2. Positron-emitter production in the proton therapy.

Reaction	Threshold [MeV]	Half-life [min]	Positron Max. energy [MeV]
$^{16}O(p,pn)^{15}O$	16.79	2.037	1.72
$^{16}O(p,2p2n)^{13}N$*	5.66***	9.965	1.19
$^{14}N(p,pn)^{13}N$	11.44	9.965	1.19
$^{12}C(p,pn)^{11}C$	20.61	20.39	0.96
$^{14}N(p,2p2n)^{11}C$*	3.22***	20.39	0.96
$^{16}O(p,3p3n)^{11}C$**	27.50***	20.39	0.96

*(p,2p2n) is inclusive of (p, α)
**(p,3p3n) is inclusive of (p, αpn)
***the listed thresholds refer to (p, α) and (p, αpn)

2.2. *Prompt Gamma Ray Emissions*

For some inelastic nuclear interactions, the produced elements are in a state of nuclear excitation. Deexcitation to the ground state of these nuclei produces gamma rays with a range of energies. These nuclear deexcitations occur within nanoseconds of original nuclear interactions, and the resulting gamma rays are named prompt gammas. The cross sections of these nuclear interactions producing prompt gamma rays have peak intensities near the nuclear interaction threshold energies and decrease dramatically with increase energy of incident protons. In contrast to positron-activity imaging, detector arrays from one side of the patient with proper collimation and shielding can detect these prompt gamma rays. Moreover, the detected signal intensity peaks are close to the distal falloff of the Bragg peak of a monoenergetic proton beam. Thus, detections of prompt gamma can be detected and used for proton beam-range verification. Since the prompted gamma rays are released within 10^{-19} to 10^{-9} seconds of the nuclear interactions, real-time range verification can be achieved using prompt gamma detection and analysis. Table 3 lists the prompt gamma rays energies by proton interaction with major elements in human tissues.[17]

3. Range Uncertainty in Proton Therapy

3.1. *Uncertainty in CT Number-to-Proton-Relative-Stopping-Power Calibration*

In modern radiation therapy, cancer patients usually receive CT scans (using kV X-rays) that include the section of the body enclosing tumors or targets. These 3-dimensional (3D) CT images are sent to a computerized treatment planning

Table 3. Gamma rays energies by proton interaction with major elements in human tissues.

E (Mev)	Transition	Reaction	Mean Life (s)
0.718	$^{10}B^{0.718} \rightarrow$g.s.	$^{12}C(p,x)^{10}B^*$	1.0×10^{-9}
		$^{12}C(p,x)^{10}C(\varepsilon)^{10}B^*$	27.8
		$^{16}O(p,x)^{10}B^*$	1.0×10^{-9}
0.937	$^{18}F^{0.937} \rightarrow$g.s.	$^{16}O(^3He,p)^{18}F^*$	6.8×10^{-11}
1.022	$^{10}B^{1.740} \rightarrow {}^{10}B^{0.718}$	$^{12}C(p,x)^{10}B^*$	7.5×10^{-15}
		$^{16}O(p,x)^{10}B^*$	7.5×10^{-15}
1.042	$^{18}F^{1.042} \rightarrow$g.s.	$^{16}O(^3He,p)^{18}F^*$	2.6×10^{-15}
1.635	$^{14}N^{3.948} \rightarrow {}^{14}N^{2.313}$	$^{14}N(p,p^*)^{14}N^*$	6.9×10^{-15}
2.000	$^{11}C^{2.000} \rightarrow$g.s.	$^{12}C(p,x)^{11}C^*$	1.0×10^{-14}
2.124	$^{11}B^{2.125} \rightarrow$g.s.	$^{12}C(p,x)^{11}B^*$	5.5×10^{-15}
2.313	$^{14}N^{2.313} \rightarrow$g.s.	$^{14}N(p,p^*)^{14}N^*$	9.8×10^{-14}
		$^{16}O(p,x)^{14}N^*$	9.8×10^{-14}
2.742	$^{16}O^{8.872} \rightarrow {}^{16}O^{6.130}$	$^{16}O(p,p^*)^{16}O^*$	1.8×10^{-13}
3.736	$^{40}Ca^{3.736} \rightarrow$g.s.	$^{40}Ca(p,p^*)^{40}Ca^*$	2.9×10^{-11}
4.438	$^{12}C^{4.439} \rightarrow$g.s.	$^{12}C(p,p^*)^{12}C^*$	6.1×10^{-14}
		$^{14}N(p,x)^{12}C^*$	6.1×10^{-14}
		$^{16}O(p,x)^{12}C^*$	6.1×10^{-14}
4.444	$^{11}B^{4.445} \rightarrow$g.s.	$^{12}C(p,2p)^{11}B$	5.6×10^{-19}
		$^{14}N(p,x)^{11}B$	5.6×10^{-19}
5.105	$^{14}N^{5.105} \rightarrow$g.s.	$^{14}N(p,p^*)^{14}N^*$	6.3×10^{-12}
		$^{16}O(p,x)^{14}N^*$	6.3×10^{-12}
5.180	$^{15}O^{5.180} \rightarrow$g.s.	$^{16}O(p,x)^{15}O^*$	$<4.9 \times 10^{-14}$
6.129	$^{16}O^{6.130} \rightarrow$g.s.	$^{16}O(p,p^*)^{16}O^*$	2.7×10^{-11}
6.916	$^{16}O^{6.917} \rightarrow$g.s.	$^{16}O(p,p^*)^{16}O^*$	6.8×10^{-15}
7.115	$^{16}O^{7.117} \rightarrow$g.s.	$^{16}O(p,p^*)^{16}O^*$	1.2×10^{-14}
15.10	$^{12}C^{15.11} \rightarrow$g.s.	$^{12}C(p,p^*)^{12}C^*$	1.5×10^{-17}

system (TPS)[18] for target and OAR delineation and treatment planning. This approach allows clinicians to visualize the tumor and its geometric relationship to the surrounding OARs and can potentially minimize the radiation dose to these OARs in the optimized treatment plan. During the treatment planning process, the planner can place a digital treatment machine (with the same properties as an actual treatment machine, Fig. 3) at different angles and directions to create a treatment plan that delivers the prescribed dose to the target while irradiating the minimum amount of health tissue. To calculate dose to the target and to the irradiated healthy tissues, the TPS has to be able to calculate the energy deposited from the radiation beams to the patient 3D CT dataset.

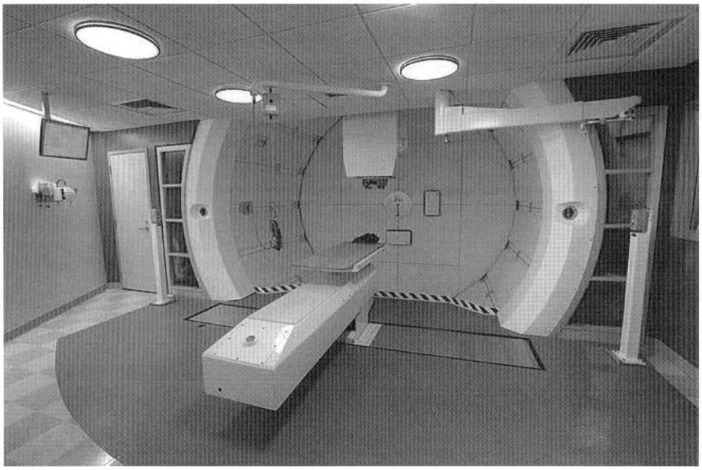

Fig. 3. Proton therapy gantry room.

The CT dataset is comprised of many voxels with different Hounsfield Unit (HU) numbers. The HU number of each voxel is proportional to the kV X-ray attenuation coefficients of the materials of that voxel. Proton stopping powers are needed to calculate the radiation dose to each voxel. The relationship between the CT HU numbers and proton relative stopping power to water of various materials has to be defined. This relationship is called CT number-to-relative-stopping-power calibration. It is an important step toward accurate proton dose and range calculation inside the patient CT dataset.[19] Schneider *et al.* proposed using a stoichiometric method for the CT number-to-proton-relative-stopping-power calibration. There are two main steps in this approach:

(1) Parameterize the HU number calculations equation using tissue substitute materials with known chemical compositions (Fig. 4).
(2) Using the obtained parameters to calculate the HU number and the relative stopping power of various human tissues with known chemical compositions (published by the ICRU), obtain the calibration curve.

Nevertheless, there are some intrinsic uncertainties existed in this calibration method. The tissue chemical compositions published by ICRU are from several specific individuals. The elemental compositions of the same type of tissues from different patients may vary. Furthermore, for the same tissue substitutes with fixed X-ray kVp of CT scanner, the obtained CT HU number also changes with phantom size and relative location of the tissue substitute inside the phantom. This variation leads to an uncertainty in the relative stopping power, thus leads to uncertainty of proton beam range inside the patient. This range uncertainty

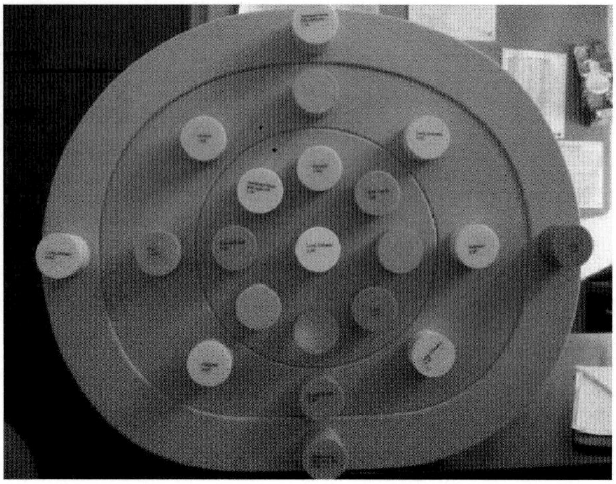

Fig. 4. CT calibration phantom with tissue substitute inserts.

can potentially lead to overdose to OARs, i.e., spinal cord or brainstem, at the distal end of the proton beams. Therefore, there are needs to either accurately monitor the beam range for each patient during treatment (prompt gamma detection) or after treatment (proton positron activation detection). The alternative is to find a more accurate relationship between patient tissues and their relative stopping power to water using proton CT.

3.2. *Anatomical Changes and Daily Setup Uncertainty*

Patient weight loss, tumor progression, and tumor shrinkage can lead to anatomical changes during a course of treatment. An individual tumor can shift in a small region relative to the bony anatomy due to various reasons, including respiratory motion that causes tumor motion inside the lungs or upper abdomen; empty/full bladder and rectal filling, which changes the prostate location in the pelvis; and voluntary motion of the head with respect to an immobilization mask in conventional head and neck radiotherapy.[20] These anatomical changes and organ motions affect the range of proton beams and can lead to tumor underdose or severe damage of OARs, the spinal cord, and heart (see Fig. 5), which can be located just beyond the distal falloff of the beam. Medial lung tumors can be close to heart, and some posterior lung tumors can be in the vicinity of the spinal cord. Thus, daily setup and tumor motion within the lungs are of great interest to clinicians. Shimizu *et al.* investigated lung tumor motion during treatment using a gold marker inserted in the tumor. During normal breathing, the marker motion was 5.5∼10.9 mm

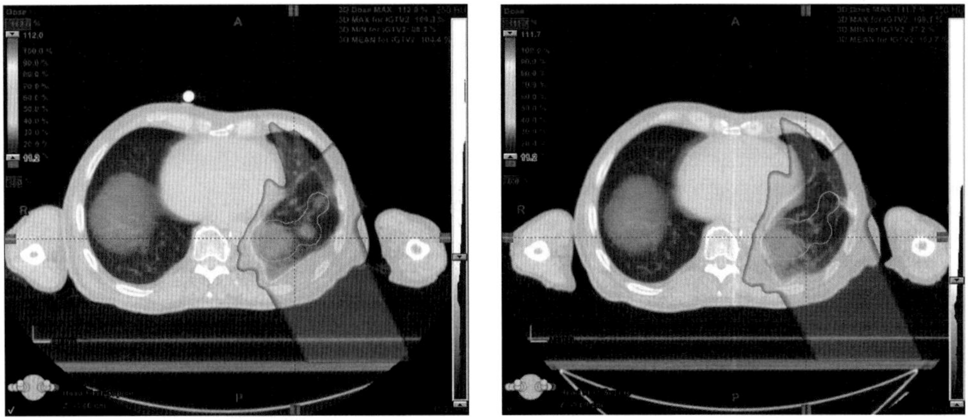

Original Treatment Plan Verification Plan after 4 weeks

Fig. 5. Tumor volume change within a treatment course and its impact on proton beam range.

along the right-left, 6.8~15.9 mm along the superior-inferior, and 8.1~14.6 along the anterior-posterior directions. Lung tumor motion was reduced to within 5.3 mm in all three directions with gating.[21] The largest movement in the lung could be up to 2.0 cm in the longitudinal direction.[22] These tumor motion and anatomical changes during a treatment course result in significant proton-range variations and have a negative dosimetric impact; consequently, they must be monitored to ensure proper treatment.

4. Advanced Imaging Technologies Addressing the Range Uncertainty

4.1. *Range Uncertainty and its Impacts*

Range uncertainty can be categorized into systematic and random types. The intrinsic uncertainty of the CT HU number-to-proton-relative-stopping-power calibration causes systematic proton range changes. Patient daily setup cannot be perfectly matched to the CT-scanned patient geometry; this is usually a small difference that follows Gaussian distribution of the setup errors and leads to random range uncertainty. When patients experience either significant body mass changes (weight loss) or tumor shrinkage during treatment, proton beam ranges inside the patient are significantly affected. This results in a gradually increased systematic range uncertainty.

Figure 5 shows the dose distributions of the original proton beam on an initial CT scan and on a verification CT scan acquired 4 weeks later. It clearly shows the proton beam overshooting the target due to tumor shrinkage. Although this significant range uncertainty can be mitigated through weekly CT scans to verify mass changes of tumors and tissues along the proton beam path, it cannot be completely eliminated. Obtaining range information for the proton beam under treatment conditions will ensure delivery of the appropriate dose to the target and minimize dose to the OARs. There are several methods to verify this range before, during, and after proton therapy. We will focus on positron emission tomography (PET), real-time prompt gamma detection, and proton CT development in addition to proton radiography and implanted proton-range detector methods.

4.2. *Positron Emission Tomography*

When a therapeutic proton beam interacts with the human body, inelastic nuclear collisions between protons and tissue nuclei (^{16}O, ^{12}C, and ^{14}N) create positron-emitting nuclei (i.e., ^{15}O, ^{11}C and ^{13}N) if the proton energies are above their nuclear interaction thresholds.[23] As the primary proton beam traverses tissue toward the distal surface of the tumor, positron-emitting nuclei are created along the beam path until the proton energy decreases below the threshold for inelastic nuclear interaction. At approximately this energy level, the proton-stopping power increases significantly and creates a Bragg peak in dose deposition. Therefore, the activity distribution of the positron emitters at the conclusion of proton treatment is highly correlated with the proton range inside the patient. Positron-activity imaging of a patient during or after treatment can provide vital information concerning the actual range of the proton beam, and proton therapy facilities use in-beam, in-room, and offline PET methods to determine this information.

However, the measured activities cannot be used to directly verify the range of the proton beam inside a patient because: (1) there are intrinsic location differences between 50% of activity level and 50% of proton distal dose falloff due to the PET activation threshold energies and their variations among different elements[24]; and (2) depending on which approach is used for PET image acquisitions (i.e., in-beam, in-room, or off-line), different parts of the exponential decay curves of ^{15}O, ^{11}C, and ^{13}N are integrated during data acquisition. Combining different physical half lives with biological washout process, the 50% activity levels can vary dramatically between PET imaging approaches.

There are two practical ways to use the acquired positron-activation images for proton-range verifications.[25,26] The first approach is to acquire the positron-activation images at the exact same time during or after proton treatment. This approach can detect range variations due to anatomical changes or significant setup errors. The second approach is to calculate the positron-activity distributions using the Monte Carlo simulation approach; the calculated activity distributions are compared to the measured activity distributions. The activity distribution differences are used to evaluate the potential proton-range discrepancies between treatment planning and actual proton beam delivery. This approach works well in low-perfusion tissues, (i.e., head and neck area), which exhibit less washout of positron activities. For high-perfusion tissues, the biological washout effect has to be modeled and incorporated into the Monte Carlo simulation process. One of the approaches to model the washout processes is to simulate three different biological half-live processes in addition to the positron decay process. The three processes have fast, intermediate, and slow components. Parodi *et al.* explains this approach in detail.[26] Zhu *et al.* propose an alternative approach using a kinetic model for the biological washout of radioactivity.[27]

4.2.1. *In-beam PET*

The in-beam PET imaging system is composed of two opposing detector matrices with pixelated scintillators and position-sensitive photomultipier/photodiode arrays (Fig. 6).[28] The system starts data acquisition during proton irradiation. However, current clinical functioning systems for in-beam PET are only associated with a synchrotron proton beam accelerator. For synchrotron-based proton/particle therapy facilities, particle beam delivery has a time structure. Protons accelerated to the desired energy are extracted from the synchrotron for patient irradiation. Between extractions, there are pauses (several seconds) during which the in-beam PET system acquires signals from patients.

The main advantages of in-beam PET approach are that the patient remains in the treatment position during the imaging process and that activities from the short-lived radionuclei (^{15}O) and other relatively longer half-life radionuclei (^{11}C and ^{13}N) are acquired. The relatively high radioactivities from these nuclei enable short image acquisition time, which has minimum impact on patient treatment throughput. On the other hand, because of the limited size of the radiation detector size, planar geometry, and the limited angle detection of the photon pairs, imaging artifacts occur. The cost of developing and integrating the in-beam detectors into the existing proton gantries or treatment portals is also significant.

4.2.2. *In-room PET*

There are two types of geometric arrangements for the in-room positron-imaging approach: (1) similar to the geometry of in-beam PET, the two

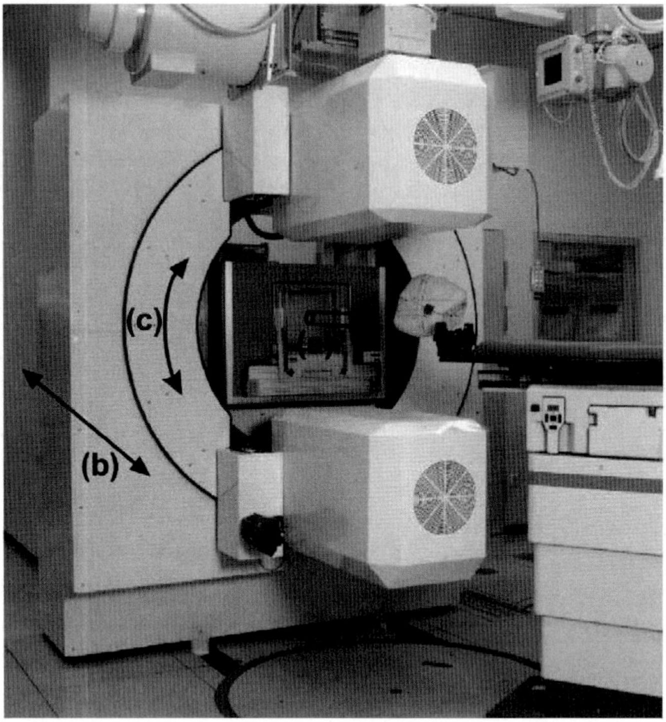

Fig. 6. In-beam PET system at GSI. (Adapted from Enghardt *et al. Nuclear Instruments and Methods in Physics Research A* **525** (2004), 284–288, with permission)

opposing detector matrices are mounted onto the treatment port or gantry (Fig. 7)[25]; and (2) a full-ring PET scanner that is set up inside the treatment room and adjacent to the treatment gantry.[29] For the first type of arrangement, immediately following irradiation, the detector pair registers the positron annihilation events while the patient remains in the treatment position and the treatment table does not move. Images with good statistics are acquired in approximately 3–5 minutes. For the second type of arrangement, the patient remains in the treatment pose while the treatment table moves toward the small, mobile full-ring PET scanner inside the treatment room. Data acquisition starts as soon as the irradiated section of patient body is within the PET field of view. The entire data-acquisition process is completed in approximately 5 minutes.

4.2.3. *Off-line PET*

The off-line PET approach removes the patient from the treatment room after proton treatment. Patients are transported to a PET/CT scanner in close vicinity to the treatment room either by walking or on a transportation vehicle.

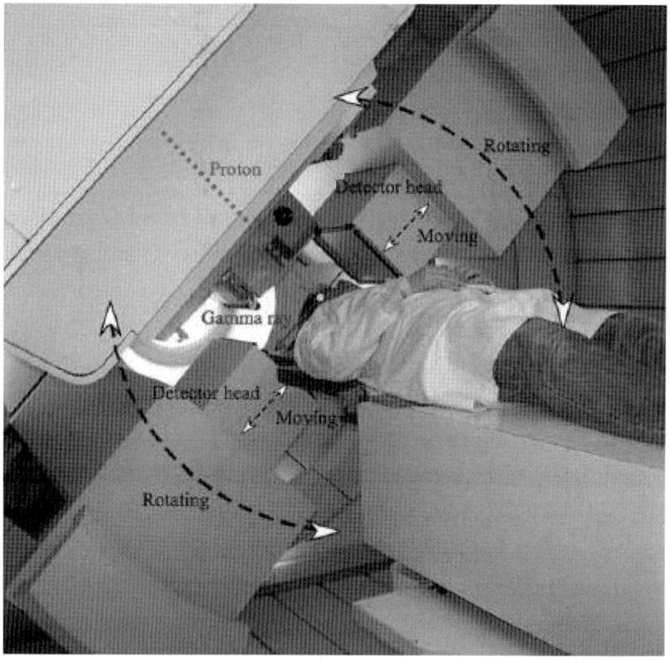

Fig. 7. In-room PET system at JNCC. (Adapted from Nishio *et al. Int J Radiat Oncol Biol Phys*, **76**(1), 277–286, with permission)

At the Heidelberg Ion-Beam Therapy Center (HIT, Heidelberg, Germany) a table-docking and transportation system is in use to transfer patients between the particle treatment and PET/CT rooms with minimum interference with treatment poses.[30]

This off-line PET approach for range verification has several advantages. From a financial point of view, there is no extra cost involved in the development of a positron-activation detection system for in-room installation. Most proton therapy clinics have PET/CT scanners available onsite; thus, this option does not require new development costs. Moreover, the full-ring PET scanner does not have the limited angle effect that is usually associated with two opposing detector matrices. However, the off-line approach also has some disadvantages. First, since patients are removed from the treatment room, CT scanning is usually required for image co-registration with the treatment planning CT. This extra imaging dose can be avoided with the in-beam or in-room approaches. Second, because of the time delay between the end of treatment and the onset of the PET acquisition, radioactivity from the positron-emitting nuclei due to natural radioactive decay and biological washout from blood flow and fluid exchange is significantly reduced. To obtain a signal level with good statistics, the PET acquisition time is much longer than those of in-beam and in-room approaches; it usually takes approximately 25–30 minutes of scan time to acquire satisfactory off-line PET images.

4.2.4. *Method comparisons and potential improvements*

Proton positron-activation imaging is used to verify range of proton beam *in vivo*. Depending on each institution's needs and available resources, these three techniques for positron-activation imaging provide different advantages (Table 4).

Currently, PET approaches are clinically feasible for particle treatment of the head and neck region, which has limited organ motion and tissue perfusion. When the treatment area has organ motion or significant biological washout of the positron activities, the Monte Carlo PET calculations have to include models of washout and evaluate the organ motion impact on the obtained PET images. Parodi *et al.* are working to improve washout modeling using carbon-irradiated mice (personal communication). Stutzer *et al.* experimentally studied the potential and limitations of time-resolved 4D PET for monitoring motion-compensated delivery of particle therapy.[31]

When comparing measured and Monte Carlo-calculated PET images, verifying proton beam-range variations is a labor intensive process for trained clinicians and medical physicists. It is very difficult for clinical particle therapy centers without extensive staff with expertise in PET image evaluation for proton range verification to adopt the PET approach as a routine practice. In an attempt to automate the proton range verification process using PET images, Helmbrecht *et al.* studied the automated range assessment from PET distributions based on profile shift analysis and/or percentage changes in fall-off in the beam eye view.[32]

There are also efforts invested in improving PET image quality to assist in PET-based proton range verification. Studies have also been performed to

Table 4. Comparisons between in-beam, in-room and off-line PET systems.

	In-beam PET	In-room PET	Off-line PET
Accelerator	Synchrotron	Synchrotron/Cyclotron	Synchrotron/Cyclotron
Patient Position	Treatment Pose	Treatment Pose	Re-setup
Image Artifact	Limited-angle	Limited-angle/None	None
Washout Effect	Very limited	Moderate	Severe
Integration Cost	High	Moderate	Low
Patient Throughput	Limited Impact	Moderate Impact	No Impact
Scan Time	Short (<1 minute)	Moderate (<5 minutes)	Long (20–30 minutes)

improve detector design and acquisition timing to increase acquired PET image quality. Current in-beam PET and some in-room PETs use two opposing planar detector matrices. The obtained images have limited-angle artifacts. Crespo *et al.* performed a simulation study for an oblique full-ring detector in-beam PET that could accommodate the treatment nozzle.[33] By doing so, the limited angle artifacts will be eliminated while patient table is still in the treatment position. They also simulated time-of-flight (TOF) image acquisition and reconstruction with various timing resolutions. The simulated positron distributions demonstrated improved image quality with finer timing resolution of TOF. Tashima *et al.* are building a small prototype full-ring scanner for in-beam PET.[34]

4.3. *Prompt Gamma Ray Imaging*

Instantaneous discrete-energy gamma ray emissions after particle nuclear interactions have been studied by particle physicists and astronomy physicists for the past few decades. The obtained knowledge and instrumentation are often used in solar missions and solar flare studies. Prompt gamma rays were first proposed for proton-range verification in a medical setting by Jongen and Stichelbaut at the annual Particle Therapy Cooperative Group Meeting (PTCOG) in 2003. Their Monte Carlo simulations demonstrated a correlation between prompt gamma-ray emissions and proton range; consequently, they proposed a general methodology for preserving this correlation. Since then, many groups and institutions have studied and prototyped prompt gamma-ray detection instruments to perform range verification in proton therapy. Since the prompt gamma ray constitutes a single photon emission from the nuclear interaction between protons and tissue nuclei and has energies ranging from 0.718 MeV to 15.1 MeV, prompt gamma-ray detection instruments are similar to those used in astronomy. Currently, there are four promising prompt gamma-ray detection instruments in development for real-time proton-range verification: the pinhole camera, electron tracking Compton camera, 3-stage Compton camera, and knife-edge-slit camera. Each instrument design has different levels of detection efficiency, and all must be improved for use in a proton therapy clinic.

4.3.1. *Pinhole camera*

Min *et al.* performed Monte Carlo simulations and developed a pinhole gamma camera for prompt gamma-based proton-range verification (Fig. 8).[35] The pinhole camera system has a CsI(Tl) scintillator detector coupled with a

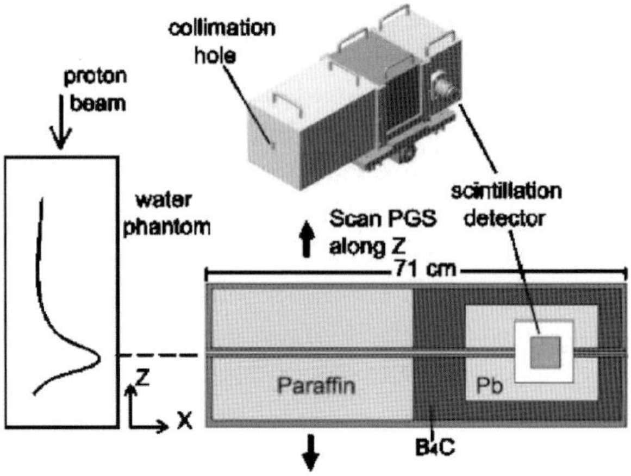

Fig. 8. Pinhole camera system setup. (Adapted from Min *et al.*, *Applied Physic Letters* **89**, 183517, 2006, with permission)

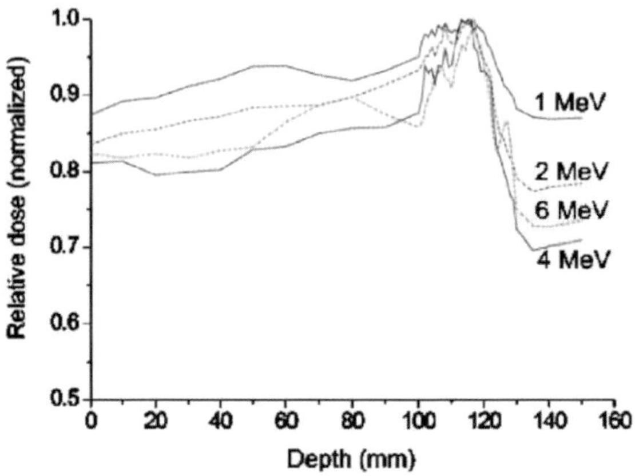

Fig. 9. Intensity profiles of prompt gamma rays with different energies. (Adapted from Min *et al.*, *Applied Physic Letters* **89**, 183517, 2006, with permission)

photomultiplier tube, corresponding electronics, and a multichannel analyzer. The scintillator is shielded by a lead enclosure with a pinhole opening. Between the lead shielding and the proton-irradiated phantom, there are paraffin plates and B_4C to moderate and capture the high-energy neutrons, respectively. Min *et al.* also studied the intensity falloff of prompt gamma rays with different energies. They concluded that higher energy prompt gamma rays led to a more distinctive correlation with distal dose falloff of proton beams (Fig. 9).

Although this experiment achieved proof of principle, many practical issues still need to be resolved before the prompt gamma-ray detection system can be used in a proton therapy clinic. First, this system can only detect the prompt gamma ray at a single location without linear motion of the entire system. Precise placement of the system relative to the patient and small range of linear motion is required to find prompt gamma-intensity falloff. Second, the most up-to-date proton therapy clinics utilize double-scattering and pencil-beam scanning techniques. Kurosawa *et al.* performed range-verification measurements using the pinhole camera system for the double-scattering and pencil-beam scanning techniques.[36] The pinhole camera system can only identify the range through sharp falloff of the prompt gamma signal for the proton pencil beam.

4.3.2. *Compton camera*

Prompt gamma rays are emitted isotropically from the proton nuclear interactions along the beam path. Determining the energy and direction of the incident prompt gamma rays is essential for the formation of 2D images of the prompt gamma intensity and for energy thresholds to improve discernability of the signal peak. Within the range of energies (~1 to 15 MeV) of prompt gamma rays in proton therapy, the Compton interaction is the dominant radiation interaction that can be used for gamma detection. Because scattered Compton photons and electrons have intrinsically related energies and emission angles relative to those of incident photons, with the proper design Compton interactions can be used to determine incident photon energies and directions. In fact, the prompt gamma-ray Compton camera is often used in astronomy to detect the energy and direction of gamma rays coming from outer space. With a design similar to that of the Compton telescope, the electron-tracking Compton and three-stage Compton cameras have been studied for prompt gamma-based range verification in proton therapy.

4.3.2.1. Electron-tracking compton camera

An electron-tracking camera (Fig. 10) (aka. a two-stage Compton camera) has two interaction stages: (1) detecting energies and scatter angles of Compton-scattered *electrons*; and (2) detecting those of the Compton-scattered photons. These stages are accomplished with an electron-tracking chamber and a pixelated scintillator array.[36] The electron-tracking chamber is filled with atmosphere-pressured Argon gas and space charge-sensing pixels or electrodes. When Compton interactions occur within the chamber, the scattered electron drifts through the chamber; the chamber electrodes can detect the electron direction and energy if it is fully stopped within the chamber. The pixelated scintillator array interacts with and absorbs the Compton-scattered photons

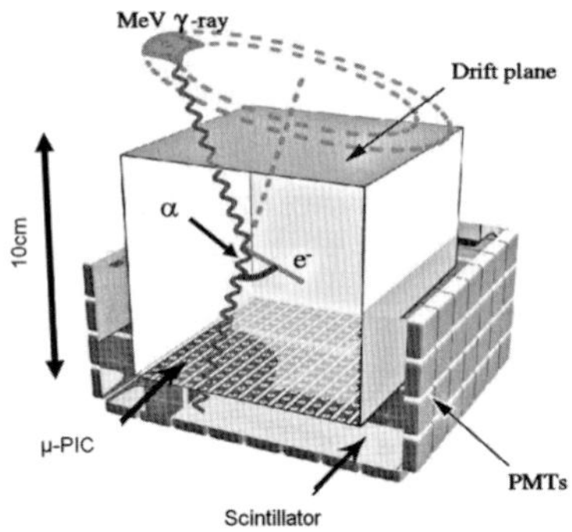

$$\cos\theta = 1 - m_e c^2\left(\frac{1}{E_{\gamma_s}} - \frac{1}{E_{\gamma_i}}\right) \quad (2)$$

$$E_{\gamma_i} = E_{\gamma_s} + E_e \quad (3)$$

$$\cos\alpha = \left[1 - \frac{m_e c^2}{E_{\gamma_s}}\right]\sqrt{\frac{E_e}{E_e + 2m_e c^2}} \quad (4)$$

Where E_{γ_i}, E_{γ_s} and E_e are energies of the incident photon, scattered photon, and scattered electron, respectively; α is the angle between the scattered photon and electron; θ is the angle between the incident and scattered photons.

Fig. 10. Illustration of electron-tracking Compton camera. (Adapted from Kurosawa *et al.* *Current Applied Physics*, **12**, 2012, 364–368, with permission)

with several Compton interactions and a final photoelectric effect, thereby providing the energy and direction of the Compton-scattered photons. If the energies and directions of the Compton-scattered photons and electrons are known, then the incident gamma-ray energies and directions within a conical area can be determined. Thus, a 2D distribution of prompt gamma rays can be reconstructed in the patient plane. Equations (2), (3), and (4) show the energy and angular relationship between the incident gamma ray and the Compton-scattered photon and electron. With the proper energy threshold in the obtained prompt gamma-ray data, the sharpest intensity falloff peak of detected prompt gamma ray can be used to perform proton-range verification.

There are several factors that can influence the reconstructed energy and direction of prompt gamma rays using the electron-tracking Compton camera system. (1) The size of the electron-tracking chamber. To accurately detect the energy of Compton-scattered electrons, they must be fully stopped within the chamber. However, for some high-energy prompt gamma rays, the Compton-scattered electrons can be very energetic; this requires the significant size of the electron-tracking chamber to prevent the electron's escape. (2) The thickness of the scintillator detector. Similar to the case of Compton-scattered electrons, accurate determination of the Compton-scattered photon energy requires that the photon is fully absorbed inside the scintillator; this necessitates a fairly thick scintillator, which is usually associated with a significant cost. (3) The spatial resolution of the electron-tracking chamber electrodes and the scintillator. Finer resolution of both detectors can reduce uncertainty of the reconstructed emission location of the prompt gamma ray. (4) The energy resolution for the electron-tracking chambers and the scintillator. Similar to the effect of spatial resolution, a finer energy resolution detector reduces location uncertainty for the reconstructed location of the prompt gamma rays.

The overall gamma-detection efficiency of the electron-tracking Compton camera is crucial for the clinical application of this proton range-verification approach. Kang *et al.* simulated an electron-tracking Compton camera system and reported approximately 10^{-7} per proton detection efficiency. For a typical 2 Gy fraction dose delivered using the double-scattering technique, this gamma-detection efficiency posed a statistical challenge for data analysis. With pencil-beam scanning, each beam spot carries 2–3 orders of magnitude fewer protons than those of double scattering; there are simply not enough recorded prompt gamma rays to verify the proton range.

4.3.2.2. Three-stage Compton camera

The electron-tracking Compton camera system requires that the Compton-scattered electrons and photons are fully stopped within their corresponding detectors to accurately calculate the incident energy and angle of the initial prompt gamma ray. This limitation can be overcome using a 3-stage Compton camera.[37–39] This camera was originally implemented in the astronomy community for the Compton telescope. In the 3-stage Compton camera design, three positions and energy-sensitive solid-state detectors are arranged in certain distances among each other (Fig. 11). The first two detectors generate single Compton-scattered photons and record the position and deposited energies of the Compton interactions. The third detector only provides

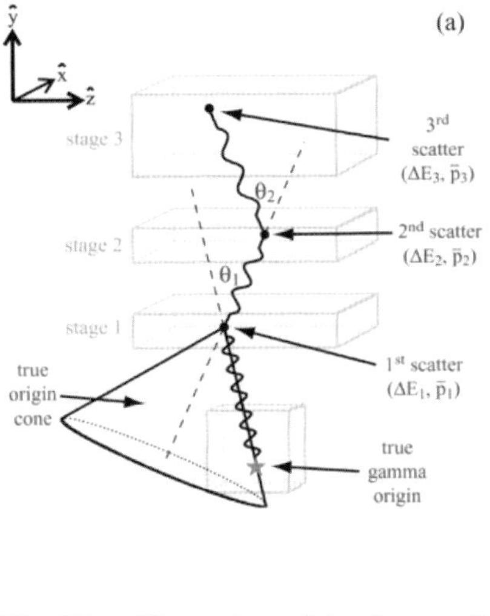

$$\cos\theta_1 = 1 + m_e c^2\left(\frac{1}{E_0} - \frac{1}{E_1}\right) \tag{5}$$

$$E_0 = \Delta E_1 + 0.5\left[\Delta E_2 + \sqrt{\Delta E_2^{\,2} + \frac{4\Delta E_2 m_e c^2}{1-\cos\theta_2}}\right] \tag{6}$$

Where E_0 and E_1 are the energies of the incident prompt gamma ray and 1st scattered photon; ΔE_1, ΔE_2 and ΔE_3 are energies deposited in 1st, 2nd and 3rd scatters, respectively; θ_1 is angle between incident prompt gamma ray and 1st scattered photon; θ_2 is angle between 1st scattered and 2nd scattered photons.

Fig. 11. Illustration of the 3-stage Compton camera system. (Adapted from Mackin *et al.*, *Medical Physics*, **40**(1), 2013, 012401-1–012402-12, with permission) the Compton interaction positions. With this information and the intrinsic relationship between the energy and scattering angle of the Compton-scattered photons, one can obtain the initial incident prompt gamma-ray energy and its incident conical cone. The intersection between the proton beam direction and this conical cone determines the prompt gamma-emission location inside patients. Equations (5) and (6) show the mathematical relationship between the scattering angles and deposited energies in the first two detectors. The third scatter provides interaction position information to decide the scattering angle (θ_2) inside the second scatter.

Peterson *et al.* performed a Monte Carlo study to optimize the detector thickness and inter-detector distances for optimal system detection efficiency of prompt gamma rays. Similar to the electron-tracking Compton camera, fine energy resolution of the detectors can reduce uncertainty in the calculation of the energy and location of the incident prompt gamma rays. Peterson's study utilized a high-purity Germanium detector for the simulation; it indicated that a trade-off exists between the thickness of the second detector and the stage-two interaction and transport efficiencies. Wider detector increases interaction efficiency in all three stages, whereas larger inter-detector distance decreases overall detection efficiency. The study determined that a realistic-sized high-purity germanium detector system should have approximately 10^{-6} to 10^{-5} per proton detection efficiency; this should provide great potential for proton-range verification. Nevertheless, practical challenges still exist for the size, cooling, cost, and compacted assembly of the high-purity germanium detector.

4.3.3. *Knife-edge-slit gamma camera*

Bom *et al.* proposed a knife-edge-slit gamma camera design and performed a Monte Carlo simulation study to determine its detection efficiency and feasibility for proton-range verification.[40] This design utilizes a position-sensitive bismuth germanium oxide (BGO) scintillator detector with a dimension of 30 cm by 50 cm. A slit made by two tungsten plates is placed near the irradiation phantom and at a relatively large distance from the BGO detector. This design utilizes the pinhole imaging principle to capture a prompt gamma-intensity profile at a spatial resolution better than that of the BGO detector due to the magnification factor. Figure 12 illustrates the clinical setup of such a system and Fig. 13 is an illustration of resolution magnification of the system. The detection system efficiency was calculated at approximately 10^{-4} per proton with a detector energy threshold at 1.5 MeV of the prompt gamma ray. This is significantly higher than the Compton camera approaches. Currently, Ion Beam Application (IBA) is prototyping this device for real-time

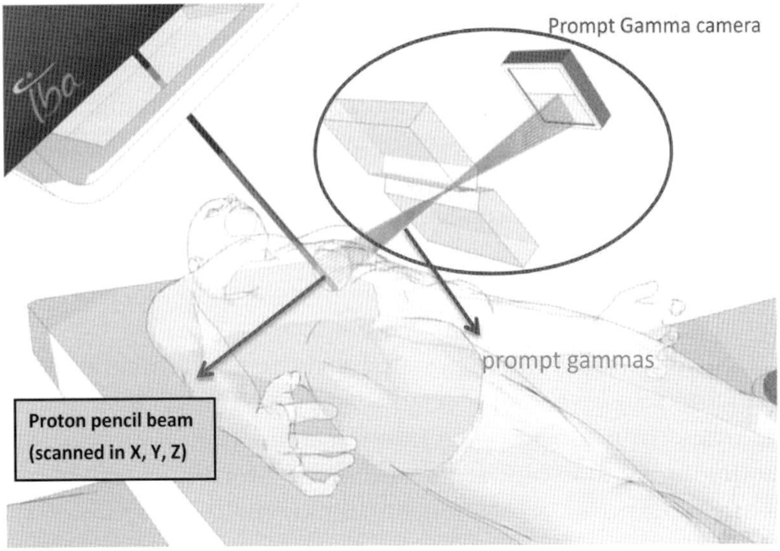

Fig. 12. Illustration of clinical setup of knife-edge-slit camera system for prompt gamma detection during pencil-beam scanning proton treatment. (Courtesy of IBA)

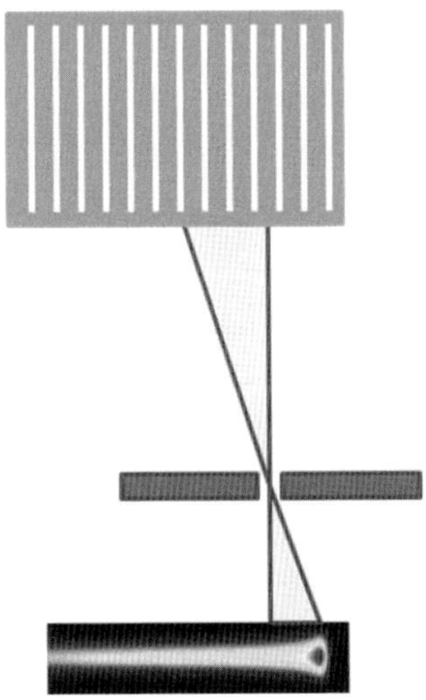

Fig. 13. Illustration of spatial resolution magnification design of knife-edge-slit camera system.

proton-range verification in proton pencil-beam scanning treatment (personal communication). Thus, the knife-edge-slit gamma camera system is potentially the most promising real-time proton-range verification system that will be introduced into clinics in the near future.

4.4. *Proton Computed Tomography*

In Section 3, we discussed the intrinsic uncertainty in proton-range determination with the current kV X-ray CT-based HU-relative stopping power calibration approach, even though the stoichiometric calibration methodology can help reduce this uncertainty. Many researchers investigated other approaches that could potentially further reduce this uncertainty (i.e., dual-energy kV CT and kV-MV CT-based calibrations).[41–43] However, the very nature of utilizing X-ray attenuation information in the proton stopping power calibration process is the limitation of all these approaches.

Nobel laureate, Alan Cormack, stated that the linear integral method used in X-ray CT can also be used for relative stopping power determination with proton particles.[44] Proton stopping power is a function of proton energy; it is a slow varying function except at the end of the proton range. However, proton mass-stopping-power-to-reference-medium (i.e., water) ratios are nearly independent of proton energy. Therefore, when a penetrating proton beam transverses a patient's anatomy, the recorded energy and direction of the exit proton combined with the energy and direction of the incident proton can help determine the linear integral of the relative stopping power of the proton. Thus, these linear integrals can be used to perform CT reconstruction. Furthermore, the proton CT reportedly has dose advantages compared to the traditional X-ray CT.

Hanson *et al.* performed preliminary research and experiments on proton CT for human tissue imaging.[45,46] In this study, the incident and exit proton beam energies and exit angles were recorded. The impact of the multiple Coulomb scattering of the proton was minimized by only using exit protons from a 2-mm area within the projected direction of the incident protons. The obtained CT images resembled the X-ray CT images, but the image resolution and accuracy of the reconstructed relative stopping power was limited by the protons' deviation from a straight path due to the multiple Coulomb scattering. The energy and spatial resolution of the proton detectors also affected the quality of the proton CT. Nevertheless, this study provided proof of feasibility for proton CT instrumentation, imaging, and reconstruction.

With improved technologies in both particle detectors and their corresponding electronics, proton CT was again a focus of some researchers. Schulte *et al.* are investigating proton CT based on single proton detection and most likely proton path concept.[47–49] Using entrance and exit pairs of silicon strip detectors, the position and direction of each individual proton can be obtained. Exit proton energy is recorded by the pixellated scintillator detectors. The most probable path of the proton transverse patient is estimated using

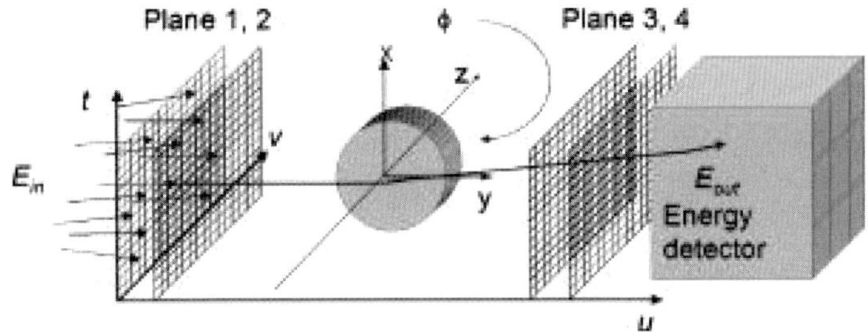

Fig. 14. Illustration of the experimental setup for proton CT data acquisition. (Adapted from Schulte *et al. Medical Physics* **32**(4), 2005, 1035–1046, with permission)

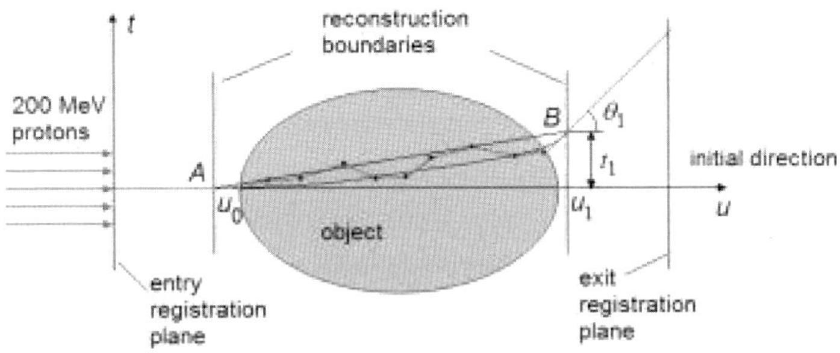

Fig. 15. Proton's path in medium due to multiple Coulomb scattering. (Adapted from Li *et al., Medical Physics* **33**(3), 2006, 699–706, with permission)

most likely path methodology that approximates effect of multiple Coulomb scattering.[50,51] Iterative reconstruction algorithm is then used to reconstruct the proton CT images of the relative stopping power. Figure 14 illustrates the experimental setup for proton CT data acquisitions. Figure 15 shows proton path deviation from straight lines between entrance and exit points due to multiple Coulomb scattering.

Currently, the proton CT is still at a research and prototyping stage. The second generation prototype of proton CT is in development by Schulte *et al.* There are still many improvements need to be made in proton detectors and their arrangement, the proton most likely path approximation as well as proton CT iterative reconstruction algorithm. Furthermore, many clinical proton centers right now have maximum proton beam energies that are not high enough to fully penetrating regular size adult patients. Thus, it is imperative to the future development of proton centers to design systems which can provide high enough proton energy to perform proton CT image acquisition.

4.5. *Other Proton-Range Verification Techniques*

Several other techniques, including proton radiography and intracavity or implanted proton detectors, have been investigated as proton beam-range verification tools for pre-treatment setup to detect either patient setup errors or anatomical changes.

Proton radiography utilizes proton detectors similar to that of proton CT to register the direction, position, and energy of the incident and exit protons.[52] Instead of acquiring multiple projected images at different angles around the patient, a single image is acquired at the proton treatment beam angle, provided that the proton detectors can be placed at both the entrance and exit beams. The proton radiograph formation requires the use of either straight-line trajectories or the most probable trajectories. Schneider *et al.* developed such a system and applied proton radiography to both phantoms and animals.[53,54] The range sensitivity of the acquired image was approximately 0.6 mm, which is applicable in pre-treatment proton beam-range verification. Moreover, the imaging dose was 1–2 orders of magnitude lower than that of the X-ray-based radiographs routinely used in pre-treatment patient setup.

Lu *et al.* developed two techniques that can be used to verify the proton beam range *in vivo*.[55–57] These techniques were developed for double-scattering proton treatment delivery modes. The first technique utilizes diodes placed on a rectal balloon inserted into patient rectum. The proposed anterior-to-posterior proton treatment beam for a prostate patient has its distal falloff in close proximity of the diodes. Double scattering delivers a SOBP proton beam using a constantly rotating range modulator. Therefore, the timing structure of the detected signal from the diode is dependent on the diode position relative to the SOBP inside the patient. This position information can be acquired using a very low dose as a testing beam at the beginning of the treatment. This technique is limited by its small number of data points and is only usable for tumor sites that have cavities at the distal falloff of the proton beam. Lu *et al.* also developed a technique that utilizes implanted wireless radiation dosimeters and a modified double-scattering proton treatment delivery method. Before the patient receives CT scans for treatment planning, a wireless radiation dosimeter is implanted into the tumor volume. The traditional SOBP has to be delivered with a pair of complimentary fields with different slope-dose profiles. Depending on the location of the dosimeter relative to the delivered SOBP, the ratios of signals acquired from the two complimentary field pair are different. Similar to the first technique, the *in vivo* range verification can be performed with a low dose as a testing beam. This technique is also limited by its point-based detection and involves more invasive procedures of implanting dosimeters into patient tumor volume.

5. Summary

Proton therapy is a form of radiation therapy that has the distinct advantage of reduced dose to healthy tissues due to the finite range of protons. Accurately determining range through either verification or treatment plan calculation is crucial to realize this advantage. Range uncertainties come from current X-ray-based CT number-to-relative-stopping-power calibration and from anatomical changes and setup errors. Successful development of proton CT would significantly reduce the intrinsic range uncertainty in proton treatment planning. Proton radiography and point-based range detection approaches are useful tools to verify patient daily treatment setup and anatomical changes before treatment. Prompt gamma detection is the most promising method of real-time monitoring the proton beam range during treatment delivery, especially for the pencil-beam scanning delivery mode. In-beam, in-room, and off-line PET are useful tools to verify the range of the delivered proton treatment beam and have already been adopted by some proton therapy clinics.

References

1. F.M. Khan, *The Physics of Radiation Therapy*, fourth edition. Baltimore, MD: Lippincott Williams & Wilkins (2009).
2. M. Baumann, C. Petersen, "TCP and NTCP: a basic introduction," *Rays* **30**, 99–104 (2005).
3. L. Xing, B. Thorndyke, E. Schreibmann, Y. Yang, T.F. Li, G.Y. Kim, G. Luxton, A Koong, "Overview of image-guided radiation therapy," *Med Dosim* **31**, 91–112 (2006).
4. D. Verellen, M. De Ridder, N. Linthout, K. Tournel, G. Soete, G. Storme, "Innovations in image-guided radiotherapy," *Nat Rev Cancer* 7, 949–960 (2007).
5. J.M. Slater, J.O. Archambeau, D.W. Miller, M.I. Notarus, W. Preston, J.D. Slater, "The proton treatment center at Loma Linda University Medical Center: rationale for and description of its development," *Int J Radiat Oncol Biol Phys* **22**, 383–389 (1992).
6. F.H. Attix, *Introduction to Radiological Physics and Radiation Dosimetry.* Hoboken, NJ: John Wiley & Sons (1991).
7. E.J. Hall, *Radiobiology for the Radiologist.* Philadelphia, PA: Lippincott Williams & Wilkins (2011).
8. C.M. Ma, K. Paskalev, "In-room CT techniques for image-guided radiation therapy," *Med Dosim* **31**, 30–39 (2006).
9. American Association of Physicists in Medicine, The Role of In-Room kV X-Ray Imaging for Patient Setup and Target Localization: 2009. Accessed at: www.aapm.org/pubs/reports/RPT_104.pdf. Report #104.

10. International Commission on Radiation Units and Measurement. Prescribing, Recording and Reporting Photon Beam Therapy: 1999. Accessed at: http://www.icru.org/home/reports/prescribing-recording-and-reporting-photon-beam-therapy-report-62. Report #62.
11. M. van Herk, "Errors and margins in radiotherapy," *Semin Radiat Oncol* **14**, 52–64 (2004).
12. D.A. Jaffray, D.G. Drake, M. Moreau, A.A. Martinez, J.W. Wong, "A radiographic and tomographic imaging system integrated into a medical linear accelerator for localization of bone and soft-tissue targets," *Int J Radiat Oncol Biol Phys* **45**, 773–789 (1999).
13. H. Paganetti, *Proton Therapy Physics.* Boca Raton, FL: CRC Press (2011).
14. T. Kanai, K. Kawachi, H. Matsuzawa, T. Inada, "Broad beam three-dimensional irradiation for proton radiotherapy," *Med Phys* **10**, 344–346 (1983).
15. E. Pedroni, R. Bacher, H. Blattmann, T. Bohringer, A. Coray, A. Lomax, S. Lin, G. Munkel, S. Scheib, U. Schneider *et al.* "The 200-MeV proton therapy project at the Paul Scherrer Institute: Conceptual design and practical realization," *Med Phys* **22**, 37–53 (1995).
16. J. Beebe-Wang, P. Vaska, F.A. Dilmanian, S.G. Peggs, D.J. Schlyer, "Simulation of proton therapy treatment verification via PET imaging of induced positron-emitters," Presented at Nuclear Science Symposium Conference Record, IEEE. Portland, OR (2003).
17. B. Kozlovsky, R.J. Murphy, R. Ramaty, "Nuclear deexcitation gamma-ray lines from accelerated particle interactions," *Astrophys J* **S141**, 523 (2002).
18. J. van Dyk, "The modern technology of radiation oncology: A compendium for medical physicists and radiation oncologists," Madison, WI: Medical Physics Pub Corp; (1999).
19. U. Schneider, E. Pedroni, A. Lomax, "The calibration of CT Hounsfield units for radiotherapy treatment planning," *Phys Med Biol* **41**, 111–124 (1996).
20. E. Soisson, "Patient Set-Up Uncertainties (Inter-fraction)," Presented at AAPM Summer School (2011).
21. S. Shimizu, H. Shirato, S. Ogura, H. Akita-Dosaka, K. Kitamura, T. Nishioka, K. Kagei, M. Nishimura, K. Miyasaka, "Detection of lung tumor movement in real-time tumor-tracking radiotherapy," *Int J Radiat Oncol Biol Phys* **51**, 304–310 (2001).
22. J. Zhou, B. Uhl, K. Dewit, M. Young, B. Taylor, D.Y. Fei, Y.C. Lo, "Analysis of daily setup variation with tomotherapy megavoltage computed tomography," *Med Dosim* **35**, 31–37 (2010).
23. M.B. Chadwick, D.T.L. Jones, G.J. Arendse, A.A. Cowley, W.A. Richter, J.J. Lawrie, R.T. Newman, J.V. Pilcher, F.D. Smit, G.F. Steyn, J.W. Koen, J.A. Stander, "Nuclear interaction cross sections for proton radiotherapy," *Nucl Phys A* **654**, 1051c–1057c (1999).
24. K. Parodi, F. Pönisch, W. Enghardt, "Experimental study on the feasibility of in-beam PET for accurate monitoring of proton therapy," *IEEE Trans Nucl Sci* **52**, 778–786 (2005).
25. T. Nishio, A. Miyatake, T. Ogino, K. Nakagawa, N. Saijo, H. Esumi, "The development and clinical use of a beam ON-LINE PET system mounted on a rotating gantry port in proton therapy," *Int J Radiat Oncol Biol Phys* **76**, 277–286 (2010).
26. K. Parodi, H. Paganetti, H.A. Shih, S. Michaud, J.S. Loeffler, T.F. DeLaney, N.J. Liebsch, J.E. Munzenrider, A.J. Fischman, A. Knopf, T. Bortfeld, "Patient study of in vivo verification of beam delivery and range, using positron emission tomography and computed tomography imaging after proton therapy," *Int J Radiat Oncol Biol Phys* **68**, 920–934 (2007).

27. X. Zhu, N. Alpert, C. Min, M. Normandin, H. Paganetti, T. Bortfeld, G. El Fakhri, "Verification of proton therapy with PET: A kinetic modeling approach," *J Nucl Med* **53**, 264 (2012).
28. W. Enghardt, P. Crespo, F. Fiedler, R. Hinz, K. Parodi, J. Pawelke, F. Pönisch, "Charged hadron tumour therapy monitoring by means of PET," *Nucl Instrum Methods Phys Res A* **525**, 284–288 (2004).
29. C.H. Min, X. Zhu, B.A. Winey, K. Grogg, M. Testa, G. El Fakhri, T.R. Bortfeld, H. Paganetti, H.A. Shih, "Clinical application of in-room positron emission tomography for in vivo treatment monitoring in proton radiation therapy," *Int J Radiat Oncol Biol Phys* **86**, 183–189 (2013).
30. K. Parodi, J. Bauer, C. Kurz, A. Mairani, F. Sommerer, D. Unholtz, T. Haberer, J. Debus, "Monte Carlo modeling and in-vivo imaging at the Heidelberg Ion Beam Therapy Center," Presented at Nuclear Science Symposium and Medical Imaging Conference, IEEE. Valencia, Spain: 2011.
31. K. Stutzer, C. Bert, W. Enghardt, S. Helmbrecht, K. Parodi, M. Priegnitz, N. Saito, F. Fiedler, "Experimental verification of a 4D MLEM reconstruction algorithm used for in-beam PET measurements in particle therapy," *Phys Med Biol* **58**, 5085–5111 (2013).
32. S. Helmbrecht, A. Santiago, W. Enghardt, P. Kuess, F. Fiedler, "On the feasibility of automatic detection of range deviations from in-beam PET data," *Phys Med Biol* **57**, 1387–1397 (2012).
33. P. Crespo, G. Shakirin, F. Fiedler, W. Enghardt, A. Wagner, "Direct time-of-flight for quantitative, real-time in-beam PET: A concept and feasibility study," *Phys Med Biol* **52**, 6795–6811 (2007).
34. H. Tashima, T. Yamaya, E. Yoshida, S. Kinouchi, M. Watanabe, E. Tanaka, "A single-ring OpenPET enabling PET imaging during radiotherapy," *Phys Med Biol* **57**, 4705–4718 (2012).
35. C.H. Min, C.H. Kim, M.Y. Youn, J.W. Kim, "Prompt gamma measurements for locating the dose falloff region in the proton therapy," *Appl Phys Lett* **89**, 183517 (2006).
36. S. Kurosawa, H. Kubo, K. Ueno, S. Kabuki, S. Iwaki, M. Takahashi, K. Taniue, N. Higashi, K. Miuchi, T. Tanimori, D. Kim, J. Kim, "Prompt gamma detection for range verification in proton therapy," *Curr Appl Phys* **12**, 364–368 (2012).
37. S.W. Peterson, D. Robertson, J. Polf, "Optimizing a three-stage Compton camera for measuring prompt gamma rays emitted during proton radiotherapy," *Phys Med Biol* **55**, 6841–6856 (2010).
38. B.H. Kang, J.W. Kim, "Monte Carlo design study of a gamma detector system to locate distal dose falloff in proton therapy," *IEEE Trans Nucl Sci* **56**, 46–50 (2009).
39. M.H. Richard, M. Chevallier, D. Dauvergne, N. Freud, P. Henriquet, F. Le Foulher, J.M. Letang, G. Montarou, C. Ray, F. Roellinghoff, E. Testa, M. Testa, A.H. Walenta, "Design guidelines for a double scattering compton camera for prompt- γ imaging during ion beam therapy: A Monte Carlo simulation study," *IEEE Trans Nucl Sci* **58**, 87–94 (2011).
40. D. Mackin, J. Polf, S. Peterson, S. Beddar, "The effects of Doppler broadening and detector resolution on the performance of three-stage Compton cameras," *Med Phys* **40**, 012402 (2013).
41. V. Bom, L. Joulaeizadeh, F. Beekman, "Real-time prompt gamma monitoring in spot-scanning proton therapy using imaging through a knife-edge-shaped slit," *Phys Med Biol* **57**, 297–308 (2012).

42. M. Yang, G. Virshup, J. Clayton, X.R. Zhu, R. Mohan, L. Dong, "Theoretical variance analysis of single- and dual-energy computed tomography methods for calculating proton stopping power ratios of biological tissues," *Phys Med Biol* **55**, 1343–1362 (2010).
43. M. Yang, G. Virshup, J. Clayton, X.R. Zhu, R. Mohan, L. Dong, "Does kV-MV dual-energy computed tomography have an advantage in determining proton stopping power ratios in patients?" *Phys Med Biol* **56**, 4499–4515 (2011).
44. M. Saito, "Potential of dual-energy subtraction for converting CT numbers to electron density based on a single linear relationship," *Med Phys* **39**, 2021–2030 (2012).
45. K.M. Hanson, J.N. Bradbury, T.M. Cannon, R.L. Hutson, D.B. Laubacher, R.J. Macek, M.A. Paciotti, C.A. Taylor, "Computed tomography using proton energy loss," *Phys Med Biol* **26**, 965–983 (1981).
46. A.M. Cormack, "Representation of a function by its line integrals, with some radiological applications," *J Appl Phys* **34**, 2722–2727 (1963).
47. K.M. Hanson, J.N. Bradbury, R.A. Koeppe, R.J. Macek, D.R. Machen, R. Morgado, M.A. Paciotti, S.A. Sandford, V.W. Steward, "Proton computed tomography of human specimens," *Phys Med Biol* **27**, 25–36 (1982).
48. R. Schulte, V. Bashkirov, T. Li, Z. Liang, K. Mueller, J. Heimann, L.R. Johnson, B. Keeney, H.F.W. Sadrozinski, A. Seiden, D.C. Williams, L. Zhang, Z. Li, S. Peggs, T. Satogata, C. Woody, "Conceptual design of a proton computed tomography system for applications in proton radiation therapy," *IEEE Trans Nucl Sci* **51**, 866–872 (2004).
49. R.W. Schulte, V. Bashkirov, M.C. Klock, T. Li, A.J. Wroe, I. Evseev, D.C. Williams, T. Satogata, "Density resolution of proton computed tomography," *Med Phys* **32**, 1035–1046 (2005).
50. D.C. Williams, "The most likely path of an energetic charged particle through a uniform medium," *Phys Med Biol* **49**, 2899–2911 (2004).
51. R.W. Schulte, A.J. Wroe, "New developments in treatment planning and verification of particle beam therapy," *Transl Cancer Res* **1**, 184–195 (2012).
52. T. Li, Z. Liang, J.V. Singanallur, T.J. Satogata, D.C. Williams, W.R. Schulte, "Reconstruction for proton computed tomography by tracing proton trajectories: a Monte Carlo study," *Med Phys* **33**, 699–706 (2006).
53. U. Schneider, E. Pedroni, "Proton radiography as a tool for quality control in proton therapy," *Med Phys* **22**, 353–363 (1995).
54. D.R. Moffett, E.P. Colton, G.A. Concaildi, E.W. Hoffman, R.D. Klem, M.J. Knott, S.L. Kramer, R.L. Martin, E.F. Parker, A.R. Passi, P.F. Schultz, R.L. Stockley, R.E. Timm, L.S. Skaggs, V.W. Steward, "Initial test of a proton radiographic system," *IEEE Trans Nucl Sci* **22**, 1749–1751 (1975).
55. U. Schneider, J. Besserer, P. Pemler, M. Dellert, M. Moosburger, E. Pedroni, B. Kaser-Hotz, "First proton radiography of an animal patient," *Med Phys* **31**, 1046–1051 (2004).
56. H.M. Lu, "A point dose method for *in vivo* range verification in proton therapy," *Phys Med Biol* **53**, N415–422 (2008).
57. H.M. Lu, "A potential method for *in vivo* range verification in proton therapy treatment," *Phys Med Biol* **53**, 1413–1424 (2008).

Chapter 19

An Automated Robust Segmentation Method for Intravascular Ultrasound Images

Prakash Manandhar, Chi Hau Chen,† Ahmet Umit Coskun‡ and Uvais A. Qidwai§*

**University of Massachusetts Dartmouth and Integra Life Sciences, Inc.*
E-mail: pmanandhar@umassd.edu

†*University of Massachusetts Dartmouth*
E-mail: cchen@umassd.edu

‡*Northeastern University, Mechanical & Industrial Engineering Department*
E-mail: acoskun@coe.neu.edu

§*Qatar University, Computer Science and Engineering Department*
E-mail: uqidwai@qu.edu.qa

It is widely known that the state of a patient's coronary heart disease can be better assessed using intravascular ultrasound (IVUS) than with more conventional angiography. Recent work has shown that segmentation and 3D reconstruction of IVUS pull-back sequence images can be used for computational fluid dynamic simulation of blood flow through the coronary arteries. This map of shear stress in the blood vessel walls can be used to predict susceptibility of a region of the arteries to future arteriosclerosis and disease. Manual segmentation of images is time consuming as well as cost prohibitive for routine diagnostic use. Current segmentation algorithms do not achieve a high enough accuracy because of the presence of speckle due to blood flow, relatively low resolution of images and presence of various artifacts including guide-wires, stents, vessel branches, and some other growth or inflammations. On the other hand, the image may be induced with additional blur due to movement distortions, as well as resolution-related mixing of closely resembling pixels thus forming a type of out-of-focus blur. Robust automated segmentation achieving high accuracy of 95% or above has been elusive despite work by a large community of researchers in the machine vision field. In this chapter, we present a comprehensive method, based on computer vision and pattern recognition, where a multitude of algorithms are applied simultaneously to the segmentation problem. The method presented is to combine algorithms using a meta-algorithmic approach. Each segmentation algorithm computes along with the segmentation a measure of confidence in the segmentation which can be biased on prior information about the presence of artifacts. A meta-algorithm then runs a library of algorithms on a sub-sequence of images to be segmented and chooses the segmentation based on computed confidence measures. Machine learning and testing is performed on a large database, that includes 2293 gated image frames that have been manually segmented for training and performance comparison, and a total of 57,098 image frames for testing the meta-algorithm to obtain reliable segmentation performance assessment.

1. Background/Literature Survey

Intravascular ultrasound (IVUS) is a vascular imaging technique that is used to study atherosclerosis since it has the ability to show the lumen and the vessel wall. As cardiovascular diseases continue to take the lives of millions each year, IVUS technology provides effective imaging methods to properly diagnose and intervene on patients who suffer from the disease. Such methods include quantitative and qualitative tools for acquiring accurate measurements of cross-sectional dimensions of the arterial lumen,[1,2] visualization and assessment of atherosclerotic plaque,[1,3] delineation of arterial wall morphology,[1] and evaluation of the outcome of an intravascular intervention.[1,2]

Overall, IVUS provides a tomographic perspective of lumen geometry and vessel wall structure that other diagnostic imaging techniques cannot. The basic task of computer analysis is the image segmentation to extract lumen and media-adventitia boundaries. Due to the ultrasound speckle, catheter artifacts, or calcification shadows, the automated analysis of large IVUS data sets represents an important challenge. The challenge is far greater, in our view, than the computer analysis of mammograms while much less research effort has been made on automated IVUS image segmentation. Manual segmentation is very time consuming and is impossible for a large IVUS data set. For any automated analysis, a very high segmentation accuracy (say within 10 pixels between manual and automated segmentation) is much needed. Such goal is far from being realized though there has been a significant number of publications in IVUS image segmentation.

Considering computer analysis of X-ray and mammograms as a first successful mile stone in medical image analysis, automated IVUS image segmentation can be considered as a second milestone yet to be achieved. It is noted that in spite of the advances of sensors such as several versions of IVUS imaging hardware available are being developed, the proposed work is useful for all IVUS systems. Also much segmentation work reported so far still relies on initialization information provided by human operator, the proposed method is a completely automated segmentation. This is treated as a basic research problem in computer vision and pattern recognition that involves fundamental studies to maximize the segmentation accuracy.

IVUS is an invasive catheter-based technique that is widely used to assess atherosclerotic plaque.[4] At the tip of an IVUS catheter, a transducer emits an ultrasound pulse and receives the reflected backscatter signal from the tissue where this backscattered signal is then processed real-time into a 2D image. The image permits accurate delineation of the vessel and lumen, dimensions, distribution and severity of coronary plaque.[4,5] The literature is rich in IVUS imaging as the technique has gained increasing acceptance in the last twenty years (see. e.g. Ref. [6]–[26]). An imaging catheter is typically inserted into the femoral artery and directed by a guide-wire into the chambers and vessels of the heart. The imaging catheter differs in length and diameter based on the vessel being imaged. At the proximal end of the catheter (end closest to physician), the catheter is connected to a motor-driven unit that is used to spin the drive cable within the catheter sheath. This drive cable is what spins the ultrasound transducer 360° and as the transducer is rotated by the drive cable at approximately 1800 rpm, the transducer generates and receives ultrasound pulses to and from the coronary tissue. The echoes, or received ultrasound pulses reflected by the tissue, are captured by the transceiver and converted from a mechanical signal (or vibration) to an electrical signal down the drive-cable. The electrical signal is then digitized and rendered onto a display, providing the physician with a 360° cross-sectional view inside the coronary vessel.

In a typical IVUS image (Fig. 1), the lumen is normally a dark echo-free area adjacent to the imaging catheter and the coronary artery vessel wall mainly appears as three layers: Intima, Media, and Adventitia. As the two inner layers are of principal concern in clinical research, segmentation of IVUS images must be able to isolate the intima-media and lumen which provides important information about the degree of vessel obstruction as well as the shape and size of plaques.

Traditionally, coronary angiography has been used to provide a two-dimensional silhouette of the lumen in coronary vessels to detect the degree and severity of stenosis. Angiography heavily relies on the positioning of the system during imaging, since it only provides a silhouette of the lumen, a physician may be incapable of properly diagnosing the severity of atherosclerosis. Coronary IVUS is most often performed in conjunction with coronary angiography. During an IVUS intervention, arteries as small in diameter as 1.5 mm can typically be visualized and typically the patient is given intravenous heparin and intracoronary nitroglycerin which prevents blood coagulation within these small coronary arteries. The procedure is typically performed by a cardiologist

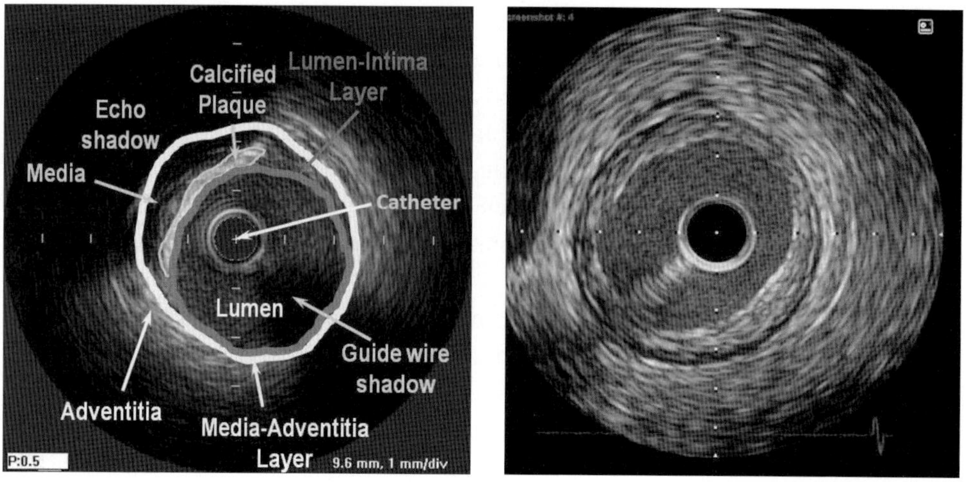

Fig. 1. IVUS images: Representation of a standard IVUS gray-scale images providing a 360° view of a coronary vessel.

or interventional cardiologist in a cardiac catheterization laboratory. IVUS imaging can complement and enhance angiographic information. When a mechanical pullback of the IVUS catheter is performed at a fixed rate, a three-dimensional (3D) reconstruction of the artery can be obtained.[17,18]

As stated earlier segmentation of IVUS images must be performed to isolate the intima-media and lumen which provides important information about the degree of vessel obstruction as well as the shape and size of plaques. Such segmentation can be performed manually by a human expert but it is very time consuming and costly also. Computer-based analysis and in fact a fully automatic image segmentation are much needed. There are several factors (artifacts) that significantly reduce the accuracy of segmentation and ultimately cause difficulty in interpretation:

1. The ever present speckle noises in the ultrasonic images of human tissues
2. Guide wire with reverberation
3. Reflection from sheath surrounding transducer
4. Barely identifiable lumen intima boundary
5. Bright echo from vessel wall being close to transducer

Other factors must be considered also, such as (a) the difference in tissues within the artery may require us to use different segmentation techniques for lumen boundary and intima-media boundary, (b) the use of stent and the bending of artery may require different consideration in segmentation. As a result a single algorithm is simply not enough to do the segmentation. Accurate automated segmentation is clearly much needed for IVUS images. There have been a large amount of efforts (e.g. Refs. [27]–[42]) including the use of automated contour model methods[27–31] and other approaches in 2D and 3D IVUS segmentations[32–51] in recent years. There are also many Ph.D. theses in the last five years that are related to computer analysis of intravascular ultrasound images (see. e.g. Refs. [52]–[56]). Our method is to employ several proven algorithms to achieve the automated segmentation results that meet the desired requirement. This is a basic research effort that involves image deconvolution to reduce the speckle noise inherent in the ultrasound images, removal of guide-wire effect, dynamic modeling of spatial temporal image sequence, feature extraction, and machine learning algorithms using neural networks and other computational intelligence methods, combining or selecting algorithms and classification problems involving identifying stent, branch and normal IVUS regions.

The speckle noise is often present in medical ultrasound images (see e.g. Ref. [57]). Blind deconvolution of IVUS images is one of the best strategies to deal with speckle noise without prior knowledge of noise. This topic will not be treated in this chapter however. A dynamic procedure for guide-wire tracking will be employed.

The contextual information in the image sequence holds key information which is often overlooked. We propose the use of statistical information from neighboring image frames, based on which textural and intensity features are extracted. As the number of features are large, several classification algorithms, each employing a feature subset, or a different training set will be used. Each segmentation algorithm carries a confidence level and the meta-algorithm makes use the weights assigned to different confidence levels or simply selects the algorithm with highest confidence level. We will work with large data sets involving a number of patients. We believe that only through testing on large data sets can our approach be fully verified for its effectiveness.

2. Preliminary Data and Studies

2.1. *Preliminary Data and Information*

There are 15 pull-out sequences from 9 patients. There are a total of 2293 gated image frames which have been manually segmented and are useful for training and validation purposes. A total of 57098 image frames provides us a large data set for algorithm testing (Table 1). Although many studies on IVUS image segmentation have been conducted with different but limited amount

Table 1. Description of our IVUS database.

Name of pullback sequence	Number of gated frames with manual segmentation	Approx. number of total frames
101-001_LAD	205	5369
101-011_RCA	92	2613
102-006_RCA	151	3464
103-007_LAD	247	4662
103-007_LCX	256	5229
106-001_LAD	62	3665
106-001_LCX	131	3848
110-001_RCA	167	3961
111-003_LAD	143	3477
111-003_LCX	131	3362
11-003_RCA	166	4611
114-001_LCX	143	3098
116-001_LAD	191	4606
116-001_LCX	108	2664
116-001_RCA	100	2469
Total	2293	57098

of success, none has employed such a large database and none has embarked on such as a comprehensive approach as presented in this proposal. We believe IVUS image segmentation is a problem in pattern recognition and computer vision. Considering the successes of many pattern recognition and computer vision problems in the last 50 years and their great impact on modern society, we are confident that the milestone of completely automated robust segmentation of IVUS images can be achieved in the near future.

2.2. *Preliminary Study Results*

The preliminary results presented here are based on our study in the last six years. It should be noted that we work with the images in polar coordinates. Our earlier effort (2007–2010) was focused on implementation of removing artifacts of IVUS images for active contour modeling (ACM) of the lumen and media-adventitia boundaries. ACM has desired characteristics of finding closed contour provided the image is free of artifacts. However, a plain ACM will distort the contours in areas where the guide-wire artefact confuses the algorithm. Additionally, when the catheter is touching or near to the vessel wall, the algorithm gets confused with the extra reverberations and distortions in the ultrasound image. Observation of the human segmentation process hinted that these artefacts are carefully avoided/ignored to create a good segmentation.

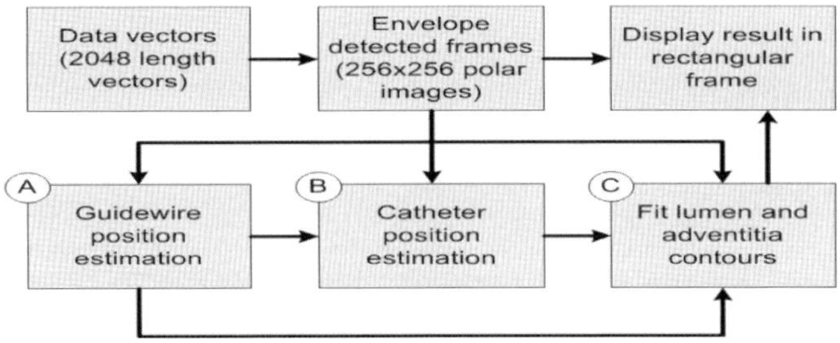

Fig. 2. Data flow block diagram of the automated segmentation process.

Additionally, the positions of the artefacts are strongly correlated between adjacent frames which provide further hints for manual segmentation process.

The guide-wire feature was carefully investigated from all frames of two different pull-back sequences consisting of about 10,000 frames in total.[58–60] Near the catheter, the guide wire produces a distinct echo-dense region with reverberations followed by a long narrow shadow region. Kalman filtering with position model and particle filtering with tunneling algorithms were developed for guide-wire tracking with very low tracking error.[60] The circular Hough transform (CHT) was employed for catheter position and vessel diameter estimates. Once the guide-wire position is estimated, the image regions distorted by the guide-wire can be ignored while performing the Hough transform. A deformable template model is then developed to refine the contour estimated by CHI so that a more accurate contour for the lumen and adventitia are produced. The block diagram showing the data flow of the automated IVUS segmentation process is given by Fig. 2. A selection of segmentation results from a pull-back sequence is shown in Fig. 3. The segmentation is mostly correct but can miss parts of the intima or EEM pointing to room for improvement.

In the last three years (2010–2013), we have made significant effort to obtain quantitative information of segmentation and to improve the segmentation process based on expanded data base. One effort adapted from Ref. [29] is to use texture and intensity information derived from Discrete Wavelet Frames Decomposition (DWFD), tested on Volcano data set.[61] The catheter induced artifacts are removed by thresholding in pre-processing of the original polar coordinate image. Four successive passes of DWFD results using both low and high pass filtering in 12 images. The average of the original and sum of DWFD images corresponding to fine texture image is used to initialize the lumen border. Significant edges are obtained by thresholding operator on such averaged image. Actual approximation of contour is obtained later by

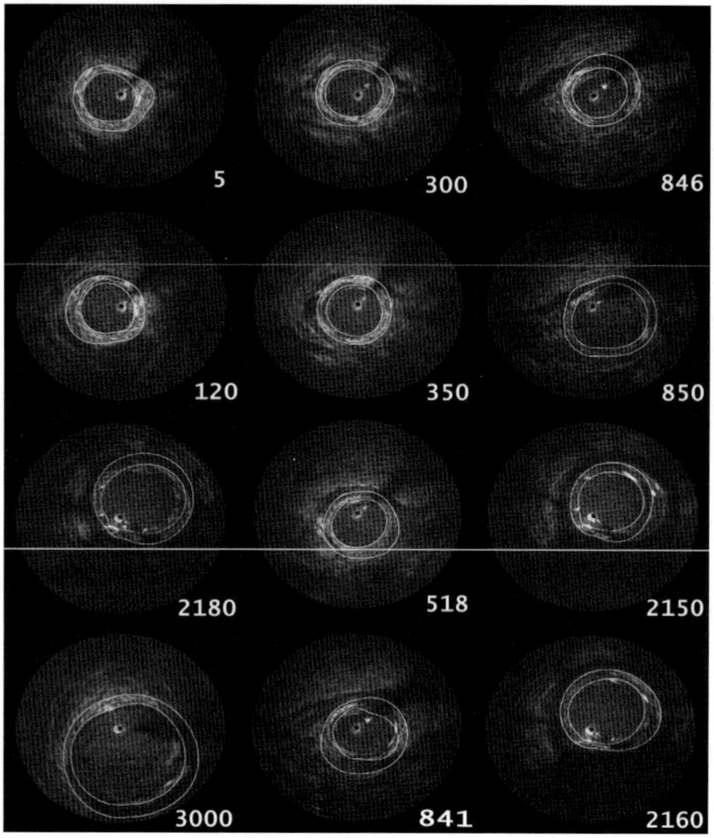

Fig. 3. A selection of segmented images.

applying radial basis functions. Once the lumen contour is initialized, we look to initialize media-adventitia border on outer side of the lumen. This saves us unnecessary computing time looking for the wall inside the lumen area. Now the average of the sum of original images after going through a series of low pass filtering contains mostly the coarse textures. In this sum image we will then look for maxima outside the lumen border. The selected pixels correspond to those on the boundary between the adventitia and media regions. Once both contours are initialized, there are multiple ways in which we can obtain the final smooth contour. The radial basis function (RBF) is selected to extract smooth and continuous contours. RBF involves a series of steps which are run on 500 continuous set of IVUS images. With combined use of texture and intensity based operations, the error area between the automatically traced contour and manually constructed contours is 1.141 ± 0.027 mm for lumen border and 1.260 ± 0.024 mm for media-adventitia border.

More recently, we employed the above method on a large data base from Brigham and Women Hospital described earlier and also take into account the temporal variation information. The images are selected by gating according to the ECG data at the same time. The image frames selected correspond to Q marker in ECG data. This will minimize the data variation. We then take the Laplacian of each pixel of the current image frame along with two previous frames and next two image frames. The resulting image frames are then processed by the composite operator that depends both on texture and temporal variation of intensity. Lumen contour can be traced based on finest texture and intensity specifics. Once we have the contour of lumen border, we can obtain the media-adventitia border by finding the coarse-most texture located outside the lumen border. Lumen could be predicted with a error of 6.9566 ± 2.2144 pixels corresponding to 0.1254 ± 0.04121 mm. EEM could be predicted with a error of 4.1915 ± 2.3017 pixels corresponding to 0.0762 ± 0.04514 mm. This is a remarkable improvement over the use of single images only, though we are dealing with two different data bases. The BWH data using Boston Scientific catheter are less noiser than the Volcano data.

We also studied the image data with stent and the prediction error is 0.048 ± 0.024 mm. We further employed the point cloud from initializations as input to the Poisson surface reconstruction algorithm to obtain a 3D visualization of coronary artery.

3. The Meta-algorithm

For this study, we have converted all available image data into polar form making it easier for research study though a rectangular display is easier for human visualization. As described above, there are a total of 2293 gated frames which have all been manually segmented and a total of 57,098 image frames from 15 pull-out image sequences coming from nine patients. The gated frames are useful for training and validation purposes in neural network classification. The entire data set is used in neural network classifications to provide us a large database for more accurate performance measurement. It is noted that some image frames have stents which must be detected, and some image frames come from branching of arteries.

A first step in pre-processing is the median filtering for each pixel and its corresponding pixels in five successive image frames. It is also possible to take the Laplacian of the five pixels, to make use of temporal image sequence information. To exploit spatial temporal information, we will consider the neighborhood of a pixel by using Gaussian Markov random field and incorporate the time sequence information to obtain a maximum a posterior estimate of the pixel. It is simplest to take median filtering though it does not remove speckle noise. The median filtered image is then deconvoled by the H-infinity method developed by Qidwai[57] which has proven to be effective to remove speckle noise in ultrasonic images.

Like many other problems in automated image segmentation, completely automated methods in segmentation of intravascular ultrasound (IVUS) images are lagging much behind segmentation by humans in terms of accuracy. It has been recognized that a particular published algorithm works well for a subset of the images in a data-set. However, the total accuracy is lowered by the presence of a large number of images where the automated algorithm fails. In the domain of brain image segmentation,[62,63] it has been recognized that the overall accuracy can be increased by using a meta-algorithm to choose a segmentation from among the outputs of multiple algorithms. A block diagram is shown in Fig. 4 which is a high level architecture for robust segmentation using a meta-algorithm with shared pre-processors. The word, "meta-algorithms" is used in different contexts with other names such as algorithm selection in the literature [see e.g. Ref. [64]–[66]]. One thing that is clear is that a single algorithm is often not sufficient to deal with a complex medical imaging problem.

An intravascular ultrasound exam produces a pull-back sequence of images. The number, K, of images in a sequence can be as large as several thousand. We

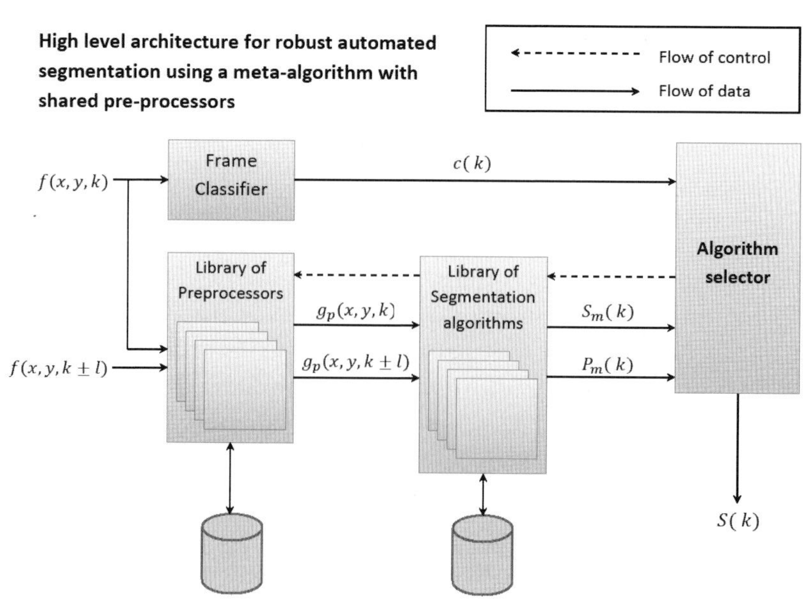

Fig. 4. Architecture of the meta-algorithm.

number the images from 0 to $K - 1$ indexed by k. Each image is of size $M \times N$, indexed by x and y. M and N can be of different sizes in different imaging systems and at different stages of processing. For example, $M \times N$ could be 1024×256 at one stage of processing which is condensed to a 256×256 image.

For the current purpose we assume a $M \times N$ image for each index k. We will call this a frame of data. In many cases, not all the pullback sequences are used. When imaging the heart, the blood vessel is moving in a rhythmic fashion and it is easy to identify a relatively stationary period during each heart beat in the data using electrocardiogram (ECG) data. The frames in this subset of the total frames are known as the gated frames. In a given pullback sequence, there are $G < K$ gated frames. The gated frames are indexed by g and the gating function maps this index to the index in the pullback sequence:

$$g = n_{gate}(k)$$

The gates in a sequence need not be uniformly spaced as the heart rate increases and decreases during the procedure. Often only the gated frames in a pullback sequence are manually segmented in data-sets to reduce the workload. Thus, evaluation of an automated algorithm is based only on the gated frames. However, it is certainly possible to have manual segmentation for the whole data-set too. The whole data for a pullback sequence is represented by $f(x; y; k)$:

$$f(x; y; k): x\varepsilon[0; M - 1]; \quad y\varepsilon[0; N - 1]; \quad k\varepsilon[0; K - 1]$$

A frame classifier algorithm takes each frame $f(-; -; k)$ and gives a classification (see Fig. 4):

$$\begin{aligned}
&c(k) = (c_1(k), c_2(k), c_3(k))) \\
&c_1(k)\ \varepsilon\ (\text{small lumen}|\text{medium lumen}|\text{large lumen}) \\
&c_2(k)\ \varepsilon\ (\text{stented}|\text{not stented}) \\
&c_3(k)\ \varepsilon\ (\text{branch}|\text{no branch})
\end{aligned}$$

For example, if the classification is $c(k) =$ (medium lumen; stented; no branch), the classifier believes that the frame indexed by k is most likely a medium sized blood vessel that is stented but without a branch. The classifier is a neural network that takes $f(-; -; k)$ and outputs three-tuple of binary classifications. Based on $c(k)$, the algorithm selector commands a subset of algorithms from a library of segmentation algorithms, indexed by m. These algorithms can draw on pre-calculated or on-demand calculated pre-processing results that are based on $f(-; -; k)$ as well as neighboring frames. Each segmentation algorithm produces along with the segmentation $S_m(k)$ a confidence metric $P_m(k)$. The algorithm selector combines $c(k)$ and $P_m(k)$ to choose the best segmentation.

If none of the initial batch of algorithms produce high confidence results, the algorithm selector can put to work a second tier of algorithms or flag the frame as a candidate for closer human analysis. A strategy for creating confidence metrics is described as follows.

Many algorithms in the literature only output the segmentation and do not produce an estimate of the algorithm's confidence on the segmentation. We have found that it is not difficult to form a confidence measure from existing algorithms. The processing of gated frames can involve neighboring frames. A method that we have found success with is the use of median of a number of frames around the gated frame. In a number of these methods, the segmentation accuracy is correlated to how fast the segmentation boundaries are changing around the gated frame. The specular reflection of sound waves from the blood is different in each IVUS image frame. When humans segment IVUS images, in areas where the segmentation is not clear, they browse the sequence of images and visually note where the pattern is changing randomly (blood) and where the patterns are changing in concert (vessel wall and other formations). The gated frames are chosen such that the movement of the vessel walls are minimal. Taking the median of the frames dramatically increases the accuracy of texture based segmentation methods. However, the segmentation can get confused when the frames are changing too fast. A simple metric to detect this has been devised:

$$\begin{aligned} m(\text{-};\ \text{-}g) &= \text{Medianlf}(\text{-};\ \text{-};\ g - l) \\ C(g) &= \text{sum of square errors of}[m(x, y, g) - f(x, y, g)] \\ &\quad \text{over } x,\ y, \text{ divided by MN.} \end{aligned}$$

where C(g), the change metric, correlates well with the mean square error.[67] Other confidence metrics we tested include: degree of smoothing of curves, closeness to threshold in thresholding steps, and neural network output.

As shown in Fig. 4, the library of preprocessors consists of all functions of pre-processing and enhancement including the use of spatial temporal information. The classification part makes use of neural networks. By going through the original gated frames, we construct the 8×8 subimages for training samples with four classes for border identification: the lumen region, the artifacts, the far field, and along the border. 10% of subimages is used for training, the next 10% is used for validation. Each subimage of 64 pixels is input to the neural network using multilayer perceptron network which now has available procedures to speed up the learning. The testing is done on all 5098 images to obtain reliable error estimate. Associated with each classification is a confidence level. Several neural networks each using different training and

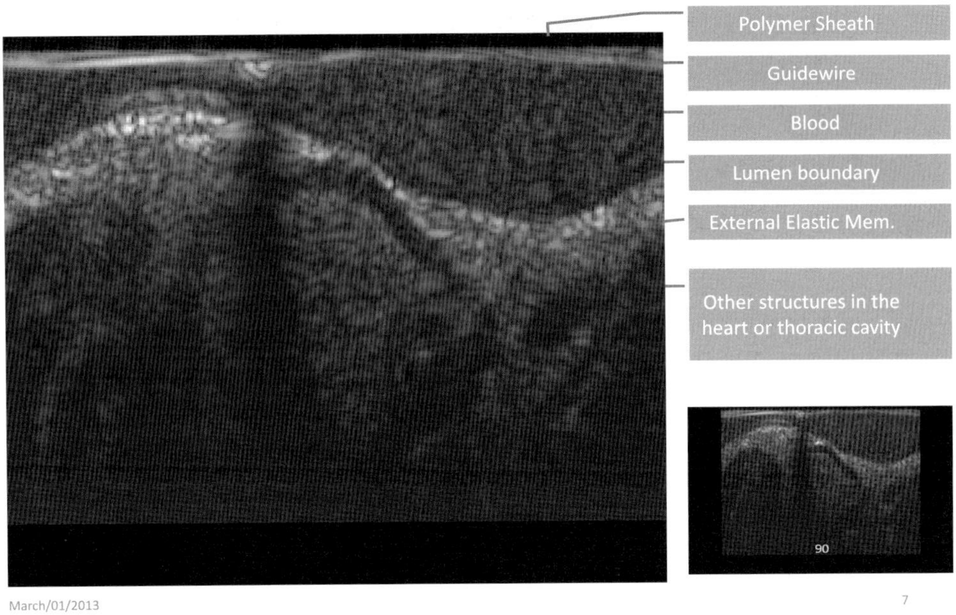

Fig. 5. A display of IVUS image in polar coordinates.

validation sets are employed for classification. Another classifier is to test the Rayleigh probability density fit of lumen area. A good fit means the subimage belongs to lumen, otherwise it may belong to lumen boundary. Sequentially the classifier with largest confidence level is selected and the lumen boundary is constructed by connecting lumen wall subimages with a local polynomial regression fitting after ignoring guide-wire artifact. Once the lumen wall is determined, we can proceed to seek for adventia-adventitia border (EEM). It is noted that for normal patient, the lumen and EEM walls can be very close. The polymer sheath may show up in some images (Fig. 5) and can be detected and largely removed by examining the first few scan lines. Figure 6 shows the lumen segmentation results. The left image shows the segmentation is accurate, and confidence is high, the middle image that has stents shows accurate segmentation but low confidence, and right image shows the segmentation is poor and confidence is low. The size of small rectangular box at lower left corner in each image denotes the confidence level.

4. Quantitative Performance Evaluation

When we looked at the computer (machine) segmented images and found that some images were with very good fidelity with respect to manual segmentation,

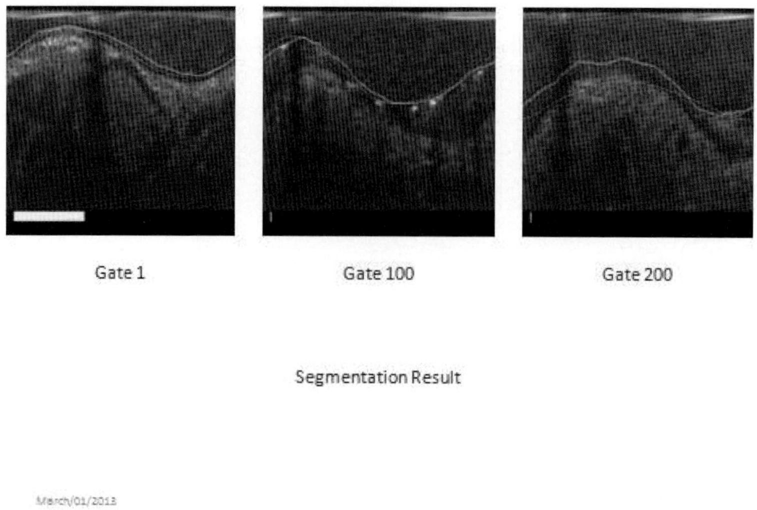

Fig. 6. A few Lumen segmentation results.

while others were medium quality and some were completely off the mark. To make this more quantitative, we decided to set a Mean Square Error of around MSE $= 12 * 12 = 144$ pixel $*$ pixel to be a threshold above which a segmentation is classified as bad. We chose 12 pixels for the error bound based on a calculation that the wavelength of the sound used is around 12 pixels. An interesting question would be how much of an error does a MSE of $12 * 12$ produce in the computational fluid dynamic simulation.

Each algorithm also computes a Confidence Metric (CM) besides the segmentation vector. Depending on the choice of the CM and a level CM0, a segmentation can be classified as good or bad. The quantitative performance measures are defined as follows.

True Positive: MSE based classification = good, CM based classification = good
False Negative: MSE based classification = good, CM based classification = bad
True Negative: MSE based classification = bad, CM based classification = bad
False Positive: MSE based classification = bad, CM based classification = good

As shown in Fig. 7 for each gated image there is a neural network segmentation error and a curve fit error with the threshold for each shown. The plot of curve fit metric versus the mean square error is shown in Fig. 8. Though the false positive is 0, the true positive is quite small. Much improvement is needed in further study.

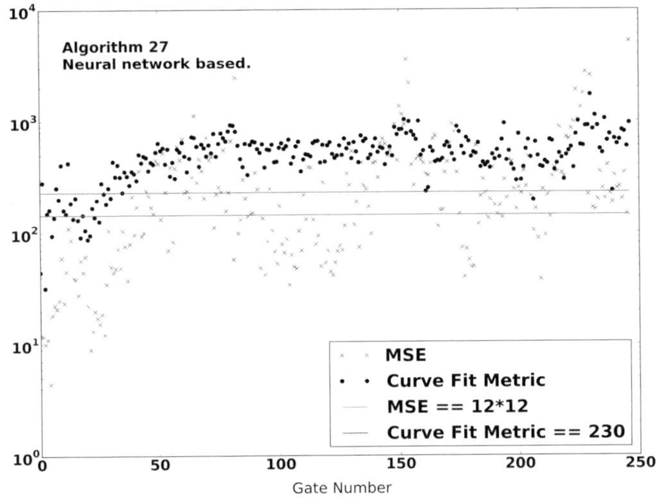

Fig. 7. A plot of segmentation error versus gate number.

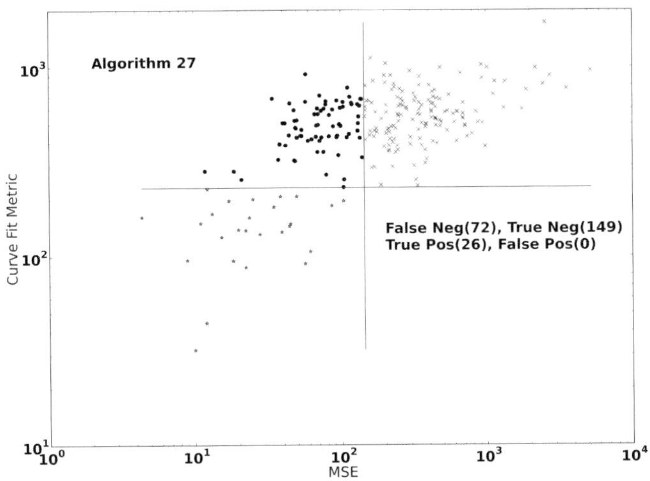

Fig. 8. A plot of curve fit error versus mean square error.

5. Concluding Remarks and Areas for Further Work

While the meta-algorithm method presented in this chapter has enormous potential to achieve a reliable fully automated IVUS image segmentation, much further work is needed to achieve the desired performance goal of say 95% correct segmentation. The combined effort[67] of image enhancement, feature extraction, meta-algorithm and the use of *a priori* knowledge about the arteries are expected to bring us much closer to the goal. For example by using properly selected features can provide effective classification with minimum neural network training time. Both texture and intensity information must be included in the features extracted. Directly inputting $8 \times 8 = 64$ pixel intensities to the neural network is clearly not effective. It is possible to use data from all five subimages in a sequence to determine the first three eigenvlaues from the 64 five dimensional vectors as input to the neural network. Other problem areas such as use of support vector machine, learning sample selection, boosting method and other machine learning methods can be explored as we proceed to make sure the desired goal can be achieved.

IVUS image segmentation results in a set of contours for all images in a long sequence. For 3D visualization, those contours need to be stacked on top of each other at regular intervals, i.e. with equal spacing between two contour sets with the assumption that the IVUS images are generated at regular intervals. Even if this is not the case, we need to perform interpolation between adjacent two contours. The interpolation procedure will be developed to reconstruct as many intermediate contours as needed to come up with a 3D tubular structure to represent the short coronary artery under consideration. The tabular structure must be rotatable to provide a 360 degree view of the structure.

References

1. S. E. Nissen, J. C. Gurley, C. L. Grines, D. C. Booth, R. McClure, M. Berk, C. Fischer, and A. N. DeMaria, "Intravascular ultrasound assessment of lumen size and wall morphology in normal subjects and patients with coronary artery disease," *Circulation* **84**, 1087–1099 (1991).
2. J. M. Tobis, J. Mallery, D. Mahon, K. Lehmann, P. Zalesky, J. Griffith, J. Gessert, M. Moriuchi, M. McRae, and M. L. Dwyer, "Intravascular ultrasound imaging of human coronary arteries *in vivo*. Analysis of tissue characterizations with comparison to in vitro histological specimens," *Circulation* **83**, 913–926 (1991).
3. A. Nair, B. D. Kuban, E. M. Tuzcu, P. Schoenhagen, S. E. Nissen, and D. G. Vince, "Coronary plaque classification with intravascular ultrasound radiofrequency data analysis," *Circulation* **106**, 2200–2206 (2002).
4. S. E. Nissen and J. C. Gurley, "Application of intravascular ultrasound for detection and quantitation of coronary atherosclerosis," *Int J Cardiac Imaging* **6**, 165–177, (1991).
5. S. K. Mehta, J. R. McCrary, A. D. Frutkin, W. J. S. Dolla, and S. P. Marso, "Intravascular ultrasound radiofrequency analysis of coronary atherosclerosis: an emerging technology for the assessment of vulnerable plaque," *Eur Heart J* **28**, 1283–1288 (2007).
6. C. Berry, P. L. L'Allier, J. Gregoire, J. Lesperance, S. Levesque, R. Ibrahim, and J. C. Tardif, "Comparison of intravascular ultrasound and quantitative coronary angiography for the assessment of coronary artery disease progression," *Circulation* **115**, 1851–1857 (2007).

7. E. Escolar, G. Weigold, A. Fuisz, and N. J. Weissman, "New imaging techniques for diagnosing coronary artery disease," *CMAJ* **174**, 487–495 (2006).
8. D. S. Baim, *Cardiac Catheterization, Angiography, and Intervention*, 7 ed Lippincott Williams & Wilkins (2005).
9. J.H. Reiber, "Accuracy and precision of quantitative digital coronary arteriography: Observer-, short-, and medium-term variabilities," *Catheter Cardiovasc Diagnosis* **28**, 187–198 (1993).
10. A. DeFranco, "Understanding the pathophysiology of the arterial wall: which method should we choose? Intra-vascular ultrasound," *Eur Heart J Suppl* **4**, F29–F40 (2002).
11. C. P. J. Blankenhorn, "The accuracy of arteriography and ultrasound imaging for atherosclerosis measurement: A review," *Arch Pathol Lab Med* 483–489 (1982).
12. F. G. Goar, F. J. Pinto, E. L. Alderman, H. A. Valantine, J. S. Schroeder, S. Z. Gao, E. B. Stinson, and R. L. Popp, "Intracoronary ultrasound in cardiac transplant recipients. *In vivo* evidence of 'angiographically silent' intimal thickening," *Circulation* **85**, 979–987 (1992).
13. E. J. Gussenhoven, C. E. Essed, C. T. Lancee, F. Mastik, P. Frietman, F. C. van Egmond, J. Reiber, H. Bosch, H. van Urk, and J. Roelandt, "Arterial wall characteristics determined by intravascular ultrasound imaging: An *in vitro* study," *J Am Coll Cardiol* **14**, 947–952 (1989).
14. J. Smith, T. E. Feldman, J. Hirshfeld, A. K. Jacobs, M. J. Kern, S. B. King III, D. A. Morrison, W. W. O'Neill, H. V. Schaff, P. L. Whitlow, D. O. Williams, E. M. Antman, J. Smith, C. D. Adams, J. 15. L. Anderson, D. P. Faxon, V. Fuster, J. L. Halperin, L. F. Hiratzka, S. A. Hunt, A. K. Jacobs, R. Nishimura, J. P. Ornato, R. L. Page, and B. Riegel, "ACC/AHA/SCAI 2005 Guideline Update for Percutaneous Coronary Intervention: A Report of the American College of Cardiology/American Heart Association Task Force on Practice Guidelines (ACC/AHA/SCAI Writing Committee to Update the 2001 Guidelines for Percutaneous Coronary Intervention)," *J Am Coll Cardiol* **47**, e1–e121 (2006).
15. B. N. ten Hoff H, "Imaging artifacts in mechanically driven ultrasound catheters," *J Cardiac Imaging* **4**, 195–199 (1989).
16. M. Dunitz, *Intravascular Ultrasound*. London: Martin Dunitz Limited (1998).
17. B. E. Zipes DP, *Braunwald's Heart Disease: A Textbook of Cardiovascular Medicine*, 7 ed. St. Louis: W.B. Saunders (2005).
18. B. J. Kimura, V. Bhargava, and A. N. DeMaria, "Value and limitations of intravascular ultrasound imaging in characterizing coronary atherosclerotic plaque," *Am Heart J* **130**, 386–396 (1995).
19. A. Coskun, Y. Yeghiazarians, S. Kinlay, M. Clark, O. Ilebbusi, A. Wahle, M. Sonka, J. Pompa, R. Kuntz, C. Feldman, and P. Stone, "Reproducibility of coronary lumen, plaque, and vessel wall reconstruction and of endothelial shear stress measurements *in vivo* in humans," *Catheter Cardiovasc Intervention* **60**, 67–78 (2003).
20. P. Stone, S. Saito, S. Takahashi, Y. Makita, Shigeru Nakarnura, T. Kawasaki, A. Takahashi, T. Katsuki, Sunano Nikarnura, A. Namiki, A. Hirohata, T. Matsumura, S. Ysmazaki, H. Yokoi, S. Tanaka, S. Otsuji, F. Yoshimachi, J. Honye, D. Harwood, M. Reitman, A. U. Coskun, M. I. Papafaklis, C. L. Feldman, "Prediction of progression of coronary artery disease and clinical outcomes using vascular profiling of endothelial shear stress and arterial plaque characteristics: The PREDICTION study," *Circulation*, 172–181 (2012).

21. P. Yock, D. Linker, O. Saether, H. Thapliyal, J. Arenson, N. White and others, "Intravascular two-dimensional catheter ultrasound: Initial clinical studies," *Circulation* **78**, 11–21 (1988).
22. M. Rosales, P. Radeva, O. Rodriguez-Leor and D. Gil, "Modelling of image-catheter motion for 3-D IVUS," *Med Image Anal* (2008).
23. D. Gil, A. Hernandez, O. Rodriguez, J. Mauri and P. Radeva, "Statistical strategy for anisotropic adventitia modelling in IVUS," *IEEE Trans Med Imaging* **25**, 768 (2006).
24. B. Godbout, J. A. de Guise, G. Soulez and G. Cloutier, "3D elastic registration of vessel structures from IVUS data on biplane angiography1," *Acad Radiol* **12**, 10–16 (2005).
25. R. Krams, J. J. Wentzel, J. A. F. Oomen, R. Vinke, J. C. H. Schuurbiers, P. J. de Feyter, P. W. Serruys and C. J. Slager, "Combining 3D reconstruction from angiography and IVUS (ANGUS) with computational fluid dynamics. *Arterioscler Thromb Vasc Biol* **17**, 2061–2065 (1997).
26. M. Rosales and P. Radeva, "A basic model for IVUS image simulation," in *Handbook of Biomedical Image Analysis* Anonymous 2005, 1–55.
27. T. McInerney and D. Terzopoulos, "Deformable models in medical image analysis: A survey," *Med Image Anal* **1**, 91–108 (1996).
28. G. D. Giannoglou, Y. S. Chatzizisis, V. Koutkias, I. Kompatsiaris, M. Papadogiorgaki, V. Mezaris, E. Parissi, P. Diamantopoulos, M. G. Strintzis and N. Maglaveras, "A novel active contour model for fully automated segmentation of intravascular ultrasound images: *In vivo* validation in human coronary arteries," *Comput Biol Med* **37**, 1292–1302 (2007).
29. M. Papadogiorgaki, V. Mexaris, Y. S. Chatzizisis, G. D. Giannoglou and I. Kompatsiaris, 'Image analysis techniques for automated IVUS contour detection," *Ultrasound Med Bio J* **34**, 1482–1498 (2008).
30. C. H. Chen, L. Potdar and R. Chittineni, "Two novel ACM (active contour model) methods for IVUS image segmentation," *Proc. Of the Review of Quantitative NDE*, (2009).
31. P. Manandhar, C. H. Chen and A. U. Coskun, "A deformable template model with feature tracking for automated IVUS segmentation," Chapter 4.3 of *Handbook of Pattern Recognition and Computer Vision*, edited by C. H. Chen, World Scientific Publishing, 497–515 (2010).
32. M. Sonka, X. Zhang, M. Siebes, M. S. Bissing, S. C. DeJong, S. M. Collins, C. R. McKay, "Segmentation of intravascular ultrasound images: A knowledge-based approach," *IEEE Trans Medical Imaging* **14**, 719–732 (1995).
33. S. Balocco, C. Gatta, C. Francesco, P. Oriol, X. Carrillo, J. Mauri, P. Radeva, "Combining growcut and temporal correlation for IVUS lumen segmentation," *Pattern Recognition and Image Analysis m Springer* **6669**, 556–563 (2011).
34. M. H Cardinal, G. Soulez, J. Tardif, J. Meunier, and G. Cloutier, "Fast-marching segmentation of three-dimensional intravascular ultrasound images: A pre- and post-intervention study," *Int J Medical Phy* **37** (2010).
35. Z. Luo, Y. Wang and W. Wang, "Estimating coronary artery lumen area with optimization-based contour detection," *IEEE Trans Medical Imaging* **22**, 564–566 (2003).
36. G. D. Giannoglou, Y. S. Chatzizisis, and G. Sianos, "*In-vivo* validation of spatially correct three- dimensional reconstruction of human coronary arteries by integrating intravascular ultrasound and biplane angiography," *Coron Artery Dis* **17**, 533–543 (2009).

37. C. Perrey, U. Scheipers, W. Bojara, M. Lindstaedt, S. Holt, and H. Ermert, "Computerized segmentation of blood and luminal borders in intravascular ultrasound," *Proc. of the 2004 IEEE Ultrasonics Symposium*, **2**, 1122–1125 (2004).
38. M. Plissiti, D. Fotiadis, L. Michalis, and L. Bozios, "An automated method for lumen and media-adventitia border detection in a sequence of IVUS frames," *IEEE Trans Infor Tech Biomed* **8** (2004).
39. C. Wentzel, J. Schuurbiers, J. Oomen, J. Kloet, and J. Krams, "True 3-dimensional reconstruction of coronary arteries in patients by fusion of angiography and IVUS (ANGUS) and its quantitative validation," *Circulation* **102**, 511–516 (2000).
40. J. Klingensmith, R. Shekhar, and D. Vince, "Evaluation of three dimensional segmentation algorithms for the identification of luminal and medial-adventitial borders in intravascular ultrasound images," *IEEE Trans Medical Imaging* **19**, 996–1011 (2000).
41. G. Beyar, R. Shofti, and R. Azhari, "Three dimensional automatic quantitative analysis of intravascular ultrasound image," *Ultrasound Med Biol* **26**, 527–537 (2000).
42. D. Gil, P. Radeva, J. Saludes and J. Mauri, "Automatic segmentation of artery wall in coronary IVUS images: a probabilistic approach," *Comp Cardiology 2000*, 687–690 (2000).
43. D. E. Ilea, C. Duffy, L. Kavanagh, A. Stanton and P. F. Whelan, "Fully automated segmentation and tracking of the intima media thickness in ultrasound video sequences of the common carotid artery," *IEEE Trans Ultrasonics Ferroelectrics Frequency Control* **60**, 158–177 (2003).
44. U. Scheipers, S. Koptenko, R. Remlinger, T. Falco and M. Lachaine, "3-D ultrasound volume reconstruction using the direct frame interpolation method," *IEEE Trans Ultrasonics Ferroelectronics Frequency Control* **57**, 2460–2470 (2010).
45. F. Destrempes, J. Meunier, M. Giroux, G. Soulez and G. Cloutier, "Segmentation of plaques in sequences of ultrasounic B-mode images of carotid arteries based on motion estimation and a Bayesian model," *IEEE Trans Biomed Eng* **58**, 2202–2211 (2011).
46. M. Sonka, M. D. Winniford and S. M. Collins, "Robust simultaneous detection of coronary borders in complex images," *IEEE Trans Medical Imaging* **14**, 151–161 (1995).
47. I. Tzovaras, D. Koutkias, and V. Strintzis, "Deformable boundary detection of stents in angiographic images," *IEEE Trans Medical Imaging* **19**, 652–662 (2000).
48. R. Krams, J. J. Wentzel, J. A. F. Oomen, R. Vinke, J. C. H. Schuurbiers, P. I. de Feyter, P. W. Serruys, and C. J. Slager, "Evaluation of endothelial shear stress and 3D geometry as factors determining the development of atherosclerosis and remodeling in human coronary arteries in-vivo: Combining 3D reconstruction from angiography and IVUS (ANGUS) with computational fluid dynamics," *Arterioscler Thromb Vasc Biol* **17**, 2061–2065 (1997).
49. A. S. Jorgensen, S. E. Schmidt, N. Staalsen, and L. R. Ostergaard, "Automatic vessel tracking and segmentation using epicardial ultrasound in bypsss surgery," *Computing Cardiol* **39**, 9–12 (2012).
50. C. V. Bourantas, I. C. Kourtis, M. E. Plissiti, D. I. Fotiadis, C. K. Katsouras and L. K. Michalis, "A method for 3D reconstruction of coronary arteries using biplane angiography and intravascular ultrasound images," *Computerized Medical Imaging Graphics* **29**, 597–606 (2005).
51. J. Anquez, E. D. Angelini, G. Grange and I. Block, "Automatic segmentation of antenatal 3-D ultrasonic images," *IEEE Trans Biomed Eng* **60**, 1388–1400 (2013).

52. S. Brugaletta, "Imaging techniques for the assessment of coronary atherosclerosis, intracoronary devices and vessel response after metallic or polymeric Scarfolds Implantation," Ph.D. Thesis, Erasmus University, Rotterdam, Advisor: Prof. Patrick Serruys (2012).
53. R. W. Downe, "Predictive analysis of coronary plaque morphology and composition on a one year timescale," Ph.D. thesis, University of Iowa. Advisor: Prof. Milan Sonka (2013).
54. S. Shivakumar, "Segmentation and 3D visualization of intravascular ultra-sound images," Ph.D Dissertation, University of Georgia, Advisor: Prof. S.M. Bhandarkar (2011).
55. M. R. Cardinal, "Segmentation d'imasges intravasculaires ultrasonores," Ph.D. thesis, University of Montreal, Advisor: Prof. Guy Cloutier (2008).
56. S. Tu, "Three-dimensional quantitative coronary angiography and the registration with intravascular ultrasound and optical coherency tomography," Ph.D. thesis, Division of Radiology, Leiden University (2012).
57. Uvais A. Qidwai and Umair A. Qidwai, "Deonvolution technique for enhancing and classifying the retinal images," Chapter 12 of *Computer Vision in Medical Imaging*, edited by C. H. Chen, World Scientific Publishing (2013).
58. P. Manandhar, "A novel IVUS segmentation method using Active Contour Models," unpublished internal report (2007).
59. P. Manandhar, "Fully automated guide-wire tracking in IVUS," unpublished internal report (2009).
60. P. Manandhar, C. H. Chen, C. L. Feldman and A. U. Coskun, "Use of guide-wire and curve tracking to augment active contour models for intravascular ultrasound," unpublished internal report (2009).
61. A. R. Gangidi and C. H. Chen, "Texture and intensity based 2D and 3D visualization of coronary arteries with IVUS imaging," unpublished internal report (2012).
62. D. E. Rex, D. W. Shattuck, R. P. Woods, K. L. Narr, E. Luders, K. Rehm, S. E. Stolzner, D. A. Rottenberg, and A. W. Toga, "A meta-algorithm for brain extraction in MRI," *NeuroImage* **23**, 625–637 (2004).
63. E. Iglesias, C. Y. Liu, P. M Thompson, and Z. Tu. "Robust brain extraction across datasets and comparison with publicly available methods," *IEEE Trans Medical Imaging* **30**, 1617–1634 (2011).
64. M. Lukac, R. Tanizawa, and M. Kameyama, "Machine learning based adaptive computer detection using algorithm selection and image splitting," *Interdisciplinary Information Sci* **18**, 123–134 (2012).
65. S. Takemoto and H. Yokota, "Algorithm selection for intracellular image segmentation based on region similarity," *Ninth International Conference Proceedings on Intelligent Systems Design and Applications*, 1413–1418 (2009).
66. L. Cruz-Reyes, C. Gomex-Santillan, J. Perex-Ortega, V. Landero, M. Quiroz and Al. Ochoa, "Algorithm selection: From meta-learning to hyper-heuristics," Chapter 4 of *Intelligent Systems*, edited by V. M. Koleshko, an INTECH publication (2012).
67. P. Manandhar, A. R. Gangidi, A. U. Coskun, and C. H. Chen, "Combining multiple algorithms for robust segmentation of intravascular ultrasound (IVUS) images," unpublished internal report (2013).

Chapter 20

Computational Methods for the Analysis of Intravascular Ultrasound Data

E. Gerardo Mendizabal-Ruiz and Ioannis A. Kakadiaris†*

**Departamento de Ciencias Computacionales*
Universidad de Guadalajara, Guadalajara, Jalisco, México
†Computational Biomedicine Lab
University of Houston, Houston, Texas, USA

Atherosclerosis is a condition in which the wall of the arteries hardens and thickens due to the accumulation of plaque. The primary cause of acute coronary events is related to the inflammation and disruption of coronary plaques. Characterization and detection of plaques vulnerable to complications (i.e., vulnerable plaque, VP) is one of the most active areas of research in cardiology. Intravascular ultrasound (IVUS) is an invasive technique that is capable of providing a real-time, high-resolution tomographic visualization of the coronary arteries which allows the accurate estimation of the morphological characteristics of the vessel. The extraction of valuable information from the IVUS data through the use of medical image analysis methods has played an important role in the detection and characterization of VP. In this chapter, we will present different computational methods developed for the analysis of IVUS data and the detection of VP.

1. Introduction

Atherosclerosis is a condition in which the wall of the arteries hardens and thickens due to the accumulation of plaque (i.e., calcium and fatty deposits such as cholesterol and triglycerides).[34,53] Coronary artery disease (CAD) is caused by atherosclerosis in the coronary arteries and is the most common type of heart disease and the cause of acute myocardial infractions. Unfortunately, the first symptoms of CAD (e.g., chest pain) may not appear until the advanced phases of the disease. Therefore, even in the severe cases, many patients remain unaware of their risk (it has been reported that for 30%–50% of individuals who suffer CAD, the first symptom of the disease is a heart attack, which commonly leads to a sudden death[41]). The primary cause of acute coronary events is related to the inflammation and disruption of coronary plaques with superimposed thrombosis. It has been shown that for up to 75% of the acute ischemic coronary syndromes (ACS), the rupture of an atherosclerotic plaque is the underlying pathological mechanism.[3,10] Pathology studies indicate that certain plaques are more prone to develop ACS than others. In this context, the field of cardiology has introduced the term "vulnerable plaque" (VP), which refers to those plaques with a high likelihood of rupture, thrombotic complications, and the consequent rapid progression to stenosis.[38,41]

Characterization and detection of VP is one of the most active areas of research in cardiology. Some of the most consistent identified histopathologic characteristics of ruptured plaques relate mainly to their morphology (e.g., outward positive remodeling, inflammatory cell infiltration, intraplaque hemorrhage, etc.) and its composition (e.g., necrotic core, fibrous cap, cholesterol crystals, etc.). Another factor that has been linked with vulnerable plaques is the presence and proliferation of microvessels at the arterial wall adventitia, and within the atherosclerotic plaque[63] (i.e., vasa vasorum, VV).

The use of medical images plays an important role towards the characterization and opportune detection of VP. Several invasive and non-invasive techniques such as angiography, thermography, magnetic resonance, optical coherence tomography, elastography, and intravascular ultrasound (IVUS) have been used for the assessment of atherosclerotic plaques.[61] In particular, IVUS is the gold-standard technique for assessing the blood vessels *in vivo*.[54]

1.1. *Intravascular Ultrasound*

IVUS is an invasive technique that is capable of providing a real-time, high-resolution tomographic visualization of the coronary arteries which allows the accurate estimation of the morphological characteristics of the vessel (e.g., lumen diameter and wall thickness), and the plaques (e.g., location, presence of intra-luminal thrombus and plaque rupture). An IVUS system consists of (1) a catheter with a miniaturized ultrasound sensor attached to its distal end, (2) a motorized pullback device, and (3) a processing unit which processes the signals received by the ultrasound transducer.

The IVUS intervention consists of steering a guidewire with a small diameter (about 0.84 mm) into the blood vessel branch to be imaged. The IVUS catheter is then percutaneously slid-in over the guidewire and positioned within a target segment of interest. For coronary imaging in humans, the entry point is typically the femoral artery in the leg.

The ultrasound probe can either be a solid-state multi array or a mechanically-rotated transducer which transmits ultrasound pulses and receives an acoustic radio frequency (RF) echo signal (i.e., A-line) at a discrete set of

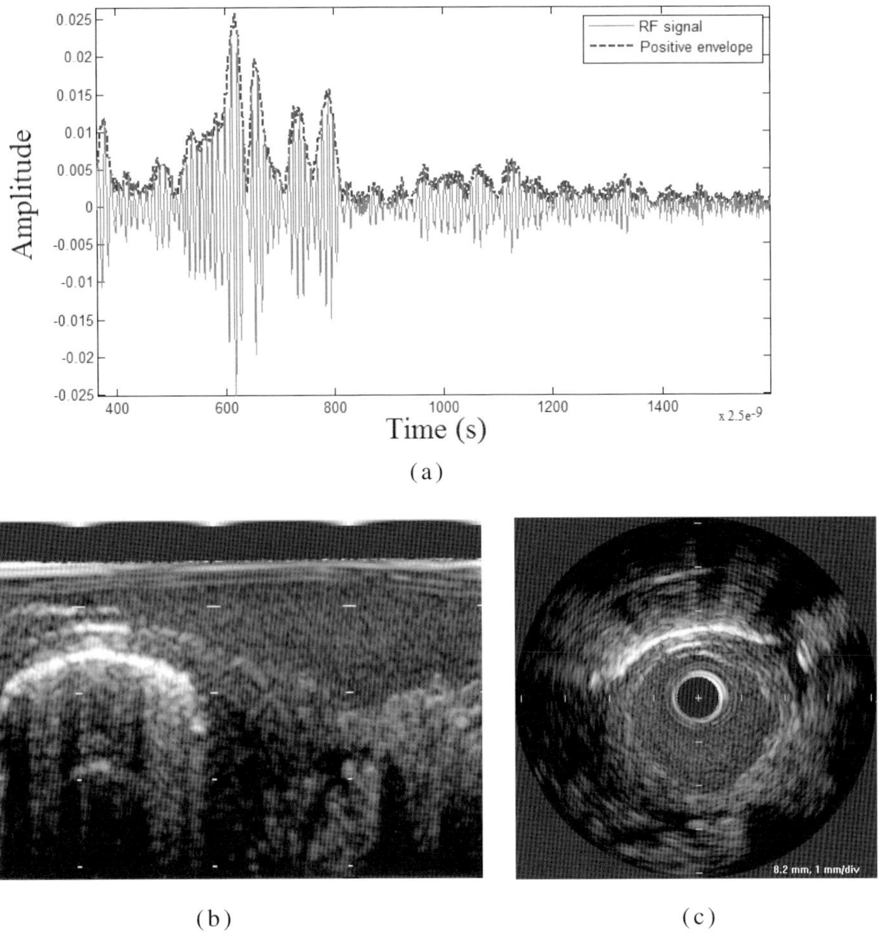

Fig. 1. Depiction of (a) an A-line signal and its envelope, and the B-Mode IVUS representations: (b) IVUS image in polar representation; (c) IVUS image in Cartesian representation.

angles. Commonly, 240 to 360 A-line RF signals are obtained per rotation. A B-mode IVUS image is obtained by the processing unit by computing the positive envelopes of each A-line. These B-mode signals are then compressed, stacked along the angular direction, and mapped into an 8-bit gray scale to form an image known as the polar B-mode image. To provide a more familiar representation of the data (to resemble the interior of a vessel), the polar B-mode image is geometrically transformed to obtain a disc-shaped image known as the Cartesian B-mode image (Fig. 1). Examples of typical normal and diseased (atherosclerotic) gray scale Cartesian IVUS images are illustrated in Fig. 2.

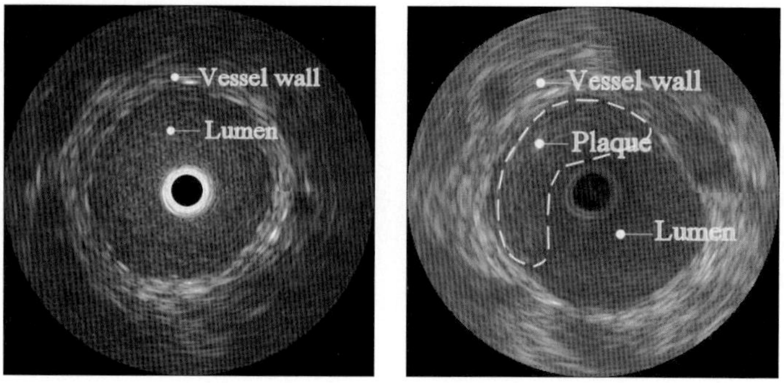

(a) (b)

Fig. 2. Examples of a typical IVUS B-mode image of (a) normal and (b) atherosclerotic vessel.

The IVUS system acquires and displays images usually at 30 frames/second. For some applications, the ultrasound catheter may be pulled back to identify and analyze the different vessel regions. The pullback can be performed either manually or using the pullback device which moves the transducer at a constant determined speed (usually 0.5 mm/s). In human coronary arteries, the target segments generally include at least 10 mm of distal vessel, the lesion site(s), and the entire proximal vessel back to the aorta.[37] If additional information about a lesion is needed, an acquisition may be performed by maintaining the IVUS catheter stationary over the region of interest. The analysis of the acquired data may be performed in real-time during the intervention or off-line after the acquisition.

The ability of the IVUS technique to provide details of the structures being imaged depends on the spatial resolution and the contrast resolution of the employed system. Spatial resolution refers to the ability of the system to discriminate small objects within the generated image and has three principal directions. The axial resolution (i.e., parallel to the beam) depends on the frequency and duration of the impulse wave employed, the size of the transducer, and the radial sampling rate. The lateral resolution (i.e., perpendicular to the beam and the catheter) depends on the wavelength of the signal, the size of the transducer employed. The out-of-plane direction (i.e., perpendicular to the axial and lateral resolution) primarily decides the slice thickness of the IVUS image and depends on the beam width. Lateral resolution degrades linearly with distance from the catheter, while axial resolution remains constant. Out-of-plane resolution improves as the distance of the beam from the catheter increases. Spatial resolution increases with transducer frequency; however, attenuation also increases with frequency. Due to the rotational tomographic nature of IVUS images, their spatial resolution is highly variable within a single image. For a 20 MHz to 40 MHz IVUS transducer, the typical resolution is considered to be 80 μm axially and 200 μm to 250 μm laterally.[37] Contrast resolution refers to the dynamic range of the generated images. An image with low dynamic range appears as black and white regions with a few intermediate gray-level values (i.e., granular), while images at high dynamic range are often softer. Contrast resolution depends directly on the hardware characteristics of the IVUS system.

1.2. *IVUS Data Analysis*

IVUS systems are very useful in situations in which angiographic imaging does not provide enough information about the morphology of the lumen or ostial lesions for a specific segment of interest, or to assess the effects of medical therapy or treatments such as angioplasty expansion with and without stents. Usually, the analysis and interpretation of the IVUS data is made by the expert physicians performing the intervention with the help of different tools implemented in the IVUS system (e.g., image correction, annotation, measurement, zoom).

However, thanks to recent advances in medical image analysis, now it is possible to process the IVUS data to automatically obtain the morphological characteristics of the vessel and plaque (i.e., IVUS segmentation), to estimate the composition of the plaque (i.e., plaque characterization), and the detection of VV within the plaque and adventitia (i.e., extra-luminal blood perfusion detection).

1.2.1. *IVUS segmentation*

Segmentation of IVUS images refers to the delineation of the lumen/intima and media/adventitia borders (Fig. 3). This process is necessary for assessing morphological characteristics of the vessel and plaque such as lumen diameter, minimum lumen cross section area, and total atheroma volume. This information is crucial for making decisions such as whether a stent is needed to restore blood flow in an artery and to determine the characteristics of the stent. Other applications of IVUS include the study of mechanical properties of the vessel wall, characteristics of the plaque, and 3D reconstruction of the vessel.

Early IVUS systems operated at frequencies in the range of 10 MHz to 20 MHz. At these frequencies, the blood presents a low acoustic impedance and speckle noise and therefore these systems produce IVUS images on which the lumen has low intensity, no texture, and a high contrast with respect to the vessel wall tissues. For this reason, many approaches for IVUS segmentation

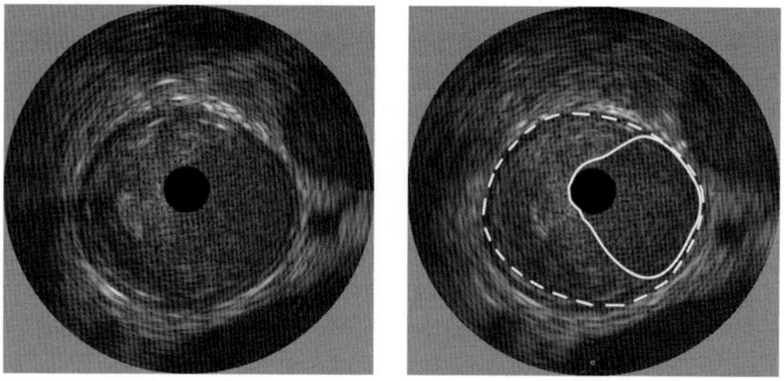

(a) (b)

Fig. 3. Example of (a) an typical IVUS image with (b) its corresponding segmentation (lumen/intima and media/adventitia interface are depicted using a solid and dotted lines, respectively).

were based on the use of local properties of the image (e.g., pixel intensity and gradient information) combined with computational methods including graph search,[56,64] active surfaces,[30] active contours,[31,35] and neural networks.[50] Modern IVUS systems operate in higher frequencies (i.e., 30 MHz to 40 MHz) and produce images with better resolution. However, the lumen on these images depicts more texture due to speckle, and lower contrast of the lumen with respect to the vessel wall tissues. For these images, edge information may not be sufficient, and therefore segmentation approaches incorporated prior knowledge using region and global information such as texture,[39] gray level variances,[20,33] statistical properties of the image,[2] temporal information,[5] (3D segmentation) and mathematical morphology techniques.[12]

Current approaches for the segmentation of IVUS images include the use of shape-driven methods,[58] 3D graph search,[13] multilevel discrete wavelet frames decomposition,[49] discrete wavelet packet transform,[25] error correcting output codes,[9] directional gradient velocity and level sets,[65] fast-marching,[6] balloon snakes,[66] morphological object reconstruction methods,[40] a method based on frequency-based harmonic information extracted by brushlet expansion,[24] a graph-based approach with an assisted manual refinement of the segmentation result,[57] an interactive segmentation method employing edge based boundary constraints,[23] and a fast-marching based method.[11]

A common characteristic of IVUS segmentation methods is that the computations are performed using the reconstructed B-mode reconstruction images either in polar, Cartesian or L-mode representations. This poses a limitation considering that, apart from the frequency of operation of the transducer, the gray level distributions of the different regions of the vessel

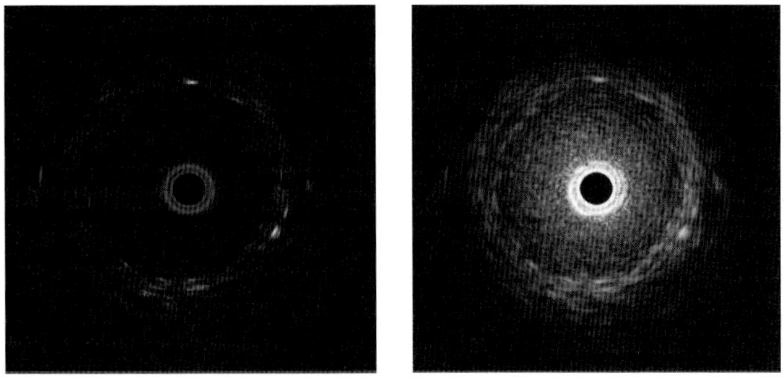

(a) (b)

Fig. 4. Example depicting a 40 MHz IVUS frame in Cartesian B-mode representation using logarithmic dynamic range compression; (b) the same frame using linear dynamic range compression with a compression factor of 0.4.

in the B-mode images depends on the reconstruction settings of the IVUS systems such as time-gain compensation (TGC), dynamic range compression and rejection, persistence, and gamma curves which are subjectively selected by the interventionist[21,37] (Fig. 4) and may change from one intervention to the next, or even during the same acquisition.[37]

To overcome this limitation our group presented a segmentation method based on the minimization of a probabilistic cost function that deforms a parametric curve which defines a probability field that is regularized with respect to the given likelihoods of the pixels belonging to blood and non-blood.[36] These likelihoods are obtained by using the prediction of a support vector machine classifier trained using texture features extracted from samples of the lumen and non-lumen regions provided by the user in the first frame of the sequence to be segmented. This enables the segmentation of IVUS images from different frequencies (i.e., 20 MHz and 40 MHz) without the need to adjust parameters, and it makes the proposed method robust to the problem of variability on the gray level distribution of the IVUS images due the B-mode image-generation parameters. Additionally, the proposed method includes a step in which possible changes in the gray level distributions of the regions of interest within a sequence are automatically detected, so that the likelihood computations are progressively adapted. This step makes the method robust with respect to a possible change of gray level distributions within an IVUS sequence caused by the blood flow and a possible sudden change in the B-mode reconstruction parameters. The results indicate that the segmentation results obtained with our method are comparable to the segmentation performed by human observers.

Due to the relevance of the IVUS segmentation problem and the variety of methods that have been presented, an evaluation framework that allows a standardized and quantitative comparison of IVUS lumen and media segmentation algorithms was introduced at the MICCAI 2011 Computing and Visualization for (Intra)Vascular Imaging (CVII) workshop[1] which compared the results of eight segmentation methods including our segmentation method.[36]

1.2.2. *Plaque characterization*

Plaque characterization from IVUS data consists of identifying the composition of the atherosclerotic plaque (e.g., fibrous, calcified, or lipid) based on the changes that occur to the sound waves as they interact with the different types of tissue.

A common approach for plaque characterization consists of computing different features from many samples of IVUS data regions identified as plaque for which the composition is known (generally by histological analysis) which are then used with supervised or unsupervised machine learning methods.

In the unsupervised methods, the features corresponding to the samples are grouped or clustered according to a given similarity criteria. In the supervised methods, a training set is built and then used to train a classifier which generates a model capable of determining the composition of a new plaque sample based on its features.

The features which allows the characterization of the plaque may be extracted from the gray-level IVUS B-mode representation (e.g., co-occurrence matrix, laws features, Gabor filters, Rayleigh mixture models).[4,26,52,55,62] However, most successful approaches compute the features directly from raw IVUS RF signal. Nair *et al.* proposed a method known as "virtual histology" (IVUS-VH)[42,43] that is based on the power spectral analysis (intercept, slope, mid-band fit, and minimum and maximum powers and their corresponding frequencies) of the IVUS RF signals combined with classification trees. Many authors have presented studies of this method reporting high correlation with the corresponding histology.[22,44,51] Other authors have proposed similar methods employing different features including the use of the integrated backscatter,[28,29] and wavelet decomposition analysis.[26,52] An extensive review in supervised and unsupervised plaque characterization methods has been presented recently.[27]

1.2.3. *Extra-luminal blood perfusion detection*

Although IVUS provides reliable cross sectional images of the coronary arteries, the *in vivo* imaging of the coronary VV microvascularization remains a great challenge due to its small size (reported diameters of human artery VV ranged from[32] 11.6 μm to 36.6 μm), echo transparency, and the presence of different IVUS artifacts.

IVUS may be used in combination with contrast agents (CE-IVUS) in the form of microbubbles of a size similar to red blood cells (diameter: 1–10 μm) that resonate in response to the pressure changes induced by the ultrasound wave making them several times more echogenic than normal body tissue. These contrast agents are injected into the bloodstream during IVUS interventions as blood tracers. Since the detection of VV can be posed as the detection of microcirculation in the plaque or vessel (i.e., extra-luminal perfusion), the detection of contrast-agent in the plaque or vessel wall (i.e., extra-luminal perfusion) may be an indication of the presence of microvasculature. The use of CE-IVUS has proven useful in imaging plaque perfusion in coronary arteries[7] and for assessing the amount and distribution of neovessels within atherosclerotic lesions.[19]

Currently, there exist two main approaches for the assessment of VV microvascularization based on the use of CE-IVUS data: (1) non-linear or harmonic response IVUS imaging and (2) differential imaging.

1.3. *Non-linear IVUS*

Depending on the energy and frequency of the ultrasound beam, the contrast agent microbubbles may present linear and nonlinear oscillations. Linear oscillations occur when equal-amplitude contraction and relaxation of the microbubbles are induced by the ultrasound signal. Nonlinear oscillations occur when the microbubbles expand above their baseline diameter at a greater scale when compared to their ability to compress below it. In the case of linear oscillations (fundamental mode), the microbubbles produce echo signals with the same frequency as the ultrasound transducer (i.e., fundamental frequency). In the case of nonlinear oscillations, the microbubbles will produce the fundamental frequency and multiples of this frequency, known as harmonics, sub-harmonics and ultra-harmonics.

The feasibility of using of harmonic and sub-harmonic IVUS for the detection of microbubbles using a prototype nonlinear IVUS system and commercially available contrast agents has been investigated.[16–18] This method is capable of providing microbubble-specific imaging by detecting non-linear signals. The prototype nonlinear IVUS system consists of a custom-built, single-element transducer that is mechanically rotated, sophisticated pulse sequences generated using pulse inversion, methods for tissue and catheter motion compensation, and specially designed signal filters for processing the received signal. A tissue harmonic imaging (THI) system which consists of a dual-frequency transducer element mounted on an IVUS catheter was also proposed.[14,15] As a result, this prototype IVUS system can operate both, in the fundamental frequency and in the second harmonic imaging modes. This system uses a conventional, continuously rotating, single-element IVUS catheter that is operated in fundamental 20 MHz, fundamental 40 MHz, and harmonic 40 MHz modes (transmit 20 MHz, receive 40 MHz). The use of a focused broadband miniature polyvinylidene fluoride-trifluoroethylene (PVDF-TrFE) ultrasonic transducer for IVUS second-harmonic imaging was also investigated.[8] This study demonstrated that focused transducers are capable of producing second harmonics faster and stronger at specific depths. The experimental results were in agreement with the modeled results, and *ex vivo* experiments in human aorta images showed the feasibility of high resolution second-harmonic imaging. Unfortunately, these methods for contrast imaging remain experimental and require non-commercially available IVUS hardware (e.g., harmonic imaging systems and catheters), non-standard contrast agents, or both.

1.4. *Differential Imaging*

The detection of extra-luminal perfusion may be performed by the comparison of the echogenicity of localized regions of a vessel wall and plaque before and after the injection of the contrast agents (Fig. 5). However, manually performing temporal analysis of variations in the echogenicity is not feasible for more than a handful of IVUS frames due to the amount of labor and

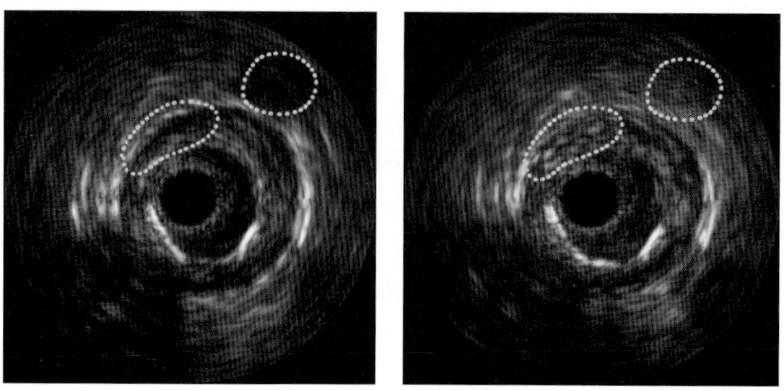

(a) (b)

Fig. 5. Example of a 20 MHz human case with enhancement. (a) Frame corresponding to the pre-contrast period and (b) frame corresponding to the post-contrast period. The annotations indicate the places where the enhancement occurred.

concentration involved in assessing changes that may be subtle to the human eye.

Computer-aided techniques may be a natural solution to this problem. However, the detection of change in echogenicity has many challenges related with a variety of motion artifacts that are consequences of cardiac and respiratory motions during acquisition within coronary arteries of living patients. Therefore, to detect enhancement in the IVUS image due to perfusion of contrast agent, it is necessary to alleviate the effect of these motion artifacts. For this goal, our group proposed a protocol and an automatic algorithm (i.e., Analysis of Contrast Enhanced Sequences, ACES) for quantification and visualization of VV in contrast-enhanced IVUS image sequences.[45] This method relies on the detection of local echogenicity changes (due to extra-luminal microbubble perfusion into the vessel wall) in stationary IVUS sequences. According to the proposed protocol, the IVUS catheter is placed in the maximally-stenotic point of a suspect plaque. The catheter is held steady and images are acquired for a time period of 10 s to 30 s. Then, a bolus injection of contrast agent is applied through the guiding catheter and proximal to the imaging catheter. After the contrast agent disappears, more images are acquired for a time period of 10 to 20 s, with the catheter kept at a steady position. The enhancement detection is performed off-line and consists of three steps:

(1) First, motion artifacts caused by the beating of the heart are eliminated from the IVUS sequence using a sequence-gating algorithm which is driven entirely by the imaging data and based on the analysis of the inter-frame correlations with a standard registration metric.[46–48] This image-based gating is accomplished by transforming the image sequence to a Euclidean multidimensional similarity space (MDS) in which each frame is represented by a particular, though not necessarily unique, point. This space is clustered using *k*-means to provide an ensemble of stabilized frames. Typically, a human operator selects the number of clusters to use from a visualization of the clusters associated with several *k* as there is a trade-off between a high value, which imposes greater restrictions on what frames are considered to be similar, and a low value, which forces some events which could be considered distinct to coalesce. The frames corresponding to the selected cluster are then used to build a new sequence for which it is assumed that the axial catheter motion has essentially been eliminated.
(2) Next, the region of interest (ROI) is defined manually by a human operator by tracing the luminal and media/adventitia contours in the first frame of the gated set of images. The ROI corresponding to each

frame in the gated sequence is located and "unwrapped" into a rectangular domain. To eliminate residual motion artifacts, the images are aligned and superimposed to obtain a pixel-wise correspondence using a two-step approach that consists of a rough, rigid alignment step followed by an elastic refinement step. A pre-contrast baseline image is computed by averaging the subset of gated frames corresponding to the period before the microbubbles' injection. The pre-contrast baseline image is subtracted from all frames in the gated sequence to form the differential images. As a result, any change that occurs due to contrast enhancement will be detected as a positive difference in the intensities in the corresponding regions of the differential images.

(3) To quantify the enhancement of a particular frame, the average of the gray intensity levels in the differential images is obtained within the ROI to produce a mean enhancement in ROI statistic (MEIR). This statistic is obtained for all the frames in the gated sequence. If perfusion occurs during the injection, the MEIR level will increase in the frames corresponding to the post-contrast injection period. If no perfusion occurs, the MEIR will return to its pre-contrast value almost immediately after the contrast agent passes through the lumen.

The feasibility of using this method for detecting perivascular blood flow, has been demonstrated in an animal study[60] and the feasibility and safety of using this technique with human patients was assessed.[59]

Currently, our group is working on alternative methods for image stabilization based on the analysis of the morphology of the lumen contour through the use of automatic segmentation methods, and novel methods to detect the changes of echogenecity in the CE-IVUS data from the B-mode reconstruction and the RF signal.

2. Conclusions

IVUS has been demonstrated to be an important tool for the understanding and treatment of CAD. Other techniques similar to IVUS, such as optical coherence tomography, have started to attract more attention mostly due to the type of data provided, which may overcome some of the limitations related to IVUS such as the presence of speckle noise which makes it challenging for physicians and computational methods to identify the different characteristics of the vessel. However, IVUS still remains the gold standard for assessing the coronary arteries. There have been important advances towards the extraction of valuable information from IVUS data by the medical image analysis scientific community. However, there are still many challenges to be overcome to develop a complete framework that will be able to provide an index for plaque vulnerability. The constant development and improvement of ultrasound transducers, contrast agents, and computational methods for the analysis of ultrasound data will contribute to achieving this goal.

Acknowledgments

E.G. Mendizabal-Ruiz is supported in part by CONACYT. I.A. Kakadiaris has been supported in part by NSF Grant DMS-0915242 and the UH Hugh Roy and Lillie Cranz Cullen Endowment Fund. Any opinions, findings, conclusions or recommendations expressed in this material are those of the authors and may not reflect the views of the sponsors.

References

1. S. Balocco, C. Gatta, F. Ciompi, A. Wahle, P. Radeva, S. Carlier, G. Unal, E. Sanidas, F. Mauri, X. Carillo, T. Kovarnik, C.-W. Wang, H.-C. Chen, T. P. Exarchos, D. I. Fotiadis, F. Destrempes, G. Cloutier, O. Pujol, M. Alberti, E. G. Mendizabal-Ruiz, M. Rivera, T. Aksoy, R. W. Downe and I. A. Kakadiaris, "Standardized evaluation methodology and reference database for evaluating ivus image segmentation," *Comp Med Imaging Graphics* **38**, 70–90 (2014).
2. E. Brusseau, C. L. de Korte, F. Mastik, J. Schaar, and A. F. W. van der Steen, "Fully automatic luminal contour segmentation in intracoronary ultrasound imaging — a statistical approach," *IEEE Trans Med Imaging* **23**, 554–566 (2004).
3. A. P. Burke, A. Farb, G. T. Malcom, Y. H. Liang, J. Smialek and R. Virmani, "Coronary risk factors and plaque morphology in men with coronary disease who died suddenly," *New Eng J Med* **336**, 1276–1282 (1997).
4. K. Caballero, J. Barajas, O. Pujol, J. Mauri and P. Radeva, "*In-vivo* IVUS tissue classification a comparison between normalized image reconstruction and RF signals analysis," *Proc. 11th Iberoamerican Congress on Pattern Recognition, Cancun, Mexico*, 137–146 (2006).
5. M. Cardinal, J. Meunier, G. Soulez, R. L. Maurice, E. Therasse and G. Cloutier, "Intravascular ultrasound image segmentation: A three-dimensional fast-marching method based on gray level distributions," *IEEE Trans Med Imaging* **25**, 590–601 (2006).
6. M. Cardinal, G. Soulez, J. C. Tardif, J. Meunier and G. Cloutier, "Fast-marching segmentation of three-dimensional intravascular ultrasound images: A pre-and post-intervention study," *Med Phy* **37**, 3633–3647 (2010).
7. S. Carlier, I. A. Kakadiaris, N. Dib, M. Vavuranakis, C. Stephanadis, S. O'Malley, C. Hartley, R. Metcalfe, R. Mehran, E. Falk, K. Gul and M. Naghavi, "Vasa vasorum imaging: A new window to the clinical detection of vulnerable atherosclerotic plaques," *Current Atherosclerosis Reports* 7, 164–169 (2005).

8. C. Chandrana, N. Kharin, G. Vince, S. Roy and A. Fleischman, "Demonstration of second-harmonic ivus feasibility with focused broadband miniature transducers," *IEEE Trans Ultrasonics, Ferroelectrics and Frequency Control* **57**, 1077–1085 (2010).
9. F. Ciompi, O. Pujol, E. Fernandez-Nofrerias, J. Mauri and P. Radeva, "ECOC random fields for lumen segmentation in radial artery IVUS sequences," *Proc. 12th International Conference on Medical Image Computing and Computer Assisted Intervention* (London, UK), 869–876 (2009).
10. P. Constantinides, "Cause of thrombosis in human atherosclerotic arteries," *Am J Cardiology* **66**, 37G–40G (1990).
11. F. Destrempes, M.-H. R. Cardinal, L. Allard, J.-C. Tardif and G. Cloutier, "Segmentation method of intravascular ultrasound images of human coronary arteries," *Comput Med Imaging Graphics* **38**, 91–103 (2014).
12. E. dos Santos Filho, M. Yoshizawa, A. Tanaka and Y. Saijo, "A study on intravascular ultrasound image processing," *Record of Electrical and Communication Engineering Conversazione, Tohoku University* **74**, 30–33 (2006).
13. R. Downe, A. Wahle, T. Kovarnik, H. Skalicka, J. Lopez, J. Horak and M. Sonka, "Segmentation of intravascular ultrasound images using graph search and a novel cost function," *Proc. 2nd MICCAI Workshop on Computer Vision for Intravascular and Intracardiac Imaging* (New York, NY), 71–79 (2008).
14. M. Frijlink, D. Goertz, L. van Damme, R. Krams and A. van der Steen, "Intravascular ultrasound tissue harmonic imaging *in vivo*," *IEEE Ultrasonics, Ferroelectrics and Frequency Control* **53**, 1844–1852 (2006a).
15. M. E. Frijlink, D. E. Goertz, H. J. Vos, E. Tesselaar, G. Blacquiere, A. Gisolf, R. Krams and A. F. van der Steen, "Harmonic intravascular ultrasound imaging with a dual-frequency catheter," *Ultrasound Med Biol* **32**, 1649–1654 (2006b).
16. D. E. Goertz, M. E. Frijlink, N. de Jong and A. F. van der Steen, "Nonlinear intravascular ultrasound contrast imaging," *Ultrasound Med Biol* **32**, 491–502 (2006a).
17. D. E. Goertz, M. E. Frijlink, D. Tempel, V. Bhagwandas, A. Gisolf, R. Krams, N. de Jong and A. van der Steen, "Subharmonic contrast intravascular ultrasound for vasa vasorum imaging," *Ultrasound Med Biol* **33**, 1859–1872 (2007).
18. D. E. Goertz, M. E. Frijlink, D. Tempel, L. C. van Damme, R. Krams, J. A. Schaar, F. J. Ten Cate, P. W. Serruys, N. de Jong and A. van der Steen, "Contrast harmonic intravascular ultrasound: A feasibility study for vasa vasorum imaging," *Investigative Radiology* **41**, 631–638 (2006b).
19. J. Granada and S. Feinstein, "Imaging of the vasa vasorum," *Nat Rev Cardiology* **5**, S18–S25 (2008).
20. C. Haas, H. Ermert, S. Holt, P. Grewe, A. Machraoui and J. Barmeyer, "Segmentation of 3D intravascular ultrasonic images based on a random field model," *Ultrasound Med Biol* **26**, 297–306 (2000).
21. T. Hiro, C. Y. Leung, R. J. Russo, H. Karimi, A. R. Farvid and J. M. Tobis, "Variability of a three-layered appearance in intravascular ultrasound coronary images: A comparison of morphometric measurements with four intravascular ultrasound systems," *Am J Cardiac Imaging* **10**, 219–227 (1996).
22. E. Hitchner, M. A. Zayed, G. Lee, D. Morrison, B. L. and W. Zhou, "Intravascular ultrasound as a clinical adjunct for carotid plaque characterization," *J Vascular Surgery* **59**, 774–780 (2014).

23. J.-L. Jones, E. Essa, X. Xie and D. Smith, "Interactive segmentation of media-adventitia border in IVUS," *Proc. 15th International Conference in Computer Analysis of Images and Patterns* **8048** (York, UK.), 466–474 (2013).
24. A. Katouzian, E. D. Angelini, B. Sturm and A. F. Laine, "Brushlet-driven segmentation framework for automatic detection of lumen borders in ivus images with comparison study," *Proc. International Symposium on Biomedical Imaging* (Barcelona, Spain.), 242–245 (2012).
25. A. Katouzian, B. Baseri, E. Konofagou and A. Laine, "Automatic detection of blood versus non-blood regions on intravascular ultrasound (IVUS) images using wavelet packet signatures," *Proc. SPIE Medical Imaging: Ultrasonic Imaging and Signal Processing* (San Diego, CA), 1–8 (2008a).
26. A. Katouzian, B. Baseri, E. E. Konofagou and A. F. Laine, "An alternative approach to spectrum-based atherosclerotic plaque characterization techniques using intravascular ultrasound (IVUS) backscattered signals," *Proc. 2nd MICCAI Workshop on Computer Vision for Intravascular and Intracardiac Imaging* (New York, NY) (2008b).
27. A. Katouzian, S. G. Carlier and A. F. Laine, *Methods in Atherosclerotic Plaque Characterization Using Intravascular Ultrasound images and Backscattered signals* (Springer New York), 121–152 (2011).
28. M. Kawasaki, H. Takatsu, T. Noda, Y. Ito, A. Kunishima, M. Arai, K. Nishigaki, G. Takemura, N. Morita, S. Minatoguchi and H. Fujiwara, "Noninvasive quantitative tissue characterization and two-dimensional color-coded map of human atherosclerotic lesions using ultrasound integrated backscatter: Comparison between histology and integrated backscatter images," *J Am College Cardiology* **38**, 486–492 (2001).
29. M. Kawasaki, H. Takatsu, T. Noda, K. Sano, Y. Ito, K. Hayakawa, K. Tsuchiya, M. Arai, K. Nishigaki, G. Takemura, S. Minatoguchi, T. Fujiwara and H. Fujiwara, "In vivo quantitative tissue characterization of human coronary arterial plaques by use of integrated backscatter intravascular ultrasound and comparison with angioscopic findings," *Circulation* **105**:2487–2492 (2002).
30. J. D. Klingensmith, R. Shekhar and D. G. Vince, "Evaluation of three-dimensional segmentation algorithms for the identification of luminal and medial-adventitial borders in intravascular ultrasound images," *IEEE Trans Med Imaging* **19**, 996–1011 (2000).
31. G. Kovalski, R. Beyar, R. Shofti and H. Azhari, "Three-dimensional automatic quantitative analysis of intravascular ultrasound images," *Ultrasound Med Biol* **26**, 527–537 (2000).
32. A. Lametschwandtner, D. Kachlik, J. Stingl and M. Setina, "Spatial analysis of vascular corrosion casts to investigate the architectonic arrangement of vasa vasorum of the human great saphenous vein in normal and pathological conditions," *Microscopy Microanalysis* **13**, 488–489 (2007).
33. Z. Luo, Y. Wang and W. Wang, "Estimating coronary artery lumen area with optimization-based contour detection," *IEEE Trans Med Imaging* **22**, 564–566 (2003).
34. A. Maton, *Human Biology and Health* (Prentice Hall) (1993).
35. E. G. Mendizabal-Ruiz, M. Rivera and I. A. Kakadiaris, "A probabilistic segmentation method for the identification of luminal borders in intravascular ultrasound images," *Proc. IEEE Computer Society Conference on Computer Vision and Pattern Recognition* (Anchorage, AK), 1–8 (2008).

36. E. G. Mendizabal-Ruiz, M. Rivera and I. A. Kakadiaris, "Segmentation of the luminal border in intravascular ultrasound b-mode images using a probabilistic approach," *Medical Image Analysis* **17**, 649–670 (2013).
37. G. S. Mintz, S. E. Nissen, W. D. Anderson, S. R. Bailey, R. Erbel, P. J. Fitzgerald, F. J. Pinto, K. Rosenfield, R. J. Siegel, E. M. Tuzcu, P. G. Yock, R. A. O'Rourke, J. Abrams, E. R. Bates, B. R. Brodie, P. S. Douglas, G. Gregoratos, M. A. Hlatky, J. S. Hochman, S. Kaul, C. M. Tracy, D. D. Waters and J. Winters and L. William, "American college of cardiology clinical expert consensus document on standards for acquisition, measurement and reporting of intravascular ultrasound studies (IVUS): A report of the american college of cardiology task force on clinical expert consensus," *J Am College Cardiology* **37**, 1478–1492 (2001).
38. A. K. Mitra, A. S. Dhume and D. K. Agrawal. "Vulnerable plaques" — ticking of the time bomb," *Canadian J Physiology Pharmacology* **82**, 860–871 (2004).
39. A. Mojsilovic, M. Popovic, N. Amodaj, R. Babic and M. Ostojic, "Automatic segmentation of intravascular ultrasound images: A texture-based approach," *Ann Biomed Eng* **25**, 1059–1071 (1997).
40. M. Moraes and S. Furuie, "Automatic coronary wall segmentation in intravascular ultrasound images using binary morphological reconstruction," *Ultrasound Med Biol* **37**, 1486–1499 (2011).
41. M. Naghavi, E. Falk, H. Hecht, M. Jamieson, S. Kaul, D. Berman, Z. Fayad, M. Budoff, J. Rumberger, T. Naqvi, L. Shaw, O. Faergeman, J. Cohn, R. Bahr, W. Koenig, J. Demirovic, D. Arking, V. Herrera, J. Badimon, J. Goldstein, Y. Rudy, J. Airaksinen, R. Schwartz, W. Riley, R. Mendes, P. Douglas and P. Shah, "From vulnerable plaque to vulnerable patient-Part III: Executive summary of the Screening for Heart Attack Prevention and Education (SHAPE) Task Force report," *Am J Cardiology* **98**, 2H–15H (2006).
42. A. Nair, B. Kuban, E. Tuzcu, P. Schoenhagen, S. Nissen and D. Vince, "Coronary plaque classification with intravascular ultrasound radiofrequency data analysis," *Circulation* **106**, 2200–2206 (2002).
43. A. Nair, M. Margolis, B. Kuban and D. Vince, "Automated coronary plaque characterisation with intravascular ultrasound backscatter: *Ex vivo* validation," *Eurointervention* **3**, 113–120 (2007).
44. K. Nasu, E. Tsuchikane, O. Katoh, D. G. Vince, R. Virmani, J. F. Surmely, A. Murata, Y. Takeda, T. Ito, M. Ehara, T. Matsubara, M. Terashima and T. Suzuki, "Accuracy of in vivo coronary plaque morphology assessment: A validation study of *in vivo* virtual histology compared with *in vitro* histopathology," *J Am College Cardiology* **47**, 2405–2412 (2006).
45. S. O'Malley, "Computational methods for contrast-enhanced intravascular ultrasound sequence analysis," Ph.D. thesis, University of Houston (2007).
46. S. O'Malley, S. Carlier, M. Naghavi and I. Kakadiaris, "Image-based frame gating of IVUS pullbacks: A surrogate for ECG," *Proc. IEEE International Conference on Acoustics, Speech and Signal Processing* (Honolulu, HI), 433–436 (2007).
47. S. O'Malley, J. Granada, S. Carlier, M. Naghavi and I. Kakadiaris, "Image-based gating of intravascular ultrasound pullback sequences," *IEEE Trans Information Techn Biomed* **12**, 299–306 (2008).
48. S. O'Malley, M. Naghavi and I. Kakadiaris, "Image-based frame gating for stationary-catheter IVUS sequences," *Proc. International Workshop on Computer Vision for Intravascular and Intracardiac Imaging* (Copenhagen, Denmark), 14–21 (2006).

49. M. Papadogiorgaki, V. Mezaris, Y. S. Chatzizisis, G. D. Giannoglou and I. Kompatsiaris, "Image analysis techniques for automated IVUS contour detection," *Ultrasound Med Biol* **34**, 1482–1498 (2008).
50. M. E. Plissiti, D. I. Fotiadis, L. K. Michalis and G. E. Bozios, "An automated method for lumen and media-adventitia border detection in a sequence of IVUS frames," *IEEE Trans Information Tech Biomed* **8**, 131–141 (2004).
51. G. A. Rodriguez-Granillo, E. P. McFadden, M. Valgimigli, C. A. van Mieghem, E. Regar, P. J. de Feyter and P. W. Serruys, "Coronary plaque composition of nonculprit lesions, assessed by in vivo intracoronary ultrasound radio frequency data analysis, is related to clinical presentation," *Am Heart J* **151**, 1020–1024 (2006).
52. A. Roodaki, A. Taki, S. K. Setarehdan and N. Navab, "Modified wavelet transform features for characterizing different plaque types in IVUS images; a feasibility study," *Proc. 9th International Conference on Signal Processing* (Beijing, China), 789–792 (2008).
53. R. Ross, "The pathogenesis of atherosclerosis: A perspective for the 1990s," *Nature* **362**, 801–809 (1993).
54. E. Sanidas, M. Vavuranakis, T. Papaioannou, I. Kakadiaris, S. Carlier, G. Syros, G. Dangas and C. Stefanadis, "Study of atheromatous plaque using intravascular ultrasound," *Hellenic J Cardiology* **49**, 415–421 (2008).
55. J. Seabra, F. Ciompi, O. Pujol, J. Mauri, P. Radeva and J. Sanches, "Rayleigh mixture model for plaque characterization in intravascular ultrasound," *IEEE Trans Biomed Eng* **58**, 1314–1324 (2011).
56. M. Sonka, X. Zhang, M. Siebes, M. S. Bissing, S. C. DeJong, S. M. Collins and R. C. McKay, "Segmentation of intravascular ultrasound images: A knowledge-based approach," *IEEE Trans Med Imaging* **14**, 719–732 (1995).
57. S. Sun, M. Sonka and R. R. Beichel, "Graph-based ivus segmentation with efficient computer-aided refinement," *Trans Med Imaging* **32**, 1536–1549 (2013).
58. G. Unal, S. Bucher, S. Carlier, G. Slabaugh, T. Fang and K. Tanaka, "Shape-driven segmentation of the arterial wall in intravascular ultrasound images," *IEEE Trans Information Tech Biomed* **12**, 335–347 (2008).
59. M. Vavuranakis, I. A. Kakadiaris, S. O'Malley, T. Papaioannou, E. Sanidas, M. Naghavi, S. Carlier, D. Tousoulis and C. Stefanadis, "A new method for assessment of plaque vulnerability based on vasa vasorum imaging, by using contrast-enhanced intravascular ultrasound and automated differential image analysis," *Int J Cardiology* **130**, 23–29 (2008).
60. M. Vavuranakis, T. Papaioannou, I. A. Kakadiaris, S. O'Malley, M. Naghavi, K. Filis, E. Sanidas, A. Papalois, I. Stamatopoulos and C. Stefanadis, "Detection of perivascular blood flow in vivo by contrast-enhanced intracoronary ultrasonography and image analysis: An animal study," *Clin Exp Pharmacology Physiology* **34**, 1319–1323 (2007a).
61. M. Vavuranakis, T. Papaioannou and C. Stefanadis, "In the search of the vulnerable plaque: Current diagnostic techniques and future directions," *Vas Dis Prevention* **4**, 21–29 (2007b).
62. D. Vince, K. Dixon, R. Cothren and J. Cornhill, "Comparison of texture analysis methods for the characterization of coronary plaques in intravascular ultrasound images," *Comp Med Imaging Graphics* **24**, 221–229 (2000).
63. R. Virmani, F. D. Kolodgie, A. P. Burke, A. V. Finn, H. K. Gold, T. N. Tulenko, S. P. Wrenn and J. Narula, "Atherosclerotic plaque progression and vulnerability to

rupture: Angiogenesis as a source of intraplaque hemorrhage," *Arteriosclerosis Throm Vas Biol* **25**, 2054–2061 (2005).

64. C. von Birgelen, C. D. Mario, W. Li, J. C. Schuurbiers, C. J. Slager, P. J. de Feyter, J. R. Roelandt and P. W. Serruys, "Morphometric analysis in three-dimensional intracoronary ultrasound: An *in vitro* and *in vivo* study using a novel system for the contour detection of lumen and plaque," *Am Heart J* **132**, 516–527 (1996).
65. M. Wennogle and W. Hoff, "Three dimensional segmentation of intravascular ultrasound data," *Proc.* 6th *International Conference on Image Analysis and Recognition*, **5627**, (Toronto, Canada), 772–781 (2009).
66. X. Zhu, P. Zhangc, J. Shaoa, Y. Chenga, Y. Zhangc and J. Bai, "A snake-based method for segmentation of intravascular ultrasound images and its *in vivo* validation," *Ultrasonics* **51**, 181–189 (2011).

Chapter 21

MEMS-based Transducers (CMUT) For Medical Ultrasound Imaging

Alessandro Stuart Savoia and Giosuè Caliano*

ACULAB, Dipartimento di Ingegneria, Università degli Studi Roma Tre, Rome, Italy
**E-mail: alessandro.savoia@uniroma3.it*

Capacitive micromachined ultrasonic transducers (CMUTs) are micro-electromechanical devices (MEMS) fabricated using silicon micromachining techniques. In the past decade, their use has proved to be attractive mainly in the field of medical ultrasound imaging as active elements in ultrasound probes. The interest of this novel technology relies on its full compatibility with standard integrated circuit technology that makes it possible to integrate, on the same chip, the transducers and the electronics, thus enabling the realization of extremely low-cost and high-performance devices. From an operational point of view, CMUTs have been widely recognized as a valuable alternative to piezoelectric transducer technology in a variety of medical imaging applications, thanks to a higher sensitivity, a wider bandwidth, and an improved thermal efficiency.

In this chapter, the design and fabrication of a 192-element linear array CMUT probe operating in the range 6–18 MHz, designed for vascular, small parts, rheumatology and anesthesiology imaging applications, is reported. The CMUT array is microfabricated and packed using a novel fabrication concept specifically conceived for imaging transducer arrays. The performance optimization of the probe is performed by connecting the CMUT array with multichannel analog front-end electronic circuits housed into the probe body. Characterization and imaging results are used to assess the performance of CMUTs with respect to conventional piezoelectric transducers.

1. Introduction

Capacitive micromachined ultrasonic transducers (CMUTs) were first researched upon at Stanford University in 1994.[1] Unlike piezoelectric transducers, which use thickness-mode vibration of piezoceramic materials, CMUTs are based on flexural vibration of electrostatically-actuated micromachined plates. Due to their intrinsically low mechanical impedance, CMUTs seemed initially to be particularly suitable for air-coupled applications.[2–5] The enhanced compatibility between micro-electro-mechanical system and standard integrated circuit technologies, with respect to piezoelectric technology, led, in a very short time, to the first CMUT on CMOS implementation.[4] Different microfabrication processes based on sacrificial release surface micromachining,[6,7] and wafer bonding[8] technologies, each having its strength and weaknesses, were experimented for CMUT fabrication. The first water-coupled operation results[9] indicated that broadband behavior and wide temperature tolerance could have made CMUTs a valid alternative to piezoelectric transducers for medical imaging applications. Since 2002, the first experimental implementations of CMUTs for conventional 2D imaging,[10,11] high frequency 2D imaging,[12] and 3D imaging[13] applications were presented, the latter being enforced by the limitations imposed by the current piezoelectric technology. The interest of some medical ultrasound imaging companies (in particular GE trough the General Electric Global Research Center, Niskayuna, NY and Esaote S.p.A., Genoa, Italy) led, in 2003, to the achievement of the first real time *in-vivo* ultrasound images[14,15] which was reached by connecting a CMUT array provided by the sole CMUT technology industrial supplier at that time (Sensant Corp., San Leandro, CA) to conventional ultrasound imaging systems. One year later, at the Acousto-Electronics Laboratory of Roma Tre University (Aculab, Università degli Studi Roma Tre, Rome, Italy) where the work here presented was carried out, the second real time *in-vivo* ultrasound images were generated[16] and successively improved[17,18] thanks to the increased sensitivity of the developed probe achieved by enhancing the CMUT microfabrication process, and by introducing previously developed electronics[19] inside the probe itself.

At the same laboratory, significant advances on the different aspects of the CMUT-related research were carried out. In particular, a new CMUT fabrication technology called "Reverse Fabrication Process" was developed, patented[20] and published.[21] Such technology led to improved ultrasound imaging[22] and permitted to realize flexible CMUTs,[23] thus enabling the adoption of CMUT technology in those imaging applications requiring curved transducer arrays. Moreover, Finite Element Modeling (FEM) was extensively used to understand non-ideal phenomena in CMUTs[24] and to design application specific devices.[25] FEM was also used to study new CMUT structures with improved sensitivity and bandwidth performance.[26,27] The use of CMUT technology was also investigated in other ultrasound imaging applications, such as volumetric imaging[28] and biometry.[29–31]

The fact that CMUT technology has been accepted by the industry as a valid alternative to the state-of-the-art piezoelectric technology is proven by the several patents filed by many companies to date. In 2008, the ultrasound probe manufacturing company Vermon (Vermon, Tours, France) compared the performance of an internally developed CMUT probe with its proprietary state-of-the-art piezoelectric technology,[32] obtaining promising results. In 2009, Hitachi (Hitachi Medical Corporation, Tokyo, Japan) announced,[33,34] the first commercial product, a linear array probe for breast imaging, based on CMUT technology. Further details on CMUT operating principle and technology can be found in Ref. [35] while a detailed review on medical applications is reported in Ref. [36]. The aim of this chapter is to present the development of a high frequency ultrasound probe for medical ultrasonography enabled by the availability of a well-established CMUT microfabrication and packaging technology. The 192-element CMUT linear array design and fabrication as well as the probe engineering and the integration in an ultrasound medical imaging system are shown. A first performance assessment of the CMUT probe is operated by electrical and acoustic measurements and benchmarking with a commercially available piezoelectric probe from Esaote. *In-vivo* ultrasound images are also generated with the two probes and compared. The work reported in this chapter was previously presented[37] and published.[38]

This chapter is organized as follows. Section 2 describes the design of the CMUT array, the microfabrication technology and the device packaging. In Section 3, the development of the ultrasound probe and the methods used to interface it to a conventional imaging system are discussed. Section 4 reports the characterization and imaging results. The discussions and conclusions are given in Section 5.

2. CMUT Array Design, Microfabrication and Packaging

2.1. *Array Design*

The linear array design parameters, such as the element number and dimensions, were chosen identical to those of the 192-element Esaote LA435 piezoelectric probe in order to easily integrate the resulting CMUT probe into the Esaote "Technos" ultrasound imaging system available at Aculab, and to fairly compare the characterization and imaging results achieved with the two probes. The main array design parameters are reported in Table 1.

The CMUT microstructure design parameters, such as the lateral dimensions of the cells and the thickness of the layers, were defined by taking into account the desired pulse-echo frequency band of operation (center frequency of 12 MHz with a −6 dB fractional bandwidth greater than 100%) as well as the dimensional constraints imposed by the element geometry. The gap height of the CMUT cells, on which the collapse voltage and consequently the maximum pulse-echo amplitude are dependant, was determined by considering

Table 1. CMUT array design parameters.

Parameter	Value
Array:	
Number of elements	192
Element pitch	200 μm
Element width (azimut)	200 μm
Element length (elevation)	3 mm
Fixed elevation focus	15 mm
CMUT Structure:	
Cell diameter	29.6 μm
Electrode diameter	20 μm
Cell-to-cell lateral distance	3.4 μm
Plate thickness	1.5 μm
Gap height	0.25 μm

the maximum excitation signal amplitude level available on the "Technos" imaging system ($\pm$80 V). With the aid of a Finite Element Modeling (FEM) CMUT design tool previously developed at Aculab,[25] it was found that the maximum pulse-echo amplitude could be obtained by driving the CMUT with the maximum signal amplitude level available and by biasing it around 70% of its collapse voltage. In order to prevent the collapse of the CMUT during operation, the sum of the bias voltage and the excitation signal positive peak voltage had to not exceed the collapse voltage. Such condition, together with the optimal biasing condition found (70%) and the maximum value of the excitation signal positive peak voltage available (80 V), led to a collapse voltage specification of 266 V. As a result of a parametric set of FEM simulations, the optimal design parameters shown in Table 1 were determined.

2.2. *Microfabrication*

The array described was fabricated using the Reverse Fabrication Process (RFP) previously developed.[21] RFP is a sacrificial release microfabrication technology for the fabrication of CMUTs on silicon wafers. In this process, CMUTs are fabricated using a top-down approach, meaning that the microfabrication is operated starting from the top layers of the structure i.e., the transducer vibrating surface, and ending with the device sealing and the definition of the electrical interconnection pads. After microfabrication, the resulting device is electrically interconnected and packed and, finally, the silicon substrate is completely removed in order to release the CMUT vibrating surface. In Fig. 1(a)–(i), the main RFP flow steps are outlined. The microfabrication starts

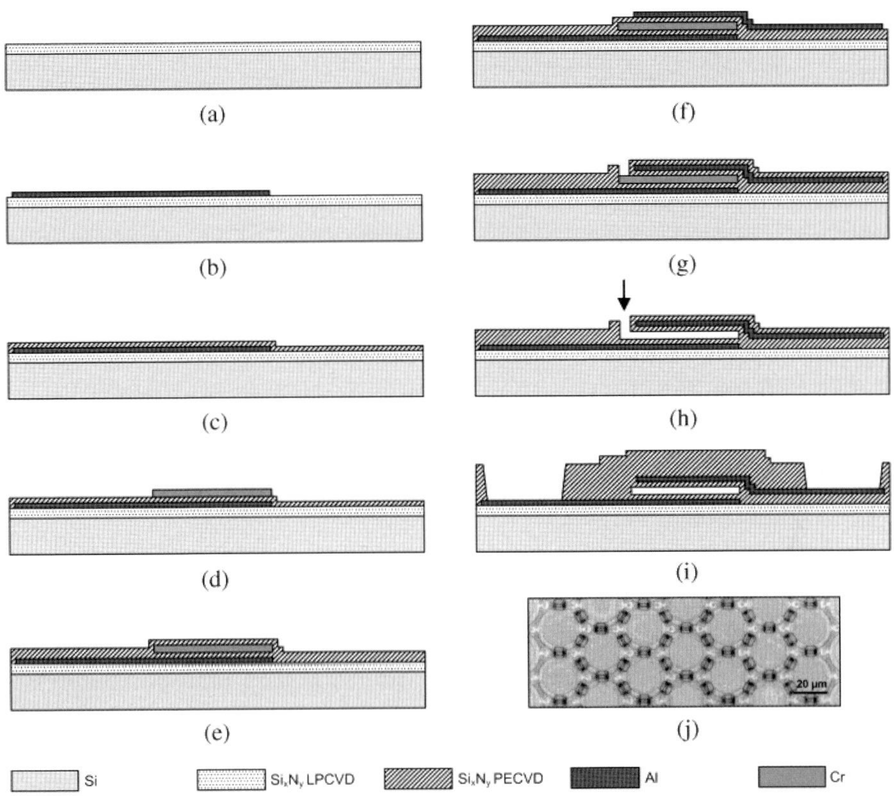

Fig. 1. (a)–(i) RFP technology flow. For clarity, only one cell is shown. (j) Picture of the cell layout of an actual microfabricated CMUT device. One array element is displayed to its full width (200 μm).

on top of a low stress and ultra precise thickness controlled LPCVD silicon nitride film grown over a silicon wafer [Fig. 1(a)]. The top electrode, made of an Al-Ti-W multilayer, is deposited and patterned [Fig. 1(b)].

The use of a thin layer of Ti-W over the Al film prevents the degradation of the metallization during the subsequent PECVD silicon nitride deposition [Fig. 1(c)], which serves as a passivation layer of the top electrode. Successively, a sacrificial Cr film is deposited and patterned [Fig. 1(d)]. A PECVD silicon nitride layer [Fig. 1(e)] is used to passivate the bottom electrode that is defined by the deposition and patterning of a second Al-Ti-W film [Fig. 1(f)]. After a further PECVD silicon nitride passivation layer is deposited, the etching holes for the evacuation of the cell cavities are created [Fig. 1(g)]. The successive step is the sacrificial release, operated by means of Cr wet etch [Fig. 1(h)]. Finally, the device is completely sealed by depositing a consistent 4-μm-thick PECVD silicon nitride film that is successively etched in order to define interconnection pads [Fig. 1(i)]. A picture of an actual CMUT device, fabricated using the RFP, is reported in Fig. 1(j) where a detail of the cell layout of one array element is shown.

Significant benefits result from the described fabrication method. Among those, the fact that the CMUT vibrating structure is almost entirely made of LPCVD silicon nitride leads to the high accuracy of its thickness over the silicon wafer resulting in a highly uniform mechanical behavior of the CMUT cells. Another important aspect is that the use of PECVD silicon nitride, which can be deposited at relatively low temperatures as compared to LPCVD silicon nitride, makes it possible to utilize Al whose electrical properties ensure low resistivity of the electrodes. Finally, thanks to the top-down nature of the fabrication method, the interconnection pads are located on the rear part of the final device. In other microfabrication approaches, this task is achievable exclusively by using through-silicon via (TSV) processes that are expensive and often unreliable.

2.3. *Packaging*

In order to provide the CMUT array with a custom backing, enable the electrical access to the elements, release the vibrating structure, and apply an acoustic lens for protection and elevation focusing, a special packaging procedure was developed and implemented. The main steps are schematically summarized in Fig. 2. The CMUT array chip is placed and held on a vacuum fixture in a way that the interconnection pads are facing upwards [Fig. 2(a)]. A rigid-flex (FR4-polyimide) PCB is placed close and aligned to the chip at a different vertical position, 0.2 mm above, and wire bonding is performed using Al wire by means of a manual Wedge Bonder 4123 (Kulicke & Soffa, Fort Washington, USA) [Fig. 2(b)]. A pre-shaped custom backing, obtained by a previously cured part of composite material made of Epotek 301 (Epoxy Technology, Bellerica, USA) epoxy filled with W and Al_2O_3 powders, is then glued on the bonded assembly [Fig. 2(c)] using the same compound that serves also as a glob top for the wire bonds. The resulting assembly is then dismounted from the vacuum fixture and placed in a PTFE case in order to perform the chemical etching of the silicon substrate [Fig. 2(d)] and release the CMUT active surface. The silicon etching is operated using a mixture of acetic, nitric and hydrofluoric acid (HNA). Finally, an acoustic lens, made of RTV silicone filled with metal oxide nano-powders, is applied to the CMUT using a stainless steel mold [Fig. 2(e)].

The described packaging process was used for the fabrication of ultrasound probe-heads. A picture of a completed probe-head prototype is shown in Fig. 2(f). In this particular prototype, pure (unfilled) transparent RTV silicone

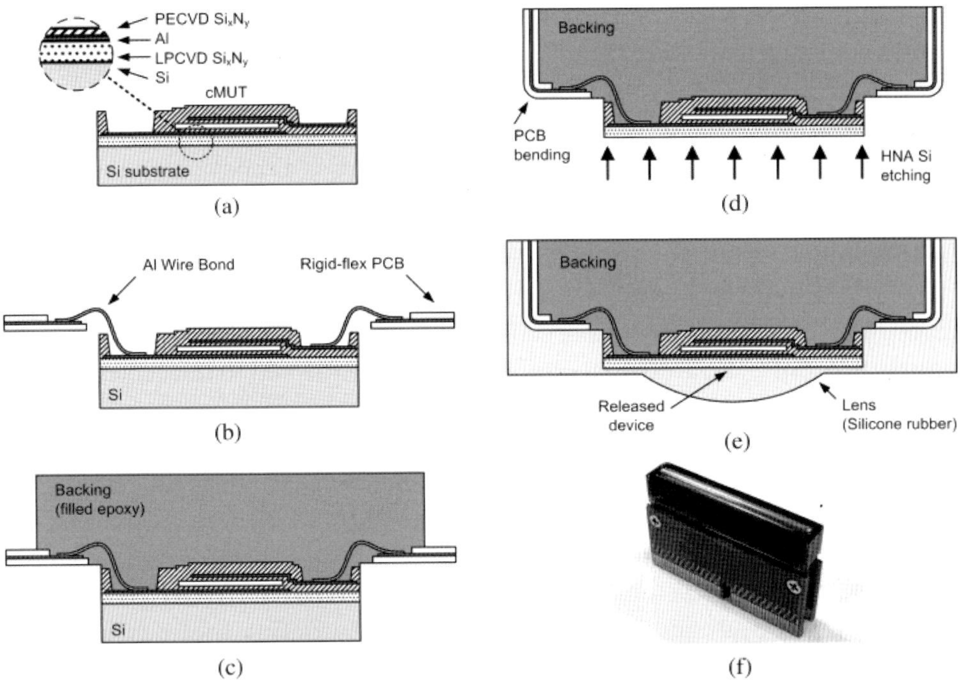

Fig. 2. RFP packaging flow. For clarity, only the flexible part of the rigid-flex PCB is shown.

has been used for the lens fabrication in order to optically evaluate the positioning accuracy achieved with the mechanical tools used to implement the packaging process. As a matter of fact, the probe-heads actually used in this work were provided with a cylindrical acoustic lens made of doped RTV silicon having a specific acoustic impedance of 1.42 MRayl, a 1100 m/s sound speed, and shaped in order to achieve elevation focusing at a 15 mm depth, resulting in a maximum thickness of 0.4 mm.

Several advantages arise from the use of the proposed packaging procedure. From a fabrication point of view, the availability of electrical interconnection pads on the rear part of the device significantly simplifies the packaging of the chip with no need to perform the wire bonding glob top protection in a dedicated step, since the same task is fulfilled during the backing application step. From an operational point of view, the use of a custom backing instead of the silicon substrate, that is normally present in CMUTs and that exhibits very poor performance as an acoustic backing,[39] improves the absorption of the acoustic energy propagated into the backing. As a matter of fact, the composite material used for the backing can be engineered in order to obtain the desired mechanical characteristics, including ultrasound attenuation. The ultrasound attenuation in the backing material applied to the probe-heads used in this work is 8 dB/mm measured at a frequency of 10 MHz and the specific acoustic impedance is 8 MRayl.

3. Probe Engineering and System Integration

In this work, a 196-channel cable provided by Esaote was used. Since each element of the CMUT array has a capacitance in the order of 20 pF whilst the capacitance of each micro-coaxial cable is 150 pF, a significant attenuation of the signal can occur if the array elements are directly connected to the cables. Therefore, the use of buffering circuits placed as close as possible to the transducer array elements is needed to preserve signal integrity during reception operation. In general, the introduction of multichannel electronics in the probe housing is challenging due to the strict requirements in terms of noise performance, power consumption, and dimensions. Recently, Maxim (Maxim Integrated Products, Sunnyvale, CA) has developed, in collaboration with Aculab, a new component, called MAX4805, designed for in-probe voltage buffering of the echo signals generated by high impedance ultrasonic transducers. A special version of this component, the MAX4805A, is optimized for the use with CMUTs (that typically have higher impedance as compared to piezoelectric transducers of the same emitting surface) through the minimization of the current noise density.

By using the MAX4805A component, a 96-channel board was developed. The circuit topology of a single channel is reported in Fig. 3. The circuit operates, in reception, the voltage buffering of the received echoes by means of a high input impedance low noise amplifier (LNA) which has a +9 dB voltage gain and an output current capability sufficient to drive the cable. The driving signals are transferred from the cable to the transducer by means of a pair of antiparallel diodes. During transmission operation, the LNA output

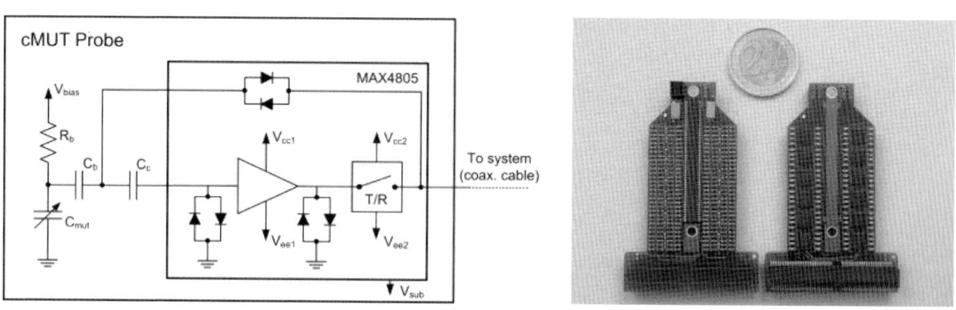

Fig. 3. Picture of the two sides of the 96-channel in-probe electronic board.

is protected by an automatically activated high voltage switch, whilst the input is protected by the external 47 pF capacitance (C_c) and by the pair of antiparallel diodes connected to ground. The board contains, in addition to the MAX4805A integrated circuits and the required external passive components, 96 bias tee networks, realized with a 10 MΩ (R_b) resistor and a 10 nF capacitor (C_b), for the voltage biasing of the CMUT array elements. The component layout and signal routing was performed on eight layers and the board prototypes were fabricated using standard FR4 PCB and SMT technology. A picture of the two sides of the board is reported in Fig. 3. Each board contains a cable connector and a probe-head connector, respectively visible on the left and on the right part of Fig. 3.

Two identical boards were fixed and thermally coupled to an aluminum frame using a conformable thermally conductive pad. The aluminum frame was coupled to the multi-coaxial cable metallic shield in order to dissipate in the same cable the heat generated by the electronics. In this way, the unwanted temperature rise of the probe-head and the probe case during operation was minimized. The whole assembly was electromagnetically shielded and housed into a plastic case. A picture of the assembled prototype is shown in Fig. 4.

The power supply voltages required by the boards, which include the five MAX4805A supplies as well as the CMUT bias voltage, were not available at the probe interface of the Esaote "Technos" imaging system. Therefore, it was necessary to provide the probe with an electronic circuit capable of generating the required six supply voltages starting from a single +5 V power supply available at the system interface. In a first step, several integrated switching regulation solutions available on the market were experimented but, in all cases, the voltage regulation performance was not good enough in relation

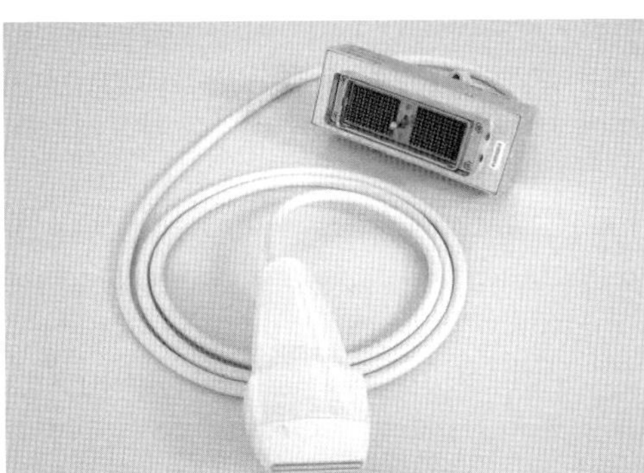

Fig. 4. Picture of the assembled CMUT probe.

to the requirements imposed by the limited power supply rejection ratio of both the MAX4805A component and the CMUT bias tee networks. A custom design of the power supply unit was then carried out. The circuit is based on the amplification, rectification and notch filtering of a pure tone generated by a 200 kHz sinusoidal oscillator. Using this approach, the five fixed supply voltages (±2 V, ±5 V and −100 V) required by the electronics as well as the adjustable CMUT bias voltage (0–300 V) were generated with inappreciable voltage ripple. The board containing the described circuit was designed to be housed into the system connector of the probe (Fig. 4). The power supply voltages were delivered to the in-probe electronic boards through six spare coaxial cables available in the multi-coaxial cable. The total power consumption of the probe was estimated to be less than 1.5 W.

4. Probe Characterization and Ultrasound Imaging

4.1. *Electrical Impedance*

All the electrical impedance measurements of the CMUT array elements were performed, using an HP4194A (Agilent Technologies, Inc., Santa Clara, CA) impedance analyzer, on a probe-head prototype without the silicone lens. At first, electrical impedance measurements were performed on a single element at different bias voltages in order to estimate the variation of the resonance frequency and extrapolate the collapse voltage. The extrapolation was obtained by fitting experimental with numerical data using the FEM model mentioned in Section 2.1. The fitted FEM model was used to compute the collapse voltage that turned out to be 280 V.

Further, electrical impedance measurements at a fixed bias voltage of 200 V were performed on all the array elements with the aim of estimating the capacitance and resonance frequency variation across the array. All the measurement data were compensated taking into account the parasitic capacitance and inductance of the cables and the fixture used for the electrical interconnection of the probe-head to the impedance analyzer. Figure 5 shows the electrical impedance measurement of the central element (96) of the CMUT array. The resonance frequency and the capacitance were computed for each array element. A smooth variation of the resonance frequency of the elements across the array was observed, indicating that the variation is mostly caused by the non-uniformity of the CMUT plate thickness. As a matter of fact, the frontal layer of the CMUT, which is made of an LPCVD silicon nitride layer, was slightly etched while being temporarily exposed to the HNA mixture during the chemical etching of the silicon substrate (see Section 2.3). Proof of this was

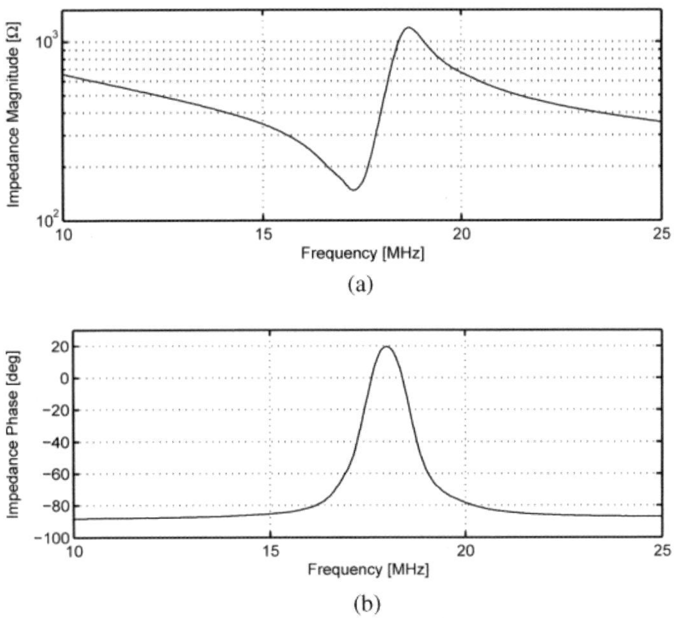

Fig. 5. Electrical impedance measurement of the central (96) CMUT array element biased at 200 V. (a) magnitude (logarithmic vertical scale) and (b) phase.

Table 2. Electrical impedance characterization.

Parameter	Value
Resonance frequency[a]	17.9 MHz
(% RSD[b])	(1.1%)
Element capacitance[a]	22.8 pF
(% RSD[b])	(2.0%)
Collapse voltage[c]	280 V

[a]Mean value
[b]Relative Standard Deviation (RSD)
[c]One element (extrapolated)

that the color of the array surface appeared slightly faded after silicon substrate removal. Furthermore, the observed capacitance variation is likely due to the parasitic capacitance of the signal traces on the rigid-flex PCB.

Table 2 summarizes the electrical impedance characterization results. The mean value and relative standard deviation of the resonance frequency and the capacitance distributions across the array elements were computed and, despite the phenomena discussed above, the uniformity assessment was considered very satisfactory.

4.2. *Pulse-echo*

All the pulse-echo measurements were performed on the same CMUT probe-head provided with the silicone lens mentioned in Section 2.3 and mounted in the probe assembly described in Section 3. In all the measurements, the probe was electrically accessed through the connector on the system side of the cable. In order to make a first performance assessment of the CMUT probe, all the pulse-echo measurements were performed also on the Esaote LA435 piezoelectric probe using exactly the same procedures.

Pulse-echo characterization was carried out by placing the probes in front of a water immersed planar reflector at a distance of 15 mm, equal to depth of the elevation focus. In all measurements, the CMUT probe was biased at 200 V. The first pulse-echo measurement was carried out with the aim to determine the center frequency and bandwidth of the two-ways transfer function as well as the pulse length. All the probe elements were excited using a −100 V negative broadband pulse generated by a Pulser/Receiver 5800 (Panametrics Inc., Waltham, MA). The echo signals received by the central element (96) of the CMUT and the piezoelectric arrays normalized to their maximum absolute value are depicted respectively in Fig. 6(a) and (b). The

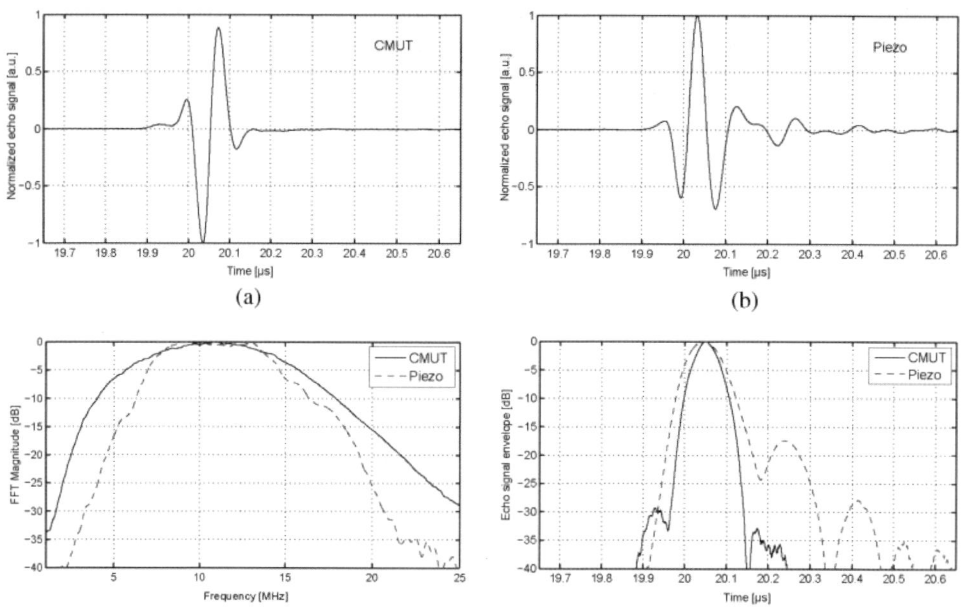

Fig. 6. Pulse-echo time-domain normalized response from the central (96) array element of the (a) CMUT probe biased at 200 V and (b) piezoelectric probe. Normalized (c) FFT magnitude and (d) time-domain envelope of the pulse-echo responses.

FFT magnitudes and the envelopes of the two echo signals are reported in Fig. 6(c) and (d). The CMUT probe shows broader bandwidth, and shorter pulse length. Among the presented results, the ones related to the envelope of the echo-signals demonstrates that, unlike the piezoelectric probe element that shows residual oscillations in its time-domain response, the CMUT probe element exhibits a nearly ideal behavior, resulting in a potentially better detail and contrast resolution during b-mode operation. The entire set of pulse-echo data was processed in order to extract, for each array element, the FFT center frequency, fractional bandwidth and amplitude variation across the array.

The second pulse-echo measurement was performed to estimate the two-ways sensitivity of the probe during the actual operative condition i.e., while being excited by a bipolar pulse by the imaging system. The elements were driven using 4-cycle, ±60 V bursts generated, at various frequencies, by a custom pulser/receiver containing the same electronic transmission modules used in the Technos imaging system front-end. The two ways sensitivity has been computed by dividing the amplitude of the received echo signal by the amplitude of the excitation signal measured at the probe connector. Since the MAX4805A introduces a voltage gain of 9 dB, the sensitivity datum obtained with the CMUT has been reduced in order to fairly compare the actual sensitivity of the CMUT and the piezoelectric transducer array elements.

Table 3 summarizes the pulse-echo characterization quantitative results for the CMUT and the piezoelectric probes. The mean value and the relative standard deviation of the center frequency, the −6 dB fractional bandwidth and the amplitude variation distributions across the array elements are reported for the two probes, together with their sensitivity estimation at various frequencies.

Table 3. Pulse-echo characterization.

Parameter	CMUT	Piezo
Center frequency[a] (−6 dB)	10.8 MHz	10.9 MHz
(% RSD[b])	(1.5%)	(1.8%)
Fractional bandwidth[a] (−6 dB)	103.9%	70.1%
(% RSD[b])	(2.1%)	(3.2%)
FFT Amplitude % RSD[b]		
(@ mean center frequency)	7.1%	11.0%
Sensitivity[c] @ 8.5 MHz	−38.4 dB	−41.7 dB
Sensitivity[c] @ 10 MHz	−37.4 dB	−41.1 dB
Sensitivity[c] @ 12 MHz	−37.0 dB	−41.2 dB

[a]Mean value

[b]Relative Standard Deviation (RSD)

[c]One element (extrapolated)

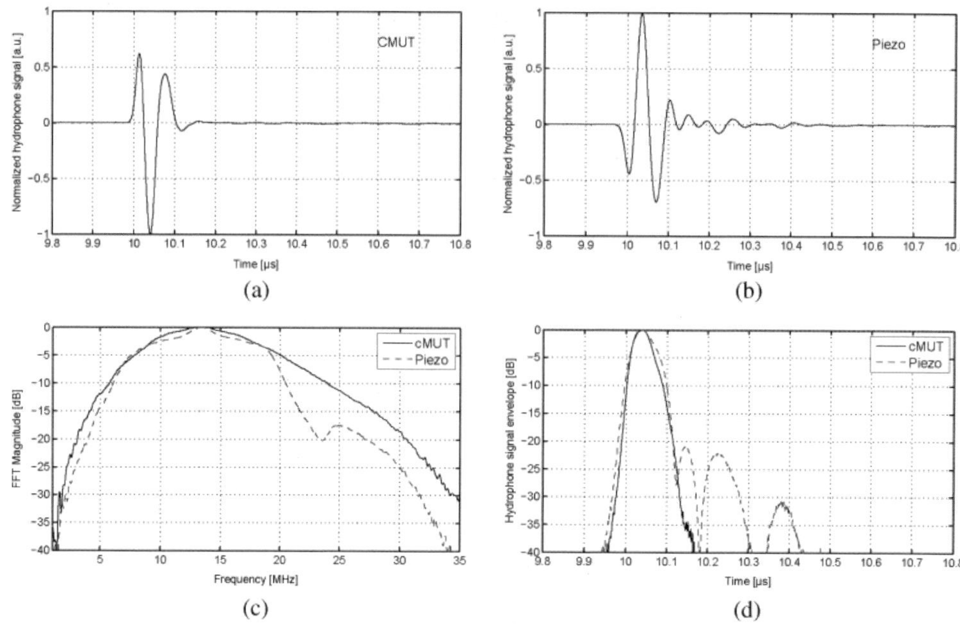

Fig. 7. Transmission time-domain normalized response from the central (96) array element of the (a) CMUT probe biased at 200 V and (b) piezoelectric probe. Normalized (c) FFT magnitude and (d) time-domain envelope of the transmission responses.

The reported results show that the CMUT probe performs better than the piezoelectric probe in terms of two-way response.

4.3. *Transmission*

Transmission measurements were carried out on a single element of the CMUT and the LA435 piezoelectric probes using the same experimental set-up described in the previous Section 4.2. A needle type MHA9-150 hydrophone (Force Technology, Brøndby, Denmark) was placed in front of the water immersed probes at a distance of 15 mm, in order to perform acoustic pressure measurements at the elevation focus depth. In all measurements, the CMUT probe was biased at 200 V.

The center frequency and bandwidth of the transmission transfer function as well as the pulse length were estimated by exciting the central element (96) of the CMUT and the piezoelectric arrays using a −100 V negative broadband pulse generated by the Panametrics Pulser/Receiver 5800. The hydrophone signals normalized to their maximum absolute value are depicted respectively in Fig. 7(a) and (b). The FFT magnitudes and the envelopes of the two hydrophone signals are reported in Fig. 7(c) and (d).

Table 4. Transmission characterization.

Parameter	CMUT	Piezo
Center frequency (−3 dB)	13.6 MHz	13.5 MHz
Fractional bandwidth (−3 dB)	67.5%	65.4%
Center frequency (−20 dB)	16.8 MHz	13.5 MHz
Fractional bandwidth (−20 dB)	163.3%	136.2%
Sensitivity @ 8.5 MHz	17.1 dB[a]	22.9 dB[a]
Sensitivity @ 10 MHz	20.9 dB[a]	25.1 dB[a]
Sensitivity @ 12 MHz	22.0 dB[a]	26.3 dB[a]
Peak-to-peak pressure @ 12 MHz	160.8 kPa	254.9 kPa

[a]Mean value
[b]Relative Standard Deviation (RSD)
[c]One element (extrapolated)

The transmission sensitivity and the acoustic pressure generated by the probe during the actual operative conditions were determined by driving the array elements using 4-cycle, ±60 V bursts generated, at different frequencies, by the custom pulser/receiver, as described in the previous section.

Table 4 summarizes the transmission characterization results for a single element of the CMUT and the piezoelectric probes. The center frequency and the fractional bandwidth at −3 dB and −20 dB are reported proving that the CMUT probe performs better than the piezoelectric probe in terms of transmission response bandwidth and pulse length. The transmission sensitivity data estimated at various frequencies as well as the peak-to-peak pressure measured at the probe nominal center frequency (12 Mhz) are also reported showing, in this case, that better results are obtained with the piezoelectric probe.

4.4. *Ultrasound Imaging*

Real time *in-vivo* ultrasound images were generated on the "Technos" imaging system, using the highest frequency linear array preset (LA424). The LA424 probe is the previous version of the LA435 probe used in this work. At first, b-mode images were generated by connecting alternately the CMUT and the piezoelectric probes to the Technos imaging system. The driving signal frequency was set at 13 MHz and the burst count at 1. Due to the maximum voltage limitation of the LA435 probe, the driving signal amplitude was set in both cases at ±60 V whilst the CMUT probe was biased at 200 V. Moreover, having the CMUT probe higher sensitivity, the b-mode gain was adjusted in order to achieve equivalent brightness of the images generated with the two

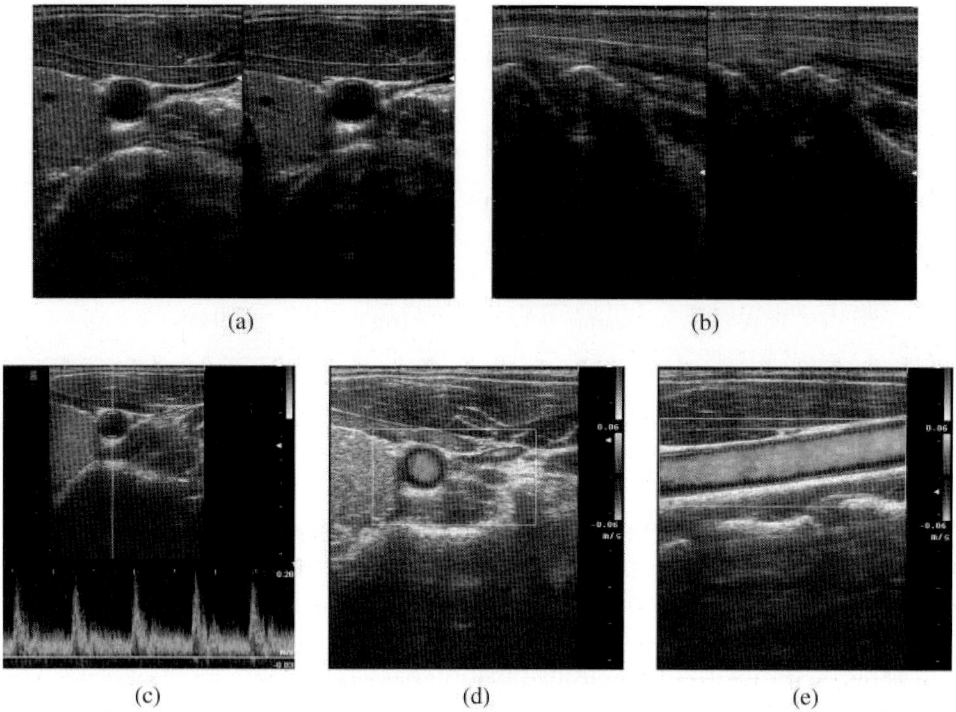

Fig. 8. *In-vivo* ultrasound images obtained with an Esaote Technos imaging system using a 13 MHz preset. B-mode images of a (a) carotid artery and (b) a forearm tendon. In (a) and (b), the images are generated using the CMUT probe (left) and the Esaote LA435 piezoelectric probe (right). (c) PW Doppler and (d)–(e) Color Doppler modes of the same carotid artery. All the images are rendered with a dynamic range of 55 dB. The image depth is 31 mm in (b) and 41 mm in (a), (c), (d) and (e). Color can be viewed in the e-book.

probes. A big effort was carried out to place the two probes in the same position in order to scan the same portion of tissue. Figure 8 reports the b-mode images of a human carotid artery [Fig. 8(a)] and a human forearm tendon [Fig. 8(b)]. In each of the two figures, the represented images were obtained with the CMUT probe (on the left) and the piezoelectric probe (on the right). A slightly improved axial resolution and penetration depth is observable in the images generated using the CMUT probe. Such improvement however, which is imputable to the CMUT larger bandwidth, was limited by the bandwidth of the reception filters implemented in the "Technos" imaging system probe preset. PW Doppler and Color Doppler modes were also experimented with the CMUT probe. In fact, being such modes more sensitive to noise as compared to b-mode, they provide an empiric but effective "testing ground" for signal-to-noise ratio and electromagnetic immunity assessment. Figure 8 reports the results achieved by successfully scanning the same carotid artery with the

CMUT probe in PW Doppler mode [Fig. 8(c)] and Color Doppler mode [Fig. 8(d) and (e)].

5. Discussion and Conclusion

This chapter presented the design, fabrication and characterization of a CMUT probe for medical ultrasound imaging. The *heart* of the probe i.e., the CMUT array, was microfabricated using the Reverse Fabrication Process, and successfully assembled in the form of a *silicon-free* ultrasound probe-head using an efficient and reliable packaging procedure. The CMUT array was provided with acoustically and thermo-mechanically engineered materials used for the fabrication of the backing and the acoustic lens designed to optimize the performance of the probe-head. The integration of the CMUT probe-head in a commercial ultrasound imaging system was supported by the introduction of electronics inside the probe that made it possible to use a standard cable and system connector, resulting in a full compatibility with the system itself. Electric and acoustic characterizations were performed to assess the probe-head fabrication process reliability and the probe performance. The results were compared with those obtained, in equivalent conditions, with a commercially available piezoelectric probe designed for the same imaging application. *In-vivo* ultrasound images using various ultrasound modes were finally generated and discussed.

The results obtained in the described framework showed the superiority of CMUT technology with respect to piezoelectric technology as regards both transmission and two-ways time and frequency response shape. The CMUT probe showed lower transmission sensitivity (−4.2 dB at the nominal center frequency) and higher two-ways sensitivity (+5 dB at the nominal center frequency) resulting from its higher reception sensitivity.

The authors would like to emphasize that the operating conditions during all tests i.e., the maximum driving voltage and the limited receiver bandwidth, were defined taking into account the limitations of the piezoelectric probe and of the imaging system. Therefore they expect to obtain even better absolute performance of the CMUT probe by overcoming such limitations.

Future work will focus on the complete characterization of the CMUT probe, that will include the measurement of the element directivity pattern, the crosstalk and the high order harmonic generation. Further, imaging capability assessment will be carried out through *in-vitro* tests on tissue-mimicking phantoms using an up-to-date imaging system capable of fully exploiting the performance provided by CMUT technology. Although Doppler mode results did not show weakness in terms of noise performance, imaging capability assessment will be fully accomplished by carrying out a deeper noise analysis of the CMUT and the in-probe electronics. Thermal efficiency will also be investigated in order to achieve a complete performance assessment of *reverse* microfabricated CMUTs.

In this work, the task to implement a device designed for an application that is already fulfilled by the current piezoelectric technology was addressed with the purpose of demonstrating that CMUT technology is mature enough and can provide added value to be used in medical ultrasound imaging applications. What is being affirmed is validated by the estimation of the industrial cost of the CMUT probe presented in this chapter, which resulted to be comparable to the industrial cost of the LA435 piezoelectric probe for a production volume of 1000 units per year.

References

1. M.I. Haller, and B.T. Khuri-Yakub, "A surface micromachined electrostatic ultrasonic air transducer," *Proc IEEE Ultrason Symp* **2**, 1241–1244 (1994).
2. I. Ladabaum, B.T. Khuri-Yakub, D. Spoliansky, and M.I. Haller, "Micromachined ultrasonic transducers (MUTs)," *Proc IEEE Ultrason Symp* **1**, 501–504 (1995).
3. D.W. Schindel, D.A. Hutchins, Zou Lichun, and M. Sayer, "The design and characterization of micromachined air-coupled capacitance transducers," *IEEE Trans Ultrason Ferroelectr Freq Contr* **42**, 42–50 (1995).
4. P.C. Eccardt, K. Niederer, T. Scheiter, and C. Hierold, "Surface micromachined ultrasound transducers in CMOS technology," *Proc IEEE Ultrason Symp* **2**, 959–962 (1996).
5. G. Caliano, V. Foglietti, E. Cianci, and M. Pappalardo, "A silicon microfabricated ultrasonic transducer: 1 MHz transmission in air and in water," *Microelectron Eng* **53**, 573–576 (2000).
6. Jin Xuecheng, I. Ladabaum, and B.T. Khuri-Yakub, "The microfabrication of capacitive ultrasonic transducers," *J Microelectromech Sys* 7, 295–302 (1998).
7. G. Caliano, F. Galanello, A. Caronti, R. Carotenuto, M. Pappalardo, V. Foglietti, and N. Lamberti, "Micromachined ultrasonic transducers using silicon nitride membrane fabricated in PECVD technology," *Proc IEEE Ultrason Symp* **1**, 963–968 (2000).
8. Yongli Huang, A.S. Ergun, E. Haeggstrom, M.H. Badi, and B.T. Khuri-Yakub, "Fabricating capacitive micromachined ultrasonic transducers with wafer-bonding technology," *J Microelectromech Sys* **12**, 128–137 (2003).
9. H.T. Soh, I. Ladabaum, A. Atalar, C.F. Quate, B.T. Khuri-Yakub, "Silicon micromachined ultrasonic immersion transducers," *Appl Phys Lett* **69**, 3674–3676 (1996).
10. Ö. Oralkan, A.S. Ergun, J.A. Johnson, M. Karaman, U. Demirci, K. Kaviani, T.H. Lee, and B.T. Khuri-Yakub, "Capacitive micromachined ultrasonic transducers: Next generation arrays for acoustic imaging?" *IEEE Trans Ultrason Ferroelectr Freq Contr* **49**, 1596–1610 (2002).
11. G. Caliano, R. Carotenuto, A. Caronti, and M. Pappalardo, "cMUT echographic probes: Design and fabrication process," *Proc IEEE Ultrason Symp* **2**, 1067–1070 (2002).

12. S. Ergun, Y. Huang, C.H. Cheng, Ö. Oralkan, J. Johnson, H. Jagannathan, U. Demirci, G.G. Yaralıoglu, M. Karaman, and B.T. Khuri-Yakub, "Broadband capacitive micromachined ultrasonic transducers ranging from 10 kHz to 60 MHz for imaging applications and more," *Proc IEEE Ultrason Symp* 1039–1043 (2002).
13. Ö. Oralkan, A.S. Ergun, C.H. Cheng, J.A. Johnson, M. Karaman, T.H. Lee, and B.T. Khuri-Yakub, "Volumetric ultrasound imaging using 2-D CMUT arrays," *IEEE Trans Ultrason Ferroelectr Freq Contr* **50**, 1581–1594 (2003).
14. D.M. Mills, and L.S. Smith, "Real-time *in-vivo* imaging with capacitive micromachined ultrasound transducer (cMUT) linear arrays," *Proc IEEE Ultrason Symp* **1**, 568–571 (2003).
15. S. Panda, C. Daft, P. Wagner, I. Ladabaum, P. Pellegretti, and F. Bertora, "Microfabricated ultrasonic transducer (cMUT) probes: Imaging advantages over PZT probes," *Proc. WFUMB (hosted by AIUM) Conference*, Montreal, Canada (2003).
16. G. Caliano, R. Carotenuto, E. Cianci, V. Foglietti, A. Caronti, and M. Pappalardo, "A cMUT linear array used as echographic probe: Fabrication, characterization, and images," *Proc IEEE Ultrason Symp* **1**, 395–398 (2004).
17. A. Savoia, G. Caliano, R. Carotenuto, C. Longo, P. Gatta, A. Caronti, E. Cianci, V. Foglietti, and M. Pappalardo, "Enhanced echographic images obtained improving the membrane structural layer of the cMUT probe," *Proc IEEE Ultrason Symp* **4**, 1960–1963 (2005).
18. A. Caronti, G. Caliano, R. Carotenuto, A. Savoia, M. Pappalardo, E. Cianci *et al.*, "Capacitive micromachined ultrasonic transducer (CMUT) arrays for medical imaging," *Microelectronics J* **37**, 770–777 (2006).
19. A. Caronti, G. Caliano, A. Savoia, M. Pappalardo, and R. Carotenuto, "A low-noise, wideband electronic system for pulse-echo ultrasound imaging with CMUT arrays," *Ultrasonics Symposium, 2004 IEEE* 2219–2222 (2004).
20. G. Caliano *et al.*, "Surface micromechanical process for manufacturing micromachined capacitive ultra-acoustic transducers and relevant micromachined capacitive ultra-acoustic transducer," United States Patent 7790490 September 7, 2010.
21. G. Caliano, A. Caronti, A. Savoia, C. Longo, M. Pappalardo, E. Cianci, and V. Foglietti, "Capacitive micromachined ultrasonic transducer (cMUT) made by a novel 'Reverse Fabrication Process'," *Proc IEEE Ultrason Symp* **1**, 479–482 (2005).
22. G. Caliano, A. Savoia, A. Caronti, C. Longo, P. Gatta, and M. Pappalardo, "Echographic images improvements with a cMUT probe," *19th International Congress on Acoustics (ICA), Madrid*, 375 (2007).
23. A. Caronti, A. Coppa, A. Savoia, C. Longo, P. Gatta, B. Mauti *et al.*, "Curvilinear capacitive micromachined ultrasonic transducer (CMUT) array fabricated using a reverse process," *Ultrasonics Symposium, 2008. IUS 2008. IEEE* 2092–2095 (2008).
24. A. Caronti, A. Savoia, G. Caliano, M. Pappalardo, "Acoustic coupling in capacitive microfabricated ultrasonic transducers: Modeling and experiments," *IEEE Trans Ultrason Ferroelectr Freq Control* **52**, 2220–2234 (2005).
25. A. Caronti, G. Caliano, P. Gatta, C. Longo, A. Savoia, and M. Pappalardo, "A finite element tool for the analysis and the design of capacitive micromachined ultrasonic transducer (cMUT) arrays for medical imaging," *J Acoust Soc Am* **123**, 3375 (2008).
26. G. Caliano, A. Savoia, A. Caronti, V. Foglietti, E. Cianci, and M. Pappalardo, "Capacitive micromachined ultrasonic transducer with an open-cells structure," *Sensors and Actuators A: Physical* **121**, 382–387 (2005).

27. A. Savoia, G. Caliano, A. Caronti, R. Carotenuto, P. Gatta, C. Longo *et al.*, "Multilayer cMUT structure for improved sensitivity and bandwidth," *Ultrasonics Symposium, 2006. IEEE* 1939–1942 (2006).
28. A. Savoia, V. Bavaro, G. Caliano, A. Caronti, R. Carotenuto, P. Gatta *et al.*, "P2B-4 crisscross 2D cMUT array: Beamforming strategy and synthetic 3D imaging results," *Ultrasonics Symposium, 2007. IEEE* 1514–1517 (2007).
29. A. Savoia, G. Caliano, A. Iula, C. Longo, A. Caronti, R. Carotenuto *et al.*, "Design and fabrication of a cmut probe for ultrasound imaging of fingerprints," *Ultrasonics Symposium (IUS), 2010 IEEE* 1877–1880 (2010).
30. A. Iula, A. Savoia, and G. Caliano, "Capacitive micro-fabricated ultrasonic transducers for biometric applications," *Microelectronic Engineering* **88**, 2278–2280 (2011).
31. N. Lamberti, G. Caliano, A. Iula, and A. S. Savoia, "A high frequency cMUT probe for ultrasound imaging of fingerprints," *Sensors and Actuators A: Physical* **172**, 561–569 (2011).
32. M. Legros, C. Meynier, R. Dufait, G. Ferin, and F. Tranquart, "Piezocomposite and CMUT arrays assessment through in vitro imaging performances," *Proc IEEE Ultrason Symp* 1142–1145 (2008).
33. "World's first practical application of medical ultrasound transducers with semiconductor process," *Hitachi Medical Corporation website*, http://www.hitachi-medical.co.jp/news/news/pdf/news090520.pdf
34. "Development of Ultrasonic Transducer "Mappie" with cMUT Technology," *Hitachi Medical Corporation website*, http://www.hitachi-medical.co.jp/medix/pdf/vol51/P31-34.pdf
35. M. Pappalardo, G. Caliano, A. S. Savoia, and A. Caronti, "Micromachined ultrasonic transducers," in *Piezoelectric and Acoustic Materials for Transducer Applications*, ed: Springer US 453–478 (2008).
36. Butrus T. Khuri-Yakub, and Ömer Oralkan, "Capacitive micromachined ultrasonic transducers for medical imaging and therapy," *J Micromechanics Microengineering* 21 (2011): 054004.
37. A. Savoia, G. Caliano, B. Mauti, and M. Pappalardo, "Performance optimization of a high frequency CMUT probe for medical imaging," presented at the *IEEE Ultrason Symp* (2011).
38. A.S. Savoia, G. Caliano, and M. Pappalardo, "A CMUT probe for medical ultrasonography: From microfabrication to system integration," *IEEE Trans Ultrason Ferroelectr Freq Control* **59**, 1127–1138 (2012).
39. I. Ladabaum, P. Wagner, C. Zanelli, J. Mould, P. Reynolds, and G. Wojcik, "Silicon substrate ringing in microfabricated ultrasonic transducers," *Proc IEEE Ultrason Symp* **1**, 943–946 (2000).

Chapter 22

Advances in Picture Archiving Communication System and Medical Imaging Cloud

Bichuan Shen[*,‡] *and Chi-Hau Chen*[†,§]

[*]4701 Monterey Oaks Blvd, Austin, TX, USA
[†]Department of Electrical and Computer Engineering, University of Massachusetts, North Dartmouth, MA, USA
[‡]E-mail: sbichuan@hotmail.com
[§]cchen@umassd.edu

Rapidly growing volumes of medical data and studies, more imaging modalities, standardization of digital imaging and communications in medicine (DICOM) and healthcare level 7 (HL7), increasingly complicated workflow and structured reports, geographically distributed storage and access, data management, and security access have driven the evolution of Picture Archiving Communication System (PACS), adoption of web-based imaging cloud for healthcare information systems. Integrated enterprise PACS and imaging cloud services facilitate archiving, sharing and exchanging of imaging studies, ubiquitous and reliable network access anytime anywhere for clinical practice and healthcare provider, and achieve smooth workflow, balanced workloads, and optimized performance.

1. Introduction

During the past decade, healthcare services are quickly evolving and becoming much more diversified due to significant advances in imaging, internet and web technologies. Widespread LANs and WANs and intranets are bridging previously separate and detached institutions and domains into inter-connected premises. Advances of PACS and cloud technologies are transforming the healthcare and clinic practice in fundamental ways, and deliver faster and better patient care. Healthcare is evolving towards more service-oriented, patient-centered, and data-driven services and models. This trend has resulted in adoption of service-based PACS model and imaging cloud with service-oriented architecture (SOA).

Medical imaging has seen rapid migration from grayscale, low resolution, single modality to support full spectrum of color, high resolution, and multi-modality. More and more imaging modalities of 1D, 2D or 3D to collect, process, analyze, archive, transmit and visualize clinical data are generating large volume data every year. For example, imaging modalities of one-dimensional signals include the electrocardiogram, invasive and noninvasive blood pressure measurement, pulse oximetry, intracardiac electrograms, and stethoscope. And two (or three)-dimensional modalities include ultrasound, coronary angiograms, and positron emission tomography (PET), magnetic resonance imaging (MRI), nuclear imaging, and computed tomography (CT).[1] According to a recent survey, in the U.S. today, about 400 million procedures a year[2] involve at least one medical image in various modalities and formats. This would create huge amount of data if we consider an average medical study with still or multi-frame DICOM images ranging from several to hundreds of Mbytes.

This trend has changed teleradiology, telemedicine, and the ecosystems of RIS/HIS/IHE drastically. Medical practice and clinical workflow call for more scalable and interoperable solutions. Physicians such as cardiologists, neurologists, oncologists, gastroenterologists, dentists, and surgeons are more and more relying on these advanced and more accurate techniques and electronic medical records (EMR) to help facilitate less or non-invasive diagnosis, consultation, prescription and treatment. They want to rapidly access images and data anytime and anywhere ubiquitously to provide better patient care. The regulation compliance of Health Insurance Portability and Accountability Act (HIPAA) on EMR retention and archive, privacy and security add to the exponential growth of massive data storage and management. Cloud computing and services facilitate archiving, sharing and exchanging of imaging studies for clinical practices. Thin client PACS and imaging cloud could offer uninterrupted across healthcare providers, departments, hospitals, institutions, and network domains without boundaries. Patient studies can be better shared by reducing unnecessary and redundant studies and data integrity can be better preserved by centralized data centers. It provides high availability, improved scalability, interoperability, portability, reliability and flexibility.

2. PACS System

2.1. *DICOM Model*

Over the past decade, telemedicine and telehealth have proliferated and evolved to an unprecedented application level. They are well-supported by DICOM as an open standard to efficiently and effectively transfer data and information between variant system components, such as imaging modalities, gateways, PACS, database management system, storage. DICOM also facilitates the healthcare workflow within and between medical departments.

Since its debut in 1993, DICOM is the widely adopted medical image standard and communication protocol introduced jointly by American College of Radiology (ACR) and the National Electrical Manufacturers Association (NEMA). DICOM format is used to collect, capture, archive, transport, process, and retrieve medical images and patient information. It is the format that most medical imaging modalities, PACS servers and clients, gateways, processing workstations, image archive and storage host, review and display stations support.

DICOM standard is quite extensive with large hierarchically predefined datasets. DICOM information model: DICOM datasets are tags-grouped. For example, the content and information objects are grouped into patient and study information, exams, reports, slices and segments, image frame and pixel data, modality and equipment manufacturer, waveforms, and annotations. These are roots respectively and more child data can be defined in the leaves of these roots. They are called as DICOM Information Object Definitions (IODs).[3–5] Each DICOM attribute is tagged by a pair of 2-byte numbers (group, element) to store the information. These include both standard and optional private attributes, which are denoted as value representation (VR) types.

DICOM format is fully compatible with variant imaging modalities through its modality tags. DICOM worklist is a scheduled sequence of procedures which can be retrieved by modality through PACS gateway. In addition, DICOM can be interfaced to PACS, and further mapped to HL7 standard messages. This facilitates transparent information workflow between modality, gateway, PACS, radiology information system (RIS), hospital information system (HIS) and Integrated Healthcare Enterprise (IHE). DICOM utilizes its C-FIND, C-GET, and C-MOVE, C-STORE protocols to realize query/retrieval of PACS and RIS.

Image tagging is a great feature for DICOM to store patient and study information, which may include anatomic structures, volumes, regions and labels, measurements, scoring and calculations. This enhances the interpretation capabilities of imaging content and data and allows physicians to add more clinical descriptions. For example, image annotations can be stored and exported by DICOM to compatible PACS and RIS.

The way how DICOM data are encoded and communicated is called transfer syntax, which is defined in the DICOM file header. In order to preserve high-fidelity of medical and diagnostic data, DICOM images use compressed standards such as lossless RLE and JPEG and lossy JPEG 2000. They use the well-known block DCT for JPEG and wavelet transform for JPEG 2000, followed by RLE and entropy coding. To increase the compression ratios further, the multi-frame DICOM files can be further compressed into AVI and other formats by using MJPEG, VC1, XVID MPEG4, and other codec including H.264 and newly emerged HEVC standards. Most advanced compression standards use hybrid encoding methods, including motion estimation and compensation, and adaptive deblock filtering.

2.2. *Medical Imaging and PACS*

Medical imaging is very important to healthcare and has been widely used in radiology, cardiology, pathology, pediatrics, obstetrics, and gynecology etc. There are many available imaging tools such as CT, MRI, PET, and ultrasonography. Visual data is collected by imaging modality, based on respective sensing physics principles and target interactive material characteristics. Accurate imaging data of patient's organs, specimens, fetus, and full body anatomy help physicians diagnose and evaluate patient's condition, prescribe suitable medication, and recommend procedures, or operations. No matter which sensing methods were used, all imaging systems consist of image capture or acquisition, high speed data transfer, processing, post-processing, converting, storage, archiving, retrieving, rendering.

In order to achieve smooth health information sharing, medical imaging workflow has been closely integrated into radiology information system (RIS) and hospital information system (HIS). As mentioned above, DICOM standard and format contain patient study information and medical imaging data, by which imaging modalities can be interfaced into PACS through gateways.

DICOM modality worklist (MWL) tags are used to schedule imaging procedures on which imaging modality patient data is sensed, captured, and acquired.

Visualizing and displaying electronic imaging records is the core functionality of rendering, for example, X-ray dental records, ultrasound fetus records. It is very critical to medical imaging not only because of the importance of presenting the massive data, but also its close relation to overall system performance. In thin or zero-footprint client model, remote rendering from PACS and cloud servers to distributed light-weighted consuming devices connected by network could greatly simplify design and maintenance of clients, and maximize system usage and minimize cost.

Besides two-dimensional data, 3D[6] or 4D volume medical data require both advanced processing and rendering algorithms, high performance optimized software, and graphics hardware. Super vectorized, parallel, and pipeline architectures and rendering engines such as GPU, multi-core CPU are quickly evolving and have been adopted widely in many clinical facilities and hospitals. By using texture and shader technologies, and employing DirectShow, DirectX, DXVA, and OpenGL, high volume and fidelity study images can be efficiently accelerated and rendered.

Usability is one of the major considerations of PACS and medical imaging system. The complexity of underlying imaging modalities, hardware, device, software stacks and protocols need to be transparent to physician users at the top application layer. Many important image manipulation functions facilitate PACS and imaging system usability. They include brightness and contrast, window level adjustment, zoom in zoom out, orientation rotation and pan translation, flip and inversion. Physicians and radiologists can mark image editing and record annotation in PACS database. Image special effects and video overlay are also desired.

In addition, advanced image processing functions can be integrated into PACS, to better understand, analyze and present medical images or volume data. Automatic extraction of key geometric features, boundary and contour detection, image segmentation have been employed in PACS. These functions allow quantitative analysis and measurement of regions and anatomic structures, volumes and mass, and facilitate clinical decision and treatment. For example, segmentation of brain images, mammograms can better reveal organs, tissues, and allows to calculate volumes in CT images. There are many segmentation and classification techniques, for instance, watershed algorithm, region grouping and growing, active contours etc. The purpose of segmentation in medical imaging is to separate and extract different regions of interest, in which the same regions contain homogeneous textures, geometrics, or features. Segmentation algorithms can be mainly divided into three groups: that is, automatic or un-supervised, semi-supervised, and supervised categories.

As PACS is archiving and warehousing of massive medical data, the capabilities to search, index, query and retrieve patient and study information are essential to PACS functionality. Query and retrieval can be performed both locally on a thick-client PACS and remotely on a thin-client PACS or web-based PACS servers. DICOM protocols provide this support through C-FIND, C-GET, and transfer and storage of data through C-MOVE, C-STORE. More than this, clinical data mining is also desirable to help physicians and radiologists extract and analyze critical data, correlate disease symptoms, clinical observations and diagnosis, and treatment and medications.

2.3. *Multimodality Imaging and PACS*

To meet growing needs of more accurate diagnosis and better patient care, more modalities are introduced to interface an integrated PACS. Different imaging characteristics, resolutions, and *in vivo* scan capabilities of noninvasive ultrasound, CT, PET, and MRI can complement each other in clinical practice. For example, whole body PET and CT to reveal more and higher level details of organs and body parts than 2D ultrasound. These 3D imaging signals and volumes can be reconstructed from well aligned sequential 2D multi-frame images. In addition, 3D volume data can be augmented to 4D volume to account for the time factor.

These joint combinations of alternate modalities generate massive medical imaging data. Therefore, higher system performance and software scalability are required. DICOM based enterprise PACS and cloud services are ideal for multimodality support.

2.4. *Cardiovascular Imaging PACS*

Cardiovascular disease is one of the most serious health problems in both developed and developing countries, threatening quite a certain portion of middle and senior aged people. This leads to significant impacts on individuals, families and communities in medication, cure, treatment, and aftermath care. Governments, societies, industries are engaged in and collaborating on research, funding, and education.

The most effective approach to control and prevent it is early diagnosis and accurate examination. For this purpose, advanced cardiac imaging modalities have evolved and been introduced to clinic practice. Cardiac imaging can be categorized into invasive and non-invasive imaging. For example, invasive modality includes cardiovascular angiography, intravascular ultrasonic imaging. Non-invasive techniques include cardiac nuclear imaging, computed tomography, and ultrasonic echocardiography.

PACS plays a significant role in cardiovascular imaging systems. Cardiovascular PACS is required to efficiently manage massive studies of coronary ultrasound, stress echocardiography (Stress Echo), coronary angiography, coronary computed tomography, and cardiac nuclear images. Support of heterogeneous imaging modalities, transfer and interpretation of massive data, switching of multiple cardiac studies, and vendor neutral archive of variant imaging data present a real challenge for enterprise cardiac PACS, and database management system.

2.5. *PACS and Models*

The models of PACS can be categorized into mainly three architectures, that is, thick-client or stand-alone model, client-server model, and web-based model.[7] In thick client model, PACS clients are designed to have large computing resources, processing capabilities, and local data center and storage to run medical applications locally, without solely depending upon the PACS server and network connection and bandwidth. Thus network disconnection, limited bandwidth, and latency do not affect the performance of thick client significantly, which is the advantage. But in this model, medical data and databases may have redundancy and resides on geographically different physical locations, so data integrity is not guaranteed and both hardware and software resources and systems are not portable and scalable.

In contrary to thick client's scenario, thin clients (also called small-footprint client) rely more on services provided through PACS servers through network connection such as VPN on LAN or WAN. In this model, clients have very limited software, storage and computing powers, and even not have a full-fledged OS, except a very small and portable browser or viewer to consume the services and data provided by the server. For example, smartphone, tablet, and any other smart portable devices can access securely to centralized PACS or cloud servers to remotely display images or review structured reports. They facilitate non-stop 24/7 medical workflow from admission and scheduling, medication, immunization, and testing, transfer and discharge, to billing and insurance. Thus, this greatly increases the availability of patient care. In addition, using the standardized interface could make it vendor neutral solution. Of course, the response time, latency and performance of these VM-based solutions are sensitive to and dependent on network connection and bandwidth. More and more thin clients are deployed in healthcare due to its light-weight characteristics, scalability and portability.

3. Medical Imaging Cloud

3.1. *Cloud Model*

Scalability is very critical not only to the service availability, software portability, system performance, and platform independency, but also has big impact to the infrastructure and architecture of hospital information system (HIS) and healthcare information exchange (HIE). In a cloud-based model, the combination of centralized data center and thin clients make it more flexible to providing more services and adding virtual machines (VM) and resources, and release them after on-demand usage. Therefore, it can leverage existing resources and power to support upgrades.

Cloud service model is also called web-based model. National Institute of Standards and Technology defines its five essential characteristics as: on demand self-service, broad network access, resource sharing, rapid elasticity, measured service.[8] In this model, available services are published by cloud servers in centralized data center and cloud repository to archive and store medical images and studies, import and export patient studies. Clients could remote access and share the healthcare services and medical contents through reliable and secure network connections. The universal viewing and displaying tools can be available to most web browsers. Light-weighted or zero-footprint medical viewers can access the provisioned services and consume the medical data on demand and on the fly. It instantiate the virtualization of software and computing resources provided in the cloud data centers and remote clients do not involve in rendering. This improves content and data interoperability, software and device portability, enhances medical workflow, ensures data security and integrity, reduces cost and improves efficiency per medical image study. Variant zero-footprint viewers including fore-mentioned AT&T medical mobile viewer fall into this category.

Cloud model make the virtualization of services and computing resources such as CPUs, processors, memory, and storage disks, data center possible and viable. When connected to advanced imaging modalities of high cost, its cost sharing of each user per usage is thus greatly reduced. Cloud model offers healthcare quick provisioning of flexible computing resources, centralized PACS server, data center and cloud storage on a pay by demand basis. It provides benefits of platform independence, and cross-department transparency.

Depending on what portions of computing resources are required locally and the other portions are provisioned from cloud, there are mainly three cloud deployment models, Software as a Service (SaaS), Platform as a Service (PaaS), and Infrastructure as a Service (IaaS).

Software as a Service (SaaS) sits at the top application layer of cloud abstract model. In SaaS, only software applications are provisioned and shared across users but not platforms and infrastructures. This simplifies management and maintenance of clients and allow for feature enhancements and updates instantly from servers. Services in this model are usually provided through web browser, and very suitable for remote diagnosis and real-time patient monitoring, in telemedicine and teleradiology. In contrast to SaaS, PaaS and IaaS models provides more computing power and resources than SaaS, including virtual platforms and infrastructures to clients respectively.

For example, modern EMR, RIS could be deployed in SaaS cloud. In this model, services and resources are provisioned on-demand per use. It helps healthcare service providers achieve scalability, flexibility, efficiency and optimal performance through virtually provisioned resources and services, at much reduced management and maintenance costs.

Cloud can be deployed in three delivery models, that is, private, public, and hybrid model. Public cloud is the most cost-effective and flexible delivery model which is open to general public through internet. Typical examples are Microsoft Azure, Google AppEngine, Apple, and Amazon Elastic Compute Cloud (EC2).[9] In this model, any user can upload certain data to the centered server. Or they can download any published applications, updates, and client data from it. This model enable maximized sharing of services and data with other authorized users across the whole cloud.

However, due to strict security and privacy policies, public cloud model cannot guarantee the total confidentiality of uploaded clinical data and content. Therefore, it is not well suitable for clinical practice. In contrast, private cloud is the most adopted model in healthcare. It is owned and operated by only one single organization. It is more proprietary and not open to public access. It can assure the privacy and confidentiality while achieving workflow integrity and performance. Hybrid cloud combines two or more of different clouds together.

In the context of imaging cloud, clients initiate request for services and medical records to the server, and server respond with either acceptance of this request or service or access deny. This is called service negotiation, and done through service requestor on the client side, and request monitor on the server side.[10] The kinds of service requests can be bundled with service level and quality specifications, or as default. Once request monitor detect such a request, it will be forwarded to service processor to process this request and request allocator will decide resource allocation and send the decision back to the requestor. Clients could always request to add, reduce, or terminate on-the-fly services and resources during the runtime of service provision.

3.2. *Case Study of Citrix Based Cloud*

Among many virtual and cloud-based computing solutions, Citrix provides a bridge connecting the presentation server and remote clients consuming the published services. This allow physicians to dynamically provision and securely access the services anytime and anywhere, deliver medical imaging and healthcare textual data transparently across networks, visualize and display the DICOM and non-DICOM images remotely. This preserve integrity for centralized and aggregated imaging data, simplify design and maintenance of thin client PACS, and optimize system runtime performance.

For example, thin client or zero-footprint client can be provided on a Citrix XenApp and MetaFrame platforms. In this solution, presentation virtualization is realized through Citrix ICA (Independent Computing Architecture) channel. This is an error-free virtual communication channel over TCP/IP and RTP/RTCP. It is also a session-based protocol in which packet is the basic data unit of transmission including both data and control packets.

To achieve and optimize high performance of services and data transfer provisioned on demand from cloud servers, Citrix servers send encoding of the display updates to clients with high compression ratio, rather than raw display data whose amount is usually very prohibitive. This model is called server push model. In this model, the protocol is responsible to allocate adaptive transmitting buffers on the service side. Besides Citrix solution, Microsoft Terminal Services fall into this category. This is different from client pull model-based solutions like AT&T VNC, in which client will initiate the request of display updates and the server will send the response instead.

By sending compressed graphics updates, web-based cloud greatly reduce its network bandwidth requirement for on demand provisioning during runtime.

In addition, most thin client protocols support memory and disk caching to further improve system performance. In this approach, small bitmaps will be cached in RAM, and large bitmaps will be on disk.

This service model is PaaS. In this model, a limited APIs and SDKs are available for development on the client, but remote desktops do not need to install full-scaled software, and can still enjoy a rich featured remote desktop. Other examples include Microsoft Remote Desktop Services, Microsoft Terminal Services, and VMware View.

3.3. *Zero-footprint Client*

Both PACS and pure web-based cloud software as a service gradually adapt to utilize universal web browser technologies, interfacing into DICOM, use advanced video compression standards, to provide cross-enterprise, scalable web services. On any HTML5 compatible mobile and handheld devices, zero-footprint client could connect and communicate with web servers, without installing a full-fledged OS and application. Zero-footprint clients based on

Citrix solution and Microsoft RDP/RFX are examples. This solution only require minimum hardware requirements such as low-end CPU/GPU, processing power, and small local storage, as compared to high-end CPU/GPU, large storage and power consumption used by thick clients. As long as compatible web browsers such as Apple Safari and Google Chrome are installed, it will be able to connect to web servers. In this model, security and management are supported by the cloud servers. It greatly reduces computing complexity and simplifies the workload of client, is cost effective and easier to maintain.

HTML5 is compatible with web browsers such as Google Chrome and Safari. It supports open video codec standards such as H.264 and MPEG-4[11]. There are many video compression and encoding standards, but not all of them are supported in HTML5 compatible web browsers. Major native players on the web browsers support playback of video files, without installing any third-party plug-ins or software components. With advanced compression techniques, thin client PACS and web-based cloud could improve performance for network bandwidth bottleneck in LAN and WAN. It could also save storage as well.

3.4. *Vendor Neutral Archive*

The trend of Medical imaging and PACS evolution has reached to a key point where scalable architecture, support of open DICOM and non-proprietary standards, and vendor neutral archive[12] are desired. The complexity of RIS/HIS/IHE systems lies not only in the large scale of heterogeneous modalities, hardware and devices, but also in different operating systems, software and applications. In addition, integration, interface, and collaboration between disparate PACSs require support of variant medical images and textual data and structured diagnostic reports, for smooth workflow and efficiency.

In an imaging cloud especially, scalable cloud provides and provisions virtualized services to multitude of remote desktops, laptops, work stations, and mobile devices including smartphone and tablet, by centralized data center and database management system. Vendor neutral imaging archive allows for scaling aggregated imaging records and data with improved performance, while preserving data integrity, and reducing system cost. Vendor neutral archive can also utilize video compression to save system requirement of data storage.

Vendor neutral PACS and archive consist of open architecture, protocols, and standards such as DICOM and HL7 to support the core functionalities of PACS and image cloud in abstract layers, separate from disparate imaging hardware and modalities, operating systems from variant vendors. It interfaces RIS/HIS/EHR systems, clinical databases, gateways, web browsers, provides beyond software dependency and limitation, proprietary formats and constraints.

4. Considerations

4.1. *Security and Performance*

As confidentiality and privacy are crucial to healthcare organizations, providers, and consumers, how to assure security in access control,[13] identity management, session confidentiality and data privacy is key to clinical services, EMR, information systems, and associated data and workflows. This is especially true as enterprise PACS and healthcare cloud provide higher availability and ubiquitous remote access. In observance of the trend in healthcare, HIPAA compliance requires strict authentication, authorization, and security to access protected health information (PHI).[14] Typical security mechanisms include security rules, digital certification, virtualization, and firewall. Data transmission utilizes encryption and decryption.[15]

High performance computing is important to healthcare and clinical practices and it means faster delivery of patient care, ubiquitous and reliable network access, and high availability of medication, treatment and services. PACS upgrades and migrations usually come with higher volume of data storage and access, larger medical image sizes. Optimization of archive storage and fault-tolerant backup, access control, compression engines, remote displaying and reviewing, and network bandwidth are very critical.

4.2. *Structured Report*

PACS, imaging cloud, and many clinical information systems typically deal with massive data in various formats, much more than just image or DICOM. Among these, some may be textual data in text or tabular form, while some are multimedia content including video and graphics, and waveforms. Some are calculation numbers and measurements, and some are electronic patient records.

In the same context of PACS and cloud, variant data and formats need to be populated together. Abstraction and summarization of large amount of data are not only an appealing feature to physicians and clinical staff, but also a critical requirement to interface to wide ranges of IHE systems and archives. By utilizing DICOM hierarchical information model and service object pairs (SOP), structured reports are capable of representing well information of patient studies and medical examinations, and bridging with the rest of HIS and RIS, which primarily employ HL7 standard for other non-image health data. The syntax of HL7 message contains multiple segments and is rather simple, by beginning with a message header (MSH) and ending with new line. In structured report, XML is widely used to convert messages and data from DICOM format to HL7 syntax. This is because XML is a flexible, extensible, and portable system-independent language with similar tag-based information model as DICOM.

4.3. *Compression*

Variant imaging modalities including two-dimensional ultrasound imaging, CT and computed radiography (CR), nuclear medicine imaging of cardiology, angiography, endoscopy, and microscopy could generate large DICOM images and files. For example, a typical Doppler study of continuous scan could consist of several to over one hundred Mbytes.

Huge volumes of high resolution imaging data require large amount of storage. They cause maintenance and scalability issues for PACS and imaging cloud. Data integrity can be potentially compromised if they are distributed on geographically disparate locations.

Traditionally, lossless and lossy JPEG and JPEG 2000 are the major native DICOM compression and transfer standards in order to achieve high fidelity and quality of medical data, but the compression ratios are usually below 5 for reversible compression, or never go beyond 10 for lossy methods. Historically in a clinical workflow and hospital contexts, this is not only acceptable and but also the very first priority. This is because that once information is lost, it will be very hard to revert back, if not impossible.

The goals of medical imaging compression depend on not only the characteristics of medical images, but also the contexts and applications. Introduction of enterprise PACS and cloud are migrating quickly to support diverse modalities, interfacing to heterogeneous components, hosts, and end devices, thus this requirement could be relaxed. For example, for remote rendering and display, a high-compression ratio encoding is desirable to tradeoff the quality loss while accommodate low transmission bandwidth and storage saving.

By using highly efficient video compression technologies, these issues can be well-controlled and they can be effectively and efficiently transported, archived, stored, and reviewed. Advanced video encoding standards such as H.263, H.263+, H.264 and MPEG-4 can be used, without losing critical information and still obtain acceptable quality of data. Originally targeting efficient and effective video transmission and streaming over lossy and error-prone channels and possible low network bandwidths, these methods employ hybrid block-based motion estimation and compensation, adaptive quantization, flexible mode optimization and selection, addressing robust error-resilient transmission.

A lot of research and development efforts have been devoted to extend DICOM's transfer syntax. For instance, MPEG-4 and H.264 encoding have been applied onto encoding medical images such as ultrasound and echocardiography data. Scalable video coding can be combined with interactive segmentation assisted with experienced physicians or automatically grouping of homogeneous regions. Multiple studies have demonstrated the effectiveness and efficiency of MPEG-4 compression for both telemedicine ultrasound and echocardiography archive and transmission, without degrading the diagnostic quality at an acceptable level. More and more compression technologies have begun to flourish across 3G, 4G LTE, WiFi, and satellite networks for mobile medical imaging applications.

5. Conclusion

The steady increase of aging population, explosive growth of clinical data, and advances in healthcare information technologies have accelerated the rapid transition of PACS and evolution of imaging cloud into a more centralized data center and more connection-based distributed architecture and deployment model. Migrated from mini-PACS and disparate image archives, large-scaled enterprise PACS and web-based imaging cloud deliver healthcare services with high scalability, availability, and flexibility, with multimodality support of ultrasound, catheterization, nuclear, MRI, and CT imaging, and compatibility with DICOM and HL7 standards. As a result, they have fostered the growth of teleradiology and telemedicine across the Globe.

Cloud computing and services facilitate archiving, sharing and exchanging of imaging studies, ubiquitous and reliable network access. It has fundamentally transformed the delivery of healthcare workflow, business models, practice and procedures, and deliver better patient care. By adopting thin client PACS and imaging cloud platform, healthcare practitioners and clinical physicians can reliably and securely access medical data and content anytime and anywhere. They can better access, switch, and share patient studies, analyze, measure, and interpret regions of interest, display and review DICOMs and images, and automate generation of structured reports. The advent of zero-foot print PACS and cloud clients provide instantaneous access to patient studies and imaging data based on universal web browsers, without installing any applications and third-party plug-ins or libraries. These solution models can largely decouple the application processes on the clients from the virtual resources and machines on the servers, reduce development efforts and costs, deployment complexity and maintenance and updates.

To achieve the full potentials of imaging cloud model and PACS, we need to understand overall workflow and workloads of different sectors within and across healthcare institutions, and information dynamics. In addition, adopt suitable deployment PACS and cloud architectures, employ open standards, establish software update and maintenance strategy, and manage business models to optimize computing resources, achieve smooth and balanced workflow, and optimized performance.

References

1. J. J. Goldberger and J. Ng, eds., *Practical Signal and Image Processing in Clinical Cardiology*, Springer (2010).
2. Medical imaging in the cloud, AT&T.
3. W. DEAN Bidgood, Jr., S. C. Horii, F. W. Prior and D. Vansyckle, "Understanding and using DICOM, the data interchange standard for biomedical imaging," *J Am Medical Informatics Assoc* **4**, 199–212 (1997).
4. B. Gibaud, "The quest for standards in medical imaging." *Eur J Radiology* **78**, 190–198 (2011).
5. O. S. Pianykh, *Digital Imaging and Communications in Medicine (DICOM): A Practical Introduction and Survival Guide*, Springer (2012).
6. A. Fenster, D. B. Downey and H. N. Cardinal, "Three-dimensional ultrasound imaging," *Phys Med Biol* **46**, R67–R99 (2001).
7. H. K. Huang, *PACS and Imaging Informatics: Basic Principles and Applications*, John Wiley & Sons (2004).
8. P. Mell and T. Grance, "The NIST definition of cloud computing," *Nat Institute Standards Tech* **53**, 50 (2009).
9. S. A. Ahson and M. Ilyas, *Cloud Computing and Software Services: Theory and Techniques*, CRC Press (2010).
10. W. T. Tsai, X. Sun and J. Balasooriya, "Service-oriented cloud computing architecture," *Information Technology: New Generations (ITNG), 2010 Seventh International Conference on. IEEE*, 684–689 (2010).
11. H. Yu, Z. Lin and F. Pan, "Applications and improvement of H. 264 in medical video compression," *Circuits and Systems I: Regular Papers, IEEE Transactions on* **52**, 2707–2716 (2005).
12. C. Bolan, "Cloud PACS and mobile apps reinvent radiology workflow," *Appl Radiology* **42**, 24–29 (2013).
13. H. A. J. Narayanan and M. H. Gunes. "Ensuring access control in cloud provisioned healthcare systems," *Consumer Communications and Networking Conference (CCNC), IEEE* **2011**, 247–251 (2011).

14. S. Yu, C. Wang, K. Ren and W. Lou, "Achieving secure, scalable, and fine-grained data access control in cloud computing," *INFOCOM, Proceedings IEEE* **2010**, 1–9 (2010).
15. L. S. Ribeiro, C. Carlos and L. O. Jose, "Current trends in archiving and transmission of Medical Images," *Medical Imaging*, Dr. Okechukwu Felix Erondu (Ed.), InTech, 89–106 (2011).

Index